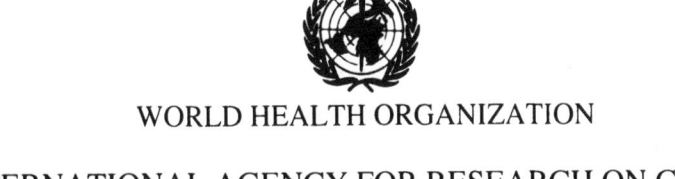

WORLD HEALTH ORGANIZATION

INTERNATIONAL AGENCY FOR RESEARCH ON CANCER

IARC MONOGRAPHS
ON THE
EVALUATION OF CARCINOGENIC RISKS TO HUMANS

Some Pharmaceutical Drugs

VOLUME 66

This publication represents the views and expert opinions
of an IARC Working Group on the
Evaluation of Carcinogenic Risks to Humans,
which met in Lyon,

13–20 February 1996

1996

IARC MONOGRAPHS

In 1969, the International Agency for Research on Cancer (IARC) initiated a programme on the evaluation of the carcinogenic risk of chemicals to humans involving the production of critically evaluated monographs on individual chemicals. The programme was subsequently expanded to include evaluations of carcinogenic risks associated with exposures to complex mixtures, life-style factors and biological agents, as well as those in specific occupations.

The objective of the programme is to elaborate and publish in the form of monographs critical reviews of data on carcinogenicity for agents to which humans are known to be exposed and on specific exposure situations; to evaluate these data in terms of human risk with the help of international working groups of experts in chemical carcinogenesis and related fields; and to indicate where additional research efforts are needed.

This project is supported by PHS Grant No. 5-UO1 CA33193-14 awarded by the United States National Cancer Institute, Department of Health and Human Services. Additional support has been provided since 1986 by the European Commission.

©International Agency for Research on Cancer, 1996

IARC Library Cataloguing in Publication Data

IARC Working Group on the Evaluation of Carcinogenic Risks to Humans
  (1996 : Lyon, France)
Some pharmaceutical drugs: views and expert opinions of an IARC Working Group on the Evaluation of Carcinogenic Risks to Humans which met in Lyon, 13–20 February 1996.

(IARC monographs on the evaluation of carcinogenic risks to humans ; 66)

1. Carcinogens – congresses   2. Drugs – congresses
3. Neoplasms – chemically induced
I. Series

ISBN 92 832 1266 5   (NLM Classification: W 1)

ISSN 0250-9555

Publications of the World Health Organization enjoy copyright protection in accordance with the provisions of Protocol 2 of the Universal Copyright Convention.

All rights reserved. Application for rights of reproduction or translation, in part or in toto, should be made to the International Agency for Research on Cancer.
Distributed by IARC*Press* (Fax: +33 72 73 83 02; E-mail: press@iarc.fr)
and by the World Health Organization Distribution and Sales, CH-1211 Geneva 27
(Fax: +41 22 791 4857)

PRINTED IN THE UNITED KINGDOM

CONTENTS

NOTE TO THE READER 1

LIST OF PARTICIPANTS 3

PREAMBLE
    Background 7
    Objective and Scope 7
    Selection of Topics for Monographs 8
    Data for Monographs 9
    The Working Group 9
    Working Procedures 9
    Exposure Data 10
    Studies of Cancer in Humans 12
    Studies of Cancer in Experimental Animals 15
    Other Data Relevant to an Evaluation of Carcinogenicity and Its Mechanisms 18
    Summary of Data Reported 19
    Evaluation 21
    References 25

GENERAL REMARKS 29

THE MONOGRAPHS

Benzodiazepines and related compounds and phenytoin 35
    Diazepam 37
    Doxefazepam 97
    Estazolam 105
    Oxazepam 115
    Prazepam 143
    Ripazepam 157
    Temazepam 161
    Phenytoin 175

Anti-oestrogenic compounds 239
    Droloxifene 241
    Tamoxifen 253
    Toremifene 367

Hypolipidaemic drugs 389
    Clofibrate 391
    Gemfibrozil 427

SUMMARY OF FINAL EVALUATIONS 445

GLOSSARY 447

APPENDIX 1. SUMMARY TABLES OF GENETIC AND RELATED EFFECTS.....451

APPENDIX 2. ACTIVITY PROFILES FOR GENETIC AND RELATED EFFECTS 467

SUPPLEMENTARY CORRIGENDA TO VOLUMES 1–65 485

CUMULATIVE INDEX TO THE *MONOGRAPHS* SERIES 487

NOTE TO THE READER

The term 'carcinogenic risk' in the *IARC Monographs* series is taken to mean the probability that exposure to an agent will lead to cancer in humans.

Inclusion of an agent in the *Monographs* does not imply that it is a carcinogen, only that the published data have been examined. Equally, the fact that an agent has not yet been evaluated in a monograph does not mean that it is not carcinogenic.

The evaluations of carcinogenic risk are made by international working groups of independent scientists and are qualitative in nature. No recommendation is given for regulation or legislation.

Anyone who is aware of published data that may alter the evaluation of the carcinogenic risk of an agent to humans is encouraged to make this information available to the Unit of Carcinogen Identification and Evaluation, International Agency for Research on Cancer, 150 cours Albert Thomas, 69372 Lyon Cedex 08, France, in order that the agent may be considered for re-evaluation by a future Working Group.

Although every effort is made to prepare the monographs as accurately as possible, mistakes may occur. Readers are requested to communicate any errors to the Unit of Carcinogen Identification and Evaluation, so that corrections can be reported in future volumes.

IARC WORKING GROUP ON THE EVALUATION OF CARCINOGENIC RISKS TO HUMANS: SOME PHARMACEUTICAL DRUGS

Lyon, 13–20 February 1996

LIST OF PARTICIPANTS

Members[1]

G.A. Boorman, Pathology Branch, National Institute of Environmental Health Sciences, 111 T.W. Alexander Drive, PO Box 12233, Research Triangle Park, NC 27709, United States

R.C. Cattley, Carcinogenesis Program, Chemical Industry Institute of Technology, 6 Davis Drive, PO Box 12137, Research Triangle Park, NC 27709, United States

D.W. Cramer, Obstetrics and Gynecology Epidemiology Center at Brigham and Women's Hospital, Harvard Medical School, 221 Longwood Avenue, Boston, MA 02115, United States

J. Cuzick, Department of Mathematics, Statistics and Epidemiology, Imperial Cancer Research Fund, PO Box 123, 61 Lincoln's Inn Fields, London WC2A 3PX, United Kingdom

A.E. Czeizel, Department of Human Genetics and Teratology, National Institute of Hygiene, Gyáli út 2-6, 1097 Budapest, Hungary

W.D. Hooper, Drug Metabolism and Neuropharmacology Group, Department of Medicine, The University of Queensland, Royal Brisbane Hospital, Brisbane, Qld 4029, Australia

M. Kirsch-Volders, Vrije Universiteit Brussel, Laboratorium voor Antropogenetica, Pleinlaan 2, 1050 Brussels, Belgium

F.E. van Leeuwen, Department of Epidemiology, The Netherlands Cancer Institute, Plesmanlaan 121, 1066 CX Amsterdam, The Netherlands

---

[1]Unable to attend: H. Wiseman, King's College London, School of Life, Basic Medical and Health Sciences, Department of Nutrition and Dietetics, Campden Hill Road, London W8 7AH, United Kingdom

J. Little, Institute of Medical Sciences, Department of Medicine and Therapeutics, University of Aberdeen Medical School, Polwarth Building, Foresterhill, Aberdeen AB9 2ZD, United Kingdom

G.W. Lucier, Environmental Toxicology Program, National Institute of Environmental Health Sciences, PO Box 12233, Research Triangle Park, NC 27709, United States (*Chairman*)

A.B. Miller, Department of Preventive Medicine and Biostatistics, Faculty of Medicine, McMurrich Building, University of Toronto, 12 Queen's Park Crescent West, Toronto, Ontario M5S 1A8, Canada (*Vice-Chairman*)

S. Olin, Risk Science Institute, International Life Sciences Institute, 1126 Sixteenth Street, NW, Washington DC 20036, United States

D.H. Phillips, Section of Molecular Carcinogenesis, The Haddow Laboratories, Institute of Cancer Research, Cotswold Road, Sutton, Surrey SM2 5NG, United Kingdom

A. Pinter, 'B. Johan' National Institute of Public Health, Gyáli út 2-6, 1097 Budapest, Hungary

K.I. Pritchard, Toronto-Sunnybrook Regional Cancer Centre, 2075 Bayview Avenue, Toronto, Ontario M4N 3M5, Canada

S. Vamvakas, Institute of Toxicology and Pharmacology, University of Würzburg, Versbacher Strasse 9, 97078 Würzburg, Germany

G.M. Williams, American Health Foundation, 1 Dana Road, Valhalla, NY 10595, United States

Representatives/Observers

Representative of the National Cancer Institute

V. Fung, Special Assistant for Environmental Cancer, National Cancer Institute, Executive Plaza North, Room 700, 6130 Executive Boulevard, Rockville, MD 20852, United States

American Industrial Health Council

M. McClain, Hoffman-La Roche, Inc., 340 Kingsland Street, Nutley, NJ 07110-1199, United States

European Federation of Pharmaceutical Industries Associations

J. Topham, Zeneca Pharmaceuticals, Mereside, Alderley Park, Macclesfield, Cheshire SK10 4TG, United Kingdom

Secretariat

R. Black, Unit of Descriptive Epidemiology
P. Boffetta, Unit of Environmental Cancer Epidemiology
J. Cheney, Editor
M. Friesen, Unit of Environmental Carcinogenesis
P. Hainaut, Unit of Mechanisms of Carcinogenesis

PARTICIPANTS

M. Lang, Programme of Molecular Toxicology
C. Malaveille, Unit of Endogenous Cancer Risk Factors
D. McGregor (Responsible Officer), Unit of Carcinogen Identification and Evaluation
A. Meneghel, Unit of Carcinogen Identification and Evaluation
D. Mietton, Unit of Carcinogen Identification and Evaluation
C. Partensky, Unit of Carcinogen Identification and Evaluation
I. Rajower, Director's Office
S. Ruiz, Unit of Carcinogen Identification and Evaluation
A. Sasco, Programme of Epidemiology for Cancer Prevention
J. Wilbourn, Unit of Carcinogen Identification and Evaluation
H. Yamasaki, Unit of Multistage Carcinogenesis

Secretarial assistance

M. Lézère
J. Mitchell
S. Reynaud

IARC MONOGRAPHS PROGRAMME ON THE EVALUATION OF CARCINOGENIC RISKS TO HUMANS[1]

PREAMBLE

1. BACKGROUND

In 1969, the International Agency for Research on Cancer (IARC) initiated a programme to evaluate the carcinogenic risk of chemicals to humans and to produce monographs on individual chemicals. The *Monographs* programme has since been expanded to include consideration of exposures to complex mixtures of chemicals (which occur, for example, in some occupations and as a result of human habits) and of exposures to other agents, such as radiation and viruses. With Supplement 6 (IARC, 1987a), the title of the series was modified from *IARC Monographs on the Evaluation of the Carcinogenic Risk of Chemicals to Humans* to *IARC Monographs on the Evaluation of Carcinogenic Risks to Humans*, in order to reflect the widened scope of the programme.

The criteria established in 1971 to evaluate carcinogenic risk to humans were adopted by the working groups whose deliberations resulted in the first 16 volumes of the *IARC Monographs series*. Those criteria were subsequently updated by further ad-hoc working groups (IARC, 1977, 1978, 1979, 1982, 1983, 1987b, 1988, 1991a; Vainio *et al.*, 1992).

2. OBJECTIVE AND SCOPE

The objective of the programme is to prepare, with the help of international working groups of experts, and to publish in the form of monographs, critical reviews and evaluations of evidence on the carcinogenicity of a wide range of human exposures. The *Monographs* may also indicate where additional research efforts are needed.

The *Monographs* represent the first step in carcinogenic risk assessment, which involves examination of all relevant information in order to assess the strength of the available evidence that certain exposures could alter the incidence of cancer in humans. The second step is quantitative risk estimation. Detailed, quantitative evaluations of epidemiological data may be made in the *Monographs*, but without extrapolation beyond

---

[1] This project is supported by PHS Grant No. 5-UO1 CA33193-14 awarded by the United States National Cancer Institute, Department of Health and Human Services. Since 1986, the programme has also been supported by the European Commission.

the range of the data available. Quantitative extrapolation from experimental data to the human situation is not undertaken.

The term 'carcinogen' is used in these monographs to denote an exposure that is capable of increasing the incidence of malignant neoplasms; the induction of benign neoplasms may in some circumstances (see p. 17) contribute to the judgement that the exposure is carcinogenic. The terms 'neoplasm' and 'tumour' are used interchangeably.

Some epidemiological and experimental studies indicate that different agents may act at different stages in the carcinogenic process, and several different mechanisms may be involved. The aim of the *Monographs* has been, from their inception, to evaluate evidence of carcinogenicity at any stage in the carcinogenesis process, independently of the underlying mechanisms. Information on mechanisms may, however, be used in making the overall evaluation (IARC, 1991a; Vainio *et al.*, 1992; see also pp. 23–25).

The *Monographs* may assist national and international authorities in making risk assessments and in formulating decisions concerning any necessary preventive measures. The evaluations of IARC working groups are scientific, qualitative judgements about the evidence for or against carcinogenicity provided by the available data. These evaluations represent only one part of the body of information on which regulatory measures may be based. Other components of regulatory decisions may vary from one situation to another and from country to country, responding to different socioeconomic and national priorities. **Therefore, no recommendation is given with regard to regulation or legislation, which are the responsibility of individual governments and/or other international organizations.**

The *IARC Monographs* are recognized as an authoritative source of information on the carcinogenicity of a wide range of human exposures. A survey of users in 1988 indicated that the *Monographs* are consulted by various agencies in 57 countries. About 4000 copies of each volume are printed, for distribution to governments, regulatory bodies and interested scientists. The Monographs are also available from the International Agency for Research on Cancer in Lyon and via the Distribution and Sales Service of the World Health Organization.

3. SELECTION OF TOPICS FOR MONOGRAPHS

Topics are selected on the basis of two main criteria: (a) there is evidence of human exposure, and (b) there is some evidence or suspicion of carcinogenicity. The term 'agent' is used to include individual chemical compounds, groups of related chemical compounds, physical agents (such as radiation) and biological factors (such as viruses). Exposures to mixtures of agents may occur in occupational exposures and as a result of personal and cultural habits (like smoking and dietary practices). Chemical analogues and compounds with biological or physical characteristics similar to those of suspected carcinogens may also be considered, even in the absence of data on a possible carcinogenic effect in humans or experimental animals.

The scientific literature is surveyed for published data relevant to an assessment of carcinogenicity. The IARC information bulletins on agents being tested for carcinogenicity (IARC, 1973–1996) and directories of on-going research in cancer epidemiology (IARC, 1976–1994) often indicate exposures that may be scheduled for future meetings. Ad-hoc working groups convened by IARC in 1984, 1989, 1991 and 1993 gave recommendations as to which agents should be evaluated in the IARC Monographs series (IARC, 1984, 1989, 1991b, 1993).

As significant new data on subjects on which monographs have already been prepared become available, re-evaluations are made at subsequent meetings, and revised monographs are published.

4. DATA FOR MONOGRAPHS

The *Monographs* do not necessarily cite all the literature concerning the subject of an evaluation. Only those data considered by the Working Group to be relevant to making the evaluation are included.

With regard to biological and epidemiological data, only reports that have been published or accepted for publication in the openly available scientific literature are reviewed by the working groups. In certain instances, government agency reports that have undergone peer review and are widely available are considered. Exceptions may be made on an ad-hoc basis to include unpublished reports that are in their final form and publicly available, if their inclusion is considered pertinent to making a final evaluation (see pp. 23–25). In the sections on chemical and physical properties, on analysis, on production and use and on occurrence, unpublished sources of information may be used.

5. THE WORKING GROUP

Reviews and evaluations are formulated by a working group of experts. The tasks of the group are: (i) to ascertain that all appropriate data have been collected; (ii) to select the data relevant for the evaluation on the basis of scientific merit; (iii) to prepare accurate summaries of the data to enable the reader to follow the reasoning of the Working Group; (iv) to evaluate the results of epidemiological and experimental studies on cancer; (v) to evaluate data relevant to the understanding of mechanism of action; and (vi) to make an overall evaluation of the carcinogenicity of the exposure to humans.

Working Group participants who contributed to the considerations and evaluations within a particular volume are listed, with their addresses, at the beginning of each publication. Each participant who is a member of a working group serves as an individual scientist and not as a representative of any organization, government or industry. In addition, nominees of national and international agencies and industrial associations may be invited as observers.

6. WORKING PROCEDURES

Approximately one year in advance of a meeting of a working group, the topics of the monographs are announced and participants are selected by IARC staff in consultation with other experts. Subsequently, relevant biological and epidemiological data are collected by IARC from recognized sources of information on carcinogenesis, including data storage and retrieval systems such as MEDLINE and TOXLINE, and EMIC and ETIC for data on genetic and related effects and reproductive and developmental effects, respectively.

For chemicals and some complex mixtures, the major collection of data and the preparation of first drafts of the sections on chemical and physical properties, on analysis, on production and use and on occurrence are carried out under a separate contract funded by the United States National Cancer Institute. Representatives from industrial associations may assist in the preparation of sections on production and use. Information on production and trade is obtained from governmental and trade publications and, in some cases, by direct contact with industries. Separate production data on some agents may not be available because their publication could disclose confidential information. Information on uses may be obtained from published sources but is often complemented by direct contact with manufacturers. Efforts are made to supplement this information with data from other national and international sources.

Six months before the meeting, the material obtained is sent to meeting participants, or is used by IARC staff, to prepare sections for the first drafts of monographs. The first drafts are compiled by IARC staff and sent, before the meeting, to all participants of the Working Group for review.

The Working Group meets in Lyon for seven to eight days to discuss and finalize the texts of the monographs and to formulate the evaluations. After the meeting, the master copy of each monograph is verified by consulting the original literature, edited and prepared for publication. The aim is to publish monographs within six months of the Working Group meeting.

The available studies are summarized by the Working Group, with particular regard to the qualitative aspects discussed below. In general, numerical findings are indicated as they appear in the original report; units are converted when necessary for easier comparison. The Working Group may conduct additional analyses of the published data and use them in their assessment of the evidence; the results of such supplementary analyses are given in square brackets. When an important aspect of a study, directly impinging on its interpretation, should be brought to the attention of the reader, a comment is given in square brackets.

7. EXPOSURE DATA

Sections that indicate the extent of past and present human exposure, the sources of exposure, the people most likely to be exposed and the factors that contribute to the exposure are included at the beginning of each monograph.

Most monographs on individual chemicals, groups of chemicals or complex mixtures include sections on chemical and physical data, on analysis, on production and use and on occurrence. In monographs on, for example, physical agents, occupational exposures and cultural habits, other sections may be included, such as: historical perspectives, description of an industry or habit, chemistry of the complex mixture or taxonomy.

Monographs on biological agents have sections on structure and biology, methods of detection, epidemiology of infection and clinical disease other than cancer.

For chemical exposures, the Chemical Abstracts Services Registry Number, the latest Chemical Abstracts Primary Name and the IUPAC Systematic Name are recorded; other synonyms are given, but the list is not necessarily comprehensive. For biological agents, taxonomy and structure are described, and the degree of variability is given, when applicable.

Information on chemical and physical properties and, in particular, data relevant to identification, occurrence and biological activity are included. For biological agents, mode of replication, life cycle, target cells, persistence and latency and host response are given. A description of technical products of chemicals includes trades names, relevant specifications and available information on composition and impurities. Some of the trade names given may be those of mixtures in which the agent being evaluated is only one of the ingredients.

The purpose of the section on analysis or detection is to give the reader an overview of current methods, with emphasis on those widely used for regulatory purposes. Methods for monitoring human exposure are also given, when available. No critical evaluation or recommendation of any of the methods is meant or implied. The IARC publishes a series of volumes, *Environmental Carcinogens: Methods of Analysis and Exposure Measurement* (IARC, 1978–93), that describe validated methods for analysing a wide variety of chemicals and mixtures. For biological agents, methods of detection and exposure assessment are described, including their sensitivity, specificity and reproducibility.

The dates of first synthesis and of first commercial production of a chemical or mixture are provided; for agents which do not occur naturally, this information may allow a reasonable estimate to be made of the date before which no human exposure to the agent could have occurred. The dates of first reported occurrence of an exposure are also provided. In addition, methods of synthesis used in past and present commercial production and different methods of production which may give rise to different impurities are described.

Data on production, international trade and uses are obtained for representative regions, which usually include Europe, Japan and the United States of America. It should not, however, be inferred that those areas or nations are necessarily the sole or major sources or users of the agent. Some identified uses may not be current or major applications, and the coverage is not necessarily comprehensive. In the case of drugs, mention of their therapeutic uses does not necessarily represent current practice nor does it imply judgement as to their therapeutic efficacy.

Information on the occurrence of an agent or mixture in the environment is obtained from data derived from the monitoring and surveillance of levels in occupational environments, air, water, soil, foods and animal and human tissues. When available, data on the generation, persistence and bioaccumulation of the agent are also included. In the case of mixtures, industries, occupations or processes, information is given about all agents present. For processes, industries and occupations, a historical description is also given, noting variations in chemical composition, physical properties and levels of occupational exposure with time and place. For biological agents, the epidemiology of infection is described.

Statements concerning regulations and guidelines (e.g., pesticide registrations, maximal levels permitted in foods, occupational exposure limits) are included for some countries as indications of potential exposures, but they may not reflect the most recent situation, since such limits are continuously reviewed and modified. The absence of information on regulatory status for a country should not be taken to imply that that country does not have regulations with regard to the exposure. For biological agents, legislation and control, including vaccines and therapy, are described.

8. STUDIES OF CANCER IN HUMANS

(a) *Types of studies considered*

Three types of epidemiological studies of cancer contribute to the assessment of carcinogenicity in humans — cohort studies, case–control studies and correlation (or ecological) studies. Rarely, results from randomized trials may be available. Case series and case reports of cancer in humans may also be reviewed.

Cohort and case–control studies relate individual exposures under study to the occurrence of cancer in individuals and provide an estimate of relative risk (ratio of incidence or mortality in those exposed to incidence or mortality in those not exposed) as the main measure of association.

In correlation studies, the units of investigation are usually whole populations (e.g., in particular geographical areas or at particular times), and cancer frequency is related to a summary measure of the exposure of the population to the agent, mixture or exposure circumstance under study. Because individual exposure is not documented, however, a causal relationship is less easy to infer from correlation studies than from cohort and case–control studies. Case reports generally arise from a suspicion, based on clinical experience, that the concurrence of two events — that is, a particular exposure and occurrence of a cancer — has happened rather more frequently than would be expected by chance. Case reports usually lack complete ascertainment of cases in any population, definition or enumeration of the population at risk and estimation of the expected number of cases in the absence of exposure. The uncertainties surrounding interpretation of case reports and correlation studies make them inadequate, except in rare instances, to form the sole basis for inferring a causal relationship. When taken together with case–control and cohort studies, however, relevant case reports or correlation studies may add materially to the judgement that a causal relationship is present.

Epidemiological studies of benign neoplasms, presumed preneoplastic lesions and other end-points thought to be relevant to cancer are also reviewed by working groups. They may, in some instances, strengthen inferences drawn from studies of cancer itself.

(b) Quality of studies considered

The Monographs are not intended to summarize all published studies. Those that are judged to be inadequate or irrelevant to the evaluation are generally omitted. They may be mentioned briefly, particularly when the information is considered to be a useful supplement to that in other reports or when they provide the only data available. Their inclusion does not imply acceptance of the adequacy of the study design or of the analysis and interpretation of the results, and limitations are clearly outlined in square brackets at the end of the study description.

It is necessary to take into account the possible roles of bias, confounding and chance in the interpretation of epidemiological studies. By 'bias' is meant the operation of factors in study design or execution that lead erroneously to a stronger or weaker association than in fact exists between disease and an agent, mixture or exposure circumstance. By 'confounding' is meant a situation in which the relationship with disease is made to appear stronger or weaker than it truly is as a result of an association between the apparent causal factor and another factor that is associated with either an increase or decrease in the incidence of the disease. In evaluating the extent to which these factors have been minimized in an individual study, working groups consider a number of aspects of design and analysis as described in the report of the study. Most of these considerations apply equally to case–control, cohort and correlation studies. Lack of clarity of any of these aspects in the reporting of a study can decrease its credibility and the weight given to it in the final evaluation of the exposure.

Firstly, the study population, disease (or diseases) and exposure should have been well defined by the authors. Cases of disease in the study population should have been identified in a way that was independent of the exposure of interest, and exposure should have been assessed in a way that was not related to disease status.

Secondly, the authors should have taken account in the study design and analysis of other variables that can influence the risk of disease and may have been related to the exposure of interest. Potential confounding by such variables should have been dealt with either in the design of the study, such as by matching, or in the analysis, by statistical adjustment. In cohort studies, comparisons with local rates of disease may be more appropriate than those with national rates. Internal comparisons of disease frequency among individuals at different levels of exposure should also have been made in the study.

Thirdly, the authors should have reported the basic data on which the conclusions are founded, even if sophisticated statistical analyses were employed. At the very least, they should have given the numbers of exposed and unexposed cases and controls in a case–control study and the numbers of cases observed and expected in a cohort study. Further tabulations by time since exposure began and other temporal factors are also important. In a cohort study, data on all cancer sites and all causes of death should have been given, to reveal the possibility of reporting bias. In a case–control study, the effects of investigated factors other than the exposure of interest should have been reported.

Finally, the statistical methods used to obtain estimates of relative risk, absolute rates of cancer, confidence intervals and significance tests, and to adjust for confounding should have been clearly stated by the authors. The methods used should preferably have been the generally accepted techniques that have been refined since the mid-1970s. These methods have been reviewed for case–control studies (Breslow & Day, 1980) and for cohort studies (Breslow & Day, 1987).

(c) Inferences about mechanism of action

Detailed analyses of both relative and absolute risks in relation to temporal variables, such as age at first exposure, time since first exposure, duration of exposure, cumulative exposure and time since exposure ceased, are reviewed and summarized when available. The analysis of temporal relationships can be useful in formulating models of carcinogenesis. In particular, such analyses may suggest whether a carcinogen acts early or late in the process of carcinogenesis, although at best they allow only indirect inferences about the mechanism of action. Special attention is given to measurements of biological markers of carcinogen exposure or action, such as DNA or protein adducts, as well as markers of early steps in the carcinogenic process, such as proto-oncogene mutation, when these are incorporated into epidemiological studies focused on cancer incidence or mortality. Such measurements may allow inferences to be made about putative mechanisms of action (IARC, 1991a; Vainio et al., 1992).

(d) Criteria for causality

After the quality of individual epidemiological studies of cancer has been summarized and assessed, a judgement is made concerning the strength of evidence that the agent, mixture or exposure circumstance in question is carcinogenic for humans. In making its judgement, the Working Group considers several criteria for causality. A strong association (a large relative risk) is more likely to indicate causality than a weak association, although it is recognized that relative risks of small magnitude do not imply lack of causality and may be important if the disease is common. Associations that are replicated in several studies of the same design or using different epidemiological approaches or under different circumstances of exposure are more likely to represent a causal relationship than isolated observations from single studies. If there are inconsistent results among investigations, possible reasons are sought (such as differences in amount of exposure), and results of studies judged to be of high quality are given more weight than those of studies judged to be methodologically less sound. When suspicion of carcinogenicity arises largely from a single study, these data are not combined with those from later studies in any subsequent reassessment of the strength of the evidence.

If the risk of the disease in question increases with the amount of exposure, this is considered to be a strong indication of causality, although absence of a graded response is not necessarily evidence against a causal relationship. Demonstration of a decline in risk after cessation of or reduction in exposure in individuals or in whole populations also supports a causal interpretation of the findings.

Although a carcinogen may act upon more than one target, the specificity of an association (an increased occurrence of cancer at one anatomical site or of one morphological type) adds plausibility to a causal relationship, particularly when excess cancer occurrence is limited to one morphological type within the same organ.

Although rarely available, results from randomized trials showing different rates among exposed and unexposed individuals provide particularly strong evidence for causality.

When several epidemiological studies show little or no indication of an association between an exposure and cancer, the judgement may be made that, in the aggregate, they show evidence of lack of carcinogenicity. Such a judgement requires first of all that the studies giving rise to it meet, to a sufficient degree, the standards of design and analysis described above. Specifically, the possibility that bias, confounding or misclassification of exposure or outcome could explain the observed results should be considered and excluded with reasonable certainty. In addition, all studies that are judged to be methodologically sound should be consistent with a relative risk of unity for any observed level of exposure and, when considered together, should provide a pooled estimate of relative risk which is at or near unity and has a narrow confidence interval, due to sufficient population size. Moreover, no individual study nor the pooled results of all the studies should show any consistent tendency for relative risk of cancer to increase with increasing level of exposure. It is important to note that evidence of lack of carcinogenicity obtained in this way from several epidemiological studies can apply only to the type(s) of cancer studied and to dose levels and intervals between first exposure and observation of disease that are the same as or less than those observed in all the studies. Experience with human cancer indicates that, in some cases, the period from first exposure to the development of clinical cancer is seldom less than 20 years; latent periods substantially shorter than 30 years cannot provide evidence for lack of carcinogenicity.

9. STUDIES OF CANCER IN EXPERIMENTAL ANIMALS

All known human carcinogens that have been studied adequately in experimental animals have produced positive results in one or more animal species (Wilbourn *et al.*, 1986; Tomatis *et al.*, 1989). For several agents (aflatoxins, 4-aminobiphenyl, azathioprine, betel quid with tobacco, BCME and CMME (technical grade), chlorambucil, chlornaphazine, ciclosporin, coal-tar pitches, coal-tars, combined oral contraceptives, cyclophosphamide, diethylstilboestrol, melphalan, 8-methoxypsoralen plus UVA, mustard gas, myleran, 2-naphthylamine, nonsteroidal oestrogens, oestrogen replacement therapy/steroidal oestrogens, solar radiation, thiotepa and vinyl chloride), carcinogenicity in experimental animals was established or highly suspected before epidemiological studies confirmed the carcinogenicity in humans (Vainio *et al.*, 1995). Although this association cannot establish that all agents and mixtures that cause cancer in experimental animals also cause cancer in humans, nevertheless, **in the absence of adequate data on humans, it is biologically plausible and prudent to regard agents and mixtures for which there is sufficient evidence (see p. 22) of carcinogenicity in experimental animals as if they presented a carcinogenic risk to humans.** The possibility that a given agent may cause cancer through a species-specific mechanism which does not operate in humans (see p. 25) should also be taken into consideration.

The nature and extent of impurities or contaminants present in the chemical or mixture being evaluated are given when available. Animal strain, sex, numbers per group, age at start of treatment and survival are reported.

Other types of studies summarized include: experiments in which the agent or mixture was administered in conjunction with known carcinogens or factors that modify carcinogenic effects; studies in which the end-point was not cancer but a defined precancerous lesion; and experiments on the carcinogenicity of known metabolites and derivatives.

For experimental studies of mixtures, consideration is given to the possibility of changes in the physicochemical properties of the test substance during collection, storage, extraction, concentration and delivery. Chemical and toxicological interactions of the components of mixtures may result in nonlinear dose–response relationships.

An assessment is made as to the relevance to human exposure of samples tested in experimental animals, which may involve consideration of: (i) physical and chemical characteristics, (ii) constituent substances that indicate the presence of a class of substances, (iii) the results of tests for genetic and related effects, including genetic activity profiles, DNA adduct profiles, proto-oncogene mutation and expression and suppressor gene inactivation. The relevance of results obtained, for example, with animal viruses analogous to the virus being evaluated in the monograph must also be considered. They may provide biological and mechanistic information relevant to the understanding of the process of carcinogenesis in humans and may strengthen the plausibility of a conclusion that the biological agent under evaluation is carcinogenic in humans.

(a) Qualitative aspects

An assessment of carcinogenicity involves several considerations of qualitative importance, including (i) the experimental conditions under which the test was performed, including route and schedule of exposure, species, strain, sex, age, duration of follow-up; (ii) the consistency of the results, for example, across species and target organ(s); (iii) the spectrum of neoplastic response, from preneoplastic lesions and benign tumours to malignant neoplasms; and (iv) the possible role of modifying factors.

As mentioned earlier (p. 11), the *Monographs* are not intended to summarize all published studies. Those studies in experimental animals that are inadequate (e.g., too short a duration, too few animals, poor survival; see below) or are judged irrelevant to the evaluation are generally omitted. Guidelines for conducting adequate long-term carcinogenicity experiments have been outlined (e.g., Montesano *et al.*, 1986).

Considerations of importance to the Working Group in the interpretation and evaluation of a particular study include: (i) how clearly the agent was defined and, in the case of mixtures, how adequately the sample characterization was reported; (ii) whether the dose was adequately monitored, particularly in inhalation experiments; (iii) whether the doses and duration of treatment were appropriate and whether the survival of treated animals was similar to that of controls; (iv) whether there were adequate numbers of animals per group; (v) whether animals of both sexes were used; (vi) whether animals were allocated randomly to groups; (vii) whether the duration of observation was adequate; and (viii) whether the data were adequately reported. If available, recent data on the incidence of specific tumours in historical controls, as well as in concurrent controls, should be taken into account in the evaluation of tumour response.

When benign tumours occur together with and originate from the same cell type in an organ or tissue as malignant tumours in a particular study and appear to represent a stage in the progression to malignancy, it may be valid to combine them in assessing tumour incidence (Huff *et al.*, 1989). The occurrence of lesions presumed to be preneoplastic may in certain instances aid in assessing the biological plausibility of any neoplastic response observed. If an agent or mixture induces only benign neoplasms that appear to be end-points that do not readily undergo transition to malignancy, it should nevertheless be suspected of being a carcinogen and requires further investigation.

(b) Quantitative aspects

The probability that tumours will occur may depend on the species, sex, strain and age of the animal, the dose of the carcinogen and the route and length of exposure. Evidence of an increased incidence of neoplasms with increased level of exposure strengthens the inference of a causal association between the exposure and the development of neoplasms.

The form of the dose–response relationship can vary widely, depending on the particular agent under study and the target organ. Both DNA damage and increased cell division are important aspects of carcinogenesis, and cell proliferation is a strong determinant of dose–response relationships for some carcinogens (Cohen & Ellwein, 1990). Since many chemicals require metabolic activation before being converted into their reactive intermediates, both metabolic and pharmacokinetic aspects are important in determining the dose–response pattern. Saturation of steps such as absorption, activation, inactivation and elimination may produce nonlinearity in the dose–response relationship, as could saturation of processes such as DNA repair (Hoel *et al.*, 1983; Gart *et al.*, 1986).

(c) Statistical analysis of long-term experiments in animals

Factors considered by the Working Group include the adequacy of the information given for each treatment group: (i) the number of animals studied and the number examined histologically, (ii) the number of animals with a given tumour type and (iii) length of survival. The statistical methods used should be clearly stated and should be the generally accepted techniques refined for this purpose (Peto *et al.*, 1980; Gart *et al.*, 1986). When there is no difference in survival between control and treatment groups, the Working Group usually compares the proportions of animals developing each tumour type in each of the groups. Otherwise, consideration is given as to whether or not appropriate adjustments have been made for differences in survival. These adjustments can include: comparisons of the proportions of tumour-bearing animals among the effective number of animals (alive at the time the first tumour is discovered), in the case where most differences in survival occur before tumours appear; life-table methods, when tumours are visible or when they may be considered 'fatal' because mortality rapidly follows tumour development; and the Mantel-Haenszel test or logistic regression, when occult tumours do not affect the animals' risk of dying but are 'incidental' findings at autopsy.

In practice, classifying tumours as fatal or incidental may be difficult. Several survival-adjusted methods have been developed that do not require this distinction (Gart et al., 1986), although they have not been fully evaluated.

10. OTHER DATA RELEVANT TO AN EVALUATION OF CARCINO-GENICITY AND ITS MECHANISMS

In coming to an overall evaluation of carcinogenicity in humans (see p. 23), the Working Group also considers related data. The nature of the information selected for the summary depends on the agent being considered.

For chemicals and complex mixtures of chemicals such as those in some occupational situations and involving cultural habits (e.g., tobacco smoking), the other data considered to be relevant are divided into those on absorption, distribution, metabolism and excretion; toxic effects; reproductive and developmental effects; and genetic and related effects.

Concise information is given on absorption, distribution (including placental transfer) and excretion in both humans and experimental animals. Kinetic factors that may affect the dose–response relationship, such as saturation of uptake, protein binding, metabolic activation, detoxification and DNA repair processes, are mentioned. Studies that indicate the metabolic fate of the agent in humans and in experimental animals are summarized briefly, and comparisons of data from humans and animals are made when possible. Comparative information on the relationship between exposure and the dose that reaches the target site may be of particular importance for extrapolation between species. Data are given on acute and chronic toxic effects (other than cancer), such as organ toxicity, increased cell proliferation, immunotoxicity and endocrine effects. The presence and toxicological significance of cellular receptors is described. Effects on reproduction, teratogenicity, fetotoxicity and embryotoxicity are also summarized briefly.

Tests of genetic and related effects are described in view of the relevance of gene mutation and chromosomal damage to carcinogenesis (Vainio et al., 1992). The adequacy of the reporting of sample characterization is considered and, where necessary, commented upon; with regard to complex mixtures, such comments are similar to those described for animal carcinogenicity tests on p. 16. The available data are interpreted critically by phylogenetic group according to the end-points detected, which may include DNA damage, gene mutation, sister chromatid exchange, micronucleus formation, chromosomal aberrations, aneuploidy and cell transformation. The concentrations employed are given, and mention is made of whether use of an exogenous metabolic system *in vitro* affected the test result. These data are given as listings of test systems, data and references; bar graphs (activity profiles) and corresponding summary tables with detailed information on the preparation of the profiles (Waters et al., 1987) are given in appendices.

Positive results in tests using prokaryotes, lower eukaryotes, plants, insects and cultured mammalian cells suggest that genetic and related effects could occur in mammals. Results from such tests may also give information about the types of genetic effect produced and about the involvement of metabolic activation. Some end-points described are clearly genetic in nature (e.g., gene mutations and chromosomal aberrations), while others are to a greater or lesser degree associated with genetic effects (e.g., unscheduled DNA synthesis). In-vitro tests for tumour-promoting activity and for cell transformation may be sensitive to changes that are not necessarily the result of genetic alterations but that may have specific relevance to the process of carcinogenesis. A critical appraisal of these tests has been published (Montesano et al., 1986).

Genetic or other activity manifest in experimental mammals and humans is regarded as being of greater relevance than that in other organisms. The demonstration that an agent or mixture can induce gene and chromosomal mutations in whole mammals indicates that it may have carcinogenic activity, although this activity may not be detectably expressed in any or all species. Relative potency in tests for mutagenicity and related effects is not a reliable indicator of carcinogenic potency. Negative results in tests for mutagenicity in selected tissues from animals treated *in vivo* provide less weight, partly because they do not exclude the possibility of an effect in tissues other than those examined. Moreover, negative results in short-term tests with genetic end-points cannot be considered to provide evidence to rule out carcinogenicity of agents or mixtures that act through other mechanisms (e.g., receptor-mediated effects, cellular toxicity with regenerative proliferation, peroxisome proliferation) (Vainio et al., 1992). Factors that may lead to misleading results in short-term tests have been discussed in detail elsewhere (Montesano et al., 1986).

When available, data relevant to mechanisms of carcinogenesis that do not involve structural changes at the level of the gene are also described.

The adequacy of epidemiological studies of reproductive outcome and genetic and related effects in humans is evaluated by the same criteria as are applied to epidemiological studies of cancer.

Structure–activity relationships that may be relevant to an evaluation of the carcinogenicity of an agent are also described.

For biological agents — viruses, bacteria and parasites — other data relevant to carcino-genicity include descriptions of the pathology of infection, molecular biology (integration and expression of viruses, and any genetic alterations seen in human tumours) and other observations, which might include cellular and tissue responses to infection, immune response and the presence of tumour markers.

11. SUMMARY OF DATA REPORTED

In this section, the relevant epidemiological and experimental data are summarized. Only reports, other than in abstract form, that meet the criteria outlined on p. 9 are considered for evaluating carcinogenicity. Inadequate studies are generally not summarized: such studies are usually identified by a square-bracketed comment in the preceding text.

(a) Exposures

Human exposure to chemicals and complex mixtures is summarized on the basis of elements such as production, use, occurrence in the environment and determinations in human tissues and body fluids. Quantitative data are given when available. Exposure to biological agents is described in terms of transmission, and prevalence of infection.

(b) Carcinogenicity in humans

Results of epidemiological studies that are considered to be pertinent to an assessment of human carcinogenicity are summarized. When relevant, case reports and correlation studies are also summarized.

(c) Carcinogenicity in experimental animals

Data relevant to an evaluation of carcinogenicity in animals are summarized. For each animal species and route of administration, it is stated whether an increased incidence of neoplasms or preneoplastic lesions was observed, and the tumour sites are indicated. If the agent or mixture produced tumours after prenatal exposure or in single-dose experiments, this is also indicated. Negative findings are also summarized. Dose–response and other quantitative data may be given when available.

(d) Other data relevant to an evaluation of carcinogenicity and its mechanisms

Data on biological effects in humans that are of particular relevance are summarized. These may include toxicological, kinetic and metabolic considerations and evidence of DNA binding, persistence of DNA lesions or genetic damage in exposed humans. Toxicological information, such as that on cytotoxicity and regeneration, receptor binding and hormonal and immunological effects, and data on kinetics and metabolism in experimental animals are given when considered relevant to the possible mechanism of the carcinogenic action of the agent. The results of tests for genetic and related effects are summarized for whole mammals, cultured mammalian cells and nonmammalian systems.

When available, comparisons of such data for humans and for animals, and particularly animals that have developed cancer, are described.

Structure–activity relationships are mentioned when relevant.

For the agent, mixture or exposure circumstance being evaluated, the available data on end-points or other phenomena relevant to mechanisms of carcinogenesis from studies in humans, experimental animals and tissue and cell test systems are summarized within one or more of the following descriptive dimensions:

(i) Evidence of genotoxicity (structural changes at the level of the gene): for example, structure–activity considerations, adduct formation, mutagenicity (effect on specific genes), chromosomal mutation/aneuploidy

(ii) Evidence of effects on the expression of relevant genes (functional changes at the intracellular level): for example, alterations to the structure or quantity of the product of a proto-oncogene or tumour-suppressor gene, alterations to metabolic activation/inactivation/DNA repair

(iii) Evidence of relevant effects on cell behaviour (morphological or behavioural changes at the cellular or tissue level): for example, induction of mitogenesis, compensatory cell proliferation, preneoplasia and hyperplasia, survival of premalignant or malignant cells (immortalization, immunosuppression), effects on metastatic potential

(iv) Evidence from dose and time relationships of carcinogenic effects and interactions between agents: for example, early/late stage, as inferred from epidemiological studies; initiation/promotion/progression/malignant conversion, as defined in animal carcinogenicity experiments; toxicokinetics

These dimensions are not mutually exclusive, and an agent may fall within more than one of them. Thus, for example, the action of an agent on the expression of relevant genes could be summarized under both the first and second dimensions, even if it were known with reasonable certainty that those effects resulted from genotoxicity.

12. EVALUATION

Evaluations of the strength of the evidence for carcinogenicity arising from human and experimental animal data are made, using standard terms.

It is recognized that the criteria for these evaluations, described below, cannot encompass all of the factors that may be relevant to an evaluation of carcinogenicity. In considering all of the relevant scientific data, the Working Group may assign the agent, mixture or exposure circumstance to a higher or lower category than a strict interpretation of these criteria would indicate.

(*a*) *Degrees of evidence for carcinogenicity in humans and in experimental animals and supporting evidence*

These categories refer only to the strength of the evidence that an exposure is carcinogenic and not to the extent of its carcinogenic activity (potency) nor to the mechanisms involved. A classification may change as new information becomes available.

An evaluation of degree of evidence, whether for a single agent or a mixture, is limited to the materials tested, as defined physically, chemically or biologically. When the agents evaluated are considered by the Working Group to be sufficiently closely related, they may be grouped together for the purpose of a single evaluation of degree of evidence.

(*i*) *Carcinogenicity in humans*

The applicability of an evaluation of the carcinogenicity of a mixture, process, occupation or industry on the basis of evidence from epidemiological studies depends on the variability over time and place of the mixtures, processes, occupations and industries. The Working Group seeks to identify the specific exposure, process or activity which is considered most likely to be responsible for any excess risk. The evaluation is focused as narrowly as the available data on exposure and other aspects permit.

The evidence relevant to carcinogenicity from studies in humans is classified into one of the following categories:

Sufficient evidence of carcinogenicity: The Working Group considers that a causal relationship has been established between exposure to the agent, mixture or exposure circumstance and human cancer. That is, a positive relationship has been observed between the exposure and cancer in studies in which chance, bias and confounding could be ruled out with reasonable confidence.

Limited evidence of carcinogenicity: A positive association has been observed between exposure to the agent, mixture or exposure circumstance and cancer for which a causal interpretation is considered by the Working Group to be credible, but chance, bias or confounding could not be ruled out with reasonable confidence.

Inadequate evidence of carcinogenicity: The available studies are of insufficient quality, consistency or statistical power to permit a conclusion regarding the presence or absence of a causal association, or no data on cancer in humans are available.

Evidence suggesting lack of carcinogenicity: There are several adequate studies covering the full range of levels of exposure that human beings are known to encounter, which are mutually consistent in not showing a positive association between exposure to the agent, mixture or exposure circumstance and any studied cancer at any observed level of exposure. A conclusion of 'evidence suggesting lack of carcinogenicity' is inevitably limited to the cancer sites, conditions and levels of exposure and length of observation covered by the available studies. In addition, the possibility of a very small risk at the levels of exposure studied can never be excluded.

In some instances, the above categories may be used to classify the degree of evidence related to carcinogenicity in specific organs or tissues.

(ii) Carcinogenicity in experimental animals

The evidence relevant to carcinogenicity in experimental animals is classified into one of the following categories:

Sufficient evidence of carcinogenicity: The Working Group considers that a causal relationship has been established between the agent or mixture and an increased incidence of malignant neoplasms or of an appropriate combination of benign and malignant neoplasms in (a) two or more species of animals or (b) in two or more independent studies in one species carried out at different times or in different laboratories or under different protocols.

Exceptionally, a single study in one species might be considered to provide sufficient evidence of carcinogenicity when malignant neoplasms occur to an unusual degree with regard to incidence, site, type of tumour or age at onset.

Limited evidence of carcinogenicity: The data suggest a carcinogenic effect but are limited for making a definitive evaluation because, e.g., (a) the evidence of carcinogenicity is restricted to a single experiment; or (b) there are unresolved questions regarding the adequacy of the design, conduct or interpretation of the study; or (c) the agent or mixture increases the incidence only of benign neoplasms or lesions of uncertain neoplastic potential, or of certain neoplasms which may occur spontaneously in high incidences in certain strains.

Inadequate evidence of carcinogenicity: The studies cannot be interpreted as showing either the presence or absence of a carcinogenic effect because of major qualitative or quantitative limitations, or no data on cancer in experimental animals are available.

Evidence suggesting lack of carcinogenicity: Adequate studies involving at least two species are available which show that, within the limits of the tests used, the agent or mixture is not carcinogenic. A conclusion of evidence suggesting lack of carcinogenicity is inevitably limited to the species, tumour sites and levels of exposure studied.

(b) *Other data relevant to the evaluation of carcinogenicity and its mechanisms*

Other evidence judged to be relevant to an evaluation of carcinogenicity and of sufficient importance to affect the overall evaluation is then described. This may include data on preneoplastic lesions, tumour pathology, genetic and related effects, structure–activity relationships, metabolism and pharmacokinetics, physicochemical parameters and analogous biological agents.

Data relevant to mechanisms of the carcinogenic action are also evaluated. The strength of the evidence that any carcinogenic effect observed is due to a particular mechanism is assessed, using terms such as weak, moderate or strong. Then, the Working Group assesses if that particular mechanism is likely to be operative in humans. The strongest indications that a particular mechanism operates in humans come from data on humans or biological specimens obtained from exposed humans. The data may be considered to be especially relevant if they show that the agent in question has caused changes in exposed humans that are on the causal pathway to carcinogenesis. Such data may, however, never become available, because it is at least conceivable that certain compounds may be kept from human use solely on the basis of evidence of their toxicity and/or carcinogenicity in experimental systems.

For complex exposures, including occupational and industrial exposures, the chemical composition and the potential contribution of carcinogens known to be present are considered by the Working Group in its overall evaluation of human carcinogenicity. The Working Group also determines the extent to which the materials tested in experimental systems are related to those to which humans are exposed.

(c) *Overall evaluation*

Finally, the body of evidence is considered as a whole, in order to reach an overall evaluation of the carcinogenicity to humans of an agent, mixture or circumstance of exposure.

An evaluation may be made for a group of chemical compounds that have been evaluated by the Working Group. In addition, when supporting data indicate that other, related compounds for which there is no direct evidence of capacity to induce cancer in humans or in animals may also be carcinogenic, a statement describing the rationale for this conclusion is added to the evaluation narrative; an additional evaluation may be made for this broader group of compounds if the strength of the evidence warrants it.

The agent, mixture or exposure circumstance is described according to the wording of one of the following categories, and the designated group is given. The categorization of an agent, mixture or exposure circumstance is a matter of scientific judgement, reflecting the strength of the evidence derived from studies in humans and in experimental animals and from other relevant data.

Group 1 — The agent (mixture) is carcinogenic to humans.
The exposure circumstance entails exposures that are carcinogenic to humans.

This category is used when there is *sufficient evidence* of carcinogenicity in humans. Exceptionally, an agent (mixture) may be placed in this category when evidence in humans is less than sufficient but there is *sufficient evidence* of carcinogenicity in experimental animals and strong evidence in exposed humans that the agent (mixture) acts through a relevant mechanism of carcinogenicity.

Group 2

This category includes agents, mixtures and exposure circumstances for which, at one extreme, the degree of evidence of carcinogenicity in humans is almost sufficient, as well as those for which, at the other extreme, there are no human data but for which there is evidence of carcinogenicity in experimental animals. Agents, mixtures and exposure circumstances are assigned to either group 2A (probably carcinogenic to humans) or group 2B (possibly carcinogenic to humans) on the basis of epidemiological and experimental evidence of carcinogenicity and other relevant data.

Group 2A — The agent (mixture) is probably carcinogenic to humans.
The exposure circumstance entails exposures that are probably carcinogenic to humans.

This category is used when there is *limited evidence* of carcinogenicity in humans and sufficient evidence of carcinogenicity in experimental animals. In some cases, an agent (mixture) may be classified in this category when there is inadequate evidence of carcinogenicity in humans and *sufficient evidence* of carcinogenicity in experimental animals and strong evidence that the carcinogenesis is mediated by a mechanism that also operates in humans. Exceptionally, an agent, mixture or exposure circumstance may be classified in this category solely on the basis of limited evidence of carcinogenicity in humans.

Group 2B — The agent (mixture) is possibly carcinogenic to humans.
The exposure circumstance entails exposures that are possibly carcinogenic to humans.

This category is used for agents, mixtures and exposure circumstances for which there is *limited evidence* of carcinogenicity in humans and less than *sufficient evidence* of carcinogenicity in experimental animals. It may also be used when there is *inadequate evidence* of carcinogenicity in humans but there is *sufficient evidence* of carcinogenicity in experimental animals. In some instances, an agent, mixture or exposure circumstance for which there is *inadequate evidence* of carcinogenicity in humans but *limited evidence* of carcinogenicity in experimental animals together with supporting evidence from other relevant data may be placed in this group.

Group 3 — The agent (mixture or exposure circumstance) is not classifiable as to its carcinogenicity to humans.

This category is used most commonly for agents, mixtures and exposure circumstances for which the evidence of carcinogenicity is inadequate in humans and inadequate or limited in experimental animals.

Exceptionally, agents (mixtures) for which the evidence of carcinogenicity is inadequate in humans but sufficient in experimental animals may be placed in this category when there is strong evidence that the mechanism of carcinogenicity in experimental animals does not operate in humans.

Agents, mixtures and exposure circumstances that do not fall into any other group are also placed in this category.

Group 4 — The agent (mixture) is probably not carcinogenic to humans.

This category is used for agents or mixtures for which there is *evidence suggesting lack of carcinogenicity* in humans and in experimental animals. In some instances, agents or mixtures for which there is *inadequate evidence* of carcinogenicity in humans but *evidence suggesting lack of carcinogenicity* in experimental animals, consistently and strongly supported by a broad range of other relevant data, may be classified in this group.

References

Breslow, N.E. & Day, N.E. (1980) *Statistical Methods in Cancer Research*, Vol. 1, *The Analysis of Case–Control Studies* (IARC Scientific Publications No. 32), Lyon, IARC

Breslow, N.E. & Day, N.E. (1987) *Statistical Methods in Cancer Research*, Vol. 2, *The Design and Analysis of Cohort Studies* (IARC Scientific Publications No. 82), Lyon, IARC

Cohen, S.M. & Ellwein, L.B. (1990) Cell proliferation in carcinogenesis. *Science*, **249**, 1007–1011

Gart, J.J., Krewski, D., Lee, P.N., Tarone, R.E. & Wahrendorf, J. (1986) *Statistical Methods in Cancer Research*, Vol. 3, *The Design and Analysis of Long-term Animal Experiments* (IARC Scientific Publications No. 79), Lyon, IARC

Hoel, D.G., Kaplan, N.L. & Anderson, M.W. (1983) Implication of nonlinear kinetics on risk estimation in carcinogenesis. *Science*, **219**, 1032–1037

Huff, J.E., Eustis, S.L. & Haseman, J.K. (1989) Occurrence and relevance of chemically induced benign neoplasms in long-term carcinogenicity studies. *Cancer Metastasis Rev.*, **8**, 1–21

IARC (1973–1996) *Information Bulletin on the Survey of Chemicals Being Tested for Carcinogenicity/Directory of Agents Being Tested for Carcinogenicity*, Numbers 1–17, Lyon

IARC (1976–1996)
  Directory of On-going Research in Cancer Epidemiology 1976. Edited by C.S. Muir & G. Wagner, Lyon

Directory of On-going Research in Cancer Epidemiology 1977 (IARC Scientific Publications No. 17). Edited by C.S. Muir & G. Wagner, Lyon

Directory of On-going Research in Cancer Epidemiology 1978 (IARC Scientific Publications No. 26). Edited by C.S. Muir & G. Wagner, Lyon

Directory of On-going Research in Cancer Epidemiology 1979 (IARC Scientific Publications No. 28). Edited by C.S. Muir & G. Wagner, Lyon

Directory of On-going Research in Cancer Epidemiology 1980 (IARC Scientific Publications No. 35). Edited by C.S. Muir & G. Wagner, Lyon

Directory of On-going Research in Cancer Epidemiology 1981 (IARC Scientific Publications No. 38). Edited by C.S. Muir & G. Wagner, Lyon

Directory of On-going Research in Cancer Epidemiology 1982 (IARC Scientific Publications No. 46). Edited by C.S. Muir & G. Wagner, Lyon

Directory of On-going Research in Cancer Epidemiology 1983 (IARC Scientific Publications No. 50). Edited by C.S. Muir & G. Wagner, Lyon

Directory of On-going Research in Cancer Epidemiology 1984 (IARC Scientific Publications No. 62). Edited by C.S. Muir & G. Wagner, Lyon

Directory of On-going Research in Cancer Epidemiology 1985 (IARC Scientific Publications No. 69). Edited by C.S. Muir & G. Wagner, Lyon

Directory of On-going Research in Cancer Epidemiology 1986 (IARC Scientific Publications No. 80). Edited by C.S. Muir & G. Wagner, Lyon

Directory of On-going Research in Cancer Epidemiology 1987 (IARC Scientific Publications No. 86). Edited by D.M. Parkin & J. Wahrendorf, Lyon

Directory of On-going Research in Cancer Epidemiology 1988 (IARC Scientific Publications No. 93). Edited by M. Coleman & J. Wahrendorf, Lyon

Directory of On-going Research in Cancer Epidemiology 1989/90 (IARC Scientific Publications No. 101). Edited by M. Coleman & J. Wahrendorf, Lyon

Directory of On-going Research in Cancer Epidemiology 1991 (IARC Scientific Publications No.110). Edited by M. Coleman & J. Wahrendorf, Lyon

Directory of On-going Research in Cancer Epidemiology 1992 (IARC Scientific Publications No. 117). Edited by M. Coleman, J. Wahrendorf & E. Démaret, Lyon

Directory of On-going Research in Cancer Epidemiology 1994 (IARC Scientific Publications No. 130). Edited by R. Sankaranarayanan, J. Wahrendorf & E. Démaret, Lyon

Directory of On-going Research in Cancer Epidemiology 1996 (IARC Scientific Publications No. 137). Edited by R. Sankaranarayanan, J. Wahrendorf & E. Démaret, Lyon

IARC (1977) *IARC Monographs Programme on the Evaluation of the Carcinogenic Risk of Chemicals to Humans*. Preamble (IARC intern. tech. Rep. No. 77/002), Lyon

IARC (1978) *Chemicals with Sufficient Evidence of Carcinogenicity in Experimental Animals* — IARC Monographs *Volumes 1–17* (IARC intern. tech. Rep. No. 78/003), Lyon

IARC (1978–1993) *Environmental Carcinogens. Methods of Analysis and Exposure Measurement*:

Vol. 1. *Analysis of Volatile Nitrosamines in Food* (IARC Scientific Publications No. 18). Edited by R. Preussmann, M. Castegnaro, E.A. Walker & A.E. Wasserman (1978)

Vol. 2. *Methods for the Measurement of Vinyl Chloride in Poly(vinyl chloride), Air, Water and Foodstuffs* (IARC Scientific Publications No. 22). Edited by D.C.M. Squirrell & W. Thain (1978)

Vol. 3. *Analysis of Polycyclic Aromatic Hydrocarbons in Environmental Samples* (IARC Scientific Publications No. 29). Edited by M. Castegnaro, P. Bogovski, H. Kunte & E.A. Walker (1979)

Vol. 4. *Some Aromatic Amines and Azo Dyes in the General and Industrial Environment* (IARC Scientific Publications No. 40). Edited by L. Fishbein, M. Castegnaro, I.K. O'Neill & H. Bartsch (1981)

Vol. 5. *Some Mycotoxins* (IARC Scientific Publications No. 44). Edited by L. Stoloff, M. Castegnaro, P. Scott, I.K. O'Neill & H. Bartsch (1983)

Vol. 6. N-*Nitroso Compounds* (IARC Scientific Publications No. 45). Edited by R. Preussmann, I.K. O'Neill, G. Eisenbrand, B. Spiegelhalder & H. Bartsch (1983)

Vol. 7. *Some Volatile Halogenated Hydrocarbons* (IARC Scientific Publications No. 68). Edited by L. Fishbein & I.K. O'Neill (1985)

Vol. 8. *Some Metals: As, Be, Cd, Cr, Ni, Pb, Se, Zn* (IARC Scientific Publications No. 71). Edited by I.K. O'Neill, P. Schuller & L. Fishbein (1986)

Vol. 9. *Passive Smoking* (IARC Scientific Publications No. 81). Edited by I.K. O'Neill, K.D. Brunnemann, B. Dodet & D. Hoffmann (1987)

Vol. 10. *Benzene and Alkylated Benzenes* (IARC Scientific Publications No. 85). Edited by L. Fishbein & I.K. O'Neill (1988)

Vol. 11. *Polychlorinated Dioxins and Dibenzofurans* (IARC Scientific Publications No. 108). Edited by C. Rappe, H.R. Buser, B. Dodet & I.K. O'Neill (1991)

Vol. 12. *Indoor Air* (IARC Scientific Publications No. 109). Edited by B. Seifert, H. van de Wiel, B. Dodet & I.K. O'Neill (1993)

IARC (1979) *Criteria to Select Chemicals for* IARC Monographs (IARC intern. tech. Rep. No. 79/003), Lyon

IARC (1982) *IARC Monographs on the Evaluation of the Carcinogenic Risk of Chemicals to Humans*, Supplement 4, *Chemicals, Industrial Processes and Industries Associated with Cancer in Humans* (IARC Monographs, Volumes 1 to 29), Lyon

IARC (1983) *Approaches to Classifying Chemical Carcinogens According to Mechanism of Action* (IARC intern. tech. Rep. No. 83/001), Lyon

IARC (1984) *Chemicals and Exposures to Complex Mixtures Recommended for Evaluation in IARC Monographs and Chemicals and Complex Mixtures Recommended for Long-term Carcinogenicity Testing* (IARC intern. tech. Rep. No. 84/002), Lyon

IARC (1987a) *IARC Monographs on the Evaluation of Carcinogenic Risks to Humans*, Supplement 6, *Genetic and Related Effects: An Updating of Selected* IARC Monographs *from Volumes 1 to 42*, Lyon

IARC (1987b) *IARC Monographs on the Evaluation of Carcinogenic Risks to Humans*, Supplement 7, *Overall Evaluations of Carcinogenicity: An Updating of* IARC Monographs *Volumes 1 to 42*, Lyon

IARC (1988) *Report of an IARC Working Group to Review the Approaches and Processes Used to Evaluate the Carcinogenicity of Mixtures and Groups of Chemicals* (IARC intern. tech. Rep. No. 88/002), Lyon

IARC (1989) *Chemicals, Groups of Chemicals, Mixtures and Exposure Circumstances to be Evaluated in Future IARC Monographs, Report of an ad hoc Working Group* (IARC intern. tech. Rep. No. 89/004), Lyon

IARC (1991a) *A Consensus Report of an IARC Monographs Working Group on the Use of Mechanisms of Carcinogenesis in Risk Identification* (IARC intern. tech. Rep. No. 91/002), Lyon

IARC (1991b) *Report of an Ad-hoc* IARC Monographs *Advisory Group on Viruses and Other Biological Agents Such as Parasites* (IARC intern. tech. Rep. No. 91/001), Lyon

IARC (1993) *Chemicals, Groups of Chemicals, Complex Mixtures, Physical and Biological Agents and Exposure Circumstances to be Evaluated in Future* IARC Monographs, *Report of an ad-hoc Working Group* (IARC intern. Rep. No. 93/005), Lyon

Montesano, R., Bartsch, H., Vainio, H., Wilbourn, J. & Yamasaki, H., eds (1986) *Long-term and Short-term Assays for Carcinogenesis — A Critical Appraisal* (IARC Scientific Publications No. 83), Lyon, IARC

Peto, R., Pike, M.C., Day, N.E., Gray, R.G., Lee, P.N., Parish, S., Peto, J., Richards, S. & Wahrendorf, J. (1980) Guidelines for simple, sensitive significance tests for carcinogenic effects in long-term animal experiments. In: *IARC Monographs on the Evaluation of the Carcinogenic Risk of Chemicals to Humans*, Supplement 2, *Long-term and Short-term Screening Assays for Carcinogens: A Critical Appraisal*, Lyon, pp. 311–426

Tomatis, L., Aitio, A., Wilbourn, J. & Shuker, L. (1989) Human carcinogens so far identified. *Jpn. J. Cancer Res.*, **80**, 795–807

Vainio, H., Magee, P.N., McGregor, D.B. & McMichael, A.J., eds (1992) *Mechanisms of Carcinogenesis in Risk Identification* (IARC Scientific Publications No. 116), Lyon, IARC

Vainio, H., Wilbourn, J.D., Sasco, A.J., Partensky, C., Gaudin, N., Heseltine, E. & Eragne, I. (1995) Identification of human carcinogenic risk in *IARC Monographs*. *Bull. Cancer*, **82**, 339–348 (in French)

Waters, M.D., Stack, H.F., Brady, A.L., Lohman, P.H.M., Haroun, L. & Vainio, H. (1987) Appendix 1. Activity profiles for genetic and related tests. In: *IARC Monographs on the Evaluation of Carcinogenic Risks to Humans*, Suppl. 6, *Genetic and Related Effects: An Updating of Selected IARC Monographs from Volumes 1 to 42*, Lyon, IARC, pp. 687–696

Wilbourn, J., Haroun, L., Heseltine, E., Kaldor, J., Partensky, C. & Vainio, H. (1986) Response of experimental animals to human carcinogens: an analysis based upon the IARC Monographs Programme. *Carcinogenesis*, **7**, 1853–1863

GENERAL REMARKS ON THE SUBSTANCES CONSIDERED

This sixty-sixth volume of *IARC Monographs* comprises evaluations on a number of pharmaceutical drugs. Pharmaceutical drugs were considered previously in Volumes 13, 24 and 50 and Supplement 7 of the *Monographs* series (IARC, 1977, 1980, 1987, 1990). Several of the compounds — diazepam, oxazepam, clofibrate and phenytoin — have been evaluated by previous working groups. All available relevant data including mechanistic data on these compounds are included in the new evaluations. The primary objective of the evaluation process in *IARC Monographs* is hazard or risk identification, although protective effects on cancer occurrence, where pertinent, have been mentioned in the monographs.

Several of the pharmaceuticals considered in this volume are benzodiazepines or benzodiazepine analogues. This class of drugs has been extensively prescribed since the late 1950s for the treatment of anxiety and as sedatives or anticonvulsants, and for other conditions. The specific drugs of this type considered in this volume are *diazepam*, *doxefazepam*, *estazolam*, *oxazepam*, *prazepam*, *ripazepam* and *temazepam*. In addition, a diphenylhydantoin, *phenytoin*, which is another anticonvulsant, was evaluated in this volume.

Three triphenylethylene antioestrogenic drugs were considered that are at various stages of development: *tamoxifen* has been used extensively since the early 1980s, *toremifene* is just being introduced and *droloxifene* is under development for the treatment of breast cancer.

Clofibrate and *gemfibrozil* are cholesterol-lowering drugs that have been used in the treatment of patients at high risk for cardiovascular disease.

Pharmaceutical drugs, in contrast to industrial chemicals or environmental contaminants, are designed to have pharmacological properties which are beneficial. Decisions on the appropriate use of these compounds may involve risk/benefit considerations that go beyond the scope of the *Monographs* programme. It is important to note that pharmaceutical agents are developed and used because of their beneficial biological properties. Sometimes, these biological properties could be also responsible for increased risk of certain diseases including cancer.

The circumstances, magnitude and routes of human exposure for pharmaceuticals are usually easier to evaluate than for environmental or occupational agents. Thus, exposure–response relationships for pharmaceuticals often have more precision. Nevertheless, there are many complicating factors for pharmaceuticals that were considered by the Working Group. A unique feature of the data available on pharmaceuticals is that there is a wealth of information on pharmacokinetic and pharmacodynamic effects in humans obtained in well-controlled studies.

Considerable attention was given to the monograph sections on 'Other Data Relevant to an Evaluation of Carcinogenicity and its Mechanisms'. Of particular interest are the mechanistic underpinnings responsible for significant cancer findings in experimental and epidemiological studies. Although complete knowledge of the mechanism of carcinogenicity of pharmaceuticals is difficult to attain, we can discern, in some cases, the mode of action. This information can lead to biologically-based comparisons which are essential for determining how best to use experimental data in identifying human risks. Comparative data on metabolism, interactions with critical cellular targets (DNA adducts, receptor binding), alterations in gene structure and expression and early tissue responses such as cell proliferation can be especially helpful in strengthening the scientific basis for overall evaluations of carcinogenic risk. Confidence in evaluations is enhanced when there is sound scientific information available from several levels: exposure, animal toxicity and cancer studies, clinical and epidemiological studies and some knowledge of mechanism derived from human, experimental animal and isolated cell systems.

Worldwide, diazepam is the most widely prescribed of the benzodiazepines. For this reason, nearly all studies on the carcinogenicity in humans of the seven benzodiazepines evaluated relate to diazepam. For the others, the evaluation of carcinogenic risk had to rest solely on cancer studies in animals. The drugs that were associated with tumours in animals generally increased only the incidence of rodent liver tumours, a response whose significance to human risk is not clear. Moreover, these effects generally occurred at exposures of the rodents well above the human therapeutic doses. Information from mechanistic studies indicated that these drugs are non-genotoxic and that, if carcinogenic, they operate through a promoting mechanism. Information from human studies to fully evaluate the likelihood that this mechanism will occur in humans was unfortunately lacking.

There were several reports indicating that tamoxifen is a potential hazard in increasing the risk of endometrial cancer. Tamoxifen is recognized as one of the most effective drugs for the treatment of breast cancer and is one of a small group of pharmaceuticals recognized by the World Health Organization as an essential drug for this disease (WHO, 1994). It is currently being evaluated in a number of chemoprevention trials to determine whether it reduces the incidence of breast cancer in otherwise healthy women judged to be at increased risk for development of breast cancer. The Working Group reviewed all the published scientific data on second primary tumours reported in patients who had been treated with tamoxifen for breast cancer. The group further weighed the evidence for carcinogenic effects of tamoxifen in experimental animals, and evaluated possible biological mechanisms of carcinogenesis. It was the totality of the evidence that had to be considered by the Working Group in reaching their final evaluation.

Clofibrate and gemfibrozil, in addition to their therapeutic effects, cause peroxisome proliferation and neoplasia in the livers of rats and mice. All data on exposure and studies of cancer in humans and experimental animals were evaluated. Furthermore, all other data relevant to mechanisms of carcinogenesis were evaluated. Specifically, data were considered, on a case-by-case basis, with regard to (a) the potential for any liver tumour response in mice or rats to be secondary to peroxisome proliferation and (b) the potential for those effects to be observed in humans. The role of peroxisome proliferation and hepatocellular proliferation induced by chemicals such as the fibrate drugs in the development of hepatic cancer was recently addressed by an IARC Working Group (IARC, 1995).

References

IARC (1977) *IARC Monographs on the Evaluation of the Carcinogenic Risk of Chemicals to Humans*, Vol. 13, *Some Miscellaneous Pharmaceutical Substances*, Lyon

IARC (1980) *IARC Monographs on the Evaluation of the Carcinogenic Risk of Chemicals to Humans*, Vol. 24, *Some Pharmaceutical Drugs*, Lyon, pp. 39-58

IARC (1987) *IARC Monographs on the Evaluation of Carcinogenic Risks to Humans*, Suppl. 7, *Overall Evaluations of Carcinogenicity: An Updating of* IARC Monographs *Volumes 1 to 42*, Lyon, pp. 161-165, pp. 171-172

IARC (1990) *IARC Monographs on the Evaluation of Carcinogenic Risks to Humans*, Volume 50, *Pharmaceutical Drugs*, Lyon

IARC (1995) *Peroxisome Proliferation and its Role in Carcinogenesis* (IARC Technical Report No. 24), Lyon

WHO Consultation (1994) Essential drugs for cancer chemotherapy. *Bull. World Health Org.*, **72**, 893-898

THE MONOGRAPHS

# BENZODIAZEPINES AND RELATED COMPOUNDS AND PHENYTOIN

DIAZEPAM

This substance was considered by previous working groups in October 1976 (IARC, 1977) and March 1987 (IARC, 1987). Since that time, new data have become available, and these have been incorporated into the monograph and taken into consideration in the evaluation.

1. Exposure Data

1.1 Chemical and physical data

1.1.1 *Nomenclature*

Chem. Abstr. Serv. Reg. No.: 439-14-5
Deleted CAS Reg. No.: 11100-37-1; 53320-84-6
Chem. Abstr. Name: 7-Chloro-1,3-dihydro-1-methyl-5-phenyl-2*H*-1,4-benzodiazepin-2-one
IUPAC Systematic Name: 7-Chloro-1,3-dihydro-1-methyl-5-phenyl-2*H*-1,4-benzodiazepin-2-one
Synonym: Methyldiazepinone

1.1.2 *Structural and molecular formulae and relative molecular mass*

$C_{16}H_{13}ClN_2O$ Relative molecular mass: 284.75

1.1.3 *Chemical and physical properties of the pure substance*

(a) *Description*: Off-white to yellow, odourless, crystalline powder (Gennaro, 1995)
(b) *Melting-point*: 125–126 °C (Budavari, 1995)
(c) *Spectroscopy data*: Infrared, ultraviolet, nuclear magnetic resonance and mass spectral data have been reported (MacDonald *et al.*, 1972).

(d) *Solubility*: Slightly soluble in water (1 g/333 mL); soluble in acetone, benzene, chloroform (1 g/2 mL), diethyl ether (1 g/39 mL), dimethylformamide and ethanol (1 g/16 mL) (Gennaro, 1995)

(e) *Stability*: Stable in air (Gennaro, 1995)

(f) *Dissociation constant*: pK_a = 3.4 (American Hospital Formulary Service, 1995)

1.1.4 *Technical products and impurities*

Diazepam is available as 2-, 5- and 10-mg tablets, 15-mg extended release capsules, 2- and 5-mg/5 mL oral solutions, 5-mg/mL concentrated oral solution, 5-mg/mL parenteral injection, 5-mg/mL emulsion injection, 2- and 4-mg/mL rectal tube solutions and 10-mg suppositories. Preparations may also contain acetylated monoglycerides, anhydrous glucose, benzoic acid, benzyl alcohol, corn starch, ethanol, flavouring, fractionated egg phospholipids, fractionated soya bean oil, glycerol, lactose, magnesium stearate, methyl hydroxypropylcellulose, polyethylene glycol, propylene glycol, saccharin, sodium benzoate, sodium hydroxide, talc, D&C Yellow 10 (Quinoline Yellow), FD&C Blue 1 (Brilliant Blue FCF) or FD&C Yellow 6 (Sunset Yellow FCF). Sodium benzoate, benzoic acid and sodium hydroxide are added to the commercially available injection products to adjust pH (Thomas, 1991; Farmindustria, 1993; British Medical Association/Royal Pharmaceutical Society of Great Britain, 1994; American Hospital Formulary Service, 1995; Medical Economics, 1996).

Trade names and designations of the chemical and its pharmaceutical preparations include: Aliseum; Alupram; Amiprol; An-Ding; Anksiyolin; Ansiolin; Ansiolisina; Antenex; Apaurin; Apozepam; Armonil; Assival; Atensine; Atilen; Avex; Bensedin; Betapam; Bialzepam; Calmocitene; Calmpose; Canazepam; Cercine; Ceregulart; Condition; Deprestop; Diacepan; Diaceplex; Dialag; Dialar; Diapam; Diatran; Diaz; Diazem; Diazemuls; Diazepam-Lipuro; Diazidem; Dienpax; Dipam; Dizac; Dizam; Domalium; Doval; Drenian; Ducene; Duksen; Duxen; E-Pam; Eridan; Erital; Eurosan; Euphorin; Evacalm; Faustan; Gewacalm; Hexalid; Horizon; Kiatrium; LA 111; Lamra; Lembrol; Levium; Liberetas; Lizan; Lorinon; Mandrozep; Metil Gobanal; Méval; Morosan; Néo-Calme; Neosorex; Nervium; Neurolytril; Noan; Notense; Novazam; Novodipam; Paceum; Pacipam; Pacitran; Pax; Paxate; Paxel; Pro-Pam; Psychopax; Q-Pam; Quétinil; Quievita; Relaminal; Relanium; Relivan; Remedium; Renborin; Rival; Ro 5-2807; Saromet; Scriptopam; Sedapam; Sedipam; Seduxen; Serenak; Serenamin; Serenzin; Servizepam; Setonil; Sibazon; Sibazone; Sico Relax; Solis; Somasedan; Sonacon; Stesolid; Stesolin; Stress-Pam; Tensium; Tensopam; Tiromne; Tranimul; Tranquase; Tranquirit; Tranquo-Puren; Tranquo-Tablinen; Umbrium; Unisedil; Valaxona; ValCaps; Valclair; Valeo; Valibrin; Valiquid; Valitran; Valium; Valrelease; Vatran; Vival; Vivol; Wy 3467; Zepam; Zetran.

1.1.5 *Analysis*

Several international pharmacopoeias specify potentiometric titration with perchloric acid as the assay for purity of diazepam, and thin-layer chromatography for determining impurities and decomposition products. Assay methods for diazepam in capsules, tablets and injection solutions include liquid chromatography or ultraviolet/visible absorption spectrometry using standards. Assays for heavy metal impurities are also specified (Society of Japanese Pharmacopoeia, 1992; British Pharmacopoeial Commission, 1993; United States Pharmacopeial Convention, 1994). Other spectrophotometric (Mañes et al., 1987; El-Brashy et al., 1993) and mass spectrometric (McCarley & Brodbelt, 1993) methods of analysis for diazepam in pharmaceutical preparations have been reported.

Diazepam and its metabolites (including oxazepam (see pp. 116–117) and temazepam (see pp. 162–163)) can be analysed in biological fluids and tissues by radioimmunoassay (Takatori et al., 1991), gas chromatography (GC) (Löscher, 1982), GC–mass spectrometry (GC/MS) (Maurer & Pfleger, 1987), GC with electron capture detection (Peat & Kopjak, 1979; Beischlag & Inaba, 1992) and high-performance liquid chromatography (Peat & Kopjak, 1979; Lensmeyer et al., 1982; Komiskey et al., 1985; Mura et al., 1987; Fernández et al., 1991; Chiba et al., 1995).

1.2 Production and use

1.2.1 Production

A method for preparing diazepam was first reported in 1961 (Sternbach & Reeder, 1961; Sternbach et al., 1961); commercial production of diazepam in the United States of America was first reported in 1963 (United States Tariff Commission, 1964).

Diazepam is prepared by reacting 2-(methylamino)-5-chlorobenzophenone in ethereal solution with bromoacetyl bromide to form 2-(2-bromo-N-methylacetamido)-5-chlorobenzophenone. The latter is then reacted with ammonia in methanol solution to form the 2-amino-N-methylacetamido compound, which is cyclized with dehydration to produce diazepam. The crude diazepam may be purified by recrystallization from diethyl ether (Gennaro, 1995).

1.2.2 Use

Diazepam is a benzodiazepine with anxiolytic, sedative, muscle-relaxant and anticonvulsant properties. The active metabolite is N-desmethyldiazepam, which has a long duration of action (Reynolds, 1993). The therapeutic effects of the benzodiazepines are believed to be due to their binding to the protein receptor complex for the inhibitory neurotransmitter, γ-aminobutyric acid (GABA). This complex has binding sites for both phenobarbital and the benzodiazepines (Barnard et al., 1984). Binding of benzodiazepines to the α subunit of the complex affects chloride conductance within long-fibre neurons and interneurons in the central nervous system and enhances the efficiency of GABAergic transmission (Richards et al., 1986). Central benzodiazepine receptors have been found in human fetal brain tissues by 18 weeks of conceptual age (Brooksbank et al., 1982). Besides this receptor in the central nervous system, there also appears to be a benzodiazepine receptor in peripheral organs (Krueger & Papadopoulos, 1992). This is a mitochondrial protein which may be involved in the regulation of steroid biosynthesis (see Section 4.2.2(c)).

Diazepam is used in the management of severe, disabling anxiety disorders, as a hypnotic in the short-term management of insomnia, in treating convulsions, particularly status epilepticus and febrile convulsions, and in controlling alcohol withdrawal symptoms. It is also used as a premedication and sedative before surgical and other procedures, and for the relief of muscle spasm as in cerebral palsy (Reynolds, 1993). Diazepam is a common adjunct in cancer therapy and may be provided as a pre-admission drug before cancer diagnosis (Derogatis et al., 1979).

The oral dose for anxiety states usually ranges from 2 mg three times daily up to 30 mg daily in divided doses. Similar doses may be sufficient for control of mild to moderate symptoms of alcohol withdrawal. A single dose of 5–30 mg before retiring is given for insomnia associated with anxiety. In muscle spasm, 2–15 mg may be given daily in divided doses and increased, in severe spastic disorders, such as cerebral palsy, to up to 60 mg daily. A similar dosage range has been recommended for the adjunctive use of diazepam in some types of epilepsy. Diazepam at 5–20 mg may be given as a single oral dose or in divided oral doses as a premedication before dental, minor surgical or other procedures. A slow-release oral formulation of diazepam is available in some countries; a dose of 15 mg daily is considered to be equivalent to 5 mg three times daily of the conventional oral formulation. A suggested initial oral dose of diazepam for children is 100–200 µg/kg bw, but up to 800 µg/kg daily has been given. Dosage recommendations are not generally given for premature infants or infants 30 days of age or younger, since safety and efficacy have not been established for these groups (Reynolds, 1993; Medical Economics, 1996).

Diazepam may be given rectally as suppositories in doses similar to the oral doses. A rectal solution of 2–4 mg/mL diazepam may be particularly useful for the control of convulsions; the dose for adults and children over three years of age is 10 mg, and the dose for children aged one to three years is 5 mg. If there is no response after five minutes, the dose may be repeated (Reynolds, 1993).

Diazepam may be given by deep intramuscular injection, although absorption is erratic and gives rise to lower blood concentrations than those obtained after oral administration. It may also be given by intravenous injection, carried out slowly into a large vein of the antecubital fossa at a recommended rate of no more than 1 mL of a 0.5% solution (5 mg) per minute. In cases of severe anxiety or acute muscle spasm, diazepam (10 mg) may be given intramuscularly or intravenously and repeated after 4 h. Higher doses may be required for the treatment of delirium tremens. Patients with tetanus may be given 100–300 µg/kg bw intravenously, repeated every 1–4 h; alternatively, a continuous infusion of 3–10 mg/kg bw every 24 h may be used or similar doses may be given by nasoduodenal tube. Considerably higher doses have been used for extremely severe cases of tetanus. For premedication or sedation before dental, surgical or other procedures, 100–200 µg/kg bw (usually 10–20 mg for adults) may be given by injection. A suggested parenteral sedative or muscle-relaxant dose for children is up to 200 µg/kg bw (Reynolds, 1993).

Diazepam may be given parenterally, preferably by the intravenous route, for the control of status epilepticus or severe recurrent or febrile convulsions. In the United

Kingdom, the usual dose is 150–250 µg/kg bw (or 10–20 mg) for adults and 200–300 µg/kg bw or 1 mg per year of life for children. These doses may be repeated after 30–60 min if required. Once the seizures are controlled, their recurrence may be prevented by intravenous administration of phenytoin sodium (see monograph, pp. 178–179) or by a slow infusion of diazepam. For adults, the maximal total dose of diazepam is 3 mg/kg bw over 24 h (Reynolds, 1993). In the United States, the initial dose for adults is 5–10 mg, repeated if required at 10–15-min intervals up to a maximum of 30 mg. Doses for children are: infants over 30 days and under five years of age, 200–500 µg every 2–5 min up to a maximum of 5 mg; children five years and older, 1 mg every 2–5 min up to a maximum of 10 mg. The above dosage regimens may be repeated after a period of 2–4 h if necessary (Medical Economics, 1996). Elderly and debilitated patients should be given no more than one half of the usual adult dose. Reduction of dosage may also be required in patients with liver or kidney dysfunction (Reynolds, 1993).

Clinical uses of diazepam and other benzodiazepines have been reviewed (Hollister *et al.*, 1993). Diazepam has been used extensively in children (Goodman Gilman *et al.*, 1990).

Worldwide, diazepam is the most widely prescribed of the benzodiazepines. Comparative data on sales of diazepam in several countries are shown in Table 1. Overall, sales declined by approximately 16% from 1990 to 1995.

Table 2 compares the number of prescriptions written in the United States for several benzodiazepines, including diazepam, and for the anticonvulsant, phenytoin, in 1990 and 1995.

Table 3 compares the total sales for these same benzodiazepines and phenytoin in 1990 and 1995 in major markets worldwide.

1.3 Occurrence

1.3.1 *Natural occurrence*

Wildmann *et al.* (1987, 1988) reported the occurrence of trace amounts of diazepam in the brain and adrenals of rats and in wheat and potato samples.

Unseld *et al.* (1989) reported finding low concentrations of diazepam in brain tissue samples from several animal species and plants using GC/MS. Diazepam concentrations ranged from 0.005 to 0.019 ng/g wet weight in brain tissue from salmon, frog, monitor lizard, rat, cat and dog. Traces of diazepam were detected in deer, bovine, adult human and stillborn human brain tissue samples. Diazepam concentrations ranged from 0.002 to 0.010 ng/g in the plant samples (potato tuber, yellow soya beans, unpealed rice, mushrooms).

Unseld *et al.* (1990) reported on the 'natural' occurrence of diazepam in human brain samples. All brain samples were examined by GC/MS and the concentrations observed ranged from 0.15 to 0.34 ng/g wet weight tissue. The human brain tissue samples had been stored before diazepam was first synthesized in 1963.

Table 1. Sales of diazepam in various countries[a] **(number of standard units**[b]**, in thousands)**

Country	1990	1991	1992	1993	1994	1995
Africa						
South Africa	8 227	7 843	7 903	6 977	7 657	7 456
North America						
Canada	119 159	104 306	100 400	80 016	84 831	82 060
Mexico	90 858	83 626	81 044	70 177	67 265	63 874
United States	775 409	711 049	667 798	678 466	697 750	764 904
South America						
Argentina	97 383	106 010	107 794	100 037	95 962	88 942
Brazil	387 216	388 859	327 549	282 044	259 621	209 231
Colombia	9 644	10 109	12 070	4 575	1 840	2 571
Venezuela	11 398	11 959	11 153	12 821	10 552	12 190
Asia						
Japan	533 690	520 677	511 530	484 280	482 458	474 676
Republic of Korea	22 647	22 903	23 253	22 990	22 356	21 310
Australia	94 309	85 418	82 738	81 212	80 203	80 653
Europe						
Belgium	21 044	21 379	21 748	21 496	21 309	20 544
France	102 252	96 216	88 013	82 141	77 222	68 051
Germany	152 300	141 334	118 695	113 702	113 156	115 477
Greece	28 691	22 454	20 476	18 719	17 557	14 291
Italy	265 153	252 443	242 370	221 544	194 035	190 047
Netherlands	45 821	48 460	48 497	46 615	45 161	44 898
Portugal	75 961	77 806	74 370	75 962	78 941	80 988
Spain	238 524	228 722	226 454	215 093	210 853	211 265
Sweden	51 830	46 781	47 085	46 296	46 255	45 552
Switzerland	11 364	11 007	10 616	7 947	7 588	7 232
Turkey	13 156	14 370	15 507	14 809	16 054	18 156
United Kingdom	238 198	235 807	227 345	230 963	224 861	232 365

[a] Data provided by IMS
[b] Standard dosage units, uncorrected for diazepam content

1.3.2 *Occupational exposure*

No quantitative data on occupational exposure levels were available to the Working Group.

The National Occupational Exposure Survey conducted between 1981 and 1983 in the United States by the National Institute of Occupational Safety and Health indicated that about 20 650 employees were potentially occupationally exposed to diazepam. The estimate is based on a survey of United States companies and did not involve measurements of actual exposure (United States National Library of Medicine, 1996).

Table 2. Use of some benzodiazepines and phenytoin in the United States[a] (numbers of prescriptions, in thousands)

Drug	1990	1995
Diazepam	13 056	12 475
Estazolam	0	598
Oxazepam	1 647	1 436
Prazepam	1 205	1
Temazepam	5 567	5 916
Phenytoin[b]	8 848	9 811

[a] Data provided by IMS. No sales of doxefazepam or ripazepam in the United States
[b] Dilantin® only

Table 3. Comparative sales of several benzodiazepines and phenytoin in major markets worldwide[a] (number of standard units[b], in millions)

	1990	1995	Countries with the highest use
Diazepam	3 394	2 857	USA, Japan, Brazil, Spain, UK
Phenytoin	2 423	2 218	USA, Japan, UK, Canada
Oxazepam	1 278	996	Germany, France, USA, Netherlands
Temazepam	706	756	UK, USA, Australia
Prazepam	361	276	France, USA, Italy
Estazolam	158	187	Japan, USA, Portugal

[a] Data provided by IMS
[b] Standard dosage units, uncorrected for content of active ingredient

1.4 Regulations and guidelines

Diazepam is listed in the following pharmacopoeias: Belgian, British, Brazilian, Chinese, Czech, Egyptian, European, French, Greek, Hungarian, Indian, International, Italian, Japanese, Mexican, Netherlands, Nordic, Portuguese, United States and former Yugoslavian (Reynolds, 1993).

2. Studies of Cancer in Humans

Worldwide, diazepam is the most widely used of the benzodiazepines. For this reason, most specific epidemiological information about potential carcinogenic effects of the benzodiazepines relates to this drug. In addition, reported use of unspecified sedatives or hypnotics probably implies principally use of diazepam. This section therefore reviews not only epidemiological studies which investigated diazepam specifically but also those which reported risk associated with unspecified psychotropics, tranquillizers or benzodiazepines.

Several potential biases in the epidemiological studies of benzodiazepines or diazepam in relation to cancer deserve mention. Control selection may be problematic in case–control studies, in that it may be difficult to select *a priori* a diagnostic category unrelated to the exposure, while general population controls may be less likely to self-report short- or long-term use. Indication for use of diazepam or other benzodiazepines has, in general, not been considered as a potential confounding factor. If anxiety or depression due to an underlying hormonal imbalance is involved in the etiological pathway of a particular cancer, the use of psychotropic drugs is merely a marker for the underlying condition, rather than indicating that the drug is the initiator or promoter of the cancer. Another, possibly most important, consideration is that diazepam is a common adjunct in cancer therapy and may be provided as a pre-admission drug before cancer diagnosis (Derogatis *et al.*, 1979). It is therefore essential to ascertain precisely the date of first use of the drug in relation to the date of diagnosis of the cancer, so that reasonable rules for censoring exposure history may be established.

2.1 Descriptive studies

A cross-sectional study examined use of psychotropic drugs for one month or more by 250 women who had been diagnosed with breast cancer at least one year previously and who were attending breast cancer clinics for follow-up visits at two general hospitals in the United Kingdom (Stoll, 1976). Hypnotics, minor tranquillizers, sedatives and antidepressants were used by 14% of the women during the 12 months before diagnosis and by 32% in the 12 months prior to the questionnaire. Among women with metastases at presentation or recurrence within 12 months, 22% had used such drugs before diagnosis, compared to 13% among women with local disease at presentation or recurrences later than 12 months ($p < 0.03$). [The Working Group noted that both the absence of comparably collected control data and a biological rationale for distinguishing the high-usage group were limitations of this descriptive study.]

2.2 Cohort studies

Since 1969, members of the Kaiser Permanente Medical Care Program (KPMCP) in northern California, United States, have been categorized according to their drug exposure, as identified from prescription records, and followed during their membership in the KPMCP. The occurrence of cancer was identified from admission records or by cross-checking against the San Francisco Bay Area Tumor Registry. Expected numbers of cancers were based upon age- and sex-specific rates for the entire cohort. In the latest report from this study with follow-up through 1984 of 12 928 diazepam users, the standardized morbidity ratio for all cancers was 1.0 ([95% confidence interval (CI), 1.0–1.1]; 807 observed versus 784 expected); for breast cancer, 1.1 ([0.9–1.3]; 155 observed versus 144 expected); for Hodgkin's disease, 0.0 ([0.0–0.79]; 0 observed versus 4.7 expected) and for colon cancer, 0.7 ([0.5–0.9]; 57 observed versus 79.9 expected) (Selby *et al.*, 1989; Friedman & Selby, 1990). [The Working Group noted that dose response was not addressed in these data, and that age and sex were the only confounding factors considered.]

In a reconstructed retrospective cohort study, breast cancer in female members of a Group Health Cooperative (GHC) in Seattle, WA was investigated (Danielson *et al.*, 1982). During the period 1977–80, 302 women, aged 35–74 years, who had been members of the GHC for at least six months and who had a newly diagnosed breast cancer were identified. Age-specific incidence rates of breast cancer for users and non-users of diazepam were calculated. Women were classified as exposed to diazepam if at least one prescription for the drug had been filled in the six months before breast cancer diagnosis; drug taken only in the two weeks before mastectomy was not considered. Of 302 women with breast cancer, 27 had taken diazepam before their breast cancer diagnosis; on the basis of 184 438 women-years of observation in total, the age-adjusted risk ratio for breast cancer was 0.9 [95% CI, 0.6–1.3]. [The Working Group noted that this study could not address the effect of long-term use of diazepam and that no confounding factors had been considered.]

2.3 Case–control studies

Table 4 summarizes case–control data on use of benzodiazepines or diazepam that were available to the Working Group. By far the most numerous studies of diazepam in relation to human cancer are case–control studies of breast cancer.

2.3.1 *Breast cancer*

Wallace *et al.* (1982) compared diazepam use in 151 newly diagnosed breast cancer cases at hospitals of the University of Iowa, United States, between 1974 and 1978 with use in a similar number of women with non-cancer conditions selected from the general medical and surgical wards. Matching variables included age and hospital payment category. All subjects were white. The crude relative risk for breast cancer associated with diazepam use was 1.0 [95% CI, 0.5–1.8]. Adjustment for other potential confounders such as age at menarche, parity, type of menopause and family history of breast cancer did not affect the association. Details on refusal rates for controls were not provided. [The Working Group noted the small number of cases and insufficient data on refusal rates for controls.]

Table 4. Case–control studies of diazepam or benzodiazepine use

Study	Location, period	No. of cases/ controls	Source of controls	Exposure	Odds ratio	95% CI	Notes
Breast cancer							
Wallace et al. (1982)	Iowa, USA, 1974–78	151/151	Non-cancer patients	Diazepam, any use	1.0	[0.5–1.8]	Response rate not reported
Kleinerman et al. (1984)	USA, 1973–77	1075/1146	Participants in screening programme	Diazepam, any use	0.7 0.9 1.1	0.6–0.9 0.6–1.3 0.8–1.6	Invasive carcinoma > 1 cm Invasive carcinoma ≤ 1 cm In-situ carcinoma
Kaufman et al. (1982)	USA, Canada, Israel, 1976–80	1236/728	Cancer patients	Diazepam, 4 times/week, during ≥ 6 months, > 18 months before interview	0.9	0.5–1.6	Similar results with 'female' cancer or other cancer controls
Kaufman et al. (1990)	USA, 1981–87	3078/1259	Cancer and non-cancer patients	Diazepam, 4 times/week, during ≥ 6 months, > 18 months before interview	1.0	0.6–1.7	Similar results with non-cancer controls
	Toronto, Canada, 1982–86	607/1214	Census records	Diazepam, 4 times/week, during ≥ 6 months, > 18 months before interview	0.8	0.5–1.3	
Rosenberg et al. (1995)	USA, 1977–91	6056/1603	Cancer patients	Benzodiazepine, sustained use[a]	1.0	0.8–1.3	Overlap with Kaufman et al. (1982, 1990). Similar results with non-cancer controls. Odds ratio for ≥ 5 years of benzodiazepine use: 0.8 (0.5–1.4)
				Diazepam, sustained use[a]	1.0	0.7–1.4	

Table 4 (contd)

Study	Location, period	No. of cases/controls	Source of controls	Exposure	Odds ratio	95% CI	Notes
Ovarian cancer							
Tzonou et al. (1993)	Athens, Greece, 1989–91	189/200	Visitors to hospitals	'Tranquillizers or hypnotics', any use	1.0	0.6–1.6	
Harlow & Cramer (1995)	Boston, MA, USA, 1978–81, 1984–87	450/454	General population	Benzodiazepine, any use	1.8	1.0–3.1	Higher risk for use before age 50 or ≥ 10 years before interview
Rosenberg et al. (1995)	USA, 1977–91	767/1603	Cancer patients	Benzodiazepine, sustained use[a]	0.9	0.6–1.4	Similar results with non-cancer controls. Odds ratio for ≥ 5 years of benzodiazepine use: 0.3 (0.1–0.9)
				Diazepam, sustained use[a]	1.0	0.6–1.6	
Malignant melanoma							
Adam & Vessey (1981)	England and Wales, 1971–76	150/496	General practitioners' patients	Diazepam, ≥ 1 month	1.2	0.6–2.2	General practitioners' records
		101/302	General practitioners' patients	Diazepam, ≥ 1 month	1.7	0.9–3.2	Self-reported use
Rosenberg et al. (1995)	USA, 1977–91	1457/3777	Cancer patients	Benzodiazepine, sustained use[a]	1.0	0.8–1.4	Similar results with non-cancer controls. Odds ratio for ≥ 5 years of benzodiazepine use: 0.9 (0.5–1.7)
				Diazepam, sustained use[a]	1.0	0.7–1.5	

Table 4 (contd)

Study	Location, period	No. of cases/ controls	Source of controls	Exposure	Odds ratio	95% CI	Notes
Multiple myeloma							
Linet et al. (1987)	Baltimore, MD, USA, 1975–82	100/100	Hospital patients	Diazepam, any use	2.0	0.4–12	
Lung cancer							
Rosenberg et al. (1995)	USA, 1977–91	1365/3777	Cancer patients	Benzodiazepine, sustained use[a]	1.0	0.7–1.4	Similar results with non-cancer controls. Odds ratio for ≥ 5 years of benzodiazepine use: 1.2 (0.6–2.6)
				Diazepam, sustained use[a]	0.8	0.5–1.2	
Colon cancer							
Rosenberg et al. (1995)	USA, 1977–91	2203/3777	Cancer patients	Benzodiazepine, sustained use[a]	0.8	0.6–1.1	Similar results with non-cancer controls. Odds ratio for ≥ 5 years of benzodiazepine use: 0.8 (0.5–1.2)
				Diazepam, sustained use[a]	0.7	0.5–1.0	
Non-Hodgkin's lymphoma							
Rosenberg et al. (1995)	USA, 1977–91	382/3777	Cancer patients	Benzodiazepine, sustained use[a]	0.8	0.5–1.4	Similar results with non-cancer controls. Odds ratio for ≥ 5 years of benzodiazepine use: 0.8 (0.3–2.1)
				Diazepam, sustained use[a]	0.8	0.4–1.6	
Hodgkin's disease							
Rosenberg et al. (1995)	USA, 1977–91	299/3777	Cancer patients	Benzodiazepine, sustained use[a]	0.6	0.3–1.4	Similar results with non-cancer controls. Odds ratio for ≥ 5 years of benzodiazepine use: 1.2 (0.3–4.5)
				Diazepam, sustained use[a]	0.9	0.4–2.0	

Table 4 (contd)

Study	Location, period	No. of cases/ controls	Source of controls	Exposure	Odds ratio	95% CI	Notes
Thyroid cancer							
Rosenberg et al. (1995)	USA, 1977–91	111/3777	Cancer patients	Benzodiazepine, sustained use[a]	0.9	0.4–2.4	Similar results with non-cancer controls. Odds ratio for ≥ 5 years of benzodiazepine use: 1.3 (0.3–6.0)
				Diazepam, sustained use[a]	0.8	0.2–2.7	
Liver cancer							
Rosenberg et al. (1995)	USA, 1977–91	37/3777	Cancer patients	Benzodiazepine, sustained use[a]	1.2	0.3–5.2	Similar results with non-cancer controls
				Diazepam, sustained use[a]	2.0	0.5–8.4	
Endometrial cancer							
Rosenberg et al. (1995)	USA, 1977–91	812/1603	Cancer patients	Benzodiazepine, sustained use[a]	1.2	0.8–1.9	Similar results with non-cancer controls. Odds ratio for ≥ 5 years of benzodiazepine use: 1.4 (0.6–2.9)
				Diazepam, sustained use[a]	1.4	0.8–2.3	
Testicular cancer							
Rosenberg et al. (1995)	USA, 1977–91	314/2174	Cancer patients	Benzodiazepine, sustained use[a]	1.2	0.5–3.1	Similar results with non-cancer controls
				Diazepam, sustained use[a]	1.4	0.4–4.7	

[a] ≥ 4 times/week, during ≥ 1 month, > 24 months before interview

Kleinerman et al. (1984) examined the association between breast cancer and diazepam use in white women participating in the Breast Cancer Detection Demonstration Project in the United States between 1973 and 1977. The study included 1075 prevalent cases who had a histologically confirmed breast cancer detected during the five-year period and 1146 controls selected from women with normal mammographic results that did not require biopsy. Controls were matched by screening centre, age and date at entry and length of continuation in the screening programme. Exposures were assessed by home interview, and participation rates were 86% for cases and 74% for controls. Only diazepam use begun at least six months before the date of the breast cancer diagnosis was considered. The relative risk associated with diazepam use for invasive tumours > 1 cm was 0.7 (95% CI, 0.6–0.9), that for invasive tumours ≤ 1 cm was 0.9 (0.6–1.3) and that for in-situ tumours was 1.1 (0.8–1.6). [The Working Group noted that some drug-exposed women with poor survival may not have been included in this study.]

Data on breast cancer in relation to diazepam use are available from a hospital-based case–control surveillance system (Kaufman et al., 1982, 1990; Rosenberg et al., 1995). [These three studies, although reported separately, may overlap in either study methodology or subjects included.] In the first report from this series, diazepam use was ascertained by personal interviews in 1236 women less than 70 years old diagnosed with primary breast cancer in the six months before admission and 728 controls admitted to metropolitan hospitals in the United States, Canada and Israel during 1976–80 (Kaufman et al., 1982). Control women had other cancers including other 'female' cancers such as endometrial or ovarian cancer. Of patients approached, 5% refused to be interviewed. The principal analyses excluded use of diazepam in the 18 months before hospital admission, to avoid the possibility of recording use begun after a diagnosis of breast cancer or because of clinical symptoms preceding the diagnosis, and also focused on 'regular' use of diazepam (defined as use of the drug for at least four days per week) and 'sustained regular' use (for a total duration of at least six months). Potential confounding factors considered were age, geographical region, education, religion, parity, age at first pregnancy, menopausal status, age at menopause, family history of breast cancer and alcohol use. The relative risk for breast cancer associated with regular use of diazepam for six months or more was 0.9 (95% CI, 0.5–1.6), with all other cancers as the control group. The relative risk for breast cancer associated with regular use of diazepam for less than six months was 0.8 (0.4–1.4), with all other cancers as the control group. The relative risks were no greater for women with metastatic disease. Similar risk estimates were found when women with either other cancers or 'other female' cancers were used as the control group.

These investigators extended their study with data from 3078 breast cancer cases, 18–69 years old, with cancer diagnosed within six months before admission, interviewed between 1981 and 1987 in hospitals in the metropolitan United States and from three separate control groups interviewed over the same time period (Kaufman et al., 1990). As in the previous study, women with other cancers (754) or with other 'female' cancers (505) were included as controls. A non-cancer control group (672) was also included, which was composed primarily of women with ectopic pregnancy (281), appendicitis

(230) or retinal detachment (100). Women admitted for trauma were not included because of the possibility that diazepam increases the risk for accidents. Of patients approached, 4% refused to be interviewed. The authors adjusted for age, geographical region, education, religion, parity, menopausal status, age at menarche, first birth and menopause, family history of breast cancer, alcohol, oral contraceptive and other benzodiazepine use. In this study, the percentage of white women varied from 64% in the non-cancer controls to 90% in the female cancer controls, and race was included as an adjustment variable. Regular use of diazepam, defined as in the previous study, was associated with a relative risk for breast cancer of 1.0 (95% CI, 0.6–1.7), compared with controls with any other cancer and 0.8 (0.4–1.8) compared with the non-cancer controls. Risks were similar for 'sporadic' use of diazepam, defined as use beginning at least 18 months before interview and lasting for less than six months or use involving fewer than four days per week. 'Recent' use of diazepam (beginning within 18 months of interview) was also associated with a significantly elevated risk for breast cancer of 1.9 (1.1–3.1), compared with controls with any other cancer and 5.6 (2.3–13.6) compared with the non-cancer controls. [With respect to 'recent use', see the comment below.]

In the same publication, results of a separate study of 607 cases of breast cancer identified between 1982 and 1986 through the Ontario Cancer Institute, Canada, were reported (Kaufman et al., 1990). Controls in this study were 1214 women selected from municipal voting and census records matched for neighbourhood and decade of age. Refusal rates were 21% among potential cases and 35% among potential controls. The relative risks for breast cancer associated with categories of diazepam use, as defined above, were 0.8 (95% CI, 0.5–1.3) for regular use, 1.1 (0.8–1.5) for sporadic use and 3.1 (1.5–6.4) for recent use. [With respect to 'recent use', see the comment below.]

In the most recent and comprehensive report using this hospital surveillance system to investigate possible effects of benzodiazepine exposure, not only breast cancer but also other cancers were analysed (Rosenberg et al., 1995). The 6056 breast cancer cases included some previously reported cases from 1977 to 1987 as well as new cases admitted between 1988 and 1991. The primary control group was 1603 women with other cancers excluding those of the endometrium or ovary. Participation rates were about 96% and adjustment was made for age at menarche, first pregnancy and menopause, parity, religion, education, race, family history of breast cancer and duration of use of oral contraceptives or oestrogen replacement therapy. In contrast to the previous reports from this series, 'recent' use was defined in relation to a two-year interval before hospital admission, rather than an 18-month interval. 'Sustained' use of diazepam for at least four days per week for one month initiated two or more years before admission was associated with a relative risk for breast cancer of 1.0 (95% CI, 0.7–1.4). For sustained use of all benzodiazepines combined, risk did not vary significantly with the number of years since last use or with a duration of use of five years or more.

[The Working Group noted that the elevated risks for breast cancer associated with benzodiazepine use within the 'recent' period before hospital admission observed in some of these studies could be attributed to drug use begun after the diagnosis of breast cancer. More precise information on the timing of the drug exposure in relation to the date of diagnosis of breast cancer rather than the interview date might have clarified this potential bias.]

2.3.2 Ovarian cancer

Tzonou et al. (1984) studied 150 women with malignant epithelial ovarian tumours newly diagnosed during 1980 and 1981 in 10 hospitals in Athens, Greece, and compared them with 250 women in the Athens Hospital for Orthopedic Disorders. No controls approached were said to have refused, but participation rates for cases were not stated. 'Frequent' use of 'psychotropic' drugs was reported by eight cases and two controls, giving a crude odds ratio of 7.0 [95% CI, 1.8–27] for ovarian cancer associated with use of these drugs. [The Working Group noted that the indications given by the authors for 'frequent' use of 'psychotropic' drugs in this study suggest that benzodiazepines may have been used infrequently.]

In a subsequent report, the same investigators compared drug use in 189 women less than 75 years old with malignant epithelial ovarian cancer diagnosed during 1989–91 in two hospitals in greater Athens with that of 200 visitors to the same hospitals (Tzonou et al., 1993). Participation rates were 90–94%. The relative risk associated with ever use of 'tranquillizers or hypnotics' over an 'extended' period was 1.0 (95% CI, 0.6–1.6) after adjustment for age, education, weight, age at menarche and menopause, parity, smoking and other study variables.

[The Working Group noted the small number of exposed subjects in both studies, a possible lack of appropriateness of the control selection and the lack of specificity of information on the agent and its duration of use.]

Benzodiazepine use was investigated in a study which combined two case–control studies conducted previously from ten hospitals in Boston, MA, United States (Harlow & Cramer, 1995). The study included 450 cases of malignant epithelial ovarian cancer diagnosed between 1978–81 and 1984–87 in women 18–80 years old and 454 controls identified from the general population during the same period and matched for age, race and precinct of residence. Participation rates for cases and controls were around 70%. Any use of a benzodiazepine tranquillizer was associated with a relative risk for ovarian cancer of 1.8 (95% CI, 1.0–3.1) after adjustment for parity, oral contraceptive use, religion, body mass, prior hysterectomy and therapeutic abortion. Risk appeared to be confined to women whose first use of the drug either was before the age of 50 years, where the relative risk was 2.7 (1.3–5.6), or occurred 10 or more years before the age at diagnosis (3.2; 1.4–7.6). [The Working Group noted that more specific data on risk for ovarian cancer by frequency or duration of drug use would have been helpful in establishing the validity of this association.]

Data on diazepam use in relation to ovarian cancer are also available from the study by Rosenberg et al. (1995), described previously. Among 767 women with ovarian cancer, sustained use of diazepam was reported by 25 (4.3%), giving a relative risk of 1.0 (95% CI, 0.6–1.6).

2.3.3 Other cancers

A case–control study of malignant melanoma in women, aged 15–49 years, in relation to diazepam use was conducted from a survey of general practitioners in southern England between 1971 and 1976 (Adam & Vessey, 1981). Controls were selected from the practice lists of the same doctors and matched by age and marital status. The relative risk for malignant melanoma associated with use of diazepam for more than one month, as assessed from the general practitioners' records, based on 150 cases and 496 controls was 1.2 (95% CI, 0.6–2.2). The risk was 1.7 (0.9–3.2) for diazepam use as assessed from postal questionnaires completed by 101 cases and 302 controls. [The Working Group noted that the poor response rates to the postal questionnaire may have accounted for the marginally greater risk for melanoma associated with diazepam use if a greater number of responding cases recalled short-term use.]

A hospital-based case–control study of multiple myeloma was conducted in Baltimore, MD, United States (Linet et al., 1987). A total of 121 cases of multiple myeloma in white patients were ascertained from seven hospitals during the period 1 January 1975 to 31 December 1982. Controls were individually matched to cases on hospital, age (± 5 years), sex and year of diagnosis. The control group included patients randomly selected from 11 categories of disease which included digestive and nervous system diseases, accidents and poisoning but excluded diagnoses of cancer, diseases of blood-forming organs, mental disorders, obstetric conditions and congenital anomalies. Information about many factors was obtained from the study subjects with a questionnaire by telephone; if the individual concerned had died or could not be interviewed for any other reason, information was sought from the closest possible relative. The response rate was 83% among cases, leaving 100 cases for analysis. Data on drug use occurring before diagnosis were analysed. The crude odds ratio associated with diazepam use, based on nine discordant pairs, was 2.0 (95% CI, 0.4–12). [The Working Group noted that the diagnostic categories for controls could have been associated with exposure to diazepam. In addition, the greater number of proxy interviews for cases than controls could not be adjusted for with diazepam as the exposure.]

The study by Rosenberg et al. (1995), described previously, addressed risk for other cancers associated with diazepam use. For sustained use of diazepam, defined as use for at least four days per week for at least one month which had been initiated at least two years before admission, relative risks for selected sites were: 0.7 (95% CI, 0.5–1.0) for cancer of the large bowel, 0.8 (0.5–1.2) for lung cancer, 0.9 (0.4–2.0) for Hodgkin's disease, 0.8 (0.2–2.7) for cancer of the thyroid, 2.0 (0.5–8.4) for liver cancer, 1.4 (0.8–2.3) for endometrial cancer and 1.4 (0.4–4.7) for testicular cancer. [See Section 2.3.1 for the Working Group's comments on this study.]

Anthony et al. (1982) surveyed general practitioners in the United Kingdom and requested information on medications used by any new patients with cancer and by age- and sex-matched controls who were the 'next' patient with a 'new' complaint not related to cancer. Six (possibly seven) of 211 male patients with cancer (mostly lung) had taken barbiturates and benzodiazepines concomitantly, compared to none of 211 male controls [$p = 0.03$]. [The Working Group noted that participation by the general practitioners was voluntary and quite variable and that the study may have included drug exposures postdating the cancer diagnosis.]

3. Studies of Cancer in Experimental Animals

3.1 Oral administration

3.1.1 *Mouse*

Diazepam was included as a reference compound in a study on the carcinogenicity of prazepam. Groups of 100 male and 100 female albino CF1 mice (control group) and 50 male and 50 female mice (diazepam group), eight weeks of age, were given 0 or 75 mg/kg bw diazepam (melting point, 131–135 °C) mixed in the diet for up to 80 weeks, when surviving animals were killed. The dose was chosen to match the high-dose level of prazepam. The diazepam concentration in the food was adjusted weekly for changes in body weight and food consumption. The diazepam/diet mixtures were prepared freshly each week. In treated mice, body-weight gains were similar to those of controls throughout the study. From graphic presentations, there appeared to be no significant effect on mortality in male mice, but the diazepam-treated females had lower survival (65–75% survival for control and diazepam-treated males, 70% for control females and 40% for diazepam-treated females) [statistics and exact numbers not given]. Major organs [not specified] and visually apparent lesions were examined histologically. By life table analysis, the incidences of benign hepatocellular tumours were (tumour-bearing mice/effective number of mice): control males, 1/93; diazepam-treated males, 2/43; control females, 1/91; and diazepam-treated females, 0/38. Those for malignant hepatocellular tumours were: control males, 7/93; diazepam-treated males, 9/43 ($p < 0.05$, chi-square test); control females, 1/91; and diazepam-treated females, 2/38 (de la Iglesia *et al.*, 1981). [The Working Group noted that diazepam was tested only as a reference chemical and that the study was terminated at 80 weeks.]

3.1.2 *Rat*

Diazepam was included as a reference compound in a study on the carcinogenicity of prazepam. Groups of 115 male and 115 female albino SPF Wistar rats (control group) and 65 male and 65 female rats (diazepam group), eight weeks of age, were given either 0 or 75 mg/kg bw diazepam (melting-point, 131–135 °C) daily mixed in the diet for up to 104 weeks, when surviving animals were killed. The diazepam concentration in the food was adjusted weekly for changes in body weight and food consumption. The diazepam/diet mixtures were prepared freshly each week. In treated rats, body weight gains were similar to those of controls throughout the study. From graphic presentations, there appeared to be no significant effect on mortality (50–60% survival for males and about 60% for females) [statistics and exact numbers not given]. Major organs [not specified] and visually apparent lesions were examined histologically. No significant increase in the incidence of tumours at any site was seen for either male or female rats. The incidences of benign hepatocellular tumours were: control males, 1/115; diazepam-treated males,

0/65; control females, 1/115; and diazepam-treated females, 0/65. Those for malignant hepatocellular tumours were: control males, 0/115; diazepam-treated males, 3/65 [$p = 0.054$, Fisher's exact test]; control females, 0/115; and diazepam-treated females, 0/65 (de la Iglesia *et al.*, 1981).

To study initiating activity, groups of 10 male Fischer 344 rats weighing 150 g [age not specified] were given 7 and 70 mg/kg bw diazepam (purity, > 99%) suspended in 10% arabic gum solution daily by gastric instillation for 14 weeks. Forty rats served as untreated controls. Neoplastic nodules and iron-excluding foci were not found in the livers of diazepam-treated animals nor in those of the controls (Mazue *et al.*, 1982; Remandet *et al.*, 1984).

3.1.3 *Hamster*

Groups of 55–56 male and 55–56 female Syrian golden hamsters were given 120 mg/kg bw diazepam mixed in the diet for 57 weeks (females) or 79 weeks (males). Approximately 110 hamsters per sex served as controls. Some intercurrent deaths, mostly after week 30, occurred from severe enteritis. No significant increase in the incidence of tumours was found (Black *et al.*, 1987). [The Working Group noted the single dose, that diazepam was used as a reference compound for a study on quazepam and that specific data on survival were not given.]

3.1.4 *Gerbil*

Groups of 15 male and 12 female gerbils [strain and age not specified] were given 10 mg diazepam [purity not specified] per animal by gastric instillation weekly. Eleven males and ten females receiving saline served as vehicle controls. Male and female controls survived 80 and 69 weeks, respectively, while gerbils receiving diazepam survived 79–81 weeks. Complete histopathology was performed as animals died or became moribund, and two ovarian granulosa-cell tumours in control females were the only tumours reported (Green & Ketkar, 1978). [The Working Group noted the small numbers of animals and the weekly administration of diazepam.]

3.2 Administration with known carcinogens

3.2.1 *Mouse*

Groups of 40 male B6C3F1 mice, five weeks of age, were given a single intraperitoneal injection of either 0 or 90 mg/kg bw *N*-nitrosodiethylamine (NDEA) in tricaprylin. At seven weeks of age, the mice received 500 or 1500 mg/kg diet (ppm) diazepam [purity unspecified] in the diet. Eight mice per group were killed at 9, 21 and 33 weeks of exposure and the remainder were killed after 53 weeks of exposure. Complete necropsy was performed on each animal, and liver, lung, spleen, thyroid, kidney and visually apparent lesions in other organs were examined histologically. Between 33 and 53 weeks of exposure, there was an increase in the incidence of hepatocellular tumours in animals treated with NDEA and diazepam compared with those given NDEA alone (see Table 5) (Diwan *et al.*, 1986).

Table 5. Incidence of liver tumours in B6C3F1 mice

Treatment	Hepatocellular adenomas	Hepatocellular carcinomas
NDEA	10/16	0/16
NDEA + 500 ppm diazepam	13/14	5/14[a]
NDEA + 1500 ppm diazepam	15/15[a]	9/15[b]
500 ppm diazepam	0/16	0/16
1500 ppm diazepam	3/15	0/15

From Diwan et al. (1986)
[a] [$p < 0.05$, Fisher's exact test compared with NDEA controls]
[b] [$p < 0.01$, Fisher's exact test compared with NDEA controls]

3.2.2 Rat

Groups of 10 or 20 male Fischer 344 rats weighing 170 g [age unspecified] were fed basal diets or diets containing 200 mg/kg (ppm) 2-acetylaminofluorene (2-AAF) for eight weeks. The daily dose was estimated to be approximately 15 mg/kg bw. In one group of 10 rats, this was followed by 12 weeks' treatment with 70 mg/kg bw diazepam in 10% arabic gum solution (purity > 99%) daily by gastric instillation. There was no significant increase in the incidence of neoplastic nodules of the liver: untreated controls (20 rats), 0 neoplastic nodule/liver; 2-AAF alone (20 rats), 0.2 neoplastic nodule/liver; and 2-AAF plus diazepam (10 rats), 0.5 neoplastic nodule/liver (Mazue et al., 1982; Remandet et al., 1984). [The Working Group noted the small number of animals and the single dose level of diazepam.]

Groups of 10 male weanling Donryu rats, 21 days of age, were fed a diet containing 600 mg/kg (ppm) 3'-methyl-4-(dimethylamino)azobenzene for three weeks, then left for a week on basal diet followed by either basal diet or a diet with 500 mg/kg diazepam [purity unspecified] (daily intake, approximately 50 mg/kg bw) for a further 12 weeks. The rat livers were scored for adenosine triphosphatase (ATPase)-deficient islands greater than 50 µm in diameter. There was no significant difference between rats on basal diet and those given diazepam in the total number of enzyme-altered islands/cm^2 (control, 9.76 ± 1.32; diazepam-treated, 8.64 ± 0.80) or in the number of enzyme-altered islands > 400 µm (control, 1.03 ± 0.24; diazepam-treated, 1.33 ± 0.34) (Hino & Kitagawa, 1982).

3.2.3 Gerbil

Groups of 24 male and 16 female gerbils [strain and age not specified] were given 10 mg diazepam [purity not specified] per animal by gastric instillation weekly plus 30 min later weekly subcutaneous injections of 23 mg/kg bw NDEA for life. Groups of 20 male and 19 female gerbils receiving weekly subcutaneous administrations of NDEA only served as positive controls. Groups of 11 male and 10 female gerbils receiving weekly subcutaneous administrations of saline served as vehicle controls. Gerbils receiving NDEA plus diazepam tended to survive approximately 20 weeks longer than gerbils receiving NDEA alone. The incidence of nasal cavity adenocarcinomas was high in both groups: 92–95% in males and 63–69% in females. In gerbils receiving NDEA alone, 85% males and 84% females had cholangiocarcinomas of the liver versus none in the NDEA plus diazepam group (75% females and 83% males had cholangiomas of the liver). Male gerbils receiving NDEA plus diazepam had three hepatocellular adenomas and one male and one female had a hepatocellular carcinoma versus none in the NDEA group (Green & Ketkar, 1978). [The Working Group noted the small number of animals and that diazepam was administered weekly.]

3.3 Carcinogenicity of metabolites

See the monographs on oxazepam (pp. 119–123) and temazepam (pp. 164–165).

4. Other Data Relevant to an Evaluation of Carcinogenicity and its Mechanisms

4.1 Absorption, distribution, metabolism and excretion

4.1.1 *Humans*

The disposition of diazepam has been reviewed (Mandelli *et al.*, 1978; Schmidt, 1995). Diazepam is rapidly and almost completely absorbed following oral doses of 5, 10 or 20 mg; peak plasma concentrations are usually obtained within 30–90 min and a secondary peak during the elimination phase has been observed in some studies (Baird & Hailey, 1972; Hillestad *et al.*, 1974; Gamble *et al.*, 1975; Kanto, 1975; Korttila & Linnoila, 1975; Schmidt, 1995). Peak plasma concentrations vary widely (30-fold range) in different subjects given the same dose of diazepam (Gamble *et al.*, 1973). Oral administration of two 5-mg tablets to 48 healthy male volunteers aged 18–44 years resulted in peak plasma concentrations after 0.9 h (range, 0.5–2.5 h) of 406 ng/mL (range, 253–586 ng/mL) (Greenblatt *et al.*, 1989). Results were similar among pregnant women receiving single 10-mg doses during the first trimester (Jørgensen *et al.*, 1988). Intravenous administration of 10 or 20 mg diazepam to volunteers gave peak plasma concentrations of 700–800 ng/mL and 1100–1607 ng/mL, respectively, within 3–15 min. Intramuscular administration is not clinically useful in adults, but, in newborn babies and children under 12 years, doses of 0.24–1 mg/kg bw give peak plasma concentrations of 206–1400 ng/mL in 10–60 min (reviewed in Schmidt, 1995). Diazepam has a low pK_a and is lipophilic and consequently distributes quickly into lipoid tissues, and rapidly crosses the blood–brain barrier. A distribution phase with a usual half-life of about 1 h following a single dose precedes the elimination phase (Kaplan *et al.*, 1973; Klotz *et al.*, 1976a,b; Mandelli *et al.*, 1978). Plasma protein binding of diazepam is about 97% (van der Kleijn *et al.*, 1971; Klotz *et al.*, 1976b). Irrespective of the route of administration, the terminal elimination half-life is usually within the range of 24–48 h, and mean values of about 32 h have been obtained in several single-dose studies (reviewed by Schmidt, 1995). Somewhat longer half-lives (mean of 44 h) were measured by Greenblatt *et al.* (1989) in healthy male volunteers, and longer half-lives are also obtained following repeated administration (Kaplan et al., 1973; Mandelli et al., 1978). Elimination half-lives were longer in premature newborn babies (75 ± 35 h) than in full-term newborn babies (31 ± 2 h) (Morselli, 1977). Plasma clearance values (CL_E) are typically 15–35 mL/min for diazepam and 7–11 mL/min for N-desmethyldiazepam. The values tend to be lower in cases of liver disease and, at least for N-desmethyldiazepam, after the age of 60 years (Schmidt, 1995).

Diazepam has two major metabolic pathways in humans (see Figure 1), involving either the loss of the N_1-methyl group, yielding N-desmethyldiazepam, which is then oxidized at C_3 to oxazepam, or the direct oxidation at C_3, yielding temazepam. The elimination of oxazepam and temazepam is reviewed in sections 4.1.1 of the respective monographs in this volume. N-Desmethyldiazepam is the major circulating metabolite of diazepam, as some 50–60% of diazepam is demethylated (Bertilsson et al., 1990). The plasma concentrations of N-desmethyldiazepam approach those of diazepam following a single dose, and typically exceed those of diazepam after multiple doses, since the elimination half-life of this metabolite is much longer (50–120 h) than that of diazepam. Thus, in the data tabulated by Schmidt (1995), the half-lives of N-desmethyldiazepam are longer than those of diazepam in every situation where both were measured (in volunteers, psychiatric patients, epileptic patients, the elderly and patients with liver disease). N-Desmethyldiazepam has a longer half-life (40–120 h) than diazepam (20–54 h) in adults (Mandelli et al., 1978; Bertilsson et al., 1990). There have been few studies of the excretion of diazepam and its metabolites, but it appears that conjugation is important before elimination. Schwartz et al. (1965) found that approximately 71% of orally administered diazepam and its metabolites is excreted in the urine and 10% in the faeces. It is not clear whether conjugated oxazepam or conjugated N-desmethyldiazepam is the more important urinary metabolite (Schwartz et al., 1965; Morselli et al., 1973; Kanto et al., 1974; Arnold, 1975). In a recent, but preliminary, study (Chiba et al., 1995), four male volunteers aged 24–40 years were given a single dose of 4 mg diazepam orally and urine was collected over 96 h. Following treatment of the urine with β-glucuronidase/sulfatase, diazepam was not detectable and the cumulative excretion of N-desmethyldiazepam, temazepam and oxazepam was 3.9 ± 0.4, 6.6 ± 1.4 and 2.8 ± 0.6% of the dose, respectively. Enterohepatic circulation might explain the long elimination half-life of diazepam and the secondary peak observed in some studies during the elimination phase, but most studies indicate that diazepam is not excreted in the bile in significant amounts (reviewed in Schmidt, 1995).

Diazepam is able to cross the placenta rapidly (deSilva et al., 1964; Idänpään-Heikkila et al., 1971a; Jørgensen et al., 1988) and accumulates in the fetus with slow elimination of its active metabolite. The fetal plasma levels of diazepam are equal to or 1.2 times higher than the maternal plasma concentrations (Cavanagh & Condo, 1964; Erkkola et al., 1974); the level of its active metabolite, N-desmethyldiazepam, is exceptionally high in fetal liver (Erkkola et al., 1974). After the use of diazepam in labour, diazepam and N-desmethyldiazepam persist in the newborn for eight days postpartum (Cree et al., 1973). Diazepam and its active metabolite also pass from the mother's blood into breast milk (Erkkola & Kanto, 1972; Cole & Hailey, 1975).

Figure 1. Postulated metabolic pathways of diazepam

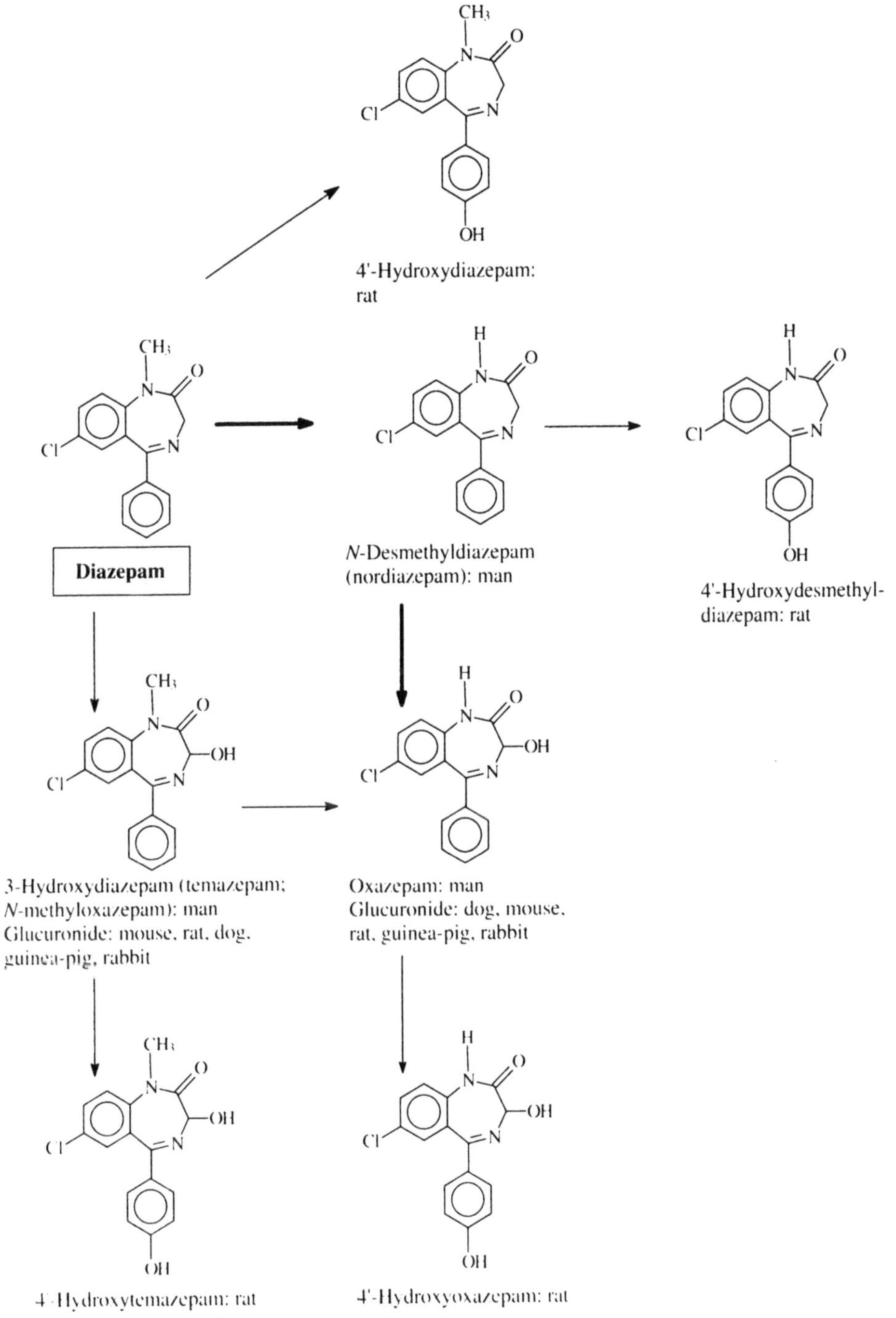

4'-Hydroxydiazepam: rat

Diazepam

N-Desmethyldiazepam (nordiazepam): man

4'-Hydroxydesmethyl-diazepam: rat

3-Hydroxydiazepam (temazepam; N-methyloxazepam): man
Glucuronide: mouse, rat, dog, guinea-pig, rabbit

Oxazepam: man
Glucuronide: dog, mouse, rat, guinea-pig, rabbit

4'-Hydroxytemazepam: rat

4'-Hydroxyoxazepam: rat

Adapted from Schmidt (1995)
Major steps are indicated by thick arrows. Note that the chlorine at the 7 position remains intact.

Diazepam clearance shows marked interindividual differences. Factors which might contribute to this phenomenon include age, sex, smoking, liver disease, enzyme induction or inhibition and genetic factors affecting the regulation of metabolism (Klotz et al., 1975, 1977; Greenblatt et al., 1980; Ochs et al., 1981a,b; Abernethy et al., 1983; Ochs et al., 1983; Alda et al., 1987; Bertilsson et al., 1989; Zhang et al., 1990; Sohn et al., 1992). With regard to the importance of the regulation of metabolism, a relationship was observed in studies of Swedish volunteers (Bertilsson et al., 1989) and Korean volunteers (Sohn et al., 1992) between more rapid elimination of diazepam and high S-mephenytoin hydroxylase activity (but see Section 4.1.2). There was no relationship with debrisoquin hydroxylation [CYP2D6] polymorphism among the Swedish subjects (Bertilsson et al., 1989). No significant difference in the clearance of diazepam was found between Chinese subjects who were extensive or poor S-mephenytoin hydroxylators (Zhang et al., 1990). Bertilsson and Kalow (1993) suggested that the racial differences can be explained in terms of the chance selection of different proportions of heterozygotes and homozygotes in these studies.

4.1.2 *Experimental systems*

In contrast to the extensive human pharmacokinetic investigations, equivalent in-vivo studies in experimental animals are rare. Garattini et al. (1973) gave rats, mice and guinea-pigs 5 mg/kg bw diazepam by intravenous injection and measured blood levels of diazepam, N-desmethyldiazepam and oxazepam at times from 1 min up to 40 h. Maximal diazepam concentrations of 2.33 ± 0.10, 1.36 ± 0.11 and 1.70 ± 0.10 µg/mL were found at 1 min in rats, mice and guinea-pigs, respectively. The blood levels were negligible by 5 h in rats and mice and by 10 h in guinea-pigs. In rats, N-desmethyldiazepam was detected only at 0.10 ± 0.01 µg/mL after 5 min, while oxazepam was not detected at all. However, in mice, N-desmethyldiazepam concentrations were significant from 1 min to 10 h, with a maximum at 30 min of 1.15 ± 0.04 µg/mL and significant oxazepam concentrations were found between 30 min and 10 h, with a maximum at 3 h of 0.22 ± 0.02 µg/mL. In guinea-pigs, concentrations of N-desmethyldiazepam were significant from 1 min to 20 h, with a maximum at 1 h of 0.37 ± 0.07 µg/mL, but no oxazepam was detected.

Lukey et al. (1991) administered a single dose of 100 µg/kg bw diazepam to six male rhesus monkeys by intramuscular injection. The maximal serum concentration of diazepam was 49.6 ± 13.9 ng/mL at 28.7 ± 3.6 min, while that of N-desmethyldiazepam was 38.4 ± 8.8 ng/mL at 169.8 ± 60.5 min. The volume of distribution and systemic clearance values were 1.5 L/kg and 19.4 mL/min/kg, respectively, assuming 100% bioavailability. Serum protein binding was about 95%.

Diazepam and N-desmethyldiazepam accumulate in adipose tissue. Garattini et al. (1973) found that adipose tissue/blood ratios in mice given 5 mg/kg bw diazepam intravenously varied from about 4 (at 5 min) to > 6 (at 5 h) while in mice given the metabolite (5 mg/kg bw), the corresponding ratios were 3 (at 5 min) and > 45 (at 5 h). Accumulation also occurred in the brain. Maximal diazepam concentrations in the brain after intravenous administration of 5 mg/kg bw were 7.04 ± 0.37 µg/g and 4.28 ± 0.14 µg/g at

1 min in mice and rats, respectively, and 6.28 ± 0.30 µg/g at 5 min in guinea-pigs. The brain : blood ratios varied from 2.6 (at 1 h) to 5.2 (at 1 min) in mice, from 1.8 (at 1 min) to 5.8 (at 3 h) in rats and from 2.8 (at 1 h) to 9.8 (at 5 min) in guinea-pigs.

The distribution of diazepam to certain tissues was examined in rats given 83 µg/kg bw by intraperitoneal injection (Takatori et al., 1991). Serum concentrations were 3.75 ± 0.62 ng/mL at 1 h and 0.28 ± 0.05 ng/mL at 4 h. Diazepam was also found in the saliva, bone marrow and brain. From 1 h to 8 h after administration, the concentration in bone marrow was higher than that in serum by factors of about 1.2–8.0. Over the period 2–8 h after dosing, concentrations in the serum, saliva and brain were similar. Transplacental transfer of diazepam occurs in mice, hamsters and monkeys (Idänpään-Heikkilä et al., 1971b).

Early studies of the metabolism of diazepam revealed substantial interspecies differences (see Figure 1), whether studied *in vivo* or by in-vitro methods using liver microsomes (Garattini et al., 1973). N-Demethylation (yielding N-desmethyldiazepam) and C_3-oxidation (yielding temazepam) occur to various extents in all species studied, but hydroxylation at the 4′-position of the 5-phenyl substituent is a major pathway in the rat. The resulting phenolic derivatives of diazepam, N-desmethyldiazepam, oxazepam and temazepam are all found in rat urine. This pathway seems to be negligible in most other species, apart from rabbits (Jommi et al., 1964). Oxazepam can be formed either from temazepam (by N-demethylation) or from N-desmethyldiazepam (by C_3-oxidation). The C_3-hydroxy compounds (oxazepam and temazepam) are eliminated in urine as glucuronides by mice (Marcucci et al., 1968), rats (Schwartz et al., 1967), guinea-pigs (Marcucci et al., 1971), rabbits (Jommi et al., 1964) and dogs (Ruelius et al., 1965). The glucuronide and/or sulfate conjugates of several metabolites have also been identified in the intestinal contents of a rat dosed intraperitoneally with 100 mg/kg bw diazepam (Schwartz et al., 1967).

In single-pass experiments with perfused male CD-1 mouse liver and an input concentration of 0.5 µM, diazepam was rapidly cleared, with a steady-state extraction ratio of 0.952 (St-Pierre & Pang, 1993). The mean hepatic clearance was 1.74 ± 0.21 mL/min/g, which was very close to the perfusate flow rate (1.82 mL/min/g). The metabolites recovered were (authors' terminology): nordiazepam (N-desmethyldiazepam) (47.7 ± 6.5%); nordiazepam conjugate (3.7 ± 2.1%); oxazepam (28.6 ± 7.1%); oxazepam glucuronide (1.7 ± 0.7%); 4′-hydroxynordiazepam (0.6 ± 0.2%); 4′-hydroxynordiazepam glucuronide (0.9 ± 0.3%); temazepam (0.7 ± 0.2%); temazepam glucuronide (0.3 ± 0.1%).

The metabolism of diazepam in cultured hepatocytes and subcellular preparations has also been studied extensively. An early study showed that diazepam undergoes both N-demethylation and C_3-hydroxylation in dog and rat liver *in vitro*, reactions that are NADPH-dependent and inducible by phenobarbital (Schwartz & Postma, 1968). Subsequently, Ackermann and Richter (1977) demonstrated that the oxidations are mediated by cytochrome P450, using human fetal liver preparations. The CYP2C11 isozyme catalyses the N-demethylation reaction, although other isozymes are also involved, while CYP3A2 is the major catalyst for C_3-hydroxylation (Reilly et al., 1990;

Neville et al., 1993; Yasumori et al., 1993). S-Mephenytoin does not inhibit either N-demethylation or C_3-hydroxylation of diazepam by human liver microsomes (Hooper et al., 1992). The human S-mephenytoin hydroxylases appear to be CYP2C9 or CYP2C18 enzymes (Nebert et al., 1989; Wilkinson et al., 1989; Romkes et al., 1991), so the apparent relationship between rapid diazepam clearance and high S-mephenytoin hydroxylase activity observed in humans (see Section 4.1.1) remains to be explained.

4.2 Toxic effects

4.2.1 Humans

(a) Acute toxicity

In a recent report on 215 lethal intoxications due to self-poisoning with diazepam alone or in combination with other substances, diazepam was associated with a higher rate of death per million prescriptions than the average for benzodiazepine anxiolytics such as lorazepam and oxazepam. However, this may not reflect a higher toxicity of diazepam, since diazepam was used more frequently together with alcohol than the other tranquillizers investigated (Serfaty & Masterton, 1993). In non-lethal intoxications, the symptoms consist mainly of an enhancement of the therapeutic effects, with severe drowsiness, oversedation and ataxia, while in some cases, particularly in elderly persons, a paradoxical excitation may be induced. Rare but severe acute adverse effects after therapeutic intravenous administration include respiratory or cardiac arrest or both (reviewed by Dollery et al., 1991).

(b) Chronic toxicity

In addition to the effects associated with psychological and physical dependence and rebound withdrawal phenomena, extremely rare but serious adverse reactions are increases in the levels of serum aminotransferase and alkaline phosphatase, jaundice (both hepatocellular and cholestatic), leukopenia, hypersensitivity reactions such as skin rashes, single cases of exfoliative dermatitis and, in predisposed persons, circulatory and respiratory depression (reviewed by Dollery et al., 1991). Taking into account the widespread use of diazepam over a long period, the virtual lack of adverse effects reported in the literature suggests the absence of organ toxicity associated with chronic administration.

4.2.2 Experimental systems

(a) Acute toxicity

Average oral LD_{50} values of 1901 and 1517 mg/kg bw in mice and rats, respectively, have been reported. The average LD_{50} values after intraperitoneal administration were 774 mg/kg bw in mice and 661 mg/kg bw in rats (Owen et al., 1970).

(b) Subchronic and chronic toxicity

Groups of 20 Charles River CD rats (10 male, 10 female) were administered 0, 600, 1250 or 2500 mg/kg diet (ppm) diazepam orally in the diet for 20–22 weeks. No deaths occurred in either control or treated rats, and neither food consumption nor body weight differed significantly between the four groups. No haematological or ophthalmological effect of diazepam was found, but kidney and pancreas weights in males and liver weights in males and females were greater at all doses. In addition to the mild renal alterations observed in males of all treated and control groups, some males of the high-dose group had histopathological traces of brown, finely granular material within the epithelial cells of the renal proximal convoluted tubules in the absence of gross toxicity. Mild alteration of the thyroid architecture was observed in some animals in each treated group, the acini appearing condensed and containing less colloid than usual (Owen et al., 1970).

Groups of four dogs were given 80, 127 or 200 mg/kg bw orally by capsule 30 min before feeding daily for four weeks (Owen et al., 1970). One dog of the high-dose group died and marked losses in weight were observed in the mid- and high-dose groups associated with decreased food consumption due to severe sedation and somnolence; in addition, increased emesis was induced in the three treated groups. The authors suggested weakness and starvation as the cause of death. Haematological examination revealed elevated haemoglobin, haematocrit, total red cell count and blood viscosity in the mid- and high-dose groups; increased weights of the kidneys and adrenal gland were also observed in these two groups. Most dogs treated with diazepam displayed histopathological and biochemical signs of hepatobiliary dysfunction and some gonadal changes, namely testicular atrophy.

[The Working Group noted that, since the study of Owen et al. (1970) focused on evaluating oxazepam toxicity, with diazepam administered only for comparison purposes, the description of the effects of diazepam is incomplete on many points and the number of animals treated with diazepam was very small.]

(c)   Effects on cell proliferation and differentiation and on steroidogenesis: the role of peripheral benzodiazepine receptors

The anxiolytic and hypnotic effects of diazepam are mediated via GABAergic receptors in the central nervous system. In addition, diazepam can affect peripheral organs, in particular the immune and endocrine system, directly through a second class of binding sites. Although the peripheral benzodiazepine receptors are ubiquitous in the organism, they are localized in very specific regions of the different organs and their density is strictly controlled by endocrine and neural mechanisms. In generalized anxiety disorders in humans and in chronically stressed or food-deprived experimental animals, the density of the peripheral benzodiazepine receptors is decreased in most organs, while diazepam administration has been reported to induce upregulation (Gavish et al., 1992; Ferrarese et al., 1993). These peripheral benzodiazepine receptors are mitochondrial proteins consisting of two subunits. The 'diazepam-binding inhibitor' peptide is a putative endogenous ligand for peripheral benzodiazepine receptors. This polypeptide has been purified from the brain and from a variety of other organs such as the liver, kidney and adrenal glands, and probably functions as a precursor of smaller biologically active neuropeptides that interact preferentially with either central or peripheral benzodiazepine receptors (Ferrarese et al., 1993).

Experimental evidence suggests that the effects of diazepam on cell proliferation and differentiation observed *in vitro* are mediated via binding to benzodiazepine receptors. Such effects include blockage of mitogenesis in Swiss 3T3 cells, induction of differentiation in murine Friend erythroleukaemia cells, acceleration of melanogenesis in mouse melanoma cells, and inhibition of proliferation of human glioma cells, rat pituitary tumour cells and cultured mouse spleen lymphocytes *in vitro* (Wang *et al.*, 1984; Pawlikowski *et al.*, 1988a,b; Kunert-Radek *et al.*, 1994). In contrast, a single subcutaneous injection of diazepam induced increased thymic mitotic activity in rats *in vivo* (Stepien *et al.*, 1988). Inhibition of plasma membrane calcium influx through voltage-dependent channels has been repeatedly discussed as a mechanism possibly involved in the inhibitory effects on cell proliferation mediated via peripheral benzodiazepine receptors (Pawlikowski *et al.*, 1988b; Ferrarese *et al.*, 1993).

In adrenocortical and testicular Leydig cells and cultured cell lines, the 'diazepam-binding inhibitor' peptide, as well as other ligands including diazepam, stimulate hormone-induced steroid biosynthesis, probably by binding to peripheral benzodiazepine receptors and thus mediating the translocation of cholesterol from the outer to the inner mitochondrial membranes and regulating cholesterol side-chain cleavage to pregnenolone (Krueger & Papadopoulos, 1990; Ferrarese *et al.*, 1993). The extent of stimulation correlates with the binding affinity of the different ligands to these peripheral receptors (Mukhin *et al.*, 1989; Ferrarese *et al.*, 1993). 'Diazepam-binding inhibitor' has been also suggested to stimulate the release of corticotropin-releasing factor from neurons and to stimulate the synthesis of neurosteroids in glial cells (Ferrarese *et al.*, 1993). Earlier studies *in vivo* demonstrated that diazepam increases corticosterone and testosterone secretion in rats, as well as plasma levels of testosterone and 11-hydrocorticoids in humans (Marc & Morselli, 1969; Argüelles & Rosner, 1975). In contrast, flunitrazepam has been reported to antagonize the stimulatory effect of purified 'diazepam-binding inhibitor' on steroidogenesis *in vitro* (Papadopoulos *et al.*, 1991).

The presence of peripheral benzodiazepine receptors in both animal and human tumours has been explored extensively. Increased density was demonstrated in various tumours, such as rat gliomas, human gliomas or astrocytomas, human colon adenocarcinomas and human ovarian and prostatic carcinomas; in contrast, peripheral benzodiazepine receptors were absent in renal carcinomas (Katz *et al.*, 1988; Ferrarese *et al.*, 1989; Gorman *et al.*, 1989; Katz *et al.*, 1989, 1990). The localization of these binding sites in the mitochondria raises the possibility that they might be involved in intermediary metabolism and in respiratory control; hence quantitative and/or qualitative changes in their function might bring about important alterations in cellular biochemistry. However, the available data are fragmentary and do not allow assessment of the role of peripheral benzodiazepine receptors in tumour formation.

(d) Effects on the immune system

The effects of diazepam on the immune functions have been studied both *in vitro* and *in vivo* with conflicting results: both stimulatory and inhibitory effects have been demonstrated. Diazepam injected one day after immunization stimulated the humoral immune response of mice to sheep red blood cells, probably as a result of T cell-dependent antigen binding to peripheral benzodiazepine receptors on macrophages (Ferrarese et al., 1993). The presence of peripheral benzodiazepine receptors on the mitochondrial and plasma membranes of peripheral lymphocytes was demonstrated immunocytochemically. Compounds that act exclusively on central GABAergic receptors do not exert immune functions (Ferrarese et al., 1992). Further studies in vitro demonstrated that binding of 'diazepam-binding inhibitor' and diazepam to the peripheral benzodiazepine receptors is involved in monocyte chemotaxis and enhances the production of interleukin-1 and tumour necrosis factor-α (Ruff et al., 1985; Taupin et al., 1991). In contrast, diazepam at micromolar concentrations, which can be achieved therapeutically in blood, inhibited phagocytosis and killing of Candida albicans cells by human polymorphonuclear cells and monocytes in vitro (Covelli et al., 1989). At similar concentrations, diazepam also suppressed the activity of natural killer cells isolated from human peripheral blood against erythroleukaemia target cells, suggesting the possibility of impairment of antiviral and antitumour defence in humans taking diazepam (Stepien et al., 1994). However, it is also possible that the demonstrated elevated levels of 'diazepam-binding inhibitor' in stress and anxiety are responsible for the reduced density of peripheral benzodiazepine receptors on lymphocytes and mediate, together with the increased levels of adrenal steroids, the immunosuppressive effects of stress (Ferrarese et al., 1993). Hence, although the involvement of peripheral receptors in immunomodulation can be considered as proven, the role of diazepam versus 'diazepam-binding inhibitor' remains to be elucidated (Zavala & Lenfant, 1987).

4.3 Reproductive and prenatal effects

4.3.1 *Humans*

The maternal metabolism of diazepam during pregnancy is discussed in Section 4.1.1.

Three kinds of developmental consequences of diazepam treatment during pregnancy can be differentiated:

(i) Congenital abnormalities, i.e., the possible classical teratogenic effect of diazepam used mainly in the first trimester of gestation.

(ii) Short-term functional alterations that are manifested postnatally and are related mainly to diazepam treatment in the perinatal period.

(iii) Long-term postnatal developmental (including behavioural) effects which in general are connected with diazepam intake in the second and third trimesters of gestation, i.e., after the development of specific brain receptors for benzodiazepines.

(a) *Possible teratogenic effect*

The possible teratogenic effects are considered according to the circumstances of exposure of the mother.

Undefined exposure circumstances

The data of the Finnish Register of Congenital Malformations (1967–71) showed a significant association between oral clefts and maternal intake of antianxiety drugs

(Saxén, 1975). Extended analysis of the Finnish case–control material (Saxén & Saxén, 1975) indicated significantly greater use of benzodiazepines (diazepam, oxazepam, nitrazepam or chlordiazepoxide) in the first trimester by the mothers of affected children (14 versus 5) among 232 children with isolated cleft palate and 226 matched controls ($p < 0.05$). Benzodiazepine use was greater, but not significantly so, in 232 children with isolated cleft lip with or without cleft palate than in 230 matched controls (11 versus 4). [The Working Group noted that benzodiazepines were not differentiated and that confounding factors such as maternal illness and use of other drugs were not controlled.]

In the Metropolitan Atlanta Congenital Defects Program monitoring the incidence of birth defects since 1967, Safra and Oakley (1975) found, by interviews of 49 women who had infants with cleft lip with or without cleft palate, a history of diazepam ingestion in the first trimester in seven, and in nine of 229 mothers of children with other congenital abnormalities (relative risk, 4.1; 95% CI, 1.5–11.5). The other abnormalities included Down's syndrome, tracheo-oesophageal fistula and/or atresia, small-bowel, rectal and anal atresia, omphalocele, diaphragmatic hernia and limb reductions. The corresponding relative risk estimate for cleft palate alone was 0.9 based on one exposed infant. Later, Safra and Oakley (1976) considered the results of their previous study to be inconclusive because there was no association between secular trends in the prevalence at birth of children with cleft lip with or without cleft palate and in drug sales.

In a hospital-based study in Norway, Aarskog (1975) evaluated retrospectively 12 (1 exposed in the first trimester) cases with cleft palate and 99 (6 exposed in the first trimester) cases with cleft lip with or without cleft palate born in 1967–71 and 362 (9 exposed in the first trimester) controls born in 1972–75. The number of subjects exposed to diazepam in the first trimester was significantly higher in the combined group with oral clefts than that of controls. [The Working Group noted that the validity of the study is uncertain in view of the different study periods for cases and controls. Moreover, cleft lip with or without cleft palate is etiologically distinct from isolated cleft palate.]

Czeizel (1976) conducted an ad-hoc population-based study using data from the Hungarian Congenital Malformation Registry for the period 1970–75. Of 413 cases with cleft lip with or without cleft palate, 121 cases with cleft palate alone and a control series comprising 843 cases with neural-tube defects, 20 (4.8%), 2 (1.7%) and 37 (4.4%), respectively, had mothers who reported having received diazepam treatment in the first trimester of pregnancy. The differences were not statistically significant.

Subsequently, Czeizel (1988) analysed the data-set of the Hungarian Case–Control Surveillance System of Congenital Abnormalities for 1980–84. Approximately 15% of pregnant Hungarian women used diazepam in the 1980s (Czeizel & Rácz, 1990). Maternal diazepam use in the first, second and third months of pregnancy did not differ significantly between 355 cases with isolated cleft lip with or without cleft palate, 167 cases with isolated cleft palate and similar numbers of matched healthy controls. A prospective follow-up study was based on women who visited genetic counselling clinics between 1973 and 1980 following exposure to potentially hazardous environmental factors during early pregnancy. Of 546 women, 33 had ingested benzodiazepines, mainly diazepam; their 26 liveborn babies had no congenital abnormality.

Rosenberg et al. (1983) compared the use of diazepam during the first four lunar months of pregnancy in 445 infants with cleft lip with or without cleft palate, in 166 infants with cleft palate alone and in 2498 controls with congenital abnormalities other than oral clefts from the birth defect surveillance system in Boston, MA, and Philadelphia, PA, United States, and Toronto, Canada, in 1976–82. The relative risk, adjusted for several confounding factors, was 0.8 (95% CI, 0.4–1.7) for cleft lip with or without cleft palate and 0.8 (0.2–2.5) for cleft palate alone.

In a prospective study of 33 249 pregnant women, in the Birth Defects Study of the National Institute of Child Health and Human Development and Kaiser-Permanente in the United States, Shiono and Mills (1984) found no increase, based on 854 cases, in the relative risk for oral clefts associated with exposure to diazepam during the first trimester (relative risk, 1.2; 95% CI, 0.17–9.0).

Exposure by attempted suicide

Two retrospective studies were carried out in Budapest and the surrounding area in 1960–79 (Czeizel et al., 1984, 1988) and 1980–84 (Czeizel & Lendvay, 1987; Lendvay & Czeizel, 1992) and one prospective study between 1985 and 1986 (Czeizel & Lendway, 1987) in self-poisoned pregnant women. [The Working Group calculated that, in these two studies, 46 pregnancies ended in births to mothers who had used diazepam for self-poisoning. Relatively low doses (25–45 mg) were used by 3 women, while higher doses of 50–95 mg were used by 11, 100–145 mg by 20 women, 150–195 mg by 3 women and more than 200 mg by 7 women. Of the children, only one was affected by congenital abnormality (Fallot tetralogy). Since the expected rate of congenital abnormalities was about 6.5% (Czeizel et al., 1993), it appears that single, extremely high doses of diazepam did not cause an increase in the rate of detectable defects in the offspring.]

Gunnarskog and Källén (1993) observed that, of 70 infants born in Sweden to mothers exposed to psychoactive drugs as a result of suicide attempts during the organ-forming period, 20 of whom were exposed to benzodiazepines, none had a congenital abnormality. [Specific drugs were not mentioned.]

Psychotherapeutic exposure

Several studies relate to the offspring of women who had psychiatric disorders for which they received high doses of benzodiazepines throughout pregnancy.

Laegreid et al. (1987) reported seven cases exposed to benzodiazepines. All offspring had intra- and extrauterine growth retardation, facial dysmorphism and central nervous system dysfunctions. Of five cases with maternal exposure to diazepam, one had submucous cleft of the hard palate and secondary hydronephrosis, another was affected with submucous cleft hard palate and a third one with microcephaly and left renal aplasia. These cases resembled, but were not identical to, the fetal alcohol syndrome but abuse of alcohol was denied by all the mothers. All the mothers had received 30–75-mg daily doses of benzodiazepines throughout pregnancy, in some cases confirmed by the examination of stored blood samples for diazepam. Laegreid et al. (1989) reported two new cases with similar findings.

In addition, Laegreid *et al.* (1990) carried out a population-based study of surviving live births born in 1985–86 in Gothenburg, Sweden. Twenty-five children were identified with one or more of (a) embryopathy-fetopathy not otherwise specified, (b) oral clefts, (c) defects of the central nervous system and (d) urinary tract malformations. It was possible to analyse maternal plasma in 18 of these cases (three were reported in previous papers) and eight samples were found to be benzodiazepine-positive, including seven for diazepam. A control series of 109 children was selected using paired sampling. Of 60 controls for whom blood analysis could be carried out, two were positive, both for diazepam. The difference in the proportion exposed to diazepam was highly significant.

Laegreid *et al.* (1992a) studied psychotropic drug use in the mothers of all 73 perinatally dead infants in the city of Gothenburg, Sweden, in 1985–86 and in control mothers of 73 surviving infants. Serum samples obtained in early pregnancy were screened for benzodiazepines. Eighteen case-mothers had used psychotropic drugs (benzodiazepines in nine) during pregnancy as documented from case-notes, compared with seven control mothers (benzodiazepines in three). The association between benzodiazepine drug use and perinatal death was significant ($p = 0.03$), but confounding due to psychiatric disorders and other drug use could not be excluded.

Bergman *et al.* (1990) evaluated the follow-up of the children of 4640 mothers in 1971–86 for their exposure to diazepam, oxazepam or nitrazepam during pregnancy. Only six of the pregnant women appeared to be regular benzodiazepine users (two diazepam, two oxazepam, one nitrazepam and one diazepam plus nitrazepam) and none of their six children had abnormalities.

Later, Bergman *et al.* (1992) examined benzodiazepine use during pregnancy in 104 339 women whose deliveries were recorded by the United States public health insurance system, Medicaid, during 1980–83. Of 80 pregnant women who had received 10 or more benzodiazepine prescriptions (63 diazepam, 36 chlordiazepoxide, 8 lorazepam, 13 flurazepam), three experienced fetal death and two infants were found to have lethal congenital abnormalities. Records of 64 surviving children could be linked to these 80 pregnancies (11 survivors could not be located), and six children had congenital abnormalities of various types. These defects differed from the pattern described by Laegreid *et al.* (1987, 1989, 1990); in particular, there were no oral clefts.

(b) *Short-term functional alterations*

There are case reports of floppy infant syndrome (namely hypotonia, hyporeflexia, apnoeic spells, reluctance to feed, a risk for inhalation of feeds, impaired metabolic responses to cold, hypothermia, low Apgar rating at birth) associated with diazepam treatment of pregnant women at doses of 30 mg or more within the 15 hours before delivery (Owen *et al.*, 1972; Cree *et al.*, 1973).

Acute withdrawal effects (namely depressed respiration, hypothermia and feeding difficulties) have been documented in neonates exposed to diazepam *in utero* for long periods (Cree *et al.*, 1973). The time of onset of the symptoms, their severity and duration were related to the dosage and fetal kinetics (including elimination) of the drug (Mazzi, 1977; Mac New & Finnigan, 1980).

(c) Human long-term postnatal studies

The behavioural development of 101 children (and their 117 siblings) of pregnant women who attempted suicide has been studied (Lendvay & Czeizel, 1992). Forty-two of the mothers had used diazepam during pregnancy. Some of the children had behavioural alterations which could be explained mainly by their familial and social problems.

Laegreid *et al.* (1992b,c) examined the neurodevelopment of 17 children born to 16 mothers who used benzodiazepines throughout pregnancy: 15 used diazepam (5–30 mg daily) or oxazepam (15–60 mg daily) alone or in combination and one mother used lorazepam. The results were compared with those for 29 children born to mothers without any known use of psychotropic drugs. A neurological investigation was performed on the second day of life. Significant differences in the frequency of pre- and perinatal complications and in neurobehaviour were found between the two groups. The benzodiazepine-exposed children recovered from their lower mean birth weight at an early stage, whereas their slightly decreased head circumference at birth remained lower. Gross motor development was retarded at six and 10 months, but was nearly normal at 18 months. Impaired fine motor functions were found on all follow-up occasions (at six, 10 and 18 months of age).

The cases studied by Laegreid *et al.* (1990, 1992b,c) were followed up prospectively in late infancy and found to have a general delay in mental development up to 18 months of age associated with prenatal exposure to benzodiazepines (Viggedal *et al.*, 1993). [The Working Group noted that all the mothers in the benzodiazepine group had psychiatric disorders, and these have an important negative effect on children's development (Cox, 1988). In addition, neuropsychological symptoms are frequent among children of abusers of psychoactive substances (Deren, 1986; Van Baar *et al.*, 1989).]

4.3.2 *Experimental systems*

Few experimental data are available concerning the effect of diazepam on reproduction. The incidence of abnormal sperm heads was significantly higher in mice after a daily oral dose of 0.5 mg diazepam (Kar & Das, 1983; Šrám & Kocišová, 1984).

Guerriero and Fox (1977) found a significant decrease in mating performance, with depressed birth weights, among Swiss-Webster mice given a diet containing 500 mg/kg diazepam.

In A/J mice given a single intramuscular dose of 100 mg/kg diazepam on day 14 of pregnancy, the frequency in the offspring of both cleft lip with or without cleft palate and cleft palate only was 3.4% (Walker & Patterson, 1974). The authors observed that this was lower than the frequency of spontaneous occurrence of these defects reported in other series.

Miller and Becker (1975) treated Swiss-Webster mice with 50, 100, 140 or 500 mg/kg bw diazepam by gastric instillation once daily for three days on gestation days 8–10 or days 11–13 or for one day only between days 8 and 15 or with 280 or 400 mg/kg bw for one day only between days 11 and 14. The highest dose was associated with a maternal mortality rate of 50%. When 140 mg/kg bw diazepam was administered on day 13, there was 21% fetal resorption. The incidence of cleft palate was significantly increased in the offspring of mice treated with 140 mg/kg bw diazepam on days 11, 12 and 13, and with single-day administrations of 400 mg/kg bw on days 11–14 and 500 mg/kg bw on days 9 and 11–15.

Tocco *et al.* (1987) reported an increase in the frequency of cleft palate in Swiss-Webster and AJ mice following two-day dosing with 400 mg/kg bw diazepam by gastric instillation on days 13.5 and 14.5. Maternal mortality was high (50% or more) but no increase in resorption was observed.

In rats, no abnormality was caused by oral administration of 20 or 80 mg/kg bw diazepam per day on days 6–15 of gestation (Beall, 1972). Saito *et al.* (1984) did not find a significant increase in any abnormalities after oral administration of 100 mg/kg bw diazepam on gestation days 8–14 in Sprague-Dawley rats.

In hamsters, exencephaly, cleft palate and limb defects were detected after a single oral dose of 30, 50, 70 or 100 mg on days 8 and 10 or single intravenous injections of 10 mg diazepam on day 11. There was no dose-related effect (Shah *et al.*, 1979). A single intraperitoneal injection of 120–980 mg/kg bw diazepam on day 8 of gestation induced a dose-related increase in the frequency of fetal malformations in hamsters, mainly exencephaly or cranioschisis, at doses of 280 mg/kg and above (Gill *et al.*, 1981).

No structural abnormality was observed in the offspring of two rhesus monkeys treated orally with diazepam (0.5–3.2 mg/kg bw) twice daily during the second and third trimesters, nor in those of three monkeys treated during the third trimester only (Jerome *et al.*, 1981). [The Working Group noted that there was no treatment during the first trimester.]

Specific receptors for benzodiazepines develop at the beginning of the fetal period in the central and peripheral nervous systems of rats (Braestrup & Nielsen, 1978). Behavioural studies have demonstrated pronounced effects in rodents following exposure to diazepam during late gestation. In rat models, prenatal exposure to diazepam and other benzodiazepines resulted in behavioural deficits in pups (Kellogg *et al.*, 1980), such as learning and memory disabilities (Gai & Grimm, 1982), the absence of acoustic startle reflexes and the impairment of conditioned avoidance response (Kellogg, 1992) which is dependent on the time of treatment (Frieder *et al.*, 1984). However, diazepam prevented the adverse effects of maternal restraint stress in postnatal development and learning in rats (Barlow *et al.*, 1979).

A chick embryotoxicity screening test did not show any teratogenic effect of diazepam (Peterka *et al.*, 1992).

4.4 Genetic and related effects (see also Table 6 for references and Appendices 1 and 2)

4.4.1 *Humans*

The first published report of a possible association between exposure to diazepam and chromosomal aberrations in the lymphocytes of patients using the drug as a tranquillizer (four patients) or for its muscle-relaxing properties (19 patients) was that of Stenchever *et al.* (1970). These patients were compared with eight controls. Although there was no

Table 6. Genetic and related effects of diazepam

Test system	Result[a] Without exogenous metabolic system	With exogenous metabolic system	Dose[b] (LED/HID)	Reference
SAD, *Salmonella typhimurium*, DNA repair	–	NT	400	Waskell (1978)
SA0, *Salmonella typhimurium* TA100, reverse mutation	–	–	500	Waskell (1978)
SA0, *Salmonella typhimurium* TA100, reverse mutation	–	–	2500	Balbi *et al.* (1980)
SA0, *Salmonella typhimurium* TA100, reverse mutation	–	–	500	Preiss *et al.* (1982)
SA0, *Salmonella typhimurium* TA100, reverse mutation	–	–	NG	Matula & Downie (1983) (abstract)
SA5, *Salmonella typhimurium* TA1535, reverse mutation	–	–	2500	Balbi *et al.* (1980)
SA5, *Salmonella typhimurium* TA1535, reverse mutation	–	–	500	Preiss *et al.* (1982)
SA7, *Salmonella typhimurium* TA1537, reverse mutation	–	–	2500	Balbi *et al.* (1980)
SA7, *Salmonella typhimurium* TA1537, reverse mutation	–	–	500	Preiss *et al.* (1982)
SA8, *Salmonella typhimurium* TA1538, reverse mutation	–	–	500	Preiss *et al.* (1982)
SA9, *Salmonella typhimurium* TA98, reverse mutation	–	–	500	Waskell (1978)
SA9, *Salmonella typhimurium* TA98, reverse mutation	–	–	2500	Balbi *et al.* (1980)
SA9, *Salmonella typhimurium* TA98, reverse mutation	–	–	500	Preiss *et al.* (1982)
SA9, *Salmonella typhimurium* TA98, reverse mutation	–	–	NG	Matula & Downie (1983) (abstract)
SCR, *Saccharomyces cerevisiae*, reverse mutation	–	NT	NG	Matula & Downie (1983) (abstract)
SCH, *Saccharomyces cerevisiae*, mitotic recombination and gene conversion	–	NT	NG	Matula & Downie (1983) (abstract)
SCN, *Saccharomyces cerevisiae*, aneuploidy	–	NT	250	Whittaker *et al.* (1990)
SCN, *Saccharomyces cerevisiae*, aneuploidy	–	NT	300	Albertini (1990)
ANN, *Aspergillus nidulans*, aneuploidy	–	NT	200	Crebelli *et al.* (1991)
URP, Unscheduled DNA synthesis, rat primary hepatocytes	–	NT	0.5	Swierenga *et al.* (1983) (abstract)
URP, Unscheduled DNA synthesis, rat primary hepatocytes	–	NT	1000	Williams *et al.* (1989)

Table 6 (contd)

Test system	Result[a] Without exogenous metabolic system	With exogenous metabolic system	Dose[b] (LED/HID)	Reference
G9H, Gene mutation, Chinese hamster lung V79 cells, *hprt* locus *in vitro*	–	–	250	Röhrborn *et al.* (1984) (abstract)
GIA, Gene mutation, rat primary hepatocytes, *hprt* locus *in vitro*	–	–	50	Swierenga *et al.* (1983) (abstract)
MIA, Micronucleus test, Chinese hamster (Cl-1) cells *in vitro*	+[c]	NT	20	Antoccia *et al.* (1991)
MIA, Micronucleus test, Chinese hamster lung V79 cells *in vitro*	+[c]	NT	NG	Bonatti *et al.* (1992)
MIA, Micronucleus test, Chinese hamster pulmonary (Luc 2) cells *in vitro*	+	NT	10	Lynch & Parry (1993)
MIA, Micronucleus test, Chinese hamster lung V79 cells *in vitro*	+[c]	NT	100	Seelbach *et al.* (1993)
CIC, Chromosomal aberrations, Chinese hamster lung CHL cells *in vitro*	–	?	1000	Matsuoka *et al.* (1979)
CIC, Chromosomal aberrations, Chinese hamster lung CHL cells *in vitro*	–	NT	125	Ishidate *et al.* (1988)
CIC, Chromosomal aberrations, Chinese hamster (CHE-3N) cells *in vitro*	?	NT	100	Lafi & Parry (1988)
AIA, Polyploidy, Chinese hamster (Don) cells *in vitro*	+	NT	100	Satya-Prakash *et al.* (1984)
AIA, Aneuploidy, Chinese hamster (Don) cells *in vitro*	NT	+	100	Hsu *et al.* (1983)
AIA, Aneuploidy, Chinese hamster (CHE-3N) cells *in vitro* (hypodiploidy)	(+)[d]	NT	100	Lafi & Parry (1988)
AIA, Aneuploidy, primary Chinese hamster embryonic cells *in vitro*	+[d]	NT	10	Natarajan *et al.* (1993)
AIA, Aneuploidy, Chinese hamster pulmonary (Luc 2p4) cells *in vitro* (hypodiploidy and polyploidy)	+	NT	10	Warr *et al.* (1993)
*, c-Mitoses, Chinese hamster (Cl-1) cells *in vitro*	+	NT	60	Antoccia *et al.* (1991)
TCL, Cell transformation, BHK 21-C13 cells *in vitro*	–	+	130	Röhrborn *et al.* (1984) (abstract)
SHF, Sister chromatid exchange, human fibroblast cell line *in vitro*	–	NT	28.5	Sasaki *et al.* (1980)
MIH, Micronucleus test, human lymphocytes *in vitro*	–	NT	75	Migliore & Nieri (1991)
MIH, Micronucleus test, human fibroblasts *in vitro*	+[c]	NT	25	Bonatti *et al.* (1992)
MIH, Micronucleus test, human lymphocytes *in vitro*	+[c]	NT	30	Ferguson *et al.* (1993)

Table 6 (contd)

Test system	Result[a] Without exogenous metabolic system	Result[a] With exogenous metabolic system	Dose[b] (LED/HID)	Reference
CHF, Chromosomal aberrations, human primary fetal fibroblasts in vitro	–	NT	50	Staiger (1969)
CHF, Chromosomal aberrations, human fibroblast cell line in vitro	–	NT	25	Staiger (1969)
CHF, Chromosomal aberrations, human fibroblast cell line in vitro	–	NT	28.5	Sasaki et al. (1980)
CHL, Chromosomal aberrations, human lymphocytes in vitro	–	NT	50	Staiger (1970)
CHL, Chromosomal aberrations, human lymphocytes in vitro	–	–	NG	Röhrborn et al. (1984) (abstract)
AIH, Aneuploidy, human primary fibroblasts in vitro	–	NT	50	Staiger (1969)
AIH, Aneuploidy, human fibroblast cell line in vitro	–[d]	NT	25	Staiger (1969)
AIH, Aneuploidy, human lymphocytes in vitro (hypodiploidy)	+	NT	25	Sbrana et al. (1993)
*, c-Mitoses, human lymphocytes in vitro	+	NT	50	Sbrana et al. (1993)
DVA, DNA strand breaks, rat liver in vitro	(+)		285 po × 1	Carlo et al. (1989)
DVA, DNA strand breaks, rat liver in vivo	–		57 po × 15	Carlo et al. (1989)
MVM, Micronucleus test, mouse bone marrow in vivo	(+)		22 po × 1	Kar & Das (1979)
MVM, Micronucleus test, mouse bone marrow in vivo	+		20 po × 2	Das & Kar (1986)
MVM, Micronucleus test, mouse bone marrow in vivo	–		150 ip × 1	Adler et al. (1991)
MVM, Micronucleus test, mouse bone marrow in vivo	–		30 ip × 1	Leopardi et al. (1993)
MVM, Micronucleus test, mouse bone marrow in vivo	(+)		10 × 1[f]	Marrazzini et al. (1994)
CBA, Chromosomal aberrations, Chinese hamster bone marrow in vivo	–		300 po × 10	Schmid & Staiger (1969)
CBA, Chromosomal aberrations, rat bone marrow in vivo	–		500 po × 10	Neda et al. (1977)
CBA, Chromosomal aberrations, mouse bone marrow in vivo	(+)		75 ip × 7	Petersen et al. (1978) (abstract)
CBA, Chromosomal aberrations, mouse bone marrow in vivo	–		0.85 ip × 1	Degraeve et al. (1985) (abstract)

Table 6 (contd)

Test system	Result[a]		Dose[b] (LED/HID)	Reference
	Without exogenous metabolic system	With exogenous metabolic system		
CBA, Chromosomal aberrations, mouse bone marrow *in vivo*	–		0.85 ip × 22	Degraeve *et al.* (1985) (abstract)
CBA, Chromosomal aberrations, mouse bone marrow *in vivo*	(+)		1000 po × 28	Kocišová & Šrám (1985) (abstract)
CBA, Chromosomal aberrations, rat bone marrow *in vivo*	–		500 po × 10	Ishimura *et al.* (1975) (abstract)
CBA, Chromosome aberrations, mouse bone marrow *in vivo*	–		100 ip × 1	Xu & Adler (1990)
CBA, Chromosomal aberrations, mouse bone marrow *in vivo*	–		10 × 1[f]	Marrazzini *et al.* (1994)
CGG, Chromosomal aberrations, mouse spermatogonia treated *in vivo*, spermatogonia observed	–		0.85 ip × 22	Degraeve *et al.* (1985) (abstract)
CCC, Chromosomal aberrations, mouse spermatocytes treated *in vivo*, spermatocytes observed	–		0.85 ip × 22	Degraeve *et al.* (1985) (abstract)
DLM, Dominant lethal test, mouse *in vivo*	(+)		22 po × 15	Kar & Das (1979)
DLM, Dominant lethal test, mouse *in vivo*	–		0.85 ip × 40	Degraeve *et al.* (1985) (abstract)
DLM, Dominant lethal test, mouse *in vivo*	–		1000 po × 28	Šrám & Kocišová (1985)
*, c-Mitoses, mouse bone marrow *in vivo*	–		150 ip × 1	Miller & Adler (1989)
AVA, Polyploidy, mouse bone marrow *in vivo*	(+)		100 ip × 1	Xu & Adler (1990)
AVA, Aneuploidy, mouse secondary spermatocytes *in vivo*	(+)		150 ip × 1	Miller & Adler (1992)
AVA, Aneuploidy, mouse bone marrow *in vivo*	–		30 ip × 1	Leopardi *et al.* (1993)
AVA, Aneuploidy, mouse secondary spermatocytes *in vivo*	–		30 ip × 1	Leopardi *et al.* (1993)
AVA, Aneuploidy, mouse oocytes *in vivo*	–		150 ip × 1	Mailhes & Marchetti (1994)

Table 6 (contd)

Test system	Result[a] Without exogenous metabolic system	Result[a] With exogenous metabolic system	Dose[b] (LED/HID)	Reference
AVA, Aneuploidy, male mouse germ cells *in vivo*	+		150 ip × 1	Gassner & Adler (1995)
AVA, Aneuploidy, mouse bone marrow *in vivo*	(+)		10 × 1[f]	Marrazzini et al. (1994)
SLH, Sister chromatid exchange, human lymphocytes *in vivo*	−		0.2 po × 1	Husum et al. (1985)
SLH, Sister chromatid exchange, human lymphocytes *in vivo*	+		NG	Huong et al. (1988)
CLH, Chromosomal aberrations, human lymphocytes *in vivo*	−		0.5 po × 1[g]	Cohen et al. (1969)
CLH, Chromosomal aberrations, human lymphocytes *in vivo*	−		0.3 po × 1[h]	Stenchever et al. (1970)
CLH, Chromosomal aberrations, human lymphocytes *in vivo*	−		0.30 iv × 1	White et al. (1974)
CLH, Chromosomal aberrations, human lymphocytes *in vivo*	+		NG	Huong et al. (1988)
CLH, Chromosomal aberrations, human lymphocytes *in vivo*	−		2.4 po × 1[i]	van Bao et al. (1992)
CLH, Chromosomal aberrations, human lymphocytes *in vivo*	−		2.4 po × 1[i]	van Bao et al. (1992)
MVH, Micronucleus test, human lymphocytes *in vivo*	+		2.4 po × 1[i]	van Bao et al. (1992)
AVH, Aneuploidy, human cells *in vivo* (hypodiploidy)	−		712	Brunner et al. (1991)
*, Inhibition of tubulin assembly *in vitro*	+		285	Wallin & Hartley-Asp (1993)
*, Inhibition of tubulin assembly *in vitro*				
ICR, Inhibition of intercellular communication, Chinese hamster lung (V79) cells *in vitro*	+		1.25	Trosko et al. (1982)
ICR, Inhibition of intercellular communication, rat liver epithelial cells	−		10	Wälder & Lützelschwab (1984)
ICR, Inhibition of intercellular communication, mouse hepatocytes *in vitro*	+		25	Diwan et al. (1989)
ICR, Inhibition of intercellular communication, Chinese hamster lung (V79) cells *in vitro*	?		20	Toraason et al. (1992)
ICH, Inhibition of intercellular communication, human hepatoma cellular carcinoma cell line (SK-HEP-1)	−		10	Rolin-Limbosch et al. (1987)

Table 6 (contd)

Test system	Result[a]		Dose[b] (LED/HID)	Reference
	Without exogenous metabolic system	With exogenous metabolic system		
SPM, Sperm morphology, mouse in vivo	+		20 po × 15	Kar & Dass (1983)
SPM, Sperm morphology, mouse in vivo	+		200 po × 28	Kocišová & Šrám (1985) (abstract)
BFA, Urine of mouse, Ames test, Salmonella typhimurium TA100	+	+	200 po × 1	Batzinger et al. (1978)
BFA, Urine of mouse, Ames test, Salmonella typhimurium TA98	+	+	200 po × 1	Batzinger et al. (1978)
BFA, Urine of mouse, Ames test, Salmonella typhimurium TA100	–		200	Matula & Downie (1983) (abstract)
BFA, Urine of mouse, Ames test, Salmonella typhimurium TA98	–		200	Matula & Downie (1983) (abstract)
*, Metabolites from canine gastric mucosa in vitro, Ames test, Salmonella typhimurium TA98	NT	+	NG	Rice et al. (1981)
*, Metabolites from human gastric mucosa in vitro, Ames test, Salmonella typhimurium TA98	NT	+	NG	Rice et al. (1981)

*Not shown on profile
[a] +, positive; (+), weak positive; –, negative; NT, not tested; ?, inconclusive
[b] LED, lowest effective dose; HID, highest ineffective dose; in-vitro tests, µg/mL; in-vivo tests, mg/kg bw/day; NG, dose not given
[c] Kinetochore-positive
[d] Negative for polyploidy
[e] Size ratio of micronuclei to main nucleus indicates aneuploidy induction
[f] Both intraperitoneal and oral routes were used when no useful indication concerning the most effective route was available from the literature.
[g] Average daily dose from six patients treated for 36–72 months
[h] Average daily dose from 23 patients teated for 0.5–36 months. One patient had a significant increase in cells with breaks following treatment (30 mg/day × 18 months)
[i] Average estimated dose from 25 self-poisoned individuals. Increase in hypodiploidy but not polyploidy 6–12 h after poisoning; no increase 3 and 30 days after poisoning

overall difference between the groups, three patients had elevated levels of chromosomal aberrations and one of these in particular showed chromosomal breakage in 15.3% of the cells examined, but, on re-examination six months after discontinuing the drug, only control levels of damage were found.

With regard to sister chromatid exchange, Torigoe (1979) studied 20 epileptic children (10 boys, 10 girls; age, 4–23 years) who had taken two to six anticonvulsant drugs for one to 18 years and 20 controls (10 boys, 10 girls; age, 6–15 years) who did not receive any drugs for at least six months; they found no significant difference between control subjects and epileptic patients. In the study of Husum *et al.* (1985), the peripheral lymphocytes of 34 persons (18 men and 16 women undergoing minor surgery) were examined before and 2–5 h after oral administration of a single 0.2 mg/kg bw dose of diazepam; possible effects of smoking were taken into account and no indication of the induction of sister chromatid exchange was found. In contrast with these observations, a cytogenetic investigation (Huong *et al.*, 1988) of 18 self-poisoned pregnant and 16 self-poisoned non-pregnant women and 31 controls (16 pregnant and 15 non-pregnant) found statistically significant differences in frequencies of sister chromatid exchange per cell between the third and seventh day after poisoning (pregnant: control, 8.55 ± 1.08; poisoned, 10.30 ± 1.63, $p < 0.01$; non-pregnant: control, 9.13 ± 1.32; poisoned, 11.26 ± 2.31, $p < 0.05$). In the same population, a very highly significant difference in the prevalence of chromosomal aberrations between self-poisoned women and controls (pregnant: control, 4.03%; poisoned, 9.56%, $p < 0.001$; non-pregnant: control, 5.99%; poisoned, 14.38%, $p < 0.001$) was also found; moreover, the frequency of chromatid aberrations was significantly lower in pregnant relative to non-pregnant women ($p < 0.05$). In contrast, the studies of White *et al.* (1974) on 20 patients given a single 20-mg intravenous injection of diazepam and of van Bao *et al.* (1992) on 25 patients 6–12 h, 3 days or 30 days after self-poisoning with diazepam failed to confirm the induction of chromosomal aberrations *in vivo* in human lymphocytes. The latter, however, reported that hypodiploidy (but neither hyperdiploidy nor polyploidy) was observed in the individuals studied 6–12 h after self-poisoning; the effects were not observed at later sampling times. [The Working Group noted that cytogenetic changes in lymphocytes disappeared six days after poisoning.]

4.4.2 *Experimental systems*

No studies have demonstrated bacterial DNA damage or mutagenicity due to diazepam itself.

No genetic effects were observed in single studies for mitotic recombination and gene conversion, in two studies for aneuploidy [no dose-dependent increase] with *Saccharomyces cerevisiae* or in a single study for chromosome malsegregation with *Aspergillus nidulans*.

Diazepam did not induce unscheduled DNA synthesis in primary cultures of rat hepatocytes in two studies or mutation at the *hprt* locus of Chinese hamster V79 cells or rat primary hepatocytes *in vitro*. Micronuclei were induced *in vitro* in Chinese hamster cell lines in four studies but the increase in chromosomal aberrations was judged to be inconclusive in two studies (one in the presence of an exogenous metabolic activation system) and negative in another study.

All studies with Chinese hamster cells aimed at the detection of aneuploidy *in vitro* were positive: moreover, in all of the micronucleus tests in which they were examined, the micronuclei contained kinetochore(s). Two studies out of four which scored for chromosome numbers detected a significant increase in hypodiploidy but not in hyperdiploidy. One study which tested the induction of polyploidy in Chinese hamster cells was positive. Meiotic delay has been observed in mouse oocytes (Stenchever & Smith, 1981) and mitotic arrest has been demonstrated in Chinese hamster Don cells (Hsu *et al.*, 1983) and human fibroblasts (Andersson *et al.*, 1981).

In a study at very low doses with human fibroblasts *in vitro*, diazepam did not induce sister chromatid exchange, whereas a significant increase in micronuclei was observed at higher dose levels. Two studies in human lymphocytes gave contradictory results. All the studies in either human fibroblasts or lymphocytes aimed at the detection of chromosomal aberrations *in vitro* were negative. c-Mitosis and hypodiploidy (but not polyploidy) were observed in single studies with human lymphocytes treated *in vitro* with diazepam. One study reported the induction of large-sized micronuclei in human lymphocytes *in vitro*.

Diazepam caused inhibition of gap-junctional intercellular communication in two out of five studies.

Urine of mice exposed *in vivo* to diazepam induced gene mutations in *Salmonella typhimurium* TA100 or TA98 in one study but not in another; metabolites from dog and human gastric mucosa incubated *in vitro* with diazepam induced a significant increase in gene mutations in *S. typhimurium* TA98.

Two mammalian studies indicated a lack of micronucleus induction in the bone marrow of mice *in vivo*; however, three other similar studies were positive at lower dose levels. [The Working Group noted that the authors reported induction of larger micronuclei taking into account neither interanimal variation nor objective criteria for micronucleus scoring.]

No increase in DNA single-strand breaks and/or alkali-labile sites was observed in the liver of rats given a single dose (1 mmol/kg) or 15 successive daily doses (0.2 mmol/kg) orally. However, predominantly negative results (seven negative studies and two inconclusive) for the induction of chromosomal aberrations have been obtained in studies of mouse or rat bone marrow. Aneuploidy, c-mitoses or polyploidy were not observed in mouse bone marrow [the Working Group noted the inadequate presentation of the results]. In mouse secondary spermatocytes, meiotic delay and aneuploidy were found at higher concentrations (150 mg/mL; Miller & Adler, 1992) but not at a lower concentration (30 mg/mL; Leopardi *et al.*, 1993); the positive effect was due to an increase in hyperploidy. At the same higher concentration, abnormalities of chromosome/spindle segregation were also reported in male mouse germ cells.

As reported in abstracts, treatment of mice with diazepam increases the proportion of sperm with abnormal head morphology.

5. Summary of Data Reported and Evaluation

5.1 Exposure data

Diazepam is the most widely used of the benzodiazepine pharmaceuticals. Produced since the 1960s, it is prescribed for the treatment of anxiety and as a sedative, muscle relaxant, and anticonvulsant.

5.2 Human carcinogenicity data

Studies investigating unspecified hypnotics or tranquillizers as well as diazepam specifically have been included in this monograph because of the dominance of this benzodiazepine among those prescribed. The risk for a variety of cancers, especially of the breast, associated with diazepam use has been investigated in two cohort studies and in six distinct and three related case–control studies.

In none of the two cohort or five case–control studies on benzodiazepine or diazepam use in relation to breast cancer was a positive association found. One case–control study of ovarian cancer reported an increased risk for diazepam use, that was not confirmed by another study. This latter study reported no association between diazepam use and the risk of several other types of cancer.

5.3 Animal carcinogenicity data

Diazepam was tested for carcinogenicity in one experiment in mice, in one experiment in rats and in one experiment in hamsters by oral administration in the diet and also in one limited study in gerbils. An increase in the incidence of hepatocellular tumours occurred in male mice. No significant increase in the incidence of tumours was observed in rats, hamsters or gerbils.

In one study in mice, oral administration of diazepam enhanced the occurrence of hepatocellular tumours induced by N-nitrosodiethylamine. In two studies in rats initiated with 2-acetylaminofluorene or 3′-methyl-4-(dimethylamino)azobenzene, there was no promoting effect of diazepam. In gerbils initiated with N-nitrosodiethylamine, simultaneous administration of diazepam decreased the incidence of cholangiocarcinomas.

5.4 Other relevant data

Diazepam is absorbed rapidly and extensively in humans. A 30-fold range of peak plasma concentrations is obtained when the same dose is given to different subjects. Diazepam is metabolized initially to N-desmethyldiazepam (nordiazepam) and temazepam, both of which may be converted to oxazepam. Diazepam clearance shows marked inter-subject variability. The mean elimination half-life is about 32 h.

There is wide inter-species variability in diazepam metabolism. While formation of N-desmethyldiazepam and temazepam occurs to some extent in all species studied, hydroxylation in the 5-phenyl ring is the major pathway in rats.

Diazepam has low acute and chronic toxicity for humans at therapeutic concentrations. The main adverse effects of chronic administration are psychological and physical dependence and withdrawal phenomena. Specific organ toxicity of diazepam to humans has not been observed.

The acute toxicity of diazepam to experimental animals can be considered as low. In subchronic toxicity assays in dogs, high doses of diazepam induced mild toxic effects in the blood, liver and gonads, while in rats, slight chemical-related histopathological changes were observed in the kidneys and thyroid gland.

The effects of diazepam on the immune system have been investigated mainly in in-vitro experiments with conflicting results: both stimulatory and inhibitory effects have been demonstrated. There are no data on immunosuppressing or immunomodulating effects in humans.

In several cultured cell systems, diazepam inhibits cell proliferation.

No consistent association between orofacial clefts and diazepam has been identified in humans. No increase in the prevalence at birth of congenital abnormalities has been found associated with attempted maternal suicide using high doses of diazepam, in some instances during the first trimester. While excesses of anomalies associated with regular psychotherapeutic benzodiazepine use have been observed, the types of developmental defects involved have not been consistent between studies.

High doses of diazepam induce cleft palate in mice, but not in rats. In hamsters, exencephaly and limb defects are seen, as well as cleft palate.

In general, diazepam did not induce gene or chromosome mutations in bacteria, yeast or cultured mammalian cells. In cultured mammalian cells, it induced micronuclei and aneuploidy, and inhibited gap-junctional intercellular communication. There are contradictory results on the induction of gene mutation in bacteria by the urinary metabolites of treated mice.

In general, diazepam did not induce micronuclei, chromosomal aberrations, aneuploidy, c-mitoses or polyploidy in bone marrow of mice *in vivo*. In rats *in vivo*, neither chromosomal aberrations in bone marrow, nor DNA strand breaks or alkali-labile sites in liver were found. In mouse spermatocytes, but not in oocytes, diazepam induced aneuploidy.

Mechanistic considerations

Diazepam does not cause gene mutations or chromosomal aberrations. One of its metabolites, oxazepam, increased the incidence of liver tumours (benign and malignant) (see Monograph on oxazepam, pp. 119–123). However, it is not clear that levels of oxazepam sufficient to induce hepatic effects are achieved in mice treated with diazepam.

5.5 Evaluation[1]

There is *evidence suggesting lack of carcinogenicity* of diazepam to the breast and *inadequate evidence* for carcinogenicity at other sites in humans.

There is *inadequate evidence* in experimental animals for the carcinogenicity of diazepam.

Overall evaluation

Diazepam is *not classifiable as to its carcinogenicity to humans (Group 3)*.

6. References

Aarskog, D. (1975) Association between maternal intake of diazepam and oral clefts (Letter to the Editor). *Lancet*, **ii**, 921

Abernethy, D.R., Greenblatt, D.J., Divoll, M., Ameer, B. & Shader, R.I. (1983) Differential effect of cimetidine on drug oxidation (antipyrine and diazepam) versus conjugation (acetaminophen and lorazepam): prevention of acetaminophen toxicity by cimetidine. *J. Pharmacol. exp. Ther.*, **224**, 508–513

Ackermann, E. & Richter, K. (1977) Diazepam metabolism in human foetal and adult liver. *Eur. J. clin. Pharmacol.*, **11**, 43–49

Adam, S. & Vessey, M. (1981) Diazepam and malignant melanoma (Letter to the Editor). *Lancet*, **ii**, 1344

Adler, I.-D., Kliesch, U., van Hummelen, P. & Kirsch-Volders, M. (1991) Mouse micronucleus tests with known and suspect spindle poisons: results from two laboratories. *Mutagenesis*, **6**, 47–53

Albertini, S. (1990) Analysis of nine known or suspected spindle poisons for mitotic chromosome malsegregation using *Saccharomyces cerevisiae* D61.M. *Mutagenesis*, **5**, 453–459

Alda, M., Dvoráková, M., Pošmurová, M., Balíková, M., Zvolský, P. & Filip, V. (1987) Pharmacogenetic study with diazepam in twins. *Neuropsychobiology*, **17**, 4–8

American Hospital Formulary Service (1995) *AHFS Drug Information® 95*, Bethesda, MD, American Society of Health-System Pharmacists, pp. 1591–1593

Andersson, L.C., Letho, V.-P., Stenman, S., Badley, R.A. & Virtanen, I. (1981) Diazepam induces mitotic arrest at prometaphase by inhibiting centriolar separation. *Nature*, **291**, 247–248

Anthony, H.M., Kenny, T.E. & MacKinnon, A.U. (1982) Drugs in the aetiology of cancer: a retrospective study. *Int. J. Epidemiol.*, **11**, 336–344

Antoccia, A., Degrassi, F., Battistoni, A., Ciliutti, P. & Tanzarella, C. (1991) In vitro micronucleus test with kinetochore staining: evaluation of test performance. *Mutagenesis*, **6**, 319–324

---

[1]For definition of the italicized terms, see Preamble, pp. 22–25.

Argüelles, A.E. & Rosner, J. (1975) Diazepam and plasma-testosterone levels (Letter to the Editor). *Lancet*, **ii**, 607

Arnold, E. (1975) A simple method for determining diazepam and its major metabolites in biological fluids: application in bioavailability studies. *Acta pharmacol. toxicol.*, **36**, 335–352

Baird, E.S. & Hailey, D.M. (1972) Delayed recovery from a sedative: correlation of the plasma levels of diazepam with clinical effects after oral and intravenous administration. *Br. J. Anaesth.*, **44**, 803–808

Balbi, A., Muscettola, G., Staiano, N., Martire, G. & De Lorenzo, F. (1980) Psychotropic drugs: evaluation of mutagenic effect. *Pharmacol. Res. Commun.*, **12**, 423–431

van Bao, T., Imreh, E. & Czeizel, A.E. (1992) Cytogenetic effects of diazepam in peripheral lymphocytes of self-poisoned persons. *Mutat. Res.*, **298**, 131–137

Barlow, S.M., Knight, A.F. & Sullivan, F.M. (1979) Prevention by diazepam of adverse effects of maternal restraint stress on postnatal development and learning in the rat. *Teratology*, **19**, 105–110

Barnard, E.A., Stephenson, F.A., Sigel, E., Mamalaki, C. & Bilbe, G. (1984) Structure and properties of the brain GABA/benzodiazepine receptor complex. *Adv. exp. Med. Biol.*, **175**, 235–254

Batzinger, R.P., Ou, S.-Y.L. & Bueding, E. (1978) Antimutagenic effects of 2(3)-*tert*-butyl-4-hydroxyanisole and of antimicrobial agents. *Cancer Res.*, **38**, 4478–4485

Beall, J.R. (1972) Study of the teratogenic potential of diazepam and SCH 12041 (Letter to the Editor). *Can. med. Assoc. J.*, **106**, 1061

Beischlag, T.V. & Inaba, T. (1992) Determination of nonderivatized *para*-hydroxylated metabolites of diazepam in biological fluids with a GC megabore column system. *J. analyt. Toxicol.*, **16**, 236–239

Bergman, U., Boethius, G., Swartling, P.G., Isacson, D. & Smedby, B. (1990) Teratogenic effects of benzodiazepine use during pregnancy (Letter to the Editor). *J. Pediatr.*, **116**, 490–491

Bergman, U., Rosa, F.W., Baum, C., Wiholm, B.-E. & Faich, G.A. (1992) Effects of exposure to benzodiazepine during fetal life. *Lancet*, **340**, 694–696

Bertilsson, L. & Kalow, W. (1993) Why are diazepam metabolism and polymorphic *S*-mephenytoin hydroxylation associated with each other in white and Korean populations but not in Chinese populations? (Letter to the Editor). *Clin. Pharmacol. Ther.*, **53**, 608–610

Bertilsson, L., Henthorn, T.K., Sanz, E., Tybring, G., Säwe, J. & Villén, T. (1989) Importance of genetic factors in the regulation of diazepam metabolism: relationship to *S*-mephenytoin, but not debrisoquin, hydroxylation phenotype. *Clin. Pharmacol. Ther.*, **45**, 348–355

Bertilsson, L., Baillie, T.A. & Reviriego, J. (1990) Factors influencing the metabolism of diazepam. *Pharmacol. Ther.*, **45**, 85–91

Black, H.E., Szot, R.J., Arthaud, L.E., Massa, T., Mylecraine, L., Klein, M., Lake, R., Fabry, A., Kaminska, G.Z., Sinha, D.P. & Schwarz, E. (1987) Preclinical safety evaluation of the benzodiazepine quazepam. *Arzneimittel-Forsch.*, **37**, 906–913

Bonatti, S., Cavalieri, Z., Viaggi, S. & Abbondandolo, A. (1992) The analysis of 10 potential spindle poisons for their ability to induce CREST-positive micronuclei in human diploid fibroblasts. *Mutagenesis*, **7**, 111–114

Braestrup, C. & Nielsen, M. (1978) Ontogenetic development of benzodiazepine receptors in the rat brain. *Brain. Res.*, **147**, 170–173

British Medical Association/Royal Pharmaceutical Society of Great Britain (1994*) British National Formulary Number 27 (March 1994)*, London, pp. 141–142, 192

British Pharmacopoeial Commission (1993) *British Pharmacopoeia 1993*, Vols. I & II, London, Her Majesty's Stationery Office, pp. 212, 874–876

Brooksbank, B.W.L., Atkinson, D.J. & Balázs, R. (1982) Biochemical development of the human brain. III. Benzodiazepine receptors, free γ-aminobutyrate (GABA) and other amino acids. *J. Neurosci. Res.*, **8**, 581–594

Brunner, M., Albertini, S. & Würgler, F.E. (1991) Effects of 10 known or suspected spindle poisons in the in vitro porcine brain tubulin assembly assay. *Mutagenesis*, **6**, 65–70

Budavari, S., ed. (1995) *The Merck Index*, 12th Ed., Rahway, NJ, Merck & Co.

Carlo, P., Finollo, R., Ledda, A. & Brambilla, G. (1989) Absence of liver DNA fragmentation in rats treated with high oral doses of 32 benzodiazepine drugs. *Fundam. appl. Toxicol.*, **1**, 34–41

Cavanagh, D. & Condo, C.S. (1964) Diazepam — A pilot study of drug concentrations in maternal blood, amniotic fluid and cord blood. *Curr. ther. Res.*, **6**, 122–126

Chiba, K., Horii, H., Chiba, T., Kato, Y., Hirano, T. & Ishizaki, T. (1995) Development and preliminary application of high-performance liquid chromatographic assay of urinary metabolites of diazepam in humans. *J. Chromatogr. B: biomed. Appl.*, **668**, 77–84

Cohen, M.M., Hirschhorn, K. & Frosch, W.A. (1969) Cytogenetic effects of tranquilizing drugs *in vivo* and *in vitro*. *J. Am. med. Assoc.*, **207**, 2425–2426

Cole, A.P. & Hailey, D.M. (1975) Diazepam and active metabolite in breast milk and their transfer to the neonate (Short report). *Arch. Dis. Child.*, **50**, 741–742

Covelli, V., Decandia, P., Altamura, M. & Jirillo, E. (1989) Diazepam inhibits phagocytosis and killing exerted by polymorphonuclear cells and monocytes from healthy donors. In vitro studies. *Immunopharmacol. Immunotoxicol.*, **11**, 701–714

Cox, A.D. (1988) Maternal depression and impact on children's development. *Arch. Dis. Child.*, **63**, 90–95

Crebelli, R., Conti, G., Conti, L. & Carere, A. (1991) In vitro studies with nine known or suspected spindle poisons: results in tests for chromosome malsegregation in *Aspergillus nidulans*. *Mutagenesis*, **6**, 131–136

Cree, J.E., Meyer, J. & Hailey, D.M. (1973) Diazepam in labour: its metabolism and effect on the clinical condition and thermogenesis of the newborn. *Br. med. J.*, **4**, 251–255

Czeizel, A.E. (1976) Diazepam, phenytoin and aetiology of cleft lip and/or cleft palate (Letter to the Editor). *Lancet*, **i**, 810

Czeizel, A.E. (1988) Lack of evidence of teratogenicity of benzodiazepine drugs in Hungary. *Reprod. Toxicol.*, **1**, 183–188

Czeizel, A.E. & Lendvay, A. (1987) In utero exposure to benzodiazepines (Letter to the Editor). *Lancet*, **i**, 628

Czeizel, A.E. & Rácz, J. (1990) Evaluation of drug intake during pregnancy in the Hungarian case–control surveillance of congenital anomalies. *Teratology*, **42**, 505–512

Czeizel, A.E., Szentesi, I., Szekeres, I., Glauber, A., Bucski, P. & Molnár, C. (1984) Pregnancy outcome and health conditions of offspring of self-poisoned pregnant women. *Acta paediat. hung.*, **25**, 209–236

Czeizel, A.E., Szentesi, I., Szekeres, I., Molnár, G., Glauber, A. & Bucski, P. (1988) A study of adverse effects on the progeny after intoxication during pregnancy. *Arch. Toxicol.*, **62**, 1–7

Czeizel, A.E., Intôdy, Z. & Modell, B. (1993) What proportion of congenital abnormalities can be prevented? *Br. med. J.*, **306**, 499–503

Danielson, D.A., Jick, H., Hunter, J.R., Stergachis, A. & Madsen, S. (1982) Nonestrogenic drugs and breast cancer. *Am. J. Epidemiol.*, **116**, 329–332

Das, R.K. & Kar, R.N. (1986) Genotoxic effects of three benzodiazepine tranquilizers in mouse bone marrow as revealed by the micronucleus test. *Caryologia*, **39**, 193–198

Degraeve, N., Chollet, C., Moutschen, J., Moutschen-Dahmen, M. & Gilet-Delhalle, J. (1985) Investigation of the potential mutagenic activity of benzodiazepines in mice (Abstract no. 23). *Mutat. Res.*, **147**, 290

Deren, S. (1986) Children of substance abusers: a review of the literature. *J. Substance Abuse Treat.*, **3**, 77–94

Derogatis, L.R., Feldstein, M., Morrow, G., Schmale, A., Schmitt, M., Gates, C., Murawski, B., Holland, J., Penman, D., Melisaratos, N., Enelow, A.J. & McKinney Adler, L. (1979) A survey of psychotropic drug prescriptions in an oncology population. *Cancer*, **44**, 1919–1929

Diwan, B.A., Rice, J.M. & Ward, J.M. (1986) Tumor-promoting activity of benzodiazepine tranquilizers, diazepam and oxazepam, in mouse liver. *Carcinogenesis*, **7**, 789–794

Diwan, B.A., Lubet, R.A., Nims, R.W., Klaunig, J.E., Weghorst, C.M., Henneman, J.R., Ward, J.M. & Rice, J.M. (1989) Lack of promoting effect of clonazepam on the development of *N*-nitrosodiethylamine-initiated hepatocellular tumors in mice is correlated with its inability to inhibit cell-to-cell communication in mouse hepatocytes. *Carcinogenesis*, **10**, 1719–1724

Dollery, C., Boobis, A.R., Burley, D., Davies, D.M., Davies, D.S., Harrison, P.I., Orme, M.E., Park, B.K. & Goldberg, L.I. (1991) *Therapeutic Drugs: Diazepam*, Edinburgh, Churchill Livingstone, pp. D86–D91

El-Brashy, A., Aly, F.A. & Belal, F. (1993) Determination of 1,4-benzodiazepines in drug dosage forms by difference spectrophotometry. *Mikrochim. Acta*, **110**, 55–60

Erkkola, R. & Kanto, J. (1972) Diazepam and breast-feeding (Letter to the Editor). *Lancet*, **i**, 1235–1236

Erkkola, R., Kanto, J. & Sellman, R. (1974) Diazepam in early human pregnancy. *Acta obstet. gynec. scand.*, **53**, 135–138

Farmindustria (1993) *Repertorio Farmaceutico Italiano* (Italian Pharmaceutical Directory), 7th Ed., Milan, Associazione Nazionale dell'Industria Farmaceutica, CEDOF S.P.A., pp. A-88–A-89, A-1606–A-1607

Ferguson, L.R., Morcombe, P. & Triggs, C.T. (1993) The size of cytokinesis-blocked micronuclei in human peripheral blood lymphocyes as a measure of aneuploidy induction by Set A compounds in the EEC trial. *Mutat. Res.*, **287**, 101–112

Fernández, P., Hermida, I., Bermejo, A.M., López-Rivadulla, M., Cruz, A. & Concheiro, L. (1991) Simultaneous determination of diazepam and its metabolites in plasma by high-performance liquid chromatography. *J. liq. Chromatogr.*, **14**, 2587–2599

Ferrarese, C., Appollonio, I., Frigo, M., Gaini, S.M., Piolti, R. & Frattola, L. (1989) Benzodiazepine receptors and diazepam-binding inhibitor in human cerebral tumors. *Ann. Neurol.*, **26**, 564–568

Ferrarese, C., Cavaletti, G., Alho, H., Pierpaoli, C., Marzorati, C., Bianchi, G., Pizzini, G. & Frattola, L. (1992) Subcellular location of peripheral benzodiazepine receptors in human lymphocytes (Abstract no. 2219). *Eur. J. Neurosci.*, **Suppl. 5**, 129

Ferrarese, C., Appollonio, I., Bianchi, G., Frigo, M., Marzorati, C., Pecora, N., Perego, M., Pierpaoli, C. & Frattola, L. (1993) Benzodiazepine receptors and diazepam binding inhibitor: a possible link between stress, anxiety and the immune system. *Psychoneuroendocrinology*, **18**, 3–22

Frieder, B., Epstein, S. & Grimm, V.E. (1984) The effects of exposure to diazepam during various stages of gestation or during lactation on the development and behavior of rat pups. *Psychopharmacology*, **83**, 51–55

Friedman, G.D. & Selby, J.V. (1990) Epidemiological screening for potentially carcinogenic drugs. In: Hoigne, R., Lawson, D.H. & Weber, E.R., eds, *Risk Factors for Adverse Drug Reactions. Epidemiological Approaches (Agents Actions Suppl. 29)*, Basel, Birkhäuser Verlag, pp. 83–96

Gai, N. & Grimm, V.E. (1982) The effect of prenatal exposure to diazepam on aspects of postnatal development and behavior in rats. *Psychopharmacology*, **78**, 225–229

Gamble, J.A.S., Mackay, J.S. & Dundee, J.W. (1973) Plasma levels of diazepam (Letter to the Editor). *Br. J. Anaesth.*, **45**, 1085

Gamble, J.A.S., Dundee, J.W. & Assaf, R.A.E. (1975) Plasma diazepam levels after single dose oral and intramuscular administration. *Anaesthesia*, **30**, 164–169

Garattini, S., Mussini, E., Marcucci, F. & Guaitani, A. (1973) Metabolic studies on benzodiazepines in various animal species. In: Garattini, S., Mussini, E. & Randall, L.O., eds, *The Benzodiazepines*, New York, Raven Press, pp. 75–97

Gassner, P. & Adler, I.-D. (1995) Analysis of chemically induced spindle aberrations in male mouse germ cells: comparison of differential and immunofluorescent staining procedures. *Mutagenesis*, **10**, 243–252

Gavish, M., Katz, Y., Bar-Ami, S. & Weizman, R. (1992) Biochemical, physiological, and pathological aspects of the peripheral benzodiazepine receptor. *J. Neurochem.*, **58**, 1589–1601

Gennaro, A.R., ed. (1995) *Remington: The Science and Practice of Pharmacy*, 19th Ed., Vol. II, Easton, PA, Mack Publishing Co., pp. 1157–1158

Gill, T.S., Guram, M.S. & Geber, W.F. (1981) Comparative study of the teratogenic effects of chlordiazepoxide and diazepam in the fetal hamster. *Life Sci.*, **29**, 2141–2147

Goodman Gilman, A., Rall, T.W., Nico, A.S. & Taylor, P., eds (1990) *Goodman and Gilman's. The Pharmacological Basis of Therapeutics*, 8th Ed., New York, Pergamon Press

Gorman, A.M.C., O'Beirne, G.B., Regan, C.M. & Williams, D.C. (1989) Antiproliferative action of benzodiazepines in cultured brain cells is not mediated through the peripheral-type benzodiazepine acceptor. *J. Neurochem.*, **53**, 849–855

Green, U. & Ketkar, M. (1978) The influence of diazepam and thiouracil upon the carcinogenic effect of diethylnitrosamine in gerbils. *Z. Krebsforsch.*, **92**, 55–62

Greenblatt, D.J., Allen, M.D., Harmatz, J.S. & Shader, R.I. (1980) Diazepam disposition determinants. *Clin. Pharmacol. Ther.*, **27**, 301–312

Greenblatt, D.J., Harmatz, J.S., Friedman, H., Locniskar, A. & Shader, R.I. (1989) A large-sample study of diazepam pharmacokinetics. *Ther. Drug Monit.*, **11**, 652–657

Guerriero, F.J. & Fox, K.A. (1977) Benzodiazepines and development of Swiss-Webster mice. *Pharmacol. Res. Comm.*, **9**, 187–196

Gunnarskog, J. & Källén, A.J.B. (1993) Drug intoxication during pregnancy: a study with central registries. *Reprod. Toxicol.*, **7**, 117–121

Harlow, B.L. & Cramer, D.W. (1995) Self-reported use of antidepressants or benzodiazepine tranquilizers and risk of epithelial ovarian cancer: evidence from two combined case–control studies (Massachusetts, United States). *Cancer Causes Control*, **6**, 130–134

Hillestad, L., Hansen, T. & Melsom, H. (1974) Diazepam metabolism in normal man. II. Serum concentration and clinical effect after oral administration and cumulation. *Clin. Pharmacol. Ther.*, **16**, 485–489

Hino, O. & Kitagawa, T. (1982) Effect of diazepam on hepatocarcinogenesis in the rat. *Toxicol. Lett.*, **11**, 155–157

Hollister, L.E., Müller-Oerlinghausen, B., Rickels, K. & Shader, R.I. (1993) Clinical uses of benzodiazepines. *J. clin. Psychopharmacol.*, **13** (Suppl. 1)

Hooper, W.D., Watt, J.A., McKinnon, G.E. & Reilly, P.E.B. (1992) Metabolism of diazepam and related benzodiazepines by human liver microsomes. *Eur. J. Drug Metab. Pharmacokinet.*, **17**, 51–59

Hsu, T.C., Liang, J.C. & Shirley, L.R. (1983) Aneuploidy induction by mitotic arrestants. Effects of diazepam on diploid Chinese hamster cells. *Mutat. Res.*, **122**, 201–209

Huong, T.T.T., Szentesi, I. & Czeizel, A.E. (1988) Lower prevalence of chromosome aberrations and SCEs in self-poisoned pregnant women. *Mutat. Res.*, **198**, 255–259

Husum, B., Wulf, H.C., Niebuhr, E. & Rasmussen, J.A. (1985) SCE in lymphocytes of patients treated with single, large doses of diazepam. *Mutat. Res.*, **155**, 71–73

IARC (1977) *IARC Monographs on the Evaluation of Carcinogenic Risk of Chemicals to Man*, Vol. 13, *Some Miscellaneous Pharmaceutical Substances*, Lyon, pp. 57–73

IARC (1987) *IARC Monographs on the Evaluation of Carcinogenic Risks to Humans*, Suppl. 7, *Overall Evaluations of Carcinogenicity: An Update of* IARC Monographs *Volumes 1 to 42*, Lyon, pp. 189–191

Idänpään-Heikkilä, J.E., Jouppila, P.I., Puolakka, J.O. & Vorne, M.S. (1971a) Placental transfer and fetal metabolism of diazepam in early human pregnancy. *Am. J. Obstet. Gynecol.*, **109**, 1011–1016

Idänpään-Heikkilä, J.E., Taska, R.J., Allen, H.A. & Schoolar, J.C. (1971b) Placental transfer of diazepam-^{14}C in mice, hamsters and monkeys. *J. Pharmacol. exp. Ther.*, **176**, 752–757

de la Iglesia, F.A., Barsoum, N., Gough, A., Mitchell, L., Martin, R.A., Di Fonzo, C. & McGuire, E.J. (1981) Carcinogenesis bioassay of prazepam (Vestran) in rats and mice. *Toxicol. appl. Pharmacol.*, **57**, 39–54

Ishidate, M., Jr, Harnois, M.C. & Sofuni, T. (1988) A comparative analysis of data on the clastogenicity of 951 chemical substances tested in mammalian cell cultures. *Mutat. Res.*, **195**, 151–213

Ishimura, K., Sawai, M., Yamamoto, K., Neda, K. & Sata, H. (1975) Studies on the chromosomes of rat bone marrow cells treated with benzodiazepine derivative *in vivo* (Abstract). *Teratology*, **12**, 199

Jerome, C.P., Golub, M.S., Cardinet, G.G., III & Hendrickx, A.G. (1981) Effects of acute and chronic diazepam administration during pregnancy on neonate rhesus monkeys (Abstract). *Teratology*, **23**, 43A

Jommi, G., Manitto, P. & Silanos, M.A. (1964) Metabolism of diazepam in rabbits. *Arch. Biochem. Biophys.*, **108**, 334–340

Jørgensen, N.P., Thurmann-Nielsen, E. & Walstad, R.A. (1988) Pharmacokinetics and distribution of diazepam and oxazepam in early pregnancy. *Acta obstet. gynecol. scand.*, **67**, 493–497

Kanto, J. (1975) Plasma concentrations of diazepam and its metabolites after peroral, intramuscular, and rectal administration. Correlation between plasma concentration and sedatory effect of diazepam. *Int. J. clin. Phramacol.*, **12**, 427–432

Kanto, J., Erkkola, R. & Sellman, R. (1974) Perinatal metabolism of diazepam (Letter to the Editor). *Br. med. J.*, **i**, 641–642

Kaplan, S.A., Jack, M.L., Alexander, K. & Weinfeld, R.E. (1973) Pharmacokinetic profile of diazepam in man following single intravenous and oral and chronic oral administrations. *J. pharm. Sci.*, **62**, 1789–1796

Kar, R.N. & Das, R.K. (1979) Dominant lethality and micronuclei in mice treated with diazepam. *Nucleus*, **22**, 192–195

Kar, R.N. & Das, R.K. (1983) Induction of sperm head abnormalities in mice by three tranquilizers. *Cytobios*, **36**, 45–51

Katz, Y., Eitan, A., Amiri, Z. & Gavish, M. (1988) Dramatic increase in peripheral benzodiazepine binding sites in human colonic adenocarcinoma as compared to normal colon. *Eur. J. Pharmacol.*, **148**, 483–484

Katz, Y., Moskovitz, B., Levin, D.R. & Gavish, M. (1989) Absence of peripheral-type benzodiazepine binding sites in renal carcinoma: a potential biochemical marker. *Br. J. Urol.*, **63**, 124–127

Katz, Y., Ben-Baruch, G., Kloog, Y., Menczer, J. & Gavish, M. (1990) Increased density of peripheral benzodiazepine-binding sites in ovarian carcinomas as compared with benign ovarian tumours and normal ovaries. *Clin. Sci. Colch.*, **78**, 155–158

Kaufman, D.W., Shapiro, S., Slone, D., Rosenberg, L., Helmrich, S.P., Miettinen, O.S., Stolley, P.D., Levy, M. & Schottenfeld, D. (1982) Diazepam and the risk of breast cancer. *Lancet*, **i**, 537–539

Kaufman, D.W., Werler, M.M., Palmer, J.R., Rosenberg, L., Stolley, P.D., Warshauer, M.E., Clarke, E.A., Miller, D.R. & Shapiro, S. (1990) Diazepam use in relation to breast cancer: results from two case–control studies. *Am. J. Epidemiol.*, **131**, 483–490

Kellogg, C.K. (1992) Benzodiazepines and the developing nervous system: laboratory findings and clinical implications. In: Zagon, I.S. & Slotkin, T.A., eds, *Maternal Substance Abuse and the Developing Nervous System*, New York, Academic Press, pp. 283–321

Kellogg, C.K., Tervo, D., Ison, J., Parisi, T. & Miller, R.K. (1980) Prenatal exposure to diazepam alters behavioral development in rats. *Science*, **207**, 205–207

van der Kleijn, E., van Rossum, J.M., Muskens, E.T.J.M. & Rijntjes, N.V.M. (1971) Pharmacokinetics of diazepam in dogs, mice and humans. *Acta pharmacol. toxicol.*, **3** (Suppl.), 109–127

Kleinerman, R.A., Brinton, L.A., Hoover, R. & Fraumeni, J.F., Jr (1984) Diazepam use and progression of breast cancer. *Cancer Res.*, **44**, 1223–1225

Klotz, U., Avant, G.R., Hoyumpa, A., Schenker, S. & Wilkinson, G.R. (1975) The effects of age and liver disease on the disposition and elimination of diazepam in adult man. *J. clin. Invest.*, **55**, 347–359

Klotz, U., Antonin, K.H. & Bieck, P.R. (1976a) Comparison of the pharmacokinetics of diazepam after single and subchronic doses. *Eur. J. clin. Pharmacol.*, **10**, 121–126

Klotz, U., Antonin, K.H. & Bieck, P.R. (1976b) Pharmacokinetics and plasma binding of diazepam in man, dog, rabbit, guinea-pig and rat. *J. Pharmacol. exp. Ther.*, **199**, 67–73

Klotz, U., Antonin, K.H., Brügel, H. & Bieck, P.R. (1977) Disposition of diazepam and its major metabolite desmethyldiazepam in patients with liver disease. *Clin. Pharmacol. Ther.*, **21**, 430–436

Kocišová, J. & Šrám, R.J. (1985) The mutagenic activity of diazepam (Abstract no. 50). *Mutat. Res.*, **147**, 304

Komiskey, H.L., Rahman, A., Weisenburger, W.P., Hayton, W.L., Zobrist, R.H. & Silvius, W. (1985) Extraction, separation and detections of ^{14}C-diazepam and ^{14}C-metabolites from brain tissue of mature and old rats. *J. analyt. Toxicol.*, **9**, 131–133

Korttila, K. & Linnoila, M. (1975) Psychomotor skills related to driving after intramuscular administration of diazepam and meperidine. *Anesthesiology*, **42**, 685–691

Krueger, K.E. & Papadopoulos, V. (1990) Peripheral-type benzodiazepine receptors mediate translocation of cholesterol from outer to inner mitochondrial membranes in adrenocortical cells. *J. biol. Chem.*, **265**, 15015–15022

Krueger, K.E. & Papadopoulos, V. (1992) Mitochondrial benzodiazepine receptors and the regulation of steroid biosynthesis. *Annu. Rev. Pharmacol. Toxicol.*, **32**, 211–237

Kunert-Radek, J., Stepien, H. & Pawlikowski, M. (1994) Inhibition of rat pituitary tumor cell proliferation by benzodiazepines *in vitro*. *Neuroendocrinology*, **59**, 92–96

Laegreid, L., Olegård, R., Wahlström, J. & Conradi, N. (1987) Abnormalities in children exposed to benzodiazepines *in utero* (Letter to the Editor). *Lancet*, **i**, 108–109

Laegreid, L., Olegård, R., Wahlström, J. & Conradi, N. (1989) Teratogenic effects of benzodiazepine use during pregnancy. *J. Pediatr.*, **114**, 126–131

Laegreid, L., Olegård, R., Conradi, N., Hagberg, G., Wahlström, J. & Abrahamsson, L. (1990) Congenital malformations and maternal consumption of benzodiazepines: a case–control study. *Dev. Med. Child Neurol.*, **32**, 432–441

Laegreid, L., Conradi, N., Hagberg, G. & Hedner, T. (1992a) Psychotropic drug use in pregnancy and perinatal death. *Acta obstet. gynecol. scand.*, **71**, 451–457

Laegreid, L., Hagberd, G. & Lundberg, A. (1992b) The effect of benzodiazepines on the fetus and the newborn. *Neuropediatrics*, **23**, 18–23

Laegreid, L., Hagberg, G. & Lundberg, A. (1992c) Neurodevelopment in late infancy after prenatal exposure to benzodiazepines — A prospective study. *Neuropediatrics*, **23**, 60–67

Lafi, A. & Parry, J.M. (1988) A study of the induction of aneuploidy and chromosome aberrations after diazepam, medazepam, midazolam and bromazepam treatment. *Mutagenesis*, **3**, 23–27

Lendvay, A. & Czeizel, A.E. (1992) A behavioural teratologic study on offspring of self-poisoned pregnant women. *Acta paediat. hung.*, **32**, 347–369

Lensmeyer, G.L., Rajani, C. & Evenson, M.A. (1982) Liquid-chromatographic procedure for simultaneous analysis for eight benzodiazepines in serum. *Clin. Chem.*, **28**, 2274–2278

Leopardi, P., Zijno, A., Bassani, B. & Pacchierotti, F. (1993) In vivo studies on chemically induced aneuploidy in mouse somatic and germinal cells. *Mutat. Res.*, **287**, 119–130

Linet, M.S., Harlow, S.D. & McLaughlin, J.K. (1987) A case–control study of multiple myeloma in whites: chronic antigenic stimulation, occupation, and drug use. *Cancer Res.*, **47**, 2978–2981

Löscher, W. (1982) Rapid gas chromatographic measurement of diazepam and its metabolites desmethyldiazepam, oxazepam and 3-hydroxydiazepam (temazepam) in small samples of plasma. *Ther. Drug Monit.*, **4**, 315–318

Lukey, B.J., Corcoran, K.D. & Solana, R.P. (1991) Pharmacokinetics of diazepam intramuscularly administered to rhesus monkeys. *J. pharm. Sci.*, **80**, 918–921

Lynch, A.M. & Parry, J.M. (1993) The cytochalasin-B micronucleus/kinetochore assay *in vitro*: studies with 10 suspected aneugens. *Mutat. Res.*, **287**, 71–86

MacDonald, A., Michaelis, A.F. & Senkowski, B.Z. (1972) Diazepam. In: Florey, K., ed., *Analytical Profiles of Drug Substances*, Vol. 1, New York, Academic Press, pp. 79–99

Mac New, B.A. & Finnegan, L.P. (1980) Identification of a benzodiazepine abstinence syndrome (BAS) using a neonatal abstinence scoring system (Abstract no. 261). *Pediatr. Res.*, **14**, 469

Mailhes, J.B. & Marchetti, F. (1994) Chemically-induced aneuploidy in mammalian oocytes. *Mutat. Res.*, **320**, 87–111

Mandelli, M., Tognoni, G. & Garattini, S. (1978) Clinical pharmacokinetics of diazepam. *Clin. Pharmacokinet.*, **3**, 72–91

Mañes, J., Civera, J., Font, G. & Bosch, F. (1987) Spectrophotometric determination of benzodiazepines in pharmaceuticals by ion pairing. *Cienc. ind. Farm.*, **6**, 333–338 (in Spanish)

Marc, V. & Morselli, P.L. (1969) Effect of diazepam on plasma corticosterone levels in the rat (Letter to the Editor). *J. Pharm. Pharmacol.*, **21**, 784–786

Marcucci, F., Guaitani, A., Kvetina, J., Mussini, E. & Garattini, S. (1968) Species difference in diazepam metabolism and anticonvulsant effect. *Eur. J. Pharmacol.*, **4**, 467–470

Marcucci, F., Guaitani, A., Fanelli, R., Mussini, E. & Garattini, S. (1971) Metabolism and anticonvulsant activity of diazepam in guinea-pigs (Short communication). *Biochem. Pharmacol.*, **20**, 1711–1713

Marrazzini, A., Betti, C., Bernacchi, F., Barrai, I. & Barale, R. (1994) Micronucleus test and metaphase analysis in mice exposed to known and suspected spindle poisons. *Mutagenesis*, **9**, 505–515

Matsuoka, A., Hayashi, M. & Ishidate, M., Jr (1979) Chromosomal aberration tests on 29 chemicals combined with S9 mix *in vitro*. *Mutat. Res.*, **66**, 277–290

Matula, T.I. & Downie, R. (1983) Evaluation of diazepam and oxazepam in in vitro microbial mutagenicity tests and in an in vivo promoter assay (Abstract no. Ee-23). *Environ. Mutag.*, **5**, 478

Maurer, H. & Pfleger, K. (1987) Identification and differentiation of benzodiazepines and their metabolites in urine by computerized gas chromatography-mass spectrometry. *J. Chromatogr.*, **422**, 85–101

Mazue, G., Remandet, B., Gouy, D., Berthe, J., Roncucci, R. & Williams, G.M. (1982) Limited in vivo bioassays on some benzodiazepines: lack of experimental initiating or promoting effect of the benzodiazepine tranquillizers diazepam, chlorazepate, oxazepam and lorazepam. *Arch. int. Pharmacodyn.*, **257**, 59–65

Mazzi, E. (1977) Possible neonatal diazepam withdrawal: a case report (Communication in brief). *Am. J. Obstet. Gynecol.*, **129**, 586–587

McCarley, T.D. & Brodbelt, J. (1993) Structurally diagnostic ion-molecule reactions and collisionally activated dissociation of 1,4-benzodiazepines in a quadrupole ion trap mass spectrometer. *Analyt. Chem.*, **65**, 2380–2388

Medical Economics (1996) *PDR®: Physicians' Desk* Reference, 50th Ed., Montvale, NJ, Medical Economics Data Production Co., pp. 1809–1810, 2169–2170, 2182–2184

Migliore, L. & Nieri, M. (1991) Evaluation of twelve potential aneuploidogenic chemicals by the in vitro human lymphocyte micronucleus assay. *Toxicol. in Vitro*, **5**, 325–336

Miller, R.P. & Becker, B.A. (1975) Teratogenicity of oral diazepam and diphenylhydantoin in mice. *Toxicol. appl. Pharmacol.*, **32**, 53–61

Miller, B.M. & Adler, I.-D. (1989) Suspect spindle poisons: analysis of c-mitotic effects in mouse bone marrow cells. *Mutagenesis*, **4**, 208–215

Miller, B.M. & Adler, I.-D. (1992) Aneuploidy induction in mouse spermatocytes. *Mutagenesis*, **7**, 69–76

Morselli, P.L. (1977) Psychotropic drugs, benzodiazepines. In: Morselli, P.L., *Drug Disposition During Development*, New York, Spectrum Publication, pp. 449–459

Morselli, P.L., Principi, N., Tognoni, G., Reali, E., Belvedere, G., Standen, S.M. & Sereni, F. (1973) Diazepam elimination in premature and full term infants, and children. *J. perinat. Med.*, **1**, 133–141

Mukhin, A.G., Papadopoulos, V., Costa, E. & Krueger, K.E. (1989) Mitochondrial benzodiazepine receptors regulate steroid biosynthesis. *Proc. natl Acad. Sci. USA*, **86**, 9813–9816

Mura, P., Piriou, A., Fraillon, P., Papet, Y. & Reiss, D. (1987) Screening procedure for benzodiazepines in biological fluids by high-performance liquid chromatography using a rapid-scanning multichannel detector. *J. Chromatogr.*, **416**, 303–310

Natarajan, A.T., Duivenvoorden, W.C.M., Meijers, W. & Zwanenburg, T.S.B. (1993) Induction of mitotic aneuploidy using Chinese hamster primary embryonic cells. Test results of 10 chemicals. *Mutat. Res.*, **287**, 47–56

Nebert, D.W., Nelson, D.R., Adesnik, M., Coon, M.J., Estabrook, R.W., Gonzalez, F.J., Guengerich, F.P., Gunsalus, I.C., Johnson, E.F., Kemper, B., Levin, W., Phillips, I.R., Sato, R. & Waterman, M.R. (1989) The P450 superfamily: updated listing of all genes and recommended nomenclature for the chromosomal loci. *DNA*, **8**, 1–13

Neda, K., Yamamoto, K., Sato, H., Sawai, M. & Ishimura, K. (1977) In vivo cytogenetic studies of 10-chloro-11b-(2-fluorophenyl)-7-(2-hydroxyethyl)-2,3,5,11b-tetrahydrooxazolo-(3,2-d)-[1,4]benzodiazepine-6-(7*H*)-one [MS-4101] on rat bone marrow cells. *Folia pharmacol. Jpn.*, **73**, 651–656 (in Japanese)

Neville, C.F., Ninomiya, S.-I., Shimada, N., Kamataki, T., Imaoka, S. & Funae, Y. (1993) Characterization of specific cytochrome P450 enzymes responsible for the metabolism of diazepam in hepatic microsomes of adult male rats. *Biochem. Pharmacol.*, **45**, 59–65

Ochs, H.R., Greenblatt, D.J., Divoll, M., Abernethy, D.R., Feyerabend, H. & Dengler, H.J. (1981a) Diazepam kinetics in relation to age and sex. *Pharmacology*, **23**, 24–30

Ochs, H.R., Greenblatt, D.J., Roberts, G.-M. & Dengler, H.J. (1981b) Diazepam interaction with antituberculosis drugs. *Clin. Pharmacol. Ther.*, **29**, 671–678

Ochs, H.R., Greenblatt, D.J., Eckardt, B., Harmatz, J.S. & Shader, R.I. (1983) Repeated diazepam dosing in cirrhotic patients: cumulation and sedation. *Clin. Pharmacol. Ther.*, **33**, 471–476

Owen, G., Smith, T.H.F. & Agersborg, H.P.K., Jr (1970) Toxicity of some benzodiazepine compounds with CNS activity. *Toxicol. appl. Pharmacol.*, **16**, 556–570

Owen, J.R., Irani, S.F. & Blair, A.W. (1972) Effect of diazepam administered to mothers during labour on temperature regulation of neonate. *Arch. Dis. Child.*, **47**, 107–110

Papadopoulos, V., Nowzari, F.B. & Krueger, K.E. (1991) Hormone-stimulated steroidogenesis is coupled to mitochondrial benzodiazepine receptors. Tropic hormone action on steroid biosynthesis is inhibited by flunitrazepam. *J. biol. Chem.*, **266**, 3682–3687

Pawlikowski, M., Kunert-Radek, J., Radek, A. & Stepien, H. (1988a) Inhibition of cell proliferation of human gliomas by benzodiazepines *in vitro*. *Acta neurol. scand.*, **77**, 231–233

Pawlikowski, M., Lyson, K., Kunert-Radek, J. & Stepien, H. (1988b) Effect of benzodiazepines on the proliferation of mouse spleen lymphocytes *in vitro*. *J. neur. Transm.*, **73**, 161–166

Peat, M.A. & Kopjak, L. (1979) Screening and quantitation of diazepam, flurazepam, chlordiazepoxide and their metabolites in blood and plasma by electron-capture gas chromatography and high-pressure liquid chromatography. *J. forensic Sci.*, **24**, 46–54

Peterka, M., Jelínek, R. & Pavlík, A. (1992) Embryotoxicity of 25 psychotropic drugs: a study using CHEST (Chick Embryotoxicity Screening). *Reprod. Toxicol.*, **6**, 367–374

Petersen, K.W., Sherwood, H.L. & Petersen, H.D. (1978) The cytogenetic effects of diazepam and chlordiazepoxide (Abstract). *Anat. Rec.*, **190**, 620

Preiss, A.M., Scheutwinkel-Reich, M., Fülle, I., Grohmann, H.G. & Stan, H.-J. (1982) Investigation with the *Salmonella*/microsome test, of psychopharmaceuticals used in meat production. *Mutat. Res.*, **104**, 333–337

Reilly, P.E.B., Thompson, D.A., Mason, S.R. & Hooper, W.D. (1990) Cytochrome P450IIIA enzymes in rat liver microsomes: involvement in C_3-hydroxylation of diazepam and nordazepam but not *N*-dealkylation of diazepam and temazepam. *Mol. Pharmacol.*, **37**, 767–774

Remandet, B., Gouy, D., Berthe, J., Mazue, G. & Williams, G.M. (1984) Lack of initiating or promoting activity of six benzodiazepine tranquilizers in rat liver limited bioassays monitored by histopathology and assay of liver and plasma enzymes. *Fund. appl. Toxicol.*, **4**, 152–163

Reynolds, J.A.F., ed. (1993) *Martindale: The Extra Pharmacopoeia*, 30th Ed., London, The Pharmaceutical Press, pp. 584–585

Rice, S., Ichinotsubo, D., Stemmermann, G., Hayashi, T., Palumbo, N., Sylvester, S., Nomura, A. & Mower, H. (1981) Nitrosation reactions of stomach mucosal tissue of the human and dog. In: Bruce, W.R., Correa, P., Lipkin, M., Tannenbaum, S.R. & Wilkins, T.D., eds, *Gastrointestinal Cancer: Endogenous Factors* (Bambury Report 7), Cold Spring Harbor, Cold Spring Harbor Laboratory, pp. 185–203

Richards, J.G., Schock, P., Möhler, H. & Haefely, W. (1986) Benzodiazepam receptors resolved. *Experientia*, **42**, 121–126

Röhrborn, G., Thiel, C., Heimbach, D., Manolache, M. & Gebauer, J. (1984) Effects of diazepam in mutation test systems *in vitro* and in the BHK21 cell transformation assay (Abstract no. II.3D.20). *Mutat. Res.*, **130**, 260

Rolin-Limbosch, S., Moens, W. & Szpirer, C. (1987) Metabolic cooperation in SK-HEP-1 human hepatoma cells following treatment with benzodiazepine tranquilizers. *Carcinogenesis*, **8**, 1013–1016

Romkes, M., Faletto, M.B., Blaisdell, J.A., Raucy, J.L. & Goldstein, J.A. (1991) Cloning and expression of complementary DNAs for multiple members of the human cytochrome P450IIC subfamily. *Biochemistry*, **30**, 3247–3255

Rosenberg, L., Mitchell, A.A., Parsells, J.L., Pashayan, H., Louik, C. & Shapiro, S. (1983) Lack of relation of oral clefts to diazepam use during pregnancy. *New Engl. J. Med.*, **309**, 1282–1285

Rosenberg, L., Palmer, J.R., Zauber, A.G., Warshauer, M.E., Strom, B.L., Harlap, S. & Shapiro, S. (1995) Relation of benzodiazepine use to the risk of selected cancers: breast, large bowel, malignant melanoma, lung, endometrium, ovary, non-Hodgkin's lymphoma, testis, Hodgkin's disease, thyroid, and liver. *Am. J. Epidemiol.*, **141**, 1153–1160

Ruelius, H.W., Lee, J.M. & Alburn, H.E. (1965) Metabolism of diazepam in dogs: transformation to oxazepam. *Arch. Biochem. Biophys.*, **11**, 376–380

Ruff, M.R., Pert, C.B., Weber, R.J., Wahl, L.M., Wahl, S.M. & Paul, S.M. (1985) Benzodiazepine receptor-mediated chemotaxis of human monocytes. *Science*, **229**, 1281–1283

Safra, M.J. & Oakley, G.P., Jr (1975) Association between cleft lip with or without cleft palate and prenatal exposure to diazepam. *Lancet*, **ii**, 478–480

Safra, M.J. & Oakley, G.P., Jr (1976) Valium: an oral cleft teratogen? *Cleft Palate J.*, **13**, 198–200

Saito, H., Kobayashi, H., Takeno, S. & Sakai, T. (1984) Fetal toxicity of benzodiazepines in rats. *Res. Comm. chem. Pathol. Pharmacol.*, **46**, 437–447

Sasaki, M., Sugimura, K., Yoshida, M.A. & Abe, S. (1980) Cytogenetic effects of 60 chemicals on cultured human and Chinese hamster cells. *Kromosomo II*, **20**, 574–584

Satya-Prakash, K.L., Hsu, T.C. & Wheeler, W.J. (1984) Metaphase arrest, anaphase recovery and aneuploidy induction in cultured Chinese hamster cells following exposure to mitotic arrestants. *Anticancer Res.*, **4**, 351–356

Saxén, I. (1975) Associations between oral clefts and drugs taken during pregnancy. *Int. J. Epidemiol.*, **4**, 37–44

Saxén, I. & Saxén, L. (1975) Association between maternal intake of diazepam and oral clefts (Letter to the Editor). *Lancet*, **ii**, 498

Sbrana, I., Di Sibio, A., Lomi, A. & Scarcelli, V. (1993) C-Mitosis and numerical chromosome aberration analyses in human lymphocytes: 10 known or suspected spindle poisons. *Mutat. Res.*, **287**, 57–70

Schmid, W. & Staiger, G.R. (1969) Chromosome studies on bone marrow from Chinese hamsters treated with benzodiazepine tranquillizers and cyclophosphamide. *Mutat. Res.*, **7**, 99–108

Schmidt, D. (1995) Benzodiazepines: diazepam. In: Levy, R.H., Mattson, R.H. & Meldrum, B.S., eds, *Antiepileptic Drugs*, 4th Ed., New York, Raven Press, pp. 705–724

Schwartz, M.A. & Postma, E. (1968) Metabolism of diazepam *in vitro*. *Biochem. Pharmacol.*, **17**, 2443–2449

Schwartz, M.A., Koechlin, B.A., Postma, E., Palmer, S. & Krol, G. (1965) Metabolism of diazepam in rat, dog, and man. *J. Pharmacol. exp. Ther.*, **149**, 423–435

Schwartz, M.A., Bommer, P. & Vane, F.M. (1967) Diazepam metabolites in the rat: characterization by high-resolution mass spectrometry and nuclear magnetic resonance. *Arch. Biochem. Biophys.*, **121**, 508–516

Seelbach, A., Fissler, B., Strohbusch, A. & Madle, S. (1993) Development of a modified micronucleus assay *in vitro* for detection of aneugenic effects. *Toxic. in Vitro*, **7**, 185–193

Selby, J.V., Friedman, G.D. & Fireman, B.H. (1989) Screening prescription drugs for possible carcinogenicity: eleven to fifteen years of follow-up. *Cancer Res.*, **49**, 5736–5747

Serfaty, M. & Masterton, G. (1993) Fatal poisonings attributed to benzodiazepines in Britain during the 1980s. *Br. J. Psychiatr.*, **163**, 386–393

Shah, R.M., Donaldson, D. & Burdett, D. (1979) Teratogenic effects of diazepam in the hamster. *Can. J. Physiol. Pharmacol.*, **57**, 556–561

Shiono, P.H. & Mills, J.L. (1984) Oral clefts and diazepam use during pregnancy (Letter to the Editor). *New Engl. J. Med.*, **311**, 919–920

deSilva, J.A.F., D'Arconte, L. & Kaplan, J. (1964) The determination of blood levels and the placental transfer of diazepam in humans. *Curr. ther. Res.*, **6**, 115–121

Society of Japanese Pharmacopoeia (1992) *The Pharmacopoeia of Japan JP XII*, 12th Ed., Tokyo, p. 257

Sohn, D.-R., Kusaka, M., Ishizaki, T., Shin, S.-G., Jang, I.-J., Shin, J.-G. & Chiba, K. (1992) Incidence of S-mephenytoin hydroxylation deficiency in a Korean population and the interphenotypic differences in diazepam pharmacokinetics. *Clin. Pharmacol. Ther.*, **52**, 160–169

Šrám, R.J. & Kocišová, J. (1984) Mutagenic activity of diazepam. *Activ. nerv. sup. (Praha)*, **26**, 251–253

Šrám, R.J. & Kocišová, J. (1985) Longterm diazepam does not induce dominant lethals in mice. *Activ. nerv. sup. (Praha)*, **27**, 314–316

Staiger, G.R. (1969) Chlordiazepoxide and diazepam: absence of effects on the chromosomes of diploid human fibroblast cells. *Mutat. Res.*, **7**, 109–115

Staiger, G.R. (1970) Studies of the chromosomes of human lymphocytes treated with diazepam *in vitro*. *Mutat. Res.*, **10**, 635–644

Stenchever, M.A. & Smith, W.D. (1981) The effect of diazepam on meiosis in the CF-1 mouse. *Teratology*, **23**, 279–281

Stenchever, M.A., Frankel, R.S. & Jarvis, J.A. (1970) Effect of diazepam on chromosomes of human leukocytes *in vivo*. *Am. J. Obstet. Gynecol.*, **107**, 456–460

Stepien, H., Pawlikowska, A. & Pawlikowski, M. (1988) Effects of benzodiazepines on thymus cell proliferation. *Thymus*, **12**, 117–121

Stepien, H., Agro, A., Padol, I. & Stanisz, A. (1994) Inhibitory effect of diazepam on human natural killer activity *in vitro*. *Cytobios*, **77**, 131–136

Sternbach, L.H. & Reeder, E. (1961) Quinazolines and 1,4-benzodiazepines. IV. Transformations of 7-chloro-2-methylamino-5-phenyl-3H-1,4-benzodiazepine 4-oxide. *J. org. Chem.*, **26**, 4936–4941

Sternbach, L.H., Reeder, E., Keller, O. & Metlesics, W. (1961) Quinazolines and 1,4-benzodiazepines. III. Substituted 2-amino-5-phenyl-3*H*-1,4-benzodiazepine 4-oxides. *J. org. Chem.*, **26**, 4488–4497

Stoll, B.A. (1976) Psychosomatic factors and tumour growth. In: Stoll, B.A., ed., *Risk Factors in Breast Cancer*, London, William Heinemann, pp. 193–203

St-Pierre, M.V. & Pang, K.S. (1993) Kinetics of sequential metabolism. II. Formation and metabolism of nordiazepam and oxazepam from diazepam in the perfused murine liver. *J. Pharmacol. exp. Ther.*, **265**, 1437–1445

Swierenga, S.H.H., Butler, S.G. & Hasnain, S.H. (1983) Activity of diazepam and oxazepam in various mammalian cell in vitro toxicity tests (Abstract no. Cd-16). *Environ. Mutag.*, **5**, 417

Takatori, T., Tomii, S., Terazawa, K., Nagao, M., Kanamori, M. & Tomaru, Y. (1991) A comparative study of diazepam levels in bone marrow versus serum, saliva and brain tissue. *Int. J. leg. Med.*, **104**, 185–188

Taupin, V., Herbelin, A., Descamps-Latscha, B. & Zavala, F. (1991) Endogenous anxiogenic peptide, ODN-diazepam-binding inhibitor, and benzodiazepines enhance the production of interleukin-1 and tumor necrosis factor by human monocytes. *Lymph. Cytokin. Res.*, **10**, 7–13

Thomas, J., ed. (1991) *Prescription Products Guide 1991*, 20th Ed., Victoria, Australian Pharmaceutical Publishing Co. Ltd., pp. 306, 635–638, 692–693, 1411, 1697–1698

Tocco, D.R., Renskers, K. & Zimmerman, E.F. (1987) Diazepam-induced cleft palate in the mouse and lack of correlation with the H-2 locus. *Teratology*, **35**, 439–445

Toraason, M., Bohrman, J.S., Krieg, E., Combes, R.D., Willington, S.E., Zajac, W. & Langenbach, R. (1992) Evaluation of the V79 cell metabolic cooperation assay as a screen *in vitro* for developmental toxicants. *Toxic. in Vitro*, **6**, 165–174

Torigoe, K. (1979) Sister chromatid exchange in children treated with anticonvulsant drugs. *Acta med. biol.*, **27**, 65–72

Trosko, J.E., Yotti, L.P., Warren, S.T., Tsushimoto, G. & Chang, C.-C. (1982) Inhibition of cell-cell communication by tumor promoters. *Carcinogenesis*, **7**, 565–585

Tzonou, A., Day, N.E., Trichopoulos, D., Walker, A., Saliaraki, M., Papapostolou, M. & Polychronopoulou, A. (1984) The epidemiology of ovarian cancer in Greece: a case–control study. *Eur. J. Cancer clin. Oncol.*, **20**, 1045–1052

Tzonou, A., Polychronopoulou, A., Hsieh, C.-C., Rebelakos, A., Karakatsani, A. & Trichopoulos, D. (1993) Hair dyes, analgesics, tranquilizers and perineal talc application as risk factors for ovarian cancer. *Int. J. Cancer*, **55**, 408–410

United States National Library of Medicine (1996) *RTECS Database*, Bethesda, MD

United States Pharmacopeial Convention (1994) *The 1995 United States Pharmacopeia*, 23rd Rev./*The National Formulary*, 18th Rev., Rockville, MD, pp. 489–492

United States Tariff Commission (1964) *Synthetic Organic Chemicals, United States Production and Sales, 1963* (TC Publication 143), Washington DC, United States Government Printing Office, p. 129

Unseld, E., Rama Krishna, D., Fischer, C. & Klotz, U. (1989) Detection of desmethyldiazepam and diazepam in brain of different species and plants. *Biochem. Pharmacol.*, **38**, 2473–2478

Unseld, E., Fischer, C., Rothemund, E. & Klotz, U. (1990) Occurrence of 'natural' diazepam in human brain. *Biochem. Pharmacol.*, **39**, 210–212

Van Baar, A.L., Fleury, P., Soepatmi, S., Ultee, C.A. & Wesselman, P.J.M. (1989) Neonatal behaviour after drug dependent pregnancy. *Arch. Dis. Child.*, **64**, 235–240

Viggedal, G., Hagberg, B.S., Laegreid, L. & Aronsson, M. (1993) Mental development in late infancy after prenatal exposure to benzodiazepines — A prospective study. *J. Child Psychol. Psychiat.*, **34**, 295–305

Wälder, J. & Lützelschwab, R. (1984) Effects of 12-O-tetradecanoylphorbol-13-acetate (TPA), retinoic acid and diazepam on intercellular communication in a monolayer of rat liver epithelial cells. *Exp. Cell Res.*, **152**, 66–76

Walker, B.E. & Patterson, A. (1974) Induction of cleft palate in mice by tranquilizers and barbiturates. *Teratology*, **10**, 159–164

Wallace, R.B., Sherman, B.M. & Bean, J.A. (1982) A case–control study of breast cancer and psychotropic drug use. *Oncology*, **39**, 279–283

Wallin, M. & Hartley-Asp, B. (1993) Effects of potential aneuploidy inducing agents on microtubule assembly *in vitro*. *Mutat. Res.*, **287**, 17–22

Wang, J.K.T., Morgan, J. & Spector, S. (1984) Differentiation of Friend erythroleukaemia cells induced by benzodiazepines. *Proc. natl Acad. Sci. USA*, **81**, 3770–3772

Warr, T.J,. Parry, E.M. & Parry, J.M. (1993) A comparison of two in vitro mammalian cell cytogenetic assays for the detection of mitotic aneuploidy using 10 known or suspected aneugens. *Mutat. Res.*, **287**, 29–46

Waskell, L. (1978) A study of the mutagenicity of anesthetics and their metabolites. *Mutat. Res.*, **57**, 141–153

White, B.J., Driscoll, E.J., Tjio, J.-H. & Smilack, Z.H. (1974) Chromosomal aberration rates and intravenously given diazepam. A negative study. *J. Am. med. Assoc.*, **230**, 414–417

Whittaker, S.G., Zimmermann, F.K., Dicus, B., Piegorsch, W.W., Resnick, M.A. & Fogel, S. (1990) Detection of induced mitotic chromosome loss in *Saccharomyces cerevisiae* — An interlaboratory assessment of 12 chemicals. *Mutat. Res.*, **241**, 225–242

Wildmann, J., Möhler, H., Vetter, W., Ranalder, U., Schmidt, K. & Maurer, R. (1987) Diazepam and N-desmethyldiazepam are found in rat brain and adrenal and may be of plant origin. *J. neural Transm.*, **70**, 383–398

Wildmann, J., Vetter, W., Ranalder, U.B., Schmidt, K., Maurer, R. & Möhler, H. (1988) Occurrence of pharmacologically active benzodiazepines in trace amounts in wheat and potato. *Biochem. Pharmacol.*, **37**, 3549–3559

Wilkinson, G.R., Guengerich, F.P. & Branch, R.A. (1989) Genetic polymorphism of S-mephenytoin hydroxylation. *Pharmacol. Ther.*, **43**, 53–76

Williams, G.M., Mori, H. & McQueen, C.A. (1989) Structure–activity relationship in the rat hepatocyte DNA-repair test for 300 chemicals. *Mutat. Res.*, **221**, 263–286

Xu, W. & Adler, I.-D. (1990) Clastogenic effects of known and suspect spindle poisons studied by chromosome analysis in mouse bone marrow cells. *Mutagenesis*, **5**, 371–374

Yasumori, T., Nagata, K., Yang, S.K., Chen, L.-S., Murayama, N., Yamazoe, Y. & Kato, R. (1993) Cytochrome P450 mediated metabolism of diazepam in human and rat: involvement of human CYP2C in N-demethylation in the substrate concentration-dependent manner. *Pharmacogenetics*, **3**, 291–301

Zavala, F. & Lenfant, M. (1987) Benzodiazepines and PK 11195 exert immunomodulating activities by binding on a specific receptor on macrophages. *Ann. NY Acad. Sci.*, **496**, 240–249

Zhang, Y., Reviriego, J., Lou, Y.-Q., Sjöqvist, F. & Bertilsson, L. (1990) Diazepam metabolism in native Chinese poor and extensive hydroxylators of *S*-mephenytoin: interethnic differences in comparison with white subjects. *Clin. Pharmacol. Ther.*, **48**, 496–502

DOXEFAZEPAM

1. Exposure Data

1.1 Chemical and physical data

1.1.1 *Nomenclature*

Chem. Abstr. Serv. Reg. No.: 40762-15-0

Chem. Abstr. Name: 7-Chloro-5-(2-fluorophenyl)-1,3-dihydro-3-hydroxy-1-(2-hydroxyethyl)-2*H*-1,4-benzodiazepin-2-one

IUPAC Systematic Name: 7-Chloro-5-(*ortho*-fluorophenyl)-1,3-dihydro-3-hydroxy-1-(2-hydroxyethyl)-2*H*-1,4-benzodiazepin-2-one

Synonym: *N*-1-Hydroxyethyl-3-hydroxyflurazepam

1.1.2 *Structural and molecular formulae and relative molecular mass*

$C_{17}H_{14}ClFN_2O_3$ Relative molecular mass: 348.76

1.1.3 *Chemical and physical properties of the pure substance*

(*a*) *Description*: Crystals (Budavari, 1995)

(*b*) *Melting-point*: 138–140 °C (Budavari, 1995)

(*c*) *Spectroscopy data*: Infrared, ultraviolet, nuclear magnetic resonance and mass spectral data have been determined (Schiapparelli Farmaceutici S.P.A., 1983).

(*d*) *Solubility*: Practically insoluble in water; soluble in acetone and chloroform; moderately soluble in ethanol; slightly soluble in diethyl ether (Schiapparelli Farmaceutici S.P.A., 1983)

1.1.4 *Technical products and impurities*

There are two enantiomeric forms of the doxefazepam structure (asymmetric centre at C_3); doxefazepam in pharmaceutical preparations was the racemic mixture (Schiapparelli Farmaceutici S.P.A., 1983).

Doxefazepam was available as 20-mg capsules, which also contained magnesium stearate, mannitol, microgranular cellulose, precipitated silica, starch, and colourants E 127, E 132, E 171 and E 172. Impurities included 7-chloro-3-hydroxy-1,3-dihydro-5-(2-fluorophenyl)-2*H*-1,4-benzodiazepin-2-one ($\leq$ 0.5%), 1-(2-hydroxyethyl)-7-chloro-1,3-dihydro-5-(2-fluorophenyl)-2*H*-1,4-benzodiazepin-2-one-4-oxide ($\leq$ 0.5%) and 1-(2-hydroxyethyl)-7-chloro-4,5-dihydro-5-(2-fluorophenyl)-2*H*-1,4-benzodiazepin-2,3-(1*H*)-dione ($\leq$ 0.2%) (Schiapparelli Farmaceutici S.P.A., 1983).

A trade name and a designation for the chemical and its pharmaceutical preparations were available: Doxans and SAS 643.

1.1.5 *Analysis*

Doxefazepam can be analysed in biological fluids and tissues by gas chromatography with electron capture detection (Marcucci *et al.*, 1980; Mardente *et al.*, 1981) and reverse-phase high-performance liquid chromatography (Mascher *et al.*, 1984; Carlucci, 1988).

1.2 Production and use

1.2.1 *Production*

Doxefazepam can be prepared by alkylation of 7-chloro-1,3-dihydro-5-(2-fluorophenyl)-2*H*-1,4-benzodiazepin-2-one-4-oxide with 2-bromoethyl acetate and sodium hydride in dimethylformamide. The product is treated with acetic anhydride to form a diester. Ammonolysis of this diester, using methanolic ammonia, yields crude doxefazepam, which can be purified by crystallizing from dichloromethane/light petroleum (Tamagnone *et al.*, 1974).

1.2.2 *Use*

Doxefazepam is a benzodiazepine hypnotic, that has been used in the short-term management of insomnia at an oral dose of 20 mg before retiring at night (Reynolds, 1993) (see monograph on diazepam, pp. 39–41, for a brief overview of the pharmacology of therapeutic action for this class of drugs).

In 1990, approximately 184 000 standard units of doxefazepam (uncorrected for content of doxefazepam) were sold in Italy, the only country in which the drug was available. By 1995, it was no longer being sold in any country (information provided by IMS).

1.3 Occurrence

Doxefazepam is not known to occur as a natural product.

Doxefazepam is an active metabolite of flurazepam (Borelli et al., 1990).

1.4 Regulations and guidelines

Doxefazepam was approved for use in Italy from the mid-1980s until 1995 (Searle Farmaceutici S.r.l., 1996).

2. Studies of Cancer in Humans

No data were available to the Working Group (see the monograph on diazepam, pp. 44–54, for a discussion of benzodiazepines).

3. Studies of Cancer in Experimental Animals

3.1 Oral administration

Rat: Groups of 50 male and 50 female Sprague-Dawley rats, six weeks of age, were given 0 (control), 3, 10 or 30 mg/kg bw doxefazepam [purity not specified] mixed in the diet for up to 104 weeks, when surviving males and females of all groups were killed. The highest dose was set at 60 times the mean daily hypnotic dose level for an adult man. Body-weight gains and mortality rates were similar in all groups. From graphic presentations, survival appeared to be greater than 60% for all groups of males and 40–50% for the females. Complete histological examinations were performed on 47–50 males per group and 49–50 females per group. The incidences of hepatocellular adenomas in females were 1/49, 0/50, 3/49 and 5/50 [$p = 0.011$, trend test] and those for hepatocellular carcinomas were 0/49, 1/50, 1/49 and 1/50 in control, low-dose, mid-dose and high-dose animals, respectively. When the numbers of liver adenoma-bearing female rats were considered in relation to the numbers of females alive at the week of first tumour appearance (control, 1/18; low-dose, 0/17; mid-dose, 3/18; high-dose, 5/18), a significant trend by the Cochran-Armitage and Peto incidental tumour test ($p < 0.01$) was seen. In the male rats, the incidences of hepatocellular adenomas were 0/48, 0/50, 1/47 and 3/50 and those for hepatocellular carcinomas were 1/48, 3/50, 3/47 and 2/50 in control, low-dose, mid-dose and high-dose animals, respectively, showing no statistically significant increase. [When adenomas and carcinomas in male rats were combined, with the assumption that adenomas and carcinomas occurred in different animals, the cumulative incidence of tumours was not significantly increased (control, 1/48; low-dose, 3/50; mid-dose, 4/47; and high-dose, 5/50 ($p = 0.09$, trend test)] (Borelli et al., 1990).

4. Other Data Relevant to an Evaluation of Carcinogenicity and its Mechanisms

4.1 Absorption, distribution, metabolism and excretion

4.1.1 *Humans*

The disposition of doxefazepam has received very little study. Mardente *et al.* (1981) reported mean plasma concentration–time profiles of total and non-conjugated doxefazepam in eight individuals given both 10-mg and 20-mg single oral doses. No pharmacokinetic data were presented, but concentrations had declined to about 10% of the peak values after 16 h [suggesting a half-life of around 3–4 h]. Means of 32% of the 10-mg dose and 50% of the 20-mg dose were recovered in urine as conjugated doxefazepam within 48 h. The N_1-dealkylated derivative and an oxidized derivative in which the N_1-substituent was -CH_2COOH were identified as urinary metabolites (see Figure 1).

Figure 1. Metabolism of doxefazepam

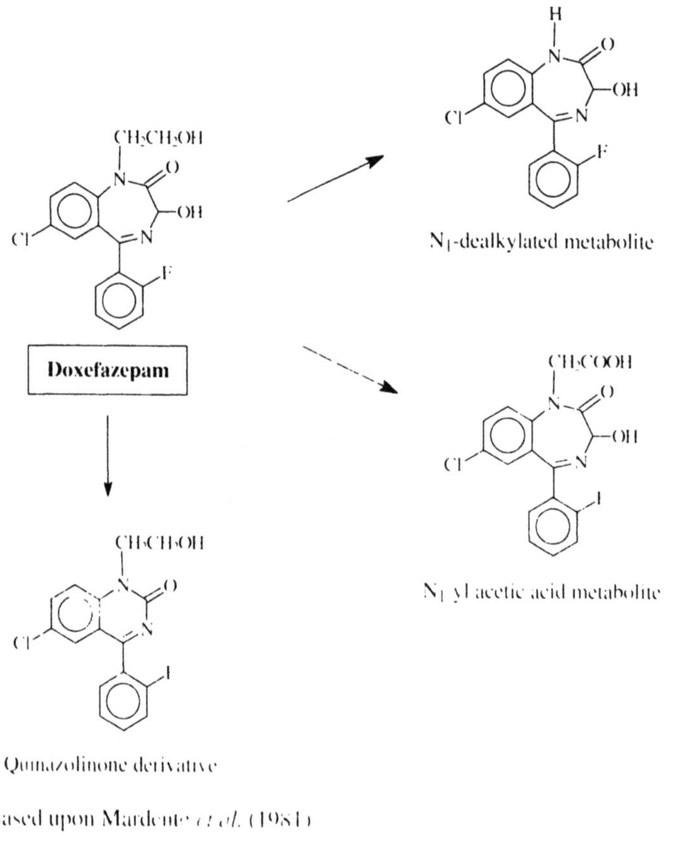

Based upon Mardente *et al.* (1981)

4.1.2 *Experimental systems*

Very few data are available. One report of an analytical method (Marcucci *et al.*, 1980) included data showing that doxefazepam is rapidly absorbed and accumulates in adipose tissue after a relatively high oral dose (5 mg/kg) administered to rats. Brain levels were approximately double the plasma concentrations. After an intravenous dose of 5 mg/kg, the elimination half-lives in rats and mice were 0.29 h and 1.32 h respectively in the blood.

4.2 Toxic effects

4.2.1 *Humans*

No data were available to the Working Group.

4.2.2 *Experimental systems*

(a) *Acute toxicity*

Doxefazepam was generally well tolerated after oral and intraperitoneal administration to rodents and beagle dogs (Bertoli *et al.*, 1989). No difference between males and females in the response to the compound was apparent. The oral LD_{50} was > 2000 mg/kg bw in Swiss mice, Charles River rats and beagle dogs. The intraperitoneal LD_{50} was estimated to be 746, 544 and > 1000 mg/kg bw in mice, rats and dogs, respectively. Deaths and/or signs of toxicity, consisting mainly of dose-dependent dyspnoea and decreased motor activity (in all species), dose-dependent prostration (in rodents) and dose-dependent tachycardia (only in dogs), occurred within 72 h after treatment.

(b) *Subacute and chronic toxicity*

Male and female Sprague-Dawley rats were given doxefazepam by gastric instillation (0, 50 or 100 mg/kg bw per day for eight weeks or 0, 15, 30 or 60 mg/kg bw per day for 26 weeks) and male and female beagle dogs were similarly treated with 0 or 10 mg/kg bw per day for 26 weeks (Bertoli *et al.*, 1989). The only symptom observed in rats for several hours after administration was ataxia, which was dose-dependent in the eight-week study and occurred only at the highest dose in the 26-week study. Liver weights were increased in rats given the highest dose in the 26-week study. There was no other clinical, haematological or histopathological sign of toxicity in either rats or dogs.

4.3 Reproductive and prenatal effects

4.3.1 *Humans*

No data were available to the Working Group.

4.3.2 *Experimental systems*

Doxefazepam did not exert any teratogenic effect in offspring of Sprague-Dawley rats treated orally with 15 or 30 mg/kg bw at gestation days 6–16 or in those of New Zealand White rabbits treated orally with 10, 20 or 30 mg/kg bw at gestation days 6–18. Moreover, it did not alter the reproductive performance of Charles-River rats treated orally with 15, 30 or 45 mg/kg bw (Bertoli et al., 1989).

4.4 Genetic and related effects

4.4.1 *Humans*

No data were available to the Working Group

4.4.2 *Experimental systems* (see also Table 1 for references and Appendices 1 and 2)

In one study, no significant response was observed in tests for mutation in *Salmonella typhimurium*, gene conversion in *Saccharomyces cerevisiae*, aneuploidy in *Aspergillus nidulans* or micronucleus induction in mouse bone-marrow cells *in vivo*. In another study, no increase in DNA strand breaks and/or alkali-labile sites was observed in the liver of rats given single or multiple oral doses of doxefazepam.

5. Summary of Data Reported and Evaluation

5.1 Exposure data

Doxefazepam is a benzodiazepine hypnotic that was used in the past to a limited extent in the short-term management of insomnia.

5.2 Human carcinogenicity data

No data were available to the Working Group.

5.3 Animal carcinogenicity data

Doxefazepam was tested for carcinogenicity in one experiment in rats by oral administration in the diet. A slight dose-related increase in the incidence of hepatocellular adenomas was observed.

5.4 Other relevant data

Doxefazepam disposition has received little study. In humans, the drug was eliminated in urine mainly as a conjugate, and two oxidative metabolites were identified. The elimination half-life was 3–4 h. No satisfactory metabolism studies in animals were available.

Data on human toxicity were not available. In rats treated with 60 mg/kg bw per day for 26 weeks, increased liver weights were reported without other clinical, haematological or histopathological signs of toxicity.

In a single study, doxefazepam was not teratogenic in rats or rabbits.

The few data available on genetic effects were negative.

Table 1. Genetic and related effects of doxefazepam

Test system	Result[a] Without exogenous metabolic system	Result[a] With exogenous metabolic system	Dose[b] (LED/HID)	Reference
SA0, *Salmonella typhimurium* TA100, reverse mutation	–	–	500	Bertoli *et al.* (1989)
SA5, *Salmonella typhimurium* TA1535, reverse mutation	–	–	500	Bertoli *et al.* (1989)
SA8, *Salmonella typhimurium* TA1538, reverse mutation	–	–	500	Bertoli *et al.* (1989)
SA9, *Salmonella typhimurium* TA98, reverse mutation	–	–	500	Bertoli *et al.* (1989)
SCG, *Saccharomyces cerevisiae*, gene conversion	–	–	10	Bertoli *et al.* (1989)
ANG, *Aspergillus nidulans*, mitotic crossing-over	–	–	8000	Bertoli *et al.* (1989)
DVA, DNA strand breaks, rat liver *in vivo*	–		349 po × 1	Carlo *et al.* (1989)
DVA, DNA strand breaks, rat liver *in vivo*	–		70 po × 15	Carlo *et al.* (1989)
MVR, Micronucleus test, mouse bone marrow *in vivo*	–		155	Bertoli *et al.* (1989)

[a] +, positive; (+), weak positive; –, negative; ?, inconclusive
[b] LED, lowest effective dose; HID, highest ineffective dose; in-vitro tests, μg/mL; in-vivo tests, mg/kg bw/day

5.5 Evaluation[1]

There is *inadequate evidence* in humans for the carcinogenicity of doxefazepam.

There is *limited evidence* in experimental animals for the carcinogenicity of doxefazepam.

Overall evaluation

Doxefazepam is *not classifiable as to its carcinogenicity to humans (Group 3)*.

6. References

Bertoli, D., Borelli, G. & Carazzone, M. (1989) Toxicological evaluations of the benzodiazepine doxefazepam. *Arzneimittel-Forsch.*, **39**, 480–484

Borelli, G., Bertoli, D. & Chieco, P. (1990) Carcinogenicity study of doxefazepam administered in the diet to Sprague-Dawley rats. *Fundam. appl. Toxicol.*, **15**, 82–92

Budavari, S., ed. (1995) *The Merck Index*, 12th Ed., Rahway, NJ, Merck & Co.

Carlo, P., Finollo, R., Ledda, A. & Brambilla, G. (1989) Absence of liver DNA fragmentation in rats treated with high oral doses of 32 benzodiazepine drugs. *Fundam. appl. Toxicology*, **12**, 34–41

Carlucci, G. (1988) High-performance liquid-chromatographic method for the determination of doxefazepam in human plasma using a solid-phase extraction column. *J. liq. Chromatogr.*, **11**, 1559–1568

Marcucci, F., Garbagna, L., Monti, F., Bonazzi, P., Canobbio, L., Zuccato, E. & Mussini, E. (1980) Gas chromatographic determination of two fluorinated benzodiazepines in rats and mice. *J. Chromatogr.*, **198**, 180–184

Mardente, S., Bicchi, C. & Nano, G.M. (1981) GLC-ECD determination of 1-(2-hydroxyethyl)-3-hydroxy-7-chloro-1,3-dihydro-5-(*o*-fluorophenyl)-2*H*-1,4-benzodiazepin-2-one (SAS 643) in plasma and urine and identification of its main biotransformation products. *Ther. Drug Monit.*, **3**, 351–356

Mascher, H., Nitsche, V. & Schütz, H. (1984) Separation, isolation and identification of optical isomers of 1,4-benzodiazepine glucuronides from biological fluids by reversed-phase high-performance liquid chromatography. *J. Chromatogr. biomed. Appl.*, **306**, 231–239

Reynolds, J.A.F., ed. (1993) *Martindale: The Extra Pharmacopoeia*, 30th Ed., London, The Pharmaceutical Press, p. 735

Schiapparelli Farmaceutici S.P.A. (1983) CMC Dossier submitted for Registration, Turin, Italy

Searle Farmaceutica S.v.l. (1996) *Doxefazepam*, Milan, Italy

Tamagnone, G.F., Torrielli, M.V. & de Marchi, F. (1974) A new benzodiazepine: 1-(2-hydroxyethyl)-3-hydroxy-7-chloro-1,3-dihydro-5-(*o*-fluorophenyl)-2*H*-1,4-benzodiazepin-2-one. *J. Pharm. Pharmacol.*, **26**, 566–567

---

[1]For definition of the italicized terms, see Preamble, pp. 22–25.

ESTAZOLAM

1. Exposure Data

1.1 Chemical and physical data

1.1.1 Nomenclature

Chem. Abstr. Serv. Reg. No.: 29975-16-4
Chem. Abstr. Name: 8-Chloro-6-phenyl-4*H*-[1,2,4]triazolo[4,3-*a*][1,4]benzodiazepine
IUPAC Systematic Name: 8-Chloro-6-phenyl-4*H*-*s*-triazolo[4,3-*a*][1,4]benzodiazepine

1.1.2 *Structural and molecular formulae and relative molecular mass*

$C_{16}H_{11}ClN_4$ Relative molecular mass: 294.74

1.1.3 *Chemical and physical properties of the pure substance*

(a) *Description*: White crystals (Gennaro, 1995)
(b) *Melting-point*: 228–229 °C (Budavari, 1995)
(c) *Solubility*: Practically insoluble in water; soluble in ethanol (American Hospital Formulary Service, 1995)

1.1.4 *Technical products and impurities*

Estazolam is available as 1- or 2-mg tablets which also may contain corn starch, hydroxypropylcellulose, iron oxide, lactose, magnesium stearate or stearic acid (Farmindustria, 1993; Medical Economics, 1996).

Trade names and designations of the chemical and its pharmaceutical preparations include: A 47631; Abbott 47631; Bay k 4200; Cannoc; D 40TA; Deprinocte; Domnamid; Esilgan; Eurodin; Hypnomat; Julodin; Kainever; Nemurel; Noctal; Nuctalon; ProSom; Sedarest; Somnatrol; Tasedan; U 33737.

1.1.5 Analysis

The Pharmacopoeia of Japan specifies potentiometric titration with perchloric acid as the assay for purity of estazolam, and thin-layer chromatography for determining impurities and decomposition products. An assay for heavy metal impurities is also specified (Society of Japanese Pharmacopoeia, 1992). Other methods of analysis in pharmaceutical preparations include polarography (Li & Ji, 1990) and spectrophotometry (Gallo et al., 1985).

Estazolam can be analysed in biological fluids by gas chromatography with electron capture detection (Kelly & Greenblatt, 1993) and high-performance liquid chromatography (di Tella et al., 1986; Mura et al., 1987; Boukhabza et al., 1991).

1.2 Production and use

1.2.1 Production

Estazolam is prepared by reacting 7-chloro-1,3-dihydro-5-phenyl-2H-benzo[1,4]-diazepine-2-thione with formylhydrazine in boiling n-butyl alcohol (Gennaro, 1995). It was first marketed in Japan in 1975 and is currently available in at least 21 countries worldwide (Abbott Laboratories, 1996).

1.2.2 Use

Estazolam is a triazolobenzodiazepine derivative used for the short-term management of insomnia (see monograph on diazepam, pp. 39–41, for a brief overview of the pharmacology of therapeutic action for this class of drugs). The usual oral dose is 1–2 mg at night; for severe insomnia, up to 4 mg has been given. In debilitated elderly patients, an initial dose of 0.5 mg is recommended (Reynolds, 1993; Medical Economics, 1996).

Clinical uses of estazolam and other benzodiazepines have been reviewed (Hollister et al., 1993).

Comparative data on sales of estazolam in several countries are shown in Table 1. Overall, sales increased by approximately 16% from 1990 to 1995.

1.3 Occurrence

Estazolam is not known to occur as a natural product.

1.4 Regulations and guidelines

Estazolam is listed in the French and Japanese pharmacopoeias (Reynolds, 1993; Vidal, 1995).

Table 1. Sales of estazolam in various countries[a] (no. of standard units[b], in thousands)

Country	1990	1995	Country	1990	1995
North America			Asia		
Canada	0	245	Japan	111 670	116 623
Mexico	1 195	1 446	Europe		
United States	0	19 372	France	15 213	9 617
South America			Italy	12 846	14 581
Argentina	837	599	Portugal	8 642	17 424
Brazil	7 958	7 253			
Colombia	0	76			

[a] Data provided by IMS
[b] Standard dosage units, uncorrected for estazolam content

2. Studies of Cancer in Humans

No data were available to the Working Group (see the monograph on diazepam, pp. 44–54, for a discussion of benzodiazepines).

3. Studies of Cancer in Experimental Animals

3.1 Oral administration

3.1.1 *Mouse*

Groups of 50 male and 50 female B6C3F1 mice, five to six weeks of age, were given 0.8, 3 or 10 mg/kg bw estazolam [purity not specified] mixed in the diet for up to 104 weeks, when surviving animals were killed. The estazolam concentration in the food was adjusted weekly for changes in body weight and food consumption. The estazolam/diet mixtures were prepared freshly each week. Controls were 100 male and 100 female B6C3F1 mice. Increased body weights were seen in the treated animals as compared to the controls. This was more prominent for the females. Food consumption was also increased in the treated mice, by 4–17% above control values over the two-year treatment period. Convulsions and hyperactivity were associated with exposure to estazolam. An increase in mortality was observed in male mice receiving 10 mg/kg bw (deaths — males: control, 13/100; low-dose, 11/50; mid-dose, 7/50; and high-dose, 21/50; females: control, 28/100; low-dose, 12/50; mid-dose, 12/50; and high-dose, 23/50). All major organs and visually apparent lesions were examined histologically. No increase in tumour incidence was found. The incidences of hepatocellular carcinomas were: males: control, 23/100; low-dose, 11/50; mid-dose, 12/50; and high-dose, 9/50;

females: control, 2/100; low-dose, 4/50; mid-dose, 4/50; and high-dose, 2/50 (Kimura *et al.*, 1984).

3.1.2 *Rat*

Groups of 50 male and 50 female Sprague-Dawley rats, five to six weeks of age, were given 0.5, 2 or 10 mg/kg bw estazolam [purity not specified] mixed in the diet for up to 104 weeks, when surviving animals were killed. The estazolam concentration in the food was adjusted weekly for changes in body weight and food consumption. The estazolam/diet mixtures were prepared freshly each week. Controls were 100 male and 100 female Sprague-Dawley rats. No significant change in body weights was seen in the treated male rats as compared to the controls. Female rats exposed to 10 mg/kg bw estazolam had depressed body weights (approximately 13%) compared to controls. There was no significant difference in mortality between control and treated rats. All major organs and visually apparent lesions were examined histologically. There was no significant increase in tumour incidence. The incidences of neoplastic nodules in the liver were: males: control, 3/100; low-dose, 2/50; mid-dose, 1/50 and high-dose, 2/50; females: control, 5/100; low-dose, 0/50; mid-dose, 2/50 and high-dose, 1/50; those of hepatocellular carcinomas were: males: control, 4/100; low-dose, 0/50; mid-dose, 1/50 and high-dose, 1/50; females: control, 0/100; low-dose, 1/50; mid-dose, 1/50 and high-dose, 0/50 (Kimura *et al.*, 1984).

4. Other Data Relevant to an Evaluation of Carcinogenicity and its Mechanisms

4.1 Absorption, distribution, metabolism and excretion

4.1.1 *Humans*

Estazolam is rapidly and almost completely absorbed after oral doses. Peak plasma concentrations of 103 ± 18 ng/mL were achieved about 0.5 h after oral dosing with 2 mg in aqueous solution (Machinist *et al.*, 1986), while 4-mg tablets gave peak plasma concentrations of 194 ± 3.5 ng/mL within 1–3 h (Mancinelli *et al.*, 1985). In an earlier study, single doses ranging from 2 to 16 mg resulted in peak plasma concentrations proportional with the dose within 6 h. Mean elimination half-lives were 14 h, 19 h and 17 h in these three studies, respectively. During three weeks of therapy with daily doses rising each week from 2 to 4 to 6 mg, plasma concentrations increased in proportion to the dose and accumulation was essentially complete within three days of each dose change. The drug is eliminated predominantly as metabolites in the urine (Allen *et al.*, 1979). Machinist *et al.* (1986) found that urinary and faecal excretion accounted for 87% and 4%, respectively, of a 2-mg [^{14}C]estazolam dose over five days. Kanai (1974) identified five metabolites in humans, 1-oxoestazolam, 4-hydroxyestazolam, 4'-hydroxyestazolam and two benzophenones (I and II) (Figure 1). Machinist *et al.* (1986) found evidence of 11 metabolites in human urine, including those identified previously; the

Figure 1. Postulated metabolic pathways of estazolam

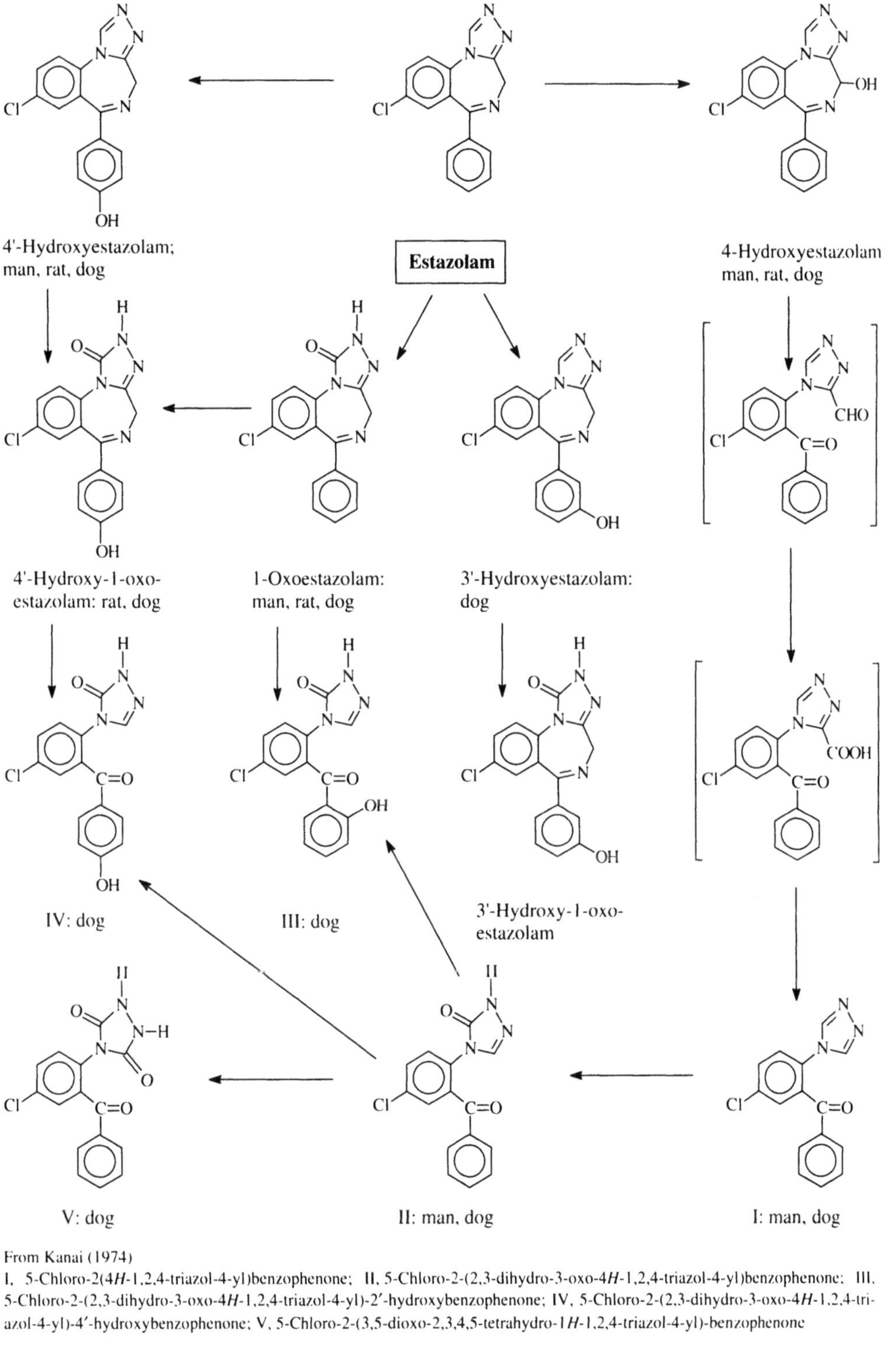

4'-Hydroxyestazolam;
man, rat, dog

Estazolam

4-Hydroxyestazolam
man, rat, dog

4'-Hydroxy-1-oxo-
estazolam: rat, dog

1-Oxoestazolam:
man, rat, dog

3'-Hydroxyestazolam:
dog

IV: dog

III: dog

3'-Hydroxy-1-oxo-
estazolam

V: dog

II: man, dog

I: man, dog

From Kanai (1974)
I, 5-Chloro-2(4H-1,2,4-triazol-4-yl)benzophenone; II, 5-Chloro-2-(2,3-dihydro-3-oxo-4H-1,2,4-triazol-4-yl)benzophenone; III, 5-Chloro-2-(2,3-dihydro-3-oxo-4H-1,2,4-triazol-4-yl)-2'-hydroxybenzophenone; IV, 5-Chloro-2-(2,3-dihydro-3-oxo-4H-1,2,4-triazol-4-yl)-4'-hydroxybenzophenone; V, 5-Chloro-2-(3,5-dioxo-2,3,4,5-tetrahydro-1H-1,2,4-triazol-4-yl)-benzophenone

major metabolite was not fully characterized but was believed to be a metabolite of 4-hydroxyestazolam.

4.1.2 *Experimental systems*

In mice given an intraperitoneal injection of 5 mg/kg bw estazolam, the plasma concentration was about 1300 ng/mL at 0.5 h, the earliest time investigated. The elimination half-life was 1.99 h, volume of distribution 3.12 L/kg and clearance 18.1 mL/min/kg (Kelly & Greenblatt, 1993).

After intravenous injection of 5 mg/kg bw into pregnant rats (Tanayama et al., 1974), the fetal/maternal blood concentration ratio one hour after dosing was approximately unity and concentrations in fetal tissues declined in parallel with the concentrations in maternal blood. Autoradiography of the fetuses showed higher concentrations in the adrenal glands, adipose tissue, liver and gastrointestinal tract wall. The compound or its metabolites also enters rat milk.

A number of studies have compared the metabolism of estazolam in different species. Tanayama and Kanai (1974) observed extensive metabolism in mice, rats, guinea-pigs, rabbits and dogs following oral administration of ^{14}C-labelled drug. The percentages of dose recovered as metabolites in the urine plus faeces were: mice, 78%; rats, 51%; guinea-pigs, 44%; rabbits, 48%; and dogs, 78%. As in humans (see Section 4.1.1), rabbits and dogs excreted more radioactivity in the urine than in faeces; in contrast, mice, rats and guinea-pigs excreted more in the faeces. The patterns of metabolites differed between species (Figure 1), but some of the metabolites were identified mainly in rats (4'-hydroxy- and 1-oxo-4'-hydroxy-) and only in dogs (two benzophenones, I and II). Kanai (1974) presented more detailed findings on rats and dogs (as well as humans): 11 metabolites identified in dog urine included six hydroxylation products and five benzophenones. The benzophenones were not observed in rats. The findings of Kanai (1974) for dogs were largely confirmed by Machinist et al. (1986).

4.2 Toxic effects

4.2.1 *Humans*

No data were available to the Working Group.

4.2.2 *Experimental systems*

Oral LD_{50}s in male mice, rats and rabbits of 740, 3200 and 300 mg/kg bw have been reported (Budavari, 1995).

4.3 Reproductive and developmental effects

4.3.1 *Humans*

No data were available to the working group.

4.3.2 *Experimental systems*

Estazolam crossed the rat placenta (Tanayama *et al.*, 1974) (see Section 4.1.2).

4.4 Genetic and related effects

4.4.1 *Humans*

No data were available to the Working Group.

4.4.2 *Experimental systems* (see also Table 2 for references and Appendices 1 and 2)

The results of the few available studies of induction of mutations in bacteria are negative. No increase in DNA single-strand breaks and/or alkali-labile sites was observed in the liver of rats receiving single or multiple doses of estazolam. In addition, estazolam does not induce chromosomal aberrations or aneuploidy in the bone-marrow cells of either rats or mice *in vivo*.

5. Summary of Data Reported and Evaluation

5.1 Exposure data

Estazolam is a triazolobenzodiazepine used since the 1970s for short-term management of insomnia.

5.2 Human carcinogenicity data

No data were available to the Working Group.

5.3 Animal carcinogenicity data

Estazolam was tested for carcinogenicity in one experiment in mice and one experiment in rats by oral administration in the diet. No increase in the incidence of tumours was found.

5.4 Other relevant data

Estazolam is rapidly and almost completely absorbed in humans. It is extensively metabolized to at least 11 metabolites and excreted mainly in the urine. The elimination half-life is 14–19 h. Metabolism is extensive in various animal species. Rabbits and dogs excrete the metabolites principally in urine, while in mice, rats and guinea-pigs the excretion is mainly in faeces. Some metabolites are species-specific.

There were no data available on reproductive effects of estazolam.

The data available on genetic effects were negative.

Table 2. Genetic and related effects of estazolam

Test system	Result[a]		Dose[b] (LED/HID)	Reference
	Without exogenous metabolic system	With exogenous metabolic system		
SA0, *Salmonella typhimurium* TA100, reverse mutation	–	–	2500	Wakisaka & Nishimoto (1987)
SA5, *Salmonella typhimurium* TA1535, reverse mutation	–	–	2500	Wakisaka & Nishimoto (1987)
SA7, *Salmonella typhimurium* TA1537, reverse mutation	–	–	2500	Wakisaka & Nishimoto (1987)
SA9, *Salmonella typhimurium* TA98, reverse mutation	–	–	2500	Wakisaka & Nishimoto (1987)
SA2, *Salmonella typhimurium* TA102, reverse mutation	–	–	2500	Wakisaka & Nishimoto (1987)
ECW, *Escherichia coli* WP2 *uvrA*, reverse mutation	–	–	2500	Wakisaka & Nishimoto (1987)
DVA, DNA strand breaks, rat liver *in vivo*	–		285 po × 1	Carlo *et al.* (1989)
DVA, DNA strand breaks, rat liver *in vivo*	–		59 po × 15	Carlo *et al.* (1989)
CBA, Chromosomal aberrations, rat (Sprague-Dawley) bone marrow *in vivo*	–		100 po × 1	Kikuchi *et al.* (1973)
CBA, Chromosomal aberrations, rat (Sprague-Dawley) bone marrow *in vivo*	–		100 po × 5	Kikuchi *et al.* (1973)
CBA, Chromosomal aberrations, mouse (CF1) bone marrow *in vivo*	–		200 po × 1	Kikuchi *et al.* (1973)
CBA, Chromosomal aberrations, mouse (CF1) bone marrow *in vivo*	–		200 po × 1	Kikuchi *et al.* (1973)
AVA, Aneuploidy, rat (Sprague-Dawley) bone marrow *in vivo*	–		100 po × 1	Kikuchi *et al.* (1973)
AVA, Aneuploidy, rat (Sprague-Dawley) bone marrow *in vivo*	–		100 po × 5	Kikuchi *et al.* (1973)
AVA, Aneuploidy, mouse (CF1) bone marrow *in vivo*	–		200 po × 1	Kikuchi *et al.* (1973)
AVA, Aneuploidy, mouse (CF1) bone marrow *in vivo*	–		200 po × 5	Kikuchi *et al.* (1973)

[a] +, positive; (+), weak positive; –, negative; ?, inconclusive
[b] LED, lowest effective dose; HID, highest ineffective dose; in-vitro tests, µg/mL; in-vivo tests, mg/kg bw/day

5.5 Evaluation[1]

There is *inadequate evidence* in humans for the carcinogenicity of estazolam.

There is *evidence suggesting a lack of carcinogenicity* in experimental animals for estazolam.

Overall evaluation

Estazolam is *not classifiable as to its carcinogenicity to humans (Group 3)*.

6. References

Abbott Laboratories (1996) *Estazolam*, North Chicago, IL

Allen, M.D., Greenblatt, D.J. & Arnold, J.D. (1979) Single- and multiple-dose kinetics of estazolam, a triazolobenzodiazepine. *Psychopharmacology*, **66**, 267–274

American Hospital Formulary Service (1995) *AHFS Drug Information*® 95, Bethesda, MD, American Society of Health-System Pharmacists, pp. 1593–1594

Boukhabza, A., Lugnier, A.A.J., Kintz, P. & Mangin, P. (1991) Simultaneous HPLC analysis of the hypnotic benzodiazepines nitrazepam, estazolam, flunitrazepam and triazolam in plasma. *J. analyt. Toxicol.*, **15**, 319–322

Budavari, S., ed. (1995) *The Merck Index*, 12th Ed., Rahway, NJ, Merck & Co., Inc.

Carlo, P., Finollo, R., Ledda, A. & Brambilla, G. (1989) Absence of liver DNA fragmentation in rats treated with high oral doses of 32 benzodiazepine drugs. *Fundam. appl. Toxicol.*, **12**, 34–41

Farmindustria (1993) *Repertorio Farmaceutico Italiano* (Italian Pharmaceutical Directory), 7th Ed., Milan, Associazione Nazionale dell'Industria Farmaceutica, CEDOF S.P.A., p. A-534

Gallo, N., Bianco, V.D. & Doronzo, S. (1985) On the spectrophotometric determination of estazolam using Ru(III) ion. *Farm. Ed. Prat.*, **40**, 77–80

Gennaro, A.R., ed. (1995) *Remington: The Science and Practice of Pharmacy*, 19th Ed., Vol. II, Easton, PA, Mack Publishing Co., p. 1158

Hollister, L.E., Müller-Oerlinghausen, B., Rickels, K. & Shader, R.I. (1993) Clinical uses of benzodiazepines. *J. clin. Psychopharmacol.*, **13** (Suppl. 1)

Kanai, Y. (1974) The biotransformation of 8-chloro-6-phenyl-4*H*-*s*-triazolo[4,3-*a*][1,4]benzodiazepine (D-40TA), a new central depressant, in man, dog and rat. *Xenobiotica*, **4**, 441–456

Kelly, J.F. & Greenblatt, D.J. (1993) Rapid and sensitive gas chromatographic determination of estazolam. *J. Chromatogr.*, **621**, 102–104

Kikuchi, Y., Hitotsumachi, S. & Suzuki, M. (1973) In vivo cytogenetic studies of 8-chloro-6-phenyl-4*H*-*s*-triazolo[4,3-*a*][1,4]benzodiazepine (D-40TA) on bone marrow cells of mice and rats. *J. Takeda Res. Lab.*, **32**, 56–61 (in Japanese)

---

[1]For definition of the italicized terms, see Preamble, pp. 22–25.

Kimura, E.T., Fort, F.L., Buratto, B., Tekeli, S., Kesterson, J.W., Heyman, I.A. & Cusick, P.K. (1984) Carcinogenic evaluation of estazolam via diet in CD strain Sprague-Dawley rats and B6C3F1 mice for 2 years. *Fundam. appl. Toxicol.*, **4**, 827–842

Li, Q.-L. & Ji, G. (1990) Studies on the polarographic behaviour of estazolam. *Talanta*, **37**, 937–940

Machinist, J.M., Bopp, B.A., Anderson D.J., Granneman, G.R., Sonders, R.C., Tolman, K., Buchi, K. & Rollins, D. (1986) Metabolism of ^{14}C-estazolam in dogs and humans. *Xenobiotica*, **16**, 11–20

Mancinelli, A., Guiso, G., Garattini, S., Urso, R. & Caccia, S. (1985) Kinetic and pharmacological studies on estazolam in mice and man. *Xenobiotica*, **15**, 257–265

Medical Economics (1996) *PDR®: Physicians' Desk* Reference, 50th Ed., Montvale, NJ, Medical Economics Data Production Co., pp. 449–451

Mura, P., Piriou, A., Fraillon, P., Papet, Y. & Reiss, D. (1987) Screening procedure for benzodiazepines in biological fluids by high-performance liquid chromatography using a rapid-scanning multichannel detector. *J. Chromatogr.*, **416**, 303–310

Reynolds, J.E.F., ed. (1993) *Martindale: The Extra Pharmacopoeia*, 30th Ed., London, The Pharmaceutical Press, p. 594

Society of Japanese Pharmacopoeia (1992) *The Pharmacopoeia of Japan JP XII*, 12th Ed., Tokyo, p. 295

Tanayama, S. & Kanai, Y. (1974) Metabolism of 8-chloro-6-phenyl-4*H*-*s*-triazolo[4,3-*a*][1,4]-benzodiazepine (D-40TA), a new central depressant. II. Species difference in metabolism. *Xenobiotica*, **4**, 49–56

Tanayama, S., Momose, S., Kanai, Y. & Shirakawa, Y. (1974) Metabolism of 8-chloro-6-phenyl-4*H*-*s*-triazolo [4,3-*a*][1,4]benzodiazepine (D-40TA), a new central depressant. IV. Placental transfer and excretion in milk in rats. *Xenobiotica*, **4**, 219–227

di Tella, A.S., Ricci, P., Di Nunzio, C. & Cassandro, P. (1986) New method for the determination in blood and urine of a novel triazolobenzodiazepine (estazolam) by HPLC. *J. analyt. Toxicol.*, **10**, 65–67

Vidal (1995) *Dictionnaire Vidal 1995*, 71st Ed., Paris, Editions du Vidal, pp. 1057–1058

Wakisaka, Y. & Nishimoto, Y. (1987) Mutagenicity study on a new sleep inducer, a 1*H*-1,2,4-triazolylbenzophenone derivative (450191-S), and its metabolite in bacteria. *Iyakuhin Kenkyu*, **18**, 12–20 (in Japanese)

OXAZEPAM

This substance was considered by previous working groups in October 1976 (IARC, 1977) and March 1987 (IARC, 1987). Since that time, new data have become available, and these have been incorporated in the monograph and taken into consideration in the evaluation.

1. Exposure Data

1.1 Chemical and physical data

1.1.1 Nomenclature

Chem. Abstr. Serv. Reg. No.: 604-75-1
Deleted CAS Reg. No.: 61036-43-9
Chem. Abstr. Name: 7-Chloro-1,3-dihydro-3-hydroxy-5-phenyl-2H-1,4-benzodiazepin-2-one
IUPAC Systematic Name: 7-Chloro-1,3-dihydro-3-hydroxy-5-phenyl-2H-1,4-benzodiazepin-2-one
Synonyms: N-Desmethyltemazepam; nortemazepam

1.1.2 Structural and molecular formulae and relative molecular mass

$C_{15}H_{11}ClN_2O_2$ Relative molecular mass: 286.72

1.1.3 Chemical and physical properties of the pure substance

(a) *Description*: Creamy white to pale-yellow powder (Gennaro, 1995)
(b) *Melting-point*: 205–206 °C (Budavari, 1995)
(c) *Spectroscopy data*: Infrared, ultraviolet, nuclear magnetic resonance and mass spectral data have been reported (Shearer & Pilla, 1974).

(d) *Solubility*: Practically insoluble in water (1 g/more than 10 000 mL); soluble in chloroform (1 g/270 mL), diethyl ether (1 g/2200 mL), ethanol (1 g/220 mL) (Gennaro, 1995) and dioxane (Budavari, 1995)

(e) *Stability*: Stable in light and nonhygroscopic (Gennaro, 1995); hydrolysed by acids (Shearer & Pilla, 1974)

(f) *Dissociation constants*: pK_as = 1.7 and 11.6 (American Hospital Formulary Service, 1995)

(g) *Octanol/water partition coefficient (P)*: log P, 1.99 (Dollery et al., 1991)

1.1.4 Technical products and impurities

There are two enantiomeric forms of the oxazepam structure (asymmetric centre at C_3); oxazepam in pharmaceutical preparations is invariably the racemic mixture (British Pharmacopoeial Commission, 1993).

Oxazepam is available as 10-, 15- and 30-mg tablets and 10-, 15- and 30-mg capsules, which may also contain gelatin, lactose, magnesium stearate, methylcellulose, polacrilin potassium, titanium dioxide, D&C Red 22 (eosine), D&C Red 28, FD&C Blue 1 (Brilliant Blue FCF), FD&C Red 40 (Allura Red AC), FD&C Yellow 5 (tartrazine) or FD&C Yellow 6 (Sunset Yellow FCF) (Thomas, 1991; British Medical Association/Royal Pharmaceutical Society of Great Britain, 1994; American Hospital Formulary Service, 1995; Medical Economics, 1996).

Trade names and designations of the chemical and its pharmaceutical preparations include: Abboxapam; Adumbran; Alepam; Alopam; Antoderin; Anxiolit; Anxiolit retard; Aplakil; Aslapax; Astress; Azutranquil; Benzotran; Bonare; Buxopax; CB 8092; Constantonin; Drimuel; Droxacepam; Durazepam; Enidrel; Hilong; Iranil; Isodin; Lederpam; Limbial; Murelax; Nesontil; Neurofren; Noctazepam; Novoxapam; Nozepam; Oxa; Oxabenz; Oxahexal; Oxa-10 L.U.T.; Oxanid; Oxa-Puren; Oxepam; Oxpam; Praxiten; Propax; Psicopax; Psiquiwas; Purata; Quen; Quilibrex; Ro 5-6789; Rondar; Sedokin; Serax; Serenal; Serenid; Serepax; Seresta; Serpax; Sigacalm; Sobile; Sobril; Tarchomin; Tazepam; Uskan; Vaben; Wy 3498; Zapex; Zaxopam.

1.1.5 Analysis

Several international pharmacopoeias specify potentiometric titration with tetrabutylammonium hydroxide or perchloric acid as the assay for purity of oxazepam, and thin-layer chromatography (TLC) or gas chromatography (GC) with flame ionization detection (FID) for determining impurities and decomposition products. Assays for oxazepam in capsules and tablets typically involve comparing ultraviolet absorbance with standards (Council of Europe, 1992; British Pharmacopoeial Commission, 1993; United States Pharmacopeial Convention, 1994). Other methods of analysis in pharmaceutical preparations include fluorimetry (Walash et al., 1994), spectrophotometry (Prada et al., 1988; El-Brashy et al., 1993), mass spectrometry (MS) (McCarley & Brodbelt, 1993) and high-performance liquid chromatography (HPLC) (Bargo, 1983).

Oxazepam and its metabolites can be analysed in biological fluids and tissues by fluorescence polarization immunoassay (Simonsson et al., 1995), fluorimetry (Walash et al.,

1994), GC (Nau et al., 1978; Peat & Kopjak, 1979; Löscher, 1982), GC/MS (Maurer & Pfleger, 1987; Langner et al., 1991) and HPLC (Peat & Kopjak, 1979; Lensmeyer et al., 1982; Komiskey et al., 1985; Mura et al., 1987; Fernández et al., 1991; Berrueta et al., 1993; Chopineau et al., 1994).

1.2 Production and use

1.2.1 *Production*

A method for preparing oxazepam was first reported in 1962 (Bell & Childress, 1962); commercial production of oxazepam in the United States of America was first reported in 1965 (United States Tariff Commission, 1967).

Oxazepam is prepared by acylating 2-amino-5-chlorobenzophenone with chloroacetyl chloride. Heating the product with sodium iodide yields the iodoacetamido compound. Treatment of the iodoacetamido compound with hydroxylamine effects dehydration and dehydrohalogenation to form a benzodiazepine derivative, which rearranges to oxazepam, with esterification, when treated with acetic anhydride. Saponification liberates oxazepam (Gennaro, 1995).

1.2.2 *Use*

Oxazepam is a benzodiazepine used in the treatment of anxiety disorders, insomnia and alcohol withdrawal symptoms (see the monograph on diazepam, pp. 39–41, for a brief overview of the pharmacology of therapeutic action for this class of drugs). The usual adult oral dose is 10–15 mg three or four times daily for the treatment of mild to moderate anxiety and 15–30 mg three or four times daily for the treatment of severe anxiety or for control of symptoms of alcohol withdrawal. A suggested initial dose for elderly or debilitated patients is 10 mg three times daily, which may be increased to 15 mg three or four times daily if necessary. Oxazepam (15–25 mg) may be given one hour before retiring for the treatment of insomnia associated with anxiety; up to 50 mg may occasionally be necessary. A dosage of oxazepam for children 6–12 years of age has not been clearly established (Reynolds, 1993; American Hospital Formulary Service, 1995; Medical Economics, 1996). Clinical uses of oxazepam and other benzodiazepines have been reviewed (Hollister et al., 1993). Oxazepam is used extensively in elderly patients and patients with impaired hepatic function (Goodman Gilman et al., 1990).

Comparative data on sales of oxazepam in several countries are shown in Table 1. Overall, sales declined by approximately 20% from 1990 to 1995. During the same period, prescriptions in the United States declined by approximately 13% (see Table 2 in the monograph on diazepam, p. 43).

Table 1. Sales of oxazepam in various countries[a] **(number of standard units**[b]**, in thousands)**

Country	1990	1995	Country	1990	1995
Africa			Europe		
South Africa	14 177	13 992	Belgium	39 581	30 502
North America			France	182 475	137 808
Canada	84 407	84 985	Germany	367 014	245 363
Mexico	5 005	0	Greece	2 870	0
United States	97 602	106 913	Italy	44 115	33 200
South America			Netherlands	94 819	104 909
Argentina	4 199	3 327	Portugal	16 205	18 431
Brazil	141	23	Spain	35 856	10 850
Venezuela	6 390	219	Sweden	99 809	64 160
Asia			Switzerland	37 824	34 404
Republic of Korea	28 316	22 942	Turkey	680	0
Australia	78 027	57 015	United Kingdom	33 365	23 406

[a] Data provided by IMS
[b] Standard dosage units, uncorrected for oxazepam content

1.3 Occurrence

1.3.1 *Natural occurrence*

Oxazepam is not known to occur as a natural product. Oxazepam is a metabolite of other benzodiazepine pharmaceuticals, including diazepam, prazepam and temazepam (Langner *et al.*, 1991).

1.3.2 *Occupational exposure*

No quantitative data on occupational exposure levels were available to the Working Group. The National Occupational Exposure Survey conducted between 1981 and 1983 in the United States by the National Institute for Occupational Safety and Health indicated that about 2650 employees were potentially occupationally exposed to oxazepam. The estimate was based on a survey of United States companies and did not involve measurements of actual exposure (United States National Library of Medicine, 1996).

1.4 Regulations and guidelines

Oxazepam is listed in the following pharmacopoeias: British, Brazilian, Czech, European, French, Italian, Nordic and United States (Reynolds, 1993; Vidal, 1995).

2. Studies of Cancer in Humans

Oxazepam, together with triazolam, was included in the 'other benzodiazepines' category in the comprehensive case–control study by Rosenberg *et al.* (1995) reviewed in detail in the monograph on diazepam (pp. 51–53). Too few subjects had used oxazepam to allow analysis of this drug as a separate category, but no elevated risk was associated with the general category 'sustained use of other benzodiazepines' for any cancer, including cancer of the large bowel (relative risk (RR), 1.5; 95% confidence interval (CI), 0.9–2.4), malignant melanoma (RR, 0.7; 95% CI, 0.3–1.6), lung cancer (RR, 1.4; 95% CI, 0.6–3.2), breast cancer (RR, 0.8; 95% CI, 0.4–1.4) and endometrial cancer (RR, 0.8; 95% CI, 0.3–2.5). Sustained use was defined as ≥ 4 days per week for at least one month that began ≥ 2 years before admission to the hospital. [See additional comments on this study in the monograph on diazepam.]

3. Studies of Cancer in Experimental Animals

3.1 Oral administration

3.1.1 *Mouse*

Groups of 14 male and 14 female Swiss-Webster mice, three months of age, were given oxazepam [purity not specified] in the diet for nine months at concentrations of 500 or 1500 mg/kg diet (ppm) or were given a control diet. After 12 months of age, all mice were given the control diet for a further two months; then, all surviving animals were killed. Selected tissues [list of organs examined not given] were evaluated histologically. In surviving animals, an increased incidence of hepatocellular adenomas (males: control, 0/13; low-dose, 3/12 (25%); high-dose, 8/13 (62%); females: controls, 0/10; low-dose, 0/10; high-dose, 5/8 (63%)) was seen (Fox & Lahcen, 1974). [The Working Group noted that the tumour incidence was given as a percentage of animals surviving at the end of the study and not of total animals.]

The incidences of liver tumours from the following two studies are presented in Table 2.

Groups of 60 male and 60 female Swiss-Webster mice, six to seven weeks of age, were given oxazepam (purity, > 99%) in the diet at concentrations of 0, 2500 or 5000 mg/kg diet (ppm) for up to 57 weeks, at which time the study was terminated due to excessive treatment-related mortality. The oxazepam/diet mixtures were prepared freshly every two weeks. Consumption of diet containing 2500 and 5000 ppm oxazepam resulted in average daily intakes of 270 and 570 mg/kg bw for males and 320 and 670 mg/kg bw for females. The body weights of the treated males were similar to those of the controls during the early weeks, but fell below those of the controls by week 17. The females had greater body weight than the controls until week 29, after which the body weights of the

Table 2. Liver tumours in oxazepam-treated mice

Strain	Sex	Dose (ppm)	No. of mice examined	No. of tumours		
				Adenomas	Carcinomas	Hepatoblastomas
Swiss-Webster (study terminated at 57 weeks)	Male	0	60	1	0	
		2500	60	35^a	5^b	
		5000	60	50^a	19^c	
	Female	0	60	0	1	
		2500	59	22^a	1	
		5000	59	47^a	11^c	
B6C3F1 (study terminated at 105 weeks)	Male	0	49	17	9	0
		125	50	18	5	2
		2500	50	34^c	45^c	21^c
		5000	50	32^c	50^c	13^c
	Female	0	50	25	9	0
		125	50	35	5	1
		2500	50	35^c	49^c	8^c
		5000	50	36^c	44^c	8^c

From United States National Toxicology Program (1993)
^{a} $p < 0.001$; logistic regression test
^{b} $p = 0.003$; life table test
^{c} $p < 0.001$; life table test

high-dose females were similar to those of the controls, while those of the low-dose females remained slightly higher. Food consumption was slightly lower in exposed males and females than in controls. At 57 weeks, there was a significant reduction in the numbers of exposed mice surviving compared with controls (males: control, 45/60; low-dose, 19/60; high-dose, 10/60; females: control, 47/60; low-dose, 28/59; high-dose, 17/59). All surviving animals were killed at 57 weeks. Complete histological examination was performed for all animals except two lost females. Systemic amyloidosis was the principal cause of death in mice dying before the study was terminated. The lower survival of mice receiving oxazepam was attributed to an increase in the extent and severity of amyloid deposits in many organs. A significant increase in the incidence of benign and malignant hepatocellular tumours was observed for male and female mice (Fisher's exact test and Cochran–Armitage linear trend test). The incidences of eosinophilic foci were also increased in exposed mice (males: control, 0/60; low-dose, 22/60 and high-dose, 22/60; females: control, 0/60; low-dose, 20/59 and high-dose, 14/59) and there was evidence of increased centrilobular hepatocyte hypertrophy (males: control, 12/60; low-dose, 46/60 and high-dose, 47/60; females: control, 3/60, low-dose, 51/59 and high-dose, 53/59) (United States National Toxicology Program, 1993; Bucher et al., 1994).

Groups of 50 male and 50 female B6C3F1 mice, six weeks of age, were given oxazepam (purity, > 99%) in the diet at concentrations of 0, 125, 2500 or 5000 mg/kg diet (ppm) for up to 105 weeks. Consumption of diets containing 125, 2500 and 5000 ppm oxazepam resulted in average daily intakes of 12, 310 and 690 mg/kg bw for males and 15, 350 and 780 mg/kg bw for females. Body-weight gain of treated males and females was similar to that of controls until about week 15, after which weight gain for mice exposed to 2500 and 5000 ppm was reduced in relation to controls, resulting in body weights 30–40% lower than those of the controls throughout the remainder of the study. Mean body weights of male mice exposed to 125 ppm oxazepam were similar to those of the controls, while those of female mice receiving 125 ppm were 10–15% lower than those of the controls after about week 45. Food consumption by exposed males and exposed females was similar to that of controls. At 105 weeks, survival of mice receiving 2500 and 5000 ppm was significantly lower than that of controls (males: control, 45/50; low-dose, 44/50; mid-dose, 15/50; high-dose, 0/50; females: 39/50, 41/50, 2/50, 0/50, respectively). All surviving animals were killed at 105 weeks. Complete histological examination was performed on all animals except one control male. The early deaths of the mice were attributed to marked increases in the incidence of hepatoblastoma, hepatocellular adenoma and hepatocellular carcinoma. Moderate hypertrophy of centrilobular hepatocytes occurred in mice receiving 2500 and 5000 ppm oxazepam (males: control, 0/49; low-dose, 2/50; mid-dose, 26/50 and high-dose, 43/50; females: control, 0/50; low-dose, 2/50; mid-dose, 11/50 and high-dose, 29/50). An increase in the incidence of follicular-cell hyperplasia of the thyroid gland occurred in all exposed groups of mice (males: control, 4/49; low-dose, 22/50; mid-dose, 49/50 and high-dose, 47/50; females: control, 16/50; low-dose, 34/50; mid-dose, 49/50 and high-dose, 44/50) and the incidence of thyroid gland follicular-cell adenoma was increased in exposed females (control, 0/50; low-dose, 4/50; mid-dose, 5/50 and high-dose, 6/50) (United States National Toxicology Program, 1993; Bucher et al., 1994). [The Working Group noted that the two highest dose levels may have been toxic.]

The hepatocellular adenomas, carcinomas and hepatoblastomas from the B6C3F1 mice exposed to oxazepam in the diet in the above study were analysed for the presence of activated *ras* proto-oncogenes (Devereux et al., 1994) (see Section 4.4.2).

3.1.2 *Rat*

To study preneoplastic events, groups of 10 male Fischer 344 rats, weighing 150 g [age not specified] were given 0 (control), 20 and 200 mg/kg bw oxazepam (> 99% pure) suspended in 10% arabic gum solution daily by gastric instillation for 14 weeks. No iron-excluding hepatocellular focus was found in the controls or the group receiving 20 mg/kg oxazepam. Four hepatocellular foci were found in one rat receiving oxazepam at the highest dose (Remandet et al., 1984).

3.2 Administration with known carcinogens

3.2.1 *Mouse*

Groups of 40 male B6C3F1 mice, five weeks of age, were given either 0 or 90 mg/kg bw *N*-nitrosodiethylamine (NDEA) in tricaprylin as a single intraperitoneal injection. At seven weeks of age, the mice were given 500 or 1500 mg/kg diet (ppm) oxazepam [purity not specified] in the diet or 500 mg/L (ppm) phenobarbital in the drinking water. Eight mice per group were killed at 9, 21 and 33 weeks of exposure and the remainder were killed after 53 weeks of exposure. Complete necropsy was performed on each animal, and liver, lung, spleen, thyroid, kidney and visually apparent lesions in other organs were examined histologically. Between 33 and 53 weeks of exposure, there was an increase in the incidence of hepatocellular tumours in animals treated with NDEA and oxazepam (see Table 3) (Diwan et al., 1986).

Table 3. Incidence of liver tumours in B6C3F1 mice

Treatment	Hepatocellular adenomas	Hepatocellular carcinomas
NDEA	10/16	0/16
NDEA + 500 ppm oxazepam	14/16^a	3/16^a
NDEA + 1500 ppm oxazepam	15/15^b	8/15^c
NDEA + 500 ppm phenobarbital	16/16	10/16
500 ppm oxazepam	2/16	0/13
1500 ppm oxazepam	0/15	0/15
500 ppm phenobarbital	0/16	0/16

From Diwan et al. (1986)
^a [$p = 0.1$; Fisher's exact test versus NDEA controls]
^b [$p = 0.01$; Fisher's exact test versus NDEA controls]
^c [$p = 0.001$; Fisher's exact test versus NDEA controls]

3.2.2 Rat

Three groups of eight male Wistar rats [age not specified] were given 200 mg/kg bw NDEA as a single intraperitoneal injection. Two weeks later, the animals were given 3000 mg/kg diet (ppm) 2-acetylaminofluorene (2-AAF) in the diet for 14 days and 2 mL/kg bw carbon tetrachloride as a single gastric instillation at the mid-point of the 2-AAF treatment. One week later, the three groups were given basal diet (control), 1000 mg/kg (ppm) oxazepam [purity unspecified] or 500 mg/kg (ppm) phenobarbital in the diet for 30 weeks. At the end of the study, livers were weighed and examined and samples from each lobe plus visually apparent tumours were examined. Both oxazepam and phenobarbital increased the incidence of hepatocellular carcinomas (controls, 0/8; oxazepam, 5/8 (62%); phenobarbital, 7/8 (87%)) (Préat et al., 1987).

Three groups of eight female Sprague-Dawley rats [age not specified] were partially hepatectomized and then given 10 mg/kg bw NDEA as a single intraperitoneal injection and held for two months. The rats were subsequently given basal diet (control), 1000 mg/kg (ppm) oxazepam [purity unspecified] or 500 mg/kg (ppm) phenobarbital in the diet for 57 weeks. At the end of the study, livers were weighed, examined and samples from each lobe as well as visually apparent tumours were examined. There was no significant increase in the incidence of hepatocellular carcinomas (controls, 0/8;

oxazepam, 2/8 (25%); phenobarbital, 0/8) (Préat *et al.*, 1987) [The Working Group noted the small numbers of animals.]

Groups of 10 or 20 male Fischer 344 rats, weighing 170 g [age not specified], were fed diets containing 200 mg/kg (ppm) 2-AAF for eight weeks. The daily dose was estimated to be approximately 15 mg/kg bw. In one group of 10 rats, this was followed by 12 weeks' treatment with 200 mg/kg bw oxazepam (purity > 99%) daily by gastric instillation. There was no significant increase in the incidence of neoplastic nodules of the liver: untreated controls (20 rats), 0 neoplastic nodule/liver; 2-AAF alone (20 rats), 0.2 neoplastic nodule/liver; and 2-AAF plus oxazepam (10 rats), 0.2 neoplastic nodule/liver (Mazue *et al.*, 1982; Remandet *et al.*, 1984). [The Working Group noted the small numbers of animals and the single dose level of oxazepam.]

4. Other Data Relevant to an Evaluation of Carcinogenicity and its Mechanisms

4.1 Absorption, distribution, metabolism and excretion

4.1.1 *Humans*

The pharmacokinetics of oxazepam have been reviewed (Greenblatt, 1981). Oxazepam is absorbed fairly rapidly, reaching peak plasma concentrations within 1–4 h, with a mean of about 2 h in most studies. Greenblatt *et al.* (1980) found that the time of maximum absorption of 30 mg oxazepam was 2.2 h (range, 0.75–4.25 h) in 18 men and 3.1 h (range, 0.5–8.0 h) in 20 women. The maximal plasma concentrations in this study were 622 ± 37 ng/mL in men and 837 ± 51 ng/mL in women. In volunteers given multiple doses (5 mg/day for 10 days), Alván *et al.* (1977) found evidence of only minimal accumulation. The bioavailability is believed to be essentially complete (93%) (Alván & Odar-Cederlöf, 1978; Sonne *et al.*, 1988). The drug is extensively (97%) bound to plasma proteins (Boudinot *et al.*, 1985). Considerable variation in the elimination half-life has been reported, with mean values ranging from about 5 to about 15 h (Greenblatt, 1981). Sonne *et al.* (1988) found values of 6.7 h (range, 5.5–9.2 h) and 5.8 h (range, 5.4–8.4 h) following intravenous and oral administration, respectively. A sex difference has been reported, with a value of 7.8 ± 0.4 h (range, 4.9–10.8 h) in men and 9.7 ± 0.8 h (range, 6.3–19.4 h) in women (Greenblatt *et al.*, 1980). In this study, the elimination half-life was not age-associated in men ($r = -0.085$), but tended to increase, although not significantly, with age in women ($r = 0.45$). Other factors which have been suggested to modify the pharmacokinetics of oxazepam are renal insufficiency (Greenblatt *et al.*, 1983) and hypothyroidism (Sonne *et al.*, 1990), which reduce clearance, while hyperthyroidism increases the rate of glucuronidation and consequently increases clearance (Scott *et al.*, 1984). However, liver disease characterized by cirrhosis or viral hepatitis has no significant effect (Shull *et al.*, 1976; Sellers *et al.*, 1979).

The percentage of dose recovered in urine as glucuronides has varied widely, which may reflect in part methodological differences (Greenblatt, 1981), but at least 60–80%

seems generally agreed. Sonne *et al.* (1988) found that, 48 h after administration of a 15-mg dose, no more than 1% was excreted in the urine as oxazepam, whereas about 70% was recovered as oxazepam glucuronide. Alván *et al.* (1977) found that the urinary recovery of conjugates was 67 ± 15% of the administered dose, with only 2.4 ± 2.4% appearing in the faeces as the parent compound. The glucuronide exists as a pair of diastereoisomers (Ruelius *et al.*, 1979), since oxazepam, like all 3-hydroxybenzodiazepines, is used clinically as a racemic mixture. In a study of these diastereoisomers, Seideman *et al.* (1981) recovered a mean of 54.6 ± 6.6 µmol total glucuronides in 24 h from the urine of six volunteers given a single oral dose of 15 mg oxazepam. The ratio of (+)/(−) isomers [(3S)/(3R) configurations] was 2.1 ± 0.8. Trace amounts of six other metabolites have been reported (Sisenwine *et al.*, 1972) (see Figure 1). It has been calculated that less than 0.1% of 10 mg given three times daily for three days would be excreted in one litre of milk of a breast-feeding mother (Wretlind, 1987). The excretion of oxazepam in breast milk has been confirmed (Dusci *et al.*, 1990).

Tomson *et al.* (1979) showed the rapid placental passage of oxazepam and the minimal capacity of the fetus to glucuronidate oxazepam even in late pregnancy. Thus, conjugated oxazepam found in fetal compartments was produced by neither the placenta nor the fetus, but was probably of maternal origin. Newborns are able to conjugate oxazepam. In early and late pregnancy, the mean ratios of the plasma concentration of total oxazepam (free and glucuronide conjugate forms) in the umbilical cord to that in a maternal vein were 0.6 and 1.1, respectively (Kangas *et al.*, 1980). The penetration of oxazepam from maternal serum to placental tissue in a 4-h period after drug administration was 49%, indicating rapid transfer (Jørgensen *et al.*, 1988).

4.1.2 *Experimental systems*

Garattini *et al.* (1973) gave rats, mice and guinea-pigs 5 mg/kg bw oxazepam by intravenous injection and measured blood levels of the drug at times from 1 min up to 10 h. Maximal oxazepam concentrations were found at the earliest sampling time in all species, the values being 1.63 ± 0.09 µg/mL at 1 min in rats, 3.16 ± 0.05 µg/mL at 1 min in mice and 1.81 ± 0.12 µg/mL at 5 min in guinea-pigs. Blood levels were < 0.05 µg/mL at 5 h in rats and 0.07 ± 0.01 µg/mL at 10 h in guinea-pigs, but were still 0.20 ± 0.01 µg/mL at 10 h in the mice. Biliary excretion of conjugated hydroxylated metabolites, expressed as percentages of the dose 3 h after administration, were 5.3 ± 0.4% in rats, 34.7 ± 3.4% in guinea-pigs and 49.7 ± 5.3% in mice. [The Working Group considered that the 'conjugated hydroxylated benzodiazepines' in this study were the glucuronides of oxazepam and not the phenolic metabolites measured in the studies of Sisenwine and Tio (1986) described below. The low recovery of the oxazepam conjugate in the rat after administration of oxazepam (5.3 ± 0.4%) is therefore consistent with the claim of Sisenwine and Tio that aromatic hydroxylation products predominate in rats.]

The plasma concentrations of oxazepam in male B6C3F1 mice fed diet containing 125 and 2500 mg/kg (ppm) oxazepam appeared to reach steady-state levels by one week of feeding. These levels were 1 µg/mL for the low-dose group and 5–10 µg/mL for the high-dose group (Yuan *et al.*, 1994).

Figure 1. Metabolism of oxazepam in man, miniature swine, rat and mouse

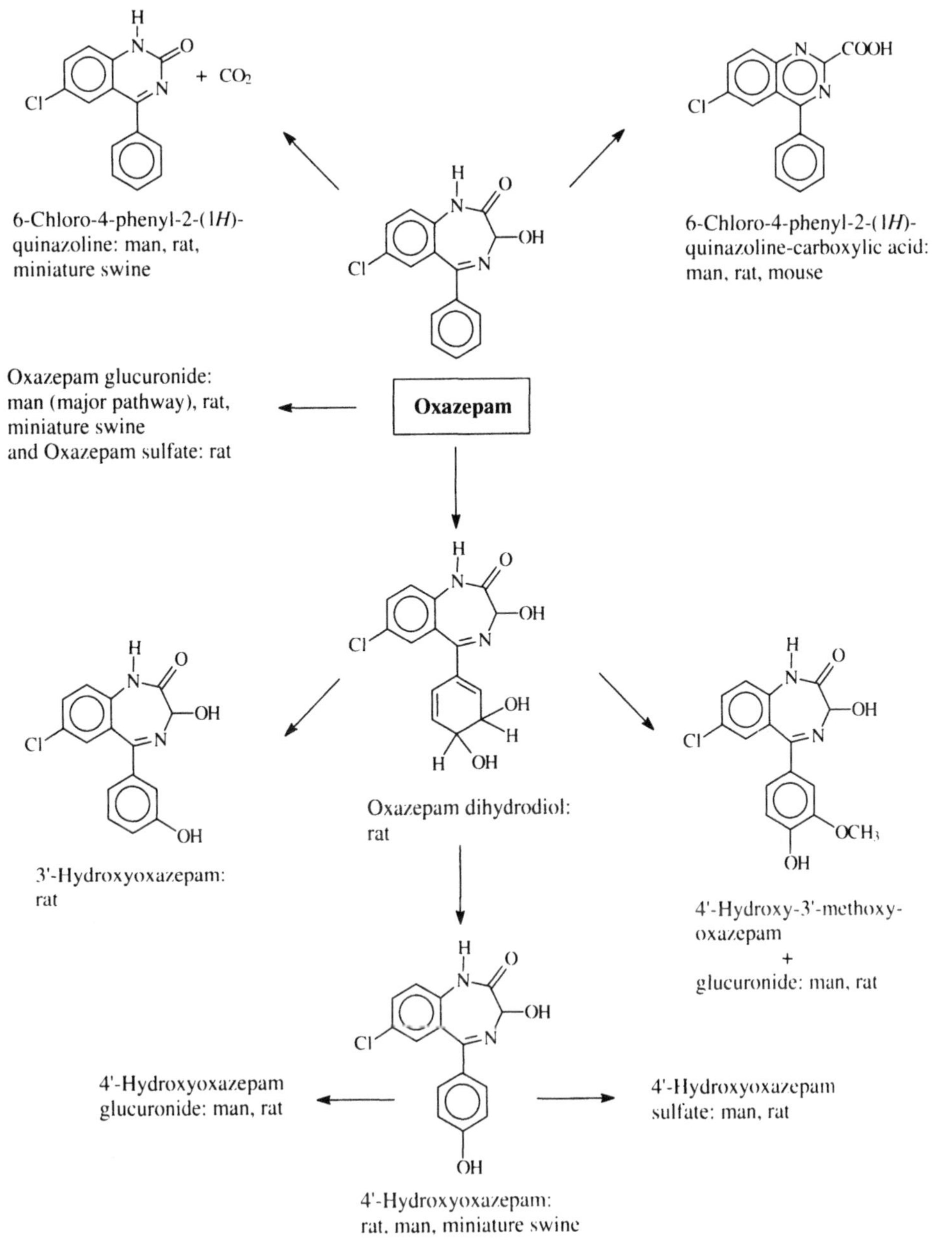

6-Chloro-4-phenyl-2-(1H)-quinazoline: man, rat, miniature swine

6-Chloro-4-phenyl-2-(1H)-quinazoline-carboxylic acid: man, rat, mouse

Oxazepam glucuronide: man (major pathway), rat, miniature swine and Oxazepam sulfate: rat

Oxazepam

3'-Hydroxyoxazepam: rat

Oxazepam dihydrodiol: rat

4'-Hydroxy-3'-methoxy-oxazepam
+
glucuronide: man, rat

4'-Hydroxyoxazepam glucuronide: man, rat

4'-Hydroxyoxazepam sulfate: man, rat

4'-Hydroxyoxazepam: rat, man, miniature swine

From Sisenwine et al. (1972); Griffin & Burka (1993, 1995)

Oxazepam accumulates in adipose tissue. Garattini *et al.* (1973) found that adipose tissue/blood ratios of the drug in mice given 5 mg/kg bw intravenously varied from 1.7 (at 5 min) to 4.9 (at 30 min). Accumulation also occurred in the brain. Maximal concentrations of oxazepam in the brain were 14.3 ± 0.17 µg/g in mice, 4.5 ± 0.03 µg/g in rats and 3.5 ± 0.47 µg/g in guinea-pigs, all at 5 min. Brain/blood drug level ratios in these species varied from 1.1 (at 1 min) to 11.3 (at 10 h) in mice, from 1.9 (at 1 min) to 6.2 (at 1 h) in rats and from 1.9 (at 5 min) to 8.9 (at 5 h) in guinea-pigs.

The disposition of oxazepam in rats and miniature swine was studied by Sisenwine *et al.* (1972). The miniature swine (like humans) eliminated oxazepam primarily as the glucuronides, while aromatic hydroxylation predominated in the rat. In rats, 70.7 ± 6.0% of a single oral dose of 20 mg/kg bw was eliminated in faeces following biliary secretion, while 18.9 ± 2.4% of the dose was found in the urine (Sisenwine & Tio, 1986). In CD-1 mice given an oral dose of 22 mg/kg bw oxazepam, 57.8% was recovered from the faeces and 27.3% was recovered from urine over five days (Sisenwine *et al.*, 1987). Reinvestigation of the metabolism of oxazepam in Swiss-Webster and B6C3F1 mice (Griffin & Burka, 1993) and in Fischer 344 rats (Griffin & Burka, 1995) confirmed the results of the earlier studies. Treatment with 2500 mg/kg diet (ppm) oxazepam in the diet for 14 days before administration of oxazepam by gastric instillation led to a shift from faecal to urinary excretion in mice, but not rats, so that the urinary excretion almost doubled.

There are three major pathways of oxazepam metabolism in mice and rats (as in humans): direct conjugation, phenyl ring oxidation and diazepine ring contraction (Sisenwine & Tio, 1986; Sisenwine *et al.*, 1987; Griffin & Burka, 1993, 1995). In mice, conjugation is mainly with glucuronide, predominantly excreted in the urine; in rats, conjugation is mainly with sulfate, which is almost entirely eliminated in the faeces. The sulfate conjugate of oxazepam, which is unstable in acidic media, may be the source of the faecal oxazepam reported by Sisenwine and Tio (1986). It has not been detected in mice. Studies with recirculating, perfused male Swiss (CD-1) mouse liver preparations showed that oxazepam glucuronides are the dominant liver metabolites in this species (St-Pierre *et al.*, 1990). Oxazepam can also be conjugated with glucuronide by the placenta of rabbits (Berte *et al.*, 1969), apparently in contrast to the human organ (Tomson *et al.*, 1979). Phenyl ring oxidation is more important in rats than in mice (or humans) and Griffin and Burka (1995) found that a dihydrodiol (probably the 3',4'-dihydrodiol, since 2'-hydroxy derivatives are not known) accounts for about 30% of the 72-h urinary metabolites in Fischer 344 rats. This metabolite, which probably forms via an arene oxide intermediate and has not been found in mice, holds implications for the toxicological properties of oxazepam. In rats, ring contraction to 6-chloro-4-phenyl-2(1*H*)-quinazoline carboxylic acid occurs to roughly one half of the extent seen in mice.

4.2 Toxic effects

4.2.1 Humans

(a) Acute toxicity

Fifteen cases of fatal poisoning due to suicidal or accidental ingestion of large doses of oxazepam, either alone or in combination with alcohol and/or other drugs, have been reported. In a review of fatal poisonings attributed to benzodiazepines in the United Kingdom during the 1980s, oxazepam had a comparatively low fatal toxicity index; that is, it caused fewer deaths per million prescriptions than temazepam, diazepam or prazepam (Serfaty & Masterton, 1993).

(b) Chronic toxicity

In addition to effects associated with psychological and physical dependence and withdrawal phenomena, chronic oxazepam administration has been associated in very rare cases with jaundice (both hepatocellular and cholestatic), nausea, skin rashes, lowering of blood pressure and, in isolated cases, with the enhancement of parkinsonism or arthritic symptoms (reviewed by Dollery *et al.*, 1991).

4.2.2 Experimental systems

(a) Acute toxicity

Oral and intraperitoneal LD_{50} values for oxazepam in carboxymethyl cellulose have been reported to range from about 1500 mg/kg bw to > 5000 mg/kg bw in various strains of mice and were greater than 5000 mg/kg bw in Wistar and Charles River CD rats (Owen *et al.*, 1970; United States National Toxicology Program, 1993). Owen *et al.* (1970) reported that oxazepam was only one third as toxic as diazepam when given by the oral route and six times less toxic after intraperitoneal administration.

Unusually high mortality rates (about 20%) were observed in Swiss albino mice within seven days after intraperitoneal injection of 60 mg/kg bw oxazepam (a hypnotic dose causing loss of righting reflex in approximately 70% of the animals) dissolved in dimethyl sulfoxide (Wong & Teo, 1992). In a diazepam-sensitive strain of Swiss albino mice developed by the same group, the mortality rate was 37.5% when 60 mg/kg bw oxazepam was administered intraperitoneally. In neither strain was there mortality among dimethyl sulfoxide-treated control animals. Gross post-mortem examination did not reveal any consistent cause of death. In contrast, with the same oxazepam treatment regimen, mortality was only 7% in BALB/c mice. [The authors did not offer any explanation for the high mortality rates in the two Swiss mouse strains; there are no other reports in the literature of such high mortality rates due to benzodiazepine administration.]

(b) Subacute and chronic toxicity

Owen *et al.* (1970) administered oxazepam in the diet to male and female Charles River CD rats at concentrations of 600, 1250, 2500 or 5000 mg/kg diet (ppm) for six weeks (20 animals per group). After six weeks, two of the high-dose rats had died, and weight gain was impaired in the males given 2500 ppm concentration. Liver, adrenal gland and kidney weights were significantly greater in the two highest-concentration groups of both sexes. The only treatment-related histopathological change was a mild to moderate increase in liver parenchymal fat; no liver necrosis or fibrosis was found. There was no increase in liver fat in animals maintained on drug-free diet for four weeks after administration of 5000 ppm oxazepam in the diet for six weeks.

Groups of 30 male and 30 female Charles River CD rats were fed diets containing 0, 150, 300, 600 or 1200 mg/kg diet (ppm) oxazepam for 55 weeks. There was no clearly treatment-related death. Except at the lowest dose, liver weights were higher compared with the controls. Kidney weights were higher at the two highest doses in oxazepam-treated males, and ventral prostate and uterine weights were lower at the highest dose level. There was no effect on body weight or haematological parameters and no significant histopathological sign of toxicity (Owen et al., 1970).

In a 14-week study, oxazepam was given to Swiss-Webster mice in the diet at concentrations of 0, 625, 1250, 2500, 5000 or 10 000 mg/kg (ppm). Consumption of these diets resulted in average daily intakes of 80, 170, 330, 680 or 1400 mg/kg bw in males and 100, 220, 440, 830 and 1620 mg/kg bw in females. The mean body weights of all groups of exposed females were greater than those of the control group. In addition to sedative effects, decreased locomotor activity and muscle strength were observed, especially at the beginning of the study. Except for the lowest-intake groups, absolute and relative liver weights were significantly greater than those of the controls; the increases were dose-related. Heart and kidney weights were increased in some male and female groups. Dose-dependent hepatocellular hypertrophy was observed in all treated animals. Foci of hepatocellular necrosis were also detected in some animals; however, the low incidence and the lack of a dose-related increase suggested that these lesions were not causally linked to oxazepam administration. In a parallel 14-week assay, the effects of oxazepam were investigated in B6C3F1 mice under similar conditions, yielding practically identical results, notably those concerning body and liver weights and liver histopathology (United States National Toxicology Program, 1993).

Groups of 10 male B6C3F1 mice were fed diet containing 0, 25, 125, 2500 or 5000 mg/kg diet (ppm) oxazepam [approximately between 2 and 400 mg/kg bw per day] for 15, 30, 45 or 90 days. The two highest doses were selected to parallel those used in the United States National Toxicology Program bioassay of oxazepam (United States National Toxicology Program, 1993) and the two lowest doses to achieve blood concentrations similar to those reported in the literature for humans at therapeutic dose levels (1.1 µg/mL) or in the course of intoxications (up to 8.0 µg/mL). During the final seven days before they were killed, the animals were exposed to bromodeoxyuridine delivered by osmotic minipumps for quantification of hepatocellular replicative DNA synthesis. Liver/body weight ratios, serum clinical chemistry and histopathology of the liver were also monitored to provide data that would permit the distinction of cytotoxic from mitogenic mechanisms of cell proliferation. The liver/body weight ratios were significantly increased in a dose-dependent manner and the major histopathological feature was dose-dependent hypertrophy of hepatocytes; neither histopathology nor serum clinical chemistry revealed clear signs of hepatotoxicity. There was a dose-related increase in replicative DNA synthesis at 15 days in the 125-, 2500- and 5000-ppm treatment groups (up to five-fold at the highest dose), but this returned to control levels in all groups by 30 days (Cunningham *et al.*, 1994). The transient mitogenic response observed might arise from initial activation followed by down-regulation of peripheral benzodiazepine receptors in the liver (Verma & Snyder, 1989). In addition to the benzodiazepine receptors in the central nervous system, there are also peripheral receptors in many organs, such as the liver, pituitary and adrenal glands, testes, heart and kidney (Ferrarese *et al.*, 1993).

Groups of male B6C3F1 mice were fed diets containing 125 mg/kg diet (ppm) (a non-carcinogenic dose in chronic studies) or 2500 mg/kg diet (ppm) (a carcinogenic dose in chronic studies [see Section 3]) oxazepam for 3, 7, 10 or 21 days. At the end of dosing, increased specific activities of various hepatic enzymes were observed, including cytochrome P450s (such as aminopyrine *N*-demethylase and aniline hydroxylase), cytochrome b5, glucuronyl transferase and glutathione *S*-transferase. At the low dose, only aminopyrine *N*-demethylase and glutathione *S*-transferase activities were significantly increased (Griffin *et al.*, 1995). The time pattern of induction was generally an early increase in the specific activities followed by a gradual decline until, by day 21, the specific activities were equivalent to or even below the control levels. The liver/body weight ratios continued to increase up to day 21.

In a continuation of these studies, labelling of hepatic cell nuclei with bromodeoxyuridine delivered by an implanted osmotic mini-pump over seven days indicated increased levels of cell proliferation by seven days on the low dose and by 10 days on the high dose. The delay observed at the higher dietary concentration probably reflects a sedative effect leading to reduced food consumption. Labelling was lower, but still above control values, after 21 days at this dose level. Hepatic cytochrome P450 and b5 protein levels and glucuronyl transferase activity were increased two-fold after 10 days of treatment with 2500 ppm oxazepam. Plasma thyroid-stimulating hormone levels were unaffected by the 125-ppm diet, but, in the mice exposed to the 2500-ppm oxazepam diet, thyroid-stimulating hormone levels increased three-fold after 10 days' treatment and returned to control levels by 21 days (Griffin *et al.*, 1996).

4.3 Reproductive and prenatal effects

4.3.1 *Humans*

Oxazepam, together with diazepam, nitrazepam and chlordiazepoxide, was included in the benzodiazepine category in a case–control study of oral clefts in Finland (Saxén & Saxén, 1975), but was not analysed as a separate category. The study is reviewed in detail in the monograph on diazepam (p. 66).

Laegreid *et al.* (1987a) reported seven cases with intra- and extrauterine growth retardation, facial dysmorphism and central nervous system dysfunction from 36 mothers (37 infants) who took benzodiazepines regularly during pregnancy. Of the seven children, two were exposed to oxazepam (75 mg daily) throughout pregnancy. One case had Moebius syndrome, including facial dysmorphism, convulsions and severe mental retardation, while another child was affected with lissencephaly, distortion of neuronal migration with cerebral pachygyria and Dandy-Walker malformation, facial dysmorphism and polycystic kidney. Later, the second case was diagnosed, following the suggestion of Winter (1987), as Zellweger syndrome (Laegreid et al., 1987b). [The Working Group noted that both Moebius and Zellweger syndromes may have a Mendelian mode of inheritance.]

The association between maternal psychotropic drug use and perinatal deaths was investigated in a case–control study in Gothenburg, Sweden (Laegreid et al., 1992a). Too few women had used oxazepam to permit analysis of the specific association with this drug. The study is reviewed in more detail in the monograph on diazepam (p. 68).

Laegreid et al. (1992b,c) examined the neurodevelopment of 17 children born to 16 mothers who used benzodiazepines throughout pregnancy: 15 used oxazepam (15–60 mg daily) or diazepam (5–30 mg daily) alone or in combination and one mother used lorazepam. The results were compared with those for 29 children born to mothers without any known use of psychotropic drugs. Significant differences in the frequency of pre- and perinatal complications, for example, intrauterine asphyxia, instrumental delivery and respiratory disturbances, and in neurobehaviour between the benzodiazepine and control groups were found.

The 17 cases studied by Laegreid et al. (1992b,c) were followed up prospectively into late infancy (Viggedal et al., 1993). A general delay in mental development up to 18 months of age associated with prenatal exposure to benzodiazepines was found. [The Working Group noted that maternal depression itself has an important negative effect on children's development (Cox, 1988). In addition, neuropsychological symptoms are frequent among children of abusers of psychoactive substances (Deren, 1986; Van Baar et al., 1989).]

A case of floppy-infant syndrome (namely muscular relaxation, respiratory depression and limpness) following treatment of pre-eclampsia with oxazepam has been reported (Drury et al., 1977).

4.3.2 *Experimental systems*

Oxazepam did not cause congenital abnormalities in mice (300 mg/kg diet (ppm)), rats (300 or 600 mg/kg diet (ppm)) or rabbits (25 or 50 mg/kg bw orally) (Owen et al., 1970). An oral dose of 400 mg/kg bw induced resorption in Swiss-Webster mice, but no increase in the frequency of malformations (Miller & Becker, 1973). However, Simon and Sulik (1992, abstract) found craniofacial malformations (agnathia, an- or microphthalmia, coloboma, exencephaly, encephalocele, holoprosencephaly) when doses of 375 mg/kg bw or 1000 mg/kg bw oxazepam were administered by gastric instillation to C57Bl/6J mice on gestational day 7 at 0 h and 4 h. However, the authors noted that human exposure to the dose range examined is unlikely.

Chronic administration of 500 or 1500 mg/kg diet (ppm) oxazepam in the diet to breeding pairs of Swiss-Webster mice resulted in a significant decrease in mating performance and in body weights at birth (Guerriero & Fox, 1976). Female mice that received oxazepam (500 mg/kg diet (ppm)) prenatally had delay in the age of vaginal opening;

however, the age of first oestrus was generally lower than that of controls due to disruption of normal hypothalamic-pituitary relations (Fox & Guerriero, 1978). Oxazepam treatment (5, 15 or 50 mg/kg bw, twice daily, orally) on days 12–16 of pregnancy also resulted in postnatal growth retardation in CD-1 mice (Alleva *et al.*, 1985). Oxazepam (100 mg/kg bw orally) showed no noteworthy fetal toxicity in Sprague-Dawley rats (Saito *et al.*, 1984).

The long-term postnatal developmental (including behavioural) effects of oxazepam have been studied. Male Swiss-Webster mice that received oxazepam (500 mg/kg diet (ppm)) prenatally and during early infancy showed enhanced performance of a Y-maze task as adults. The drug produced its greatest effect (enhanced learning) when given prenatally (Fox *et al.*, 1977). The main effect of prenatal oxazepam treatment (5, 15 or 50 mg/kg bw, twice daily, orally) in CD-1 mice on days 12–16 of pregnancy was an impairment of active avoidance response, while effects on overall discrimination performance were less marked and limited to later stages of training (Alleva *et al.*, 1985).

CD-1 mice were exposed to oxazepam (15 mg/kg bw, twice daily, orally) on days 12–16 of fetal life (at a critical ontogenetic stage of type II benzodiazepine receptor increase) or to vehicle alone. Reduced locomotor activity on postnatal day 14 and modified profiles of muscimol effects (faster recovery from the initial depression) at 21 and 28 days were observed. These effects might be explained either by accelerated development of a GABAergic regulatory mechanism or by changes in the monoaminergic system — changes which may account for other effects of prenatal benzodiazepine exposure (Laviola *et al.*, 1992a). The eight-arm maze performance and neophobia were studied in prenatally exposed mice at 7–8 weeks of age. Overall, the oxazepam-exposed mice were much less efficient in the radial arm maze task than the vehicle-exposed animals. In addition, the latency of first approach to a novel stimulus object was considerably increased and a deficit of habituation in the course of the subsequent exploratory period was found (Laviola *et al.*, 1992b).

This mouse model was used to study typical responses of lactating dams; oxazepam enhanced maternal aggression towards the offspring (Laviola *et al.*, 1991).

4.4 Genetic and related effects

4.4.1 *Humans*

No data were available to the Working Group.

4.4.2 *Experimental systems* (see also Table 4 for references and Appendices 1 and 2)

Oxazepam does not cause mutations in either *Salmonella typhimurium* or *Saccharomyces cerevisiae*. Furthermore, it does not cause mitotic recombination in *S. cerevisiae* or either non-disjunction or crossing-over in *Aspergillus nidulans*. No chromosomal damage was observed in *Nigella damascena*.

In cultured mammalian cells, oxazepam did not cause unscheduled DNA synthesis (in primary hepatocyte cultures) or mutation at either the *tk* or the *hprt* locus. Consistently positive responses have been observed in cultured mammalian (including human) cell

Table 4. Genetic and related effects of oxazepam

Test system	Result[a] Without exogenous metabolic system	Result[a] With exogenous metabolic system	Dose[b] (LED/HID)	Reference
SA0, *Salmonella typhimurium* TA100, reverse mutation	–	–	2500	Balbi *et al.* (1980)
SA0, *Salmonella typhimurium* TA100, reverse mutation	–	–	NG	Matula & Downie (1983) (abstract)
SA5, *Salmonella typhimurium* TA1535, reverse mutation	–	–	2500	Balbi *et al.* (1980)
SA7, *Salmonella typhimurium* TA1537, reverse mutation	–	–	2500	Balbi *et al.* (1980)
SA9, *Salmonella typhimurium* TA98, reverse mutation	–	–	2500	Balbi *et al.* (1980)
SA9, *Salmonella typhimurium* TA98, reverse mutation	–	–	NG	Matula & Downie (1983) (abstract)
SCH, *Saccharomyces cerevisiae*, mitotic recombination	–	NT	NG	Matula & Downie (1983) (abstract)
SCR, *Saccharomyces cerevisiae*, reverse mutation	–	NT	NG	Matula & Downie (1983) (abstract)
ANG, *Aspergillus nidulans*, non-disjunction and crossing-over	–	NT	NG	Bignami *et al.* (1974)
PLC, *Nigella damascena*, chromosomal aberrations	–	NT	50	Moutschen *et al.* (1987)
URP, Unscheduled DNA synthesis, rat primary hepatocytes	–	NT	0.5	Swierenga *et al.* (1983) (abstract)
G5T, Gene mutation, mouse lymphoma L5178Y cells, *tk* locus *in vitro*	–	NT	250	Stopper *et al.* (1993)
GIA, Gene mutation, rat primary hepatocytes, *hprt* locus *in vitro*	–	–	50	Swierenga *et al.* (1983) (abstract)
MIA, Micronucleus test, Syrian hamster embryo fibroblast (SHE) cells *in vitro*	+[c]	NT	75	Stopper *et al.* (1993)
MIA, Micronucleus test, mouse lymphoma L5178Y cells *in vitro*	+[c]	NT	50	Stopper *et al.* (1993)
MIH, Micronucleus test, human amniotic fluid fibroblast-like (AFFL) cells *in vitro*	+[c]	NT	75	Stopper *et al.* (1993)
DVA, DNA strand breaks, rat liver *in vivo*	–		287 po × 1	Carlo *et al.* (1989)

Table 4 (contd)

Test system	Result[a]		Dose[b] (LED/HID)	Reference
	Without exogenous metabolic system	With exogenous metabolic system		
DVA, DNA strand breaks, rat liver *in vivo*	–		57 po × 15	Carlo *et al.* (1989)
GVA, Gene mutation (H-*ras*), mouse liver tumours *in vivo*	–		600 diet 2 yrs	Devereux *et al.* (1994)
ICH, Inhibition of gap-junctional intercellular communication, human hepatoma cells (SK-HEP-1) *in vitro*	+	NT	10	Rolin-Limbosch *et al.* (1987)

[a] +, positive; (+), weak positive; –, negative; NT, not tested; ?, inconclusive
[b] LED, lowest effective dose; HID, highest ineffective dose; in-vitro tests, µg/mL; in-vivo tests, mg/kg bw/day
[c] Kinetochore-positive; L5178Y cells *in situ* also positive for centromeric DNA

assays for the induction of micronuclei and aneuploidy (as indicated by micronucleus tests with kinetochore staining).

Gap-junctional intercellular communication was inhibited by oxazepam in a human cell line.

No increase in DNA single-strand breaks and/or alkali-labile sites was observed in the liver of rats given single or multiple oral doses of oxazepam. Hepatocellular adenomas and carcinomas which developed in male and female B6C3F1 mice fed 0, 125, 2500 or 5000 mg/kg diet (ppm) oxazepam for up to two years (see Section 3.1.1) were examined for activated *ras* proto-oncogenes (Devereux *et al.*, 1994). Thirteen of 37 (35%) adenomas and carcinomas from the 125-ppm group carried codon 61 mutations in H-*ras*, while mutations were detected in two of 25 (8%) of the liver tumours from the 2500-ppm group and in none of 22 liver tumours in the 5000-ppm group. These figures compare with 80/126 (63%) historical controls and 11/20 (55%) concurrent control tumours. In addition, 12 hepatoblastomas from the two highest-dose groups were examined for codon 61 mutations, but none was found. These data imply that H-*ras* mutations in codon 61 do not appear to be involved in the formation of hepatocellular tumours or hepatoblastomas induced by oxazepam. This further suggests that promotion of hepatic tumours by oxazepam in mice involves a mechanism independent of that for spontaneous hepatic tumour formation. No tumour in the exposed groups had a mutation in codons 12, 13 or 117 of H-*ras* or in codons 12 or 13 of K-*ras* genes.

5. Summary of Data Reported and Evaluation

5.1 Exposure data

Oxazepam is a benzodiazepine used extensively since the 1960s for the treatment of anxiety and insomnia and in the control of symptoms of alcohol withdrawal. It is a metabolite of diazepam, prazepam and temazepam, among the benzodiazepines considered in this volume.

5.2 Human carcinogenicity data

In one case–control study evaluating benzodiazepine use, subjects using oxazepam were included, but were too few to analyse as a separate category.

5.3 Animal carcinogenicity data

Oxazepam was tested for carcinogenicity in three experiments in two strains of mice by oral administration in the diet. Significant increases in the incidence of benign and malignant liver tumours were found in two of the studies. The incidence of an uncommon malignant liver tumour, hepatoblastoma, was also increased in one strain of mice. In the third study, an increased incidence of liver adenomas was found. In one of the studies, a small increase in the incidence of thyroid gland adenomas was observed in females of one strain of mice.

Oxazepam promoted liver tumour development in one two-stage model in mice and in one of three studies in rats.

5.4 Other relevant data

Oxazepam is rapidly and completely absorbed in humans and is largely eliminated in urine conjugated with glucuronic acid. The half-life averages 5–6 h.

Oxazepam is also extensively metabolized in animals. In some species (miniature swine), conjugation predominates, while in others (rats) oxidative metabolism is the major route.

Oxazepam has low acute and chronic toxicity for humans at therapeutic concentrations. The main adverse effects of chronic administration are psychological and physical dependence and withdrawal phenomena; specific organ toxicity of oxazepam to humans has not been observed.

The acute toxicity of oxazepam to experimental animals is also low. Short-term, high-dose administration of oxazepam to mice and rats resulted in increased liver weights. A transient increase in cell proliferation was observed in oxazepam-treated mice.

Perinatal death and neurodevelopmental retardation have been reported in the offspring of women who were exposed to oxazepam during pregnancy (see the monograph on diazepam for further discussion relating to cleft palate). However, confounding factors could not be controlled adequately in these studies.

Malformations have been observed following high doses of oxazepam in mice, but not at moderate doses in this species or in rats or rabbits.

Oxazepam is inactive in most genetic toxicity assays, although it has been shown to cause micronuclei and aneuploidy *in vitro* and to inhibit gap-junctional intercellular communication in human hepatoma cells *in vitro*. No data were available on humans.

Mechanistic considerations

There is no evidence that oxazepam interacts with DNA. Evidence of mutagenic activity is limited to aneuploidy in cell culture systems.

The induction of hepatocellular proliferation and hepatic cytochrome P450s by oxazepam was observed in mice at doses that were carcinogenic following long-term exposure. These adaptive effects are typical of several non-genotoxic compounds with promoting activity that are carcinogenic in mouse liver. Oxazepam has demonstrated promoting activity. Furthermore, the formation of hepatocellular tumours and hepatoblastomas by oxazepam does not involve the H-*ras* codon 61 pathway. Similarities have been observed between the hepatic effects of oxazepam and those of phenobarbital, which also promotes development of hepatocellular tumours in mice. Taken together, these data support the conclusion that liver tumours are produced in mice by a promoting mechanism.

The implications of these findings with respect to potential cancer risk of oxazepam exposure in humans are unclear. Specifically, information on the relevant effects of oxazepam in human groups or systems is not available. In general, the sensitivity of human liver to tumour formation, even if induction of cytochrome P450s and hepatocellular proliferation at levels comparable to those in mice were to occur, has not been established.

Levels of thyroid-stimulating hormone were increased in mice fed oxazepam at doses that induced adenomas and hyperplasia following long-term exposure. Sustained thyroid stimulation has been implicated as a mechanism of thyroid tumorigenesis in rodents.

5.5 Evaluation[1]

There is *inadequate evidence* in humans for the carcinogenicity of oxazepam.

There is *sufficient evidence* in experimental animals for the carcinogenicity of oxazepam.

Overall evaluation

Oxazepam is *possibly carcinogenic to humans (Group 2B)*.

In making the overall evaluation, the Working Group took into account that:

(i) uncertainty exists regarding the formation of mouse liver tumours by oxazepam as a relevant end-point for evaluation of carcinogenic risks to humans.

(ii) appropriate mechanistic information in humans is lacking.

6. References

Alleva, E., Laviola, G., Tirelli, E. & Bignami, G. (1985) Short-, medium-, and long-term effects of prenatal oxazepam on neurobehavioural development of mice. *Psychopharmacology*, **87**, 434–441

Alván, G. & Odar-Cederlöf, I. (1978) The pharmacokinetic profiles of oxazepam. *Acta psychiat. scand.*, **Suppl 274**, 47–55

Alván, G., Siwers, B. & Vessman, J. (1977) Pharmacokinetics of oxazepam in healthy volunteers. *Acta pharmacol. toxicol.*, **40** (Suppl. 1), 40–51

American Hospital Formulary Service (1995) *AHFS Drug Information*® *95*, Bethesda, MD, American Society of Health-System Pharmacists, pp. 1602–1603

Balbi, A., Muscettola, G., Staiano, N., Martire, G. & De Lorenzo, F. (1980) Psychotropic drugs: evaluation of mutagenic effect. *Pharmacol. Res. Commun.*, **12**, 423–431

Bargo, E.S. (1983) High pressure liquid chromatographic determination of oxazepam dosage forms: collaborative study. *J. Assoc. off. analyt. Chem.*, **66**, 864–866

---

[1] For definition of the italicized terms, see Preamble, pp. 22–25.

Bell, S.C. & Childress, S.J. (1962) A rearrangement of 5-aryl-1,3-dihydro-2*H*-1,4-benzodiazepine-2-one 4-oxides. *J. org. Chem.*, **27**, 1691–1695

Berrueta, L.A., Gallo, B. & Vicente, F. (1993) Analysis of oxazepam in urine using solid-phase extraction and high-performance liquid chromatography with fluorescence detection by postcolumn derivatization. *J. Chromatogr.*, **616**, 344–348

Berte, F., Manzo, L., De Bernardi, M. & Benzi, G. (1969) Ability of the placenta to metabolize oxazepam and aminopyrine before and after drug stimulation. *Arch. int. Pharmacodyn.*, **182**, 182–185

Bignami, M., Morpurgo, G., Pagliani, R., Carere, A., Conti, G. & Di Giuseppe, G. (1974) Nondisjunction and crossing-over induced by pharmaceutical drugs in *Aspergillus nidulans*. *Mutat. Res.*, **26**, 159–170

Boudinot, F.D., Homon, C.A., Jusko, W.J. & Ruelius, H.W. (1985) Protein binding of oxazepam and its glucuronide conjugates to human albumin. *Biochem. Pharmacol.*, **34**, 2115–2121

British Medical Association/Royal Pharmaceutical Society of Great Britain (1994) *British National Formulary Number 27 (March 1994)*, London, p. 143

British Pharmacopoeial Commission (1993) *British Pharmacopoeia 1993*, Vols. I and II, London, Her Majesty's Stationery Office, pp. 467–468, 1037–1038

Bucher, J.R., Shackelford, C.C., Haseman, J.K., Johnson, J.D., Kurtz, P.J. & Persing, R.L. (1994) Carcinogenicity studies of oxazepam in mice. *Fundam. appl. Toxicol.*, **23**, 280–297

Budavari, S., ed. (1995) *The Merck Index*, 12th Ed., Rahway, NJ, Merck & Co.

Carlo, P., Finollo, R., Ledda, A. & Brambilla, G. (1989) Absence of liver DNA fragmentation in rats treated with high oral doses of 32 benzodiazepine drugs. *Fundam. appl. Toxicol.*, **12**, 34–41

Chopineau, J., Rivault, F., Sautou, V. & Sommier, M.F. (1994) Determination of temazepam and its active metabolite, oxazepam in plasma, urine and dialysate using solid-phase extraction followed by high-performance liquid chromatography. *J. liq. Chromatogr.*, **17**, 373–383

Council of Europe (1992) *European Pharmacopoeia*, 2nd Ed., Sainte-Ruffine, France, Maisonneuve S.A., pp. 778-1–778-3

Cox, A.D. (1988) Maternal depression and impact on children's development. *Arch. Dis. Child.*, **63**, 90–95

Cunningham, M.L., Maronpot, R.R., Thompson, M. & Bucher, J.R. (1994) Early responses of the liver of B6C3F1 mice to the hepatocarcinogen oxazepam. *Toxicol. appl. Pharmacol.*, **124**, 31–38

Deren, S. (1986) Children of substance abusers: a review of the literature. *J. Substance Abuse Treat.*, **3**, 77–94

Devereux, T.R., White, C.M., Sills, R.C., Bucher, J.R., Maronpot, R.R. & Anderson, M.W. (1994) Low frequency of H-*ras* mutations in hepatocellular adenomas and carcinomas and in hepatoblastomas from B6C3F1 mice exposed to oxazepam in the diet. *Carcinogenesis*, **15**, 1083–1087

Diwan, B.A., Rice, J.M. & Ward, J.M. (1986) Tumor-promoting activity of benzodiazepine tranquilizers, diazepam and oxazepam, in mouse liver. *Carcinogenesis*, **7**, 789–794

Dollery, C., Boobis, A.R., Burley, D., Davies, D.M., Davies, D.S., Harrison, P.I., Orme, M.E., Park, B.K. & Goldberg, L.I. (1991) *Therapeutic Drugs: Oxazepam*, Edinburgh, Churchill Livingstone, pp. O46–O50

Drury, K.A.D., Spalding, E., Donaldson, D. & Rutherford, D. (1977) Floppy-infant syndrome: is oxazepam the answer? (Letter to the Editor). *Lancet*, **ii**, 1126–1127

Dusci, L.J., Good, S.M., Hall, R.W. & Ilett, K.F. (1990) Excretion of diazepam and its metabolites in human milk during withdrawal from combination high dose diazepam and oxazepam. *Br. J. clin. Pharmacol.*, **29**, 123–126

El-Brashy, A., Aly, F.A. & Belal, F. (1993) Determination of 1,4-benzodiazepines in drug dosage forms by difference spectrophotometry. *Mikrochim. Acta*, **110**, 55–60

Fernández, P., Hermida, I., Bermejo, A.M., López-Rivadulla, M., Cruz, A. & Concheiro, L. (1991) Simultaneous determination of diazepam and its metabolites in plasma by high-performance liquid chromatography. *J. liq. Chromatogr.*, **14**, 2587–2599

Ferrarese, C., Appolonio, I., Bianchi, G., Frigo, M., Marzorati, C., Pecora, N., Perego, M., Pierpaoli, C. & Frattola, L. (1993) Benzodiazepine receptors and diazepam binding inhibitor: a possible link between stress, anxiety and the immune system. *Psychoneuroendocrinology*, **18**, 3–22

Fox, K.A. & Guerriero, F.J. (1978) Effect of benzodiazepines on age of vaginal perforation and first estrus in mice. *Res. Comm. chem. Pathol. Pharmacol.*, **21**, 181–184

Fox, K.A. & Lahcen, R.B. (1974) Liver-cell adenomas and peliosis hepatis in mice associated with oxazepam. *Res. Comm. chem. Pathol. Pharmacol.*, **8**, 481–488

Fox, K.A., Abendschein, D.R. & Lahcen, R.B. (1977) Effects of benzodiazepines during gestation and infancy on Y-maze performance of mice. *Pharmacol. Res. Comm.*, **9**, 325–338

Garattini, S., Mussini, E., Marcucci, F. & Guaitani, A. (1973) Metabolic studies on benzodiazepines in various animal species. In Garattini, S., Mussini, E. & Randall, L.O., eds, *The Benzodiazepines*, New York, Raven Press, pp. 75–97

Gennaro, A.R., ed. (1995) *Remington: The Science and Practice of Pharmacy*, 19th Ed., Easton, PA, Mack Publishing Co., pp. 1159–1160

Goodman Gilman, A., Rall, T.W., Nies, A.S. & Taylor, P., eds (1990) *Goodman and Gilman's. The Pharmacological Basis of Therapeutics*, 8th Ed., New York, Pergamon Press

Greenblatt, D.J. (1981) Clinical pharmacokinetics of oxazepam and lorazepam. *Clin. Pharmacokinet.*, **6**, 89–105

Greenblatt, D.J., Divoll, M., Harmatz, J.S. & Shader, R.I. (1980) Oxazepam kinetics: effects of age and sex. *J. Pharmacol. exp. Ther.*, **215**, 86–91

Greenblatt, D.J., Murray, T.G., Audet, P.R., Locniskar, A., Koepke, H.H. & Walker, B.R. (1983) Multiple-dose kinetics and dialyzability of oxazepam in renal insufficiency. *Nephron*, **34**, 234–238

Griffin, R.J. & Burka, L.T. (1993) Metabolism and elimination of oxazepam in B6C3F1 and Swiss-Webster mice. *Drug Metab. Dispos.*, **21**, 918–926

Griffin, R.J. & Burka, L.T. (1995) Metabolism and elimination of oxazepam in F344 rats. *Drug Metab. Dispos.*, **23**, 232–239

Griffin, R.J., Burka, L.T. & Cunningham, M.L. (1995) Activity of hepatic drug metabolizing enzymes following oxazepam-dosed feed treatment in B6C3F1 mice. *Toxicol. Lett.*, **76**, 251–256

Griffin, R.J., Dudley, C.N. & Cunningham, M.L. (1996) Biochemical effects of the mouse hepatocarcinogen oxazepam: similarities to phenobarbital. *Fundam. appl. Toxicol.*, **29**, 147–154

Guerriero, F.J. & Fox, K.A. (1976) Benzodiazepines and reproduction of Swiss-Webster mice. *Res. Comm. chem. Pathol. Pharmacol.*, **13**, 601–610

Hollister, L.E., Müller-Oerlinghausen, B., Rickels, K. & Shader, R.I. (1993) Clinical uses of benzodiazepines. *J. clin. Psychopharmacol.*, **13** (Suppl. 1)

IARC (1977) *IARC Monographs on the Evaluation of Carcinogenic Risk of Chemicals to Man*, Vol. 13, *Some Miscellaneous Pharmaceutical Substances*, Lyon, pp. 57–73

IARC (1987) *IARC Monographs on the Evaluation of Carcinogenic Risks to Humans*, Suppl. 7, *Overall Evaluations of Carcinogenicity: An Updating of* IARC Monographs *Volumes 1–42*, Lyon, p. 69

Jørgensen, N.P., Thurmann-Nielsen, E. & Walstad, R.A. (1988) Pharmacokinetics and distribution of diazepam and oxazepam in early pregnancy. *Acta obstet. gynecol. scand.*, **67**, 493–497

Kangas, L., Erkkola, R., Kanto, J. & Eronen, M. (1980) Transfer of free and conjugated oxazepam across the human placenta. *Eur. J. clin. Pharmacol.*, **17**, 301–304

Komiskey, H.L., Rahman, A., Weisenburger, W.P., Hayton, W.L., Zobrist, R.H. & Silvius, W. (1985) Extraction, separation and detections of ^{14}C-diazepam and ^{14}C-metabolites from brain tissue of mature and old rats. *J. analyt. Toxicol.*, **9**, 131–133

Laegreid, L., Olegård, R., Wahlström, J. & Conradi, N. (1987a) Abnormalities in children exposed to benzodiazepines *in utero* (Letter to the Editor). *Lancet*, **i**, 108–109

Laegreid, L., Olegård, R., Wahlström, J., Conradi, N. & Sisfontes, L. (1987b) Benzodiazepine overconsumption in pregnancy (Letter to the Editor). *Lancet*, **ii**, 1405–1406

Laegreid, L., Conradi, N., Hagberg, G. & Hedner, T. (1992a) Psychotropic drug use in pregnancy and perinatal death. *Acta obstet. gynecol. scand.*, **71**, 451–457

Laegreid, L., Hagberg, G. & Lundberg, A. (1992b) The effect of benzodiazepines on the fetus and the newborn. *Neuropediatrics*, **23**, 18–23

Laegreid, L., Hagberg, G. & Lundberg, A. (1992c) Neurodevelopment in late infancy after prenatal exposure to benzodiazepines — A prospective study. *Neuropediatrics*, **23**, 60–67

Langner, J.G., Gan, B.K., Liu, R.H., Baugh, L.D., Chand, P., Weng, J.-L., Edwards, C. & Walia, A.S. (1991) Enzymatic digestion, solid-phase extraction, and gas chromatography/mass spectrometry of derivatized intact oxazepam in urine. *Clin. Chem.*, **37**, 1595–1601

Laviola, G., De Acetis, L., Bignami, G. & Alleva, E. (1991) Prenatal oxazepam enhances mouse maternal aggression in the offspring, without modifying acute chlordiazepoxide effects. *Neurotoxicol. Teratol.*, **13**, 75–81

Laviola, G., Chiarotti, F. & Alleva, E. (1992a) Development of GABAergic modulation of mouse locomotor activity and pain sensitivity after prenatal benzodiazepine exposure. *Neurotoxicol. Teratol.*, **14**, 1–5

Laviola, G., Pick, C.G., Yanai, J. & Alleva, E. (1992b) Eight-arm maze performance, neophobia, and hippocampal cholinergic alterations after prenatal oxazepam in mice. *Brain Res. Bull.*, **29**, 609–616

Lensmeyer, G.L., Rajani, C. & Evenson, M.A. (1982) Liquid-chromatographic procedure for simultaneous analysis for eight benzodiazepines in serum. *Clin. Chem.*, **28**, 2274–2278

Löscher, W. (1982) Rapid gas-chromatographic measurement of diazepam and its metabolites desmethyldiazepam, oxazepam and 3-hydroxydiazepam (temazepam) in small samples of plasma. *Ther. Drug Monit.*, **4**, 315–318

Matula, T.I. & Downie, R. (1983) Evaluation of diazepam and oxazepam in in vitro microbial mutagenicity tests and in an in vivo promoter assay (Abstract no. Ee-23). *Environ. Mutag.*, **5**, 478

Maurer, H. & Pfleger, K. (1987) Identification and differentiation of benzodiazepines and their metabolites in urine by computerized gas chromatography-mass spectrometry. *J. Chromatogr.*, **422**, 85–101

Mazue, G., Remandet, B., Gouy, D., Berthe, J. & Roncucci, R. (1982) Limited in vivo bioassays on some benzodiazepines: lack of experimental initiating or promoting effect of the benzodiazepine tranquillizers diazepam, chlorazepate, oxazepam and lorazepam. *Arch. int. Pharmacodyn.*, **257**, 59–65

McCarley, T.D. & Brodbelt, J. (1993) Structurally diagnostic ion-molecule reactions and collisionally activated dissociation of 1,4-benzodiazepines in a quadrupole ion trap mass spectrometer. *Analyt. Chem.*, **65**, 2380–2388

Medical Economics (1996) *PDR®: Physicians' Desk Reference*, 50th Ed., Montvale, NJ, Medical Economics Data Production Co., pp. 2810–2811

Miller, R.P. & Becker, B.A. (1973) The teratogenicity of diazepam metabolites in Swiss-Webster mice (Abstract no. 37). *Toxicol. appl. Pharmacol.*, **25**, 453

Moutschen, J., Gilot-Delhalle, J. & Moutschen-Dahmen, M. (1987) Clastogenic effects of benzodiazepines in a *Nigella damascena* seed test. *Environ. exp. Botany*, **27**, 227–231

Mura, P., Piriou, A., Fraillon, P., Papet, Y. & Reiss, D. (1987) Screening procedure for benzodiazepines in biological fluids by high-performance liquid chromatography using a rapid-scanning multichannel detector. *J. Chromatogr.*, **416**, 303–310

Nau, H., Liddiard, C., Jesdinsky, D., Wittfoht, W. & Brendel, K. (1978) Quantitative analysis of prazepam and its metabolites by electron capture gas chromatography and selected ion monitoring. Application to diaplacental passage and fetal hepatic metabolism in early human pregnancy. *J. Chromatogr.*, **146**, 227–239

Owen, G., Smith, T.H.F. & Agersborg, H.P.K., Jr (1970) Toxicity of some benzodiazepine compounds with CNS activity. *Toxicol. appl. Pharmacol.*, **16**, 556–570

Peat, M.A. & Kopjak, L. (1979) Screening and quantitation of diazepam, flurazepam, chlordiazepoxide and their metabolites in blood and plasma by electron-capture gas chromatography and high-pressure liquid chromatography. *J. forensic Sci.*, **24**, 46–54

Prada, D., Vincente, J., Lorenzo, E., Blanco, M.H. & Hernández, L. (1988) Determination of 1,4-benzodiazepines by flow-injection analysis with spectrophotometric detection. *Quím. Anal. (Barcelona)*, **7**, 323–329 (in Spanish)

Préat, V., de Gerlache, J., Lans, M. & Roberfroid, M. (1987) Promoting effect of oxazepam in rat hepatocarcinogenesis. *Carcinogenesis*, **8**, 97–100

Remandet, B., Gouy, D., Berthe, J., Mazue, G. & Williams, G.M. (1984) Lack of initiating or promoting activity of six benzodiazepine tranquilizers in rat liver limited bioassays monitored by histopathology and assay of liver and plasma enzymes. *Fundam. appl. Toxicol.*, **4**, 152–163

Reynolds, J.E.F. (1993) *Martindale: The Extra Pharmacopoeia*, 30th Ed., London, The Pharmaceutical Press, pp. 607–608

Rolin-Limbosch, S., Moens, W. & Szpirer, C. (1987) Metabolic cooperation in SK-HEP-1 human hepatoma cells following treatment with benzodiazepine tranquilizers. *Carcinogenesis*, **8**, 1013–1016

Rosenberg, L., Palmer, J.R., Zauber, A.G., Warshauer, M.E., Strom, B.L., Harlap, S. & Shapiro, S. (1995) Relation of benzodiazepine use to the risk of selected cancers: breast, large bowel, malignant melanoma, lung, endometrium, ovary, non-Hodgkin's lymphoma, testis, Hodgkin's disease, thyroid, and liver. *Am. J. Epidemiol.*, **141**, 1153–1160

Ruelius, H.W., Tio, C.O., Knowles, J.A., McHugh, S.L., Schillings, R.T. & Sisenwine, S.F. (1979) Diastereoisomeric glucuronides of oxazepam. Isolation and stereoselective enzymic hydrolysis. *Drug Metab. Dispos.*, **7**, 40–43

Saito, H., Kobayashi, H., Takeno, S. & Sakai, T. (1984) Fetal toxicity of benzodiazepines in rats. *Res. Comm. chem. Pathol. Pharmacol.*, **46**, 437–447

Saxén, I. & Saxén, L. (1975) Association between maternal intake of diazepam and oral clefts (Letter to the Editor). *Lancet*, **ii**, 498

Scott, A.K., Khir, A.S.M., Bewsher, P.D. & Hawksworth, G.M. (1984) Oxazepam pharmacokinetics in thyroid disease. *Br. J. clin. Pharmacol.*, **17**, 49–53

Seideman, P., Ericsson, Ö., Gröningsson, K. & von Bahr, C. (1981) Effect of pentobarbital on the formation of diastereomeric oxazepam glucuronides in man: analysis by high performance liquid chromatography. *Acta pharmacol. toxicol.*, **49**, 200–204

Sellers, E.M., Greenblatt, D.J., Giles, H.G., Naranjo, C.A., Kaplan, H. & MacLeod, S.M. (1979) Chlordiazepoxide and oxazepam disposition in cirrhosis. *Clin. Pharmacol. Ther.*, **26**, 240–246

Serfaty, M. & Masterton, G. (1993) Fatal poisonings attributed to benzodiazepines in Britain during the 1980s. *Br. J. Psychiatr.*, **163**, 386–393

Shearer, C.M. & Pilla, C.R. (1974) Oxazepam. In: Florey, K., ed., *Analytical Profiles of Drug Substances*, Vol. 3, New York, Academic Press, pp. 441–464

Shull, H.J., Jr, Wilkinson, G.R., Johnson, R. & Schenker, S. (1976) Normal disposition of oxazepam in acute viral hepatitis and cirrhosis. *Ann. intern. Med.*, **84**, 420–425

Simon, A.R. & Sulik, K.K. (1992) Teratogenicity of oxazepam in C57Bl/6J mice (Abstract no. 204). *J. dent. Res.*, **71** (AADR Abstracts), 131

Simonsson, P., Lidén, A. & Lindberg, S. (1995) Effect of β-glucuronidase on urinary benzodiazepine concentrations determined by fluorescence polarization immunoassay. *Clin. Chem.*, **41**, 920–923

Sisenwine, S.F. & Tio, C.O. (1986) The metabolic disposition of oxazepam in rats. *Drug Metab. Dispos.*, **14**, 41–45

Sisenwine, S.F., Tio, C.O., Shrader, S.R. & Ruelius, H.W. (1972) The biotransformation of oxazepam (7-chloro-1,3-dihydro-3-hydroxy-5-phenyl-2*H*-1,4-benzodiazepin-2-one) in man, miniature swine and rat. *Arzneimittel-Forsch.*, **22**, 682–687

Sisenwine, S.F., Tio, C.O., Liu, A.L. & Politowski, J.F. (1987) The metabolic fate of oxazepam in mice. *Drug Metab. Dispos.*, **15**, 579–580

Sonne, J., Loft, S., Døssing, M., Vollmer-Larsen, A., Olesen, K.L., Victor, M., Andreasen, F. & Andreasen, P.B. (1988) Bioavailability and pharmacokinetics of oxazepam. *Eur. J. clin. Pharmacol.*, **35**, 385–389

Sonne, J., Boesgaard, S., Enghusen Poulsen, H., Loft, S., Mølholm Hansen, J., Døssing, M. & Andreasen, F. (1990) Pharmacokinetics and pharmacodynamics of oxazepam and metabolism of paracetamol in severe hypothyroidism. *Br. J. clin. Pharmacol.*, **30**, 737–742

Stopper, H., Körber, C., Spencer, D.L., Kirchner, S., Caspary, W.J. & Schiffmann, D. (1993) An investigation of micronucleus and mutation induction by oxazepam in mammalian cells. *Mutagenesis*, **8**, 449–455

St-Pierre, M.V., van den Berg, D. & Pang, K.S. (1990) Physiological modeling of drug and metabolite: disposition of oxazepam and oxazepam glucuronides in the recirculating perfused mouse liver preparation. *J. Pharmacokinet. Biopharmaceut.*, **18**, 423–448

Swierenga, S.H.H., Butler, S.G. & Hasnain, S.H. (1983) Activity of diazepam and oxazepam in various mammalian cell in vitro toxicity tests (Abstract no. Cd-16). *Environ. Mutag.*, **5**, 417

Thomas, J., ed. (1991) *Prescription Products Guide 1991*, 20th Ed., Victoria, Australian Pharmaceutical Publishing Co., pp. 248, 1160–1161, 1521

Tomson, G., Lunell, N.-O., Sundwall, A. & Rane, A. (1979) Placental passage of oxazepam and its metabolism in mother and newborn. *Clin. Pharmacol. Ther.*, **25**, 74–81

United States National Library of Medicine (1996) *RTECS Database*, Bethesda, MD

United States Pharmacopeial Convention (1994) *The 1995 US Pharmacopeia*, 23rd Rev./*The National Formulary*, 18th Rev., Rockville, MD, pp. 1123–1124

United States Tariff Commission (1967) *Synthetic Organic Chemicals, United States Production and Sales, 1965*, TC Publication 206, Washington DC, US Government Printing Office, p. 123

United States National Toxicology Program (1993) *Toxicology and Carcinogenesis Studies of Oxazepam (CAS No. 604-75-1) in Swiss-Webster and B6C3F1 Mice* (NTP TR No. 443; NIH Publication No. 93-3359), Research Triangle Park, NC, United States Department of Health and Human Services, National Institutes of Health

Van Baar, A.L., Fleury, P., Soepatmi, S., Ultee, C.A. & Wesselman, P.J.M. (1989) Neonatal behaviour after drug dependent pregnancy. *Arch. Dis. Child.*, **64**, 235–240

Verma, A. & Snyder, S.H. (1989) Peripheral type benzodiazepine receptors. *Annu. Rev. Pharmacol. Toxicol.*, **29**, 307–322

Vidal (1995) *Dictionnaire Vidal*, 71st Ed., Paris, Editions du Vidal, pp. 1347–1348

Viggedal, G., Hagberg, B.S., Laegreid, L. & Aronsson, M. (1993) Mental development in late infancy after prenatal exposure to benzodiazepines — A prospective study. *J. Child Psychol. Psychiat.*, **34**, 295–305

Walash, M.I., Belal, F., Metwally, M.E. & Hefnawy, M.M. (1994) A selective fluorimetric method for the determination of some 1,4-benzodiazepine drugs containing a hydroxyl group at C-3. *J. pharm. biomed. Anal.*, **12**, 1417–1423

Winter, R.M. (1987) In-utero exposure to benzodiazepines (Letter to the Editor). *Lancet*, **i**, 627

Wong, P.T.H. & Teo, W.L. (1992) Mortality in Swiss albino mice after i.p. injection of oxazepam in dimethyl sulphoxide. *Exp. Anim.*, **41**, 247–249

Wretlind, M. (1987) Excretion of oxazepam in breast milk. *Eur. J. clin. Pharmacol.*, **33**, 209–210

Yuan, J., Goehl, T.J., Hong, L., Clark, J., Murrill, E. & Moore, R. (1994) Toxicokinetics of oxazepam in rats and mice. *J. pharm. Sci.*, **83**, 1373–1379

PRAZEPAM

1. Exposure Data

1.1 Chemical and physical data

1.1.1 Nomenclature

Chem. Abstr. Serv. Reg. No.: 2955-38-6

Chem. Abstr. Name: 7-Chloro-1-(cyclopropylmethyl)-1,3-dihydro-5-phenyl-2H-1,4-benzodiazepin-2-one

IUPAC Systematic Name: 7-Chloro-1-(cyclopropylmethyl)-1,3-dihydro-5-phenyl-2H-1,4-benzodiazepin-2-one

1.1.2 Structural and molecular formulae and relative molecular mass

$C_{19}H_{17}ClN_2O$ Relative molecular mass: 324.81

1.1.3 Chemical and physical properties of the pure substance

(a) *Description*: Colourless crystalline powder (Gennaro, 1995)

(b) *Melting-point*: 145–146 °C (Budavari, 1995)

(c) *Solubility*: Practically insoluble in water [1 g/more than 10 000 mL]; sparingly soluble in anhydrous ethanol and diethyl ether; soluble in acetone, chloroform and acetic anhydride (Society of Japanese Pharmacopoeia, 1992; Gennaro, 1995)

(d) *Octanol/water partition coefficient (P)*: log P, 3.7 (Dollery *et al.*, 1991)

1.1.4 Technical products and impurities

Prazepam is available as 10- and 20-mg tablets, 16.5-mg 'drops' and 5-, 10- and 20-mg capsules which also may contain anhydrous ethanol, corn starch, flavouring, lactose, magnesium stearate, microgranular cellulose, polyethylene glycol 400, precipitated silica, propylene glycol, sodium saccharin, sodium lauryl sulfate, colloidal silicon dioxide, titanium dioxide, E 132 (Indigo carmine), D&C Yellow no. 10 (Quinoline Yellow), FD&C Blue no. 1 (Brilliant Blue FCF), FD&C Yellow 6 (Sunset Yellow FCF), FD&C green no. 3 (Fast Green FCF) (Farmindustria, 1993; Medical Economics, 1996).

Trade names and designations of the chemical and its pharmaceutical preparations include: Centrax; Demetrin; Equipaz; K 373; Lysanxia; Mono Demetrin; Prazene; Reapam; Sedapran; Settima; Trepidan; Verstran; W-4020.

1.1.5 *Analysis*

Several international pharmacopoeias specify potentiometric titration with perchloric acid as the assay for purity of prazepam and thin-layer chromatography for determining impurities and decomposition products. The assays for prazepam in capsules and tablets apply liquid chromatography or potentiometric titration with perchloric acid using standards. An assay for heavy metal impurities is also specified (Society of Japanese Pharmacopoeia, 1992; United States Pharmacopeial Convention, 1994). Spectrophotometry has also been used in the analysis for prazepam in pharmaceutical preparations (El-Yazbi *et al.*, 1986; Mañes *et al.*, 1987; Prada *et al.*, 1988).

Prazepam and its metabolites (including oxazepam) can be analysed in biological fluids by radioimmunoassay (Köhler-Schmidt & Bohn, 1983), electron capture gas chromatography (Nau *et al.*, 1978, Peat & Kopjak, 1979), gas chromatography with flame ionization detection (Quaglio & Bellini, 1984), gas chromatography–mass spectrometry (Maurer & Pfleger, 1987) and high-performance liquid chromatography (Peat & Kopjak, 1979; Lensmeyer *et al.*, 1982).

1.2 Production and use

1.2.1 *Production*

Prazepam is prepared by acylating 2-amino-5-chlorobenzophenone with cyclopropanecarbonyl chloride using triethylamine as an acid-receptor. The product is reduced with lithium aluminium hydride to give 2-cyclopropylmethylamino-5-chlorobenzhydrol, which is then oxidized with manganese dioxide to the corresponding benzophenone. This is acylated with phthalimidoacetyl chloride and the product cyclized with hydrazine hydrate to produce prazepam (Gennaro, 1995).

1.2.2 *Use*

Prazepam is a benzodiazepine used for the treatment of anxiety disorders (see the monograph on diazepam, pp. 39–41, for a brief overview of the pharmacology of therapeutic action for this class of drugs). The optimal dosage in adults, adjusted to the response of the patient, is usually 20–40 mg daily in divided doses or as a single nightly dose. In severe conditions, up to 60 mg daily has been given. In elderly or debilitated patients, treatment should be initiated with a daily dose of 10–15 mg (Reynolds, 1993).

Clinical uses of prazepam and other benzodiazepines have been reviewed (Hollister et al., 1993). Prazepam was approved for use in the United States of America in 1976 and, in France, it was first marketed in 1979 (Parke-Davis, 1996).

Comparative data on sales of prazepam in several countries are shown in Table 1. Overall, sales worldwide declined by approximately 24% from 1990 to 1995 and prescriptions in the United States dropped to almost nil (see Table 2 in the monograph on diazepam, p. 43).

Table 1. Sales of prazepam in various countries^a (no. of standard units^b, in thousands)

Country	1990	1995	Country	1990	1995
Africa			Europe		
South Africa	2 492	1 819	Belgium	10 913	9 900
North America			France	185 801	190 175
United States	65 399	1	Germany	15 246	8 702
South America			Greece	9 908	6 002
Argentina	480	239	Italy	45 244	41 032
Colombia	0	24	Netherlands	2 582	2 036
Asia			Portugal	206	962
Japan	14 161	8 074	Spain	1 515	1 165
Republic of Korea	4 205	2 947	Switzerland	3 454	2 836

^{a} Data provided by IMS
^{b} Standard dosage units, uncorrected for prazepam content

1.3 Occurrence

Prazepam is not known to occur as a natural product.

No quantitative data on occupational exposure levels were available to the Working Group.

The National Occupational Exposure Survey conducted between 1981 and 1983 in the United States by the National Institute for Occupational Safety and Health indicated that about 100 employees were potentially occupationally exposed to prazepam. The estimate was based on a survey of United States companies and did not involve measurements of actual exposure (United States National Library of Medicine, 1996).

1.4 Regulations and guidelines

Prazepam is listed in the French, Japanese and United States pharmacopoeias (Reynolds, 1993; Vidal, 1995).

2. Studies of Cancer in Humans

No data were available to the Working Group (see the monograph on diazepam, pp. 44–54, for a discussion of benzodiazepines).

3. Studies of Cancer in Experimental Animals

3.1 Oral administration

3.1.1 *Mouse*

Groups of 100 male and 100 female albino CF1 (control) or 50 male and 50 female mice (treated), eight weeks of age, were given 0, 8, 25 or 75 mg/kg bw prazepam (99% pure) mixed in the diet for up to 80 weeks. The prazepam concentration in the food was adjusted weekly for changes in body weight and food consumption. The prazepam/diet mixtures were prepared freshly each week. In treated mice, body-weight gains were similar to those of controls throughout the study. From graphic presentations, there appeared to be no significant effect on mortality (60–70% survival for males and females) [statistics and exact numbers not given.] All surviving animals were killed at 80 weeks. Major organs [unspecified] and visually apparent lesions were examined histologically. No significant increase in the incidence of tumours at any site was seen for either male or female mice. Data on incidence of hepatocellular tumours are presented in Table 2 (de la Iglesia *et al.*, 1981). [The Working Group noted that the study was terminated at 80 weeks.]

3.1.2 *Rat*

Groups of 115 male and 115 female SPF albino Wistar rats (control) or 65 male and 65 female rats (treated), eight weeks of age, were given 0, 8, 25 or 75 mg/kg bw prazepam (99% purity) mixed in the diet for up to 104 weeks. The prazepam concentration in the food was adjusted weekly for changes in body weight and food consumption. The prazepam/diet mixtures were prepared freshly each week. In treated rats, body-weight gains were similar to those of controls throughout the study. There appeared to be no significant effect on mortality (50–60% survival for males and about 60% for females) [statistics and exact numbers not given]. All surviving animals were killed at 104 weeks. Major organs [not specified] and visually apparent lesions were examined histologically. No significant increase in the incidence of tumours was seen for either male or female rats. Data on incidences of hepatocellular tumours are presented in Table 2 (de la Iglesia *et al.*, 1981).

3.2 Carcinogenicity of metabolites

See the monograph on oxazepam (pp. 119–123).

Table 2. Incidence of benign and malignant hepatocellular tumours in mice and rats treated with prazepam

Dose (mg/kg bw)	Mouse				Rat			
	Benign		Malignant		Benign		Malignant	
	Male	Female	Male	Female	Male	Female	Male	Female
0	1/100	1/100	7/100	1/100	1/115	1/115	0/115	0/115
8	0/50	1/50	5/50	0/50	0/65	0/65	0/65	0/65
25	1/50	2/50	4/50	1/50	2/65	1/65	1/65	0/65
75	1/50	0/50	4/50	0/50	1/65	3/65	1/65	0/65

From de la Iglesia *et al.* (1981)

4. Other Data Relevant to an Evaluation of Carcinogenicity and its Mechanisms

4.1 Absorption, distribution, metabolism and excretion

4.1.1 *Humans*

Prazepam is rapidly absorbed after oral administration, the peak plasma concentration of the unchanged compound appearing within 0.5 h. While some authors have not seen measurable concentrations of prazepam in plasma after dosing with tablets, Smith *et al.* (1979) detected low concentrations (> 2.5 ng/mL) for brief periods in four of nine subjects after ingestion of tablets and in all nine subjects after ingestion of a solution. The bioavailability from tablets relative to the solution was 86%. The elimination half-life of the parent drug was approximately 1 h. The major non-conjugated compound in plasma was the N-dealkylated metabolite, N-desmethyldiazepam. Peak plasma concentrations of N-desmethyldiazepam following oral administration of prazepam tablets have been reported to be 321 ± 76 ng/mL at 4.25 ± 1.75 h (30-mg dose; Smith *et al.*, 1979), 235 ± 68 ng/mL at 12 h (30-mg dose; Chasseaud *et al.*, 1980) and 105 ± 12 ng/mL at 9.2 ± 3 h (20-mg dose; Greenblatt *et al.*, 1988). Allen *et al.* (1980) reported differences according to age and sex, with average peak plasma levels of 92–142 ng/mL being reached in an average of 10–20 h. The elimination half-life of N-desmethyldiazepam in these studies was reported to be 96 ± 34 h (Smith *et al.*, 1979), 82 [± 23 h] (Chasseaud *et al.*, 1980) and ranging from 29 to 224 h (Allen *et al.*, 1980). In this last study, the elimination half-life increased with age in men, but not in women. The major metabolic pathways of prazepam are N-dealkylation (Allen *et al.*, 1979; Chasseaud *et al.*, 1980) and 3-hydroxylation (DiCarlo *et al.*, 1970). The glucuronides of 3-hydroxyprazepam and oxazepam are the main metabolites eliminated in urine (Figure 1). Neither prazepam nor N-desmethyldiazepam was detected in 24-h urine samples of women given three 10-mg prazepam capsules (Chasseaud *et al.*, 1980).

Figure 1. Postulated metabolic pathways of prazepam

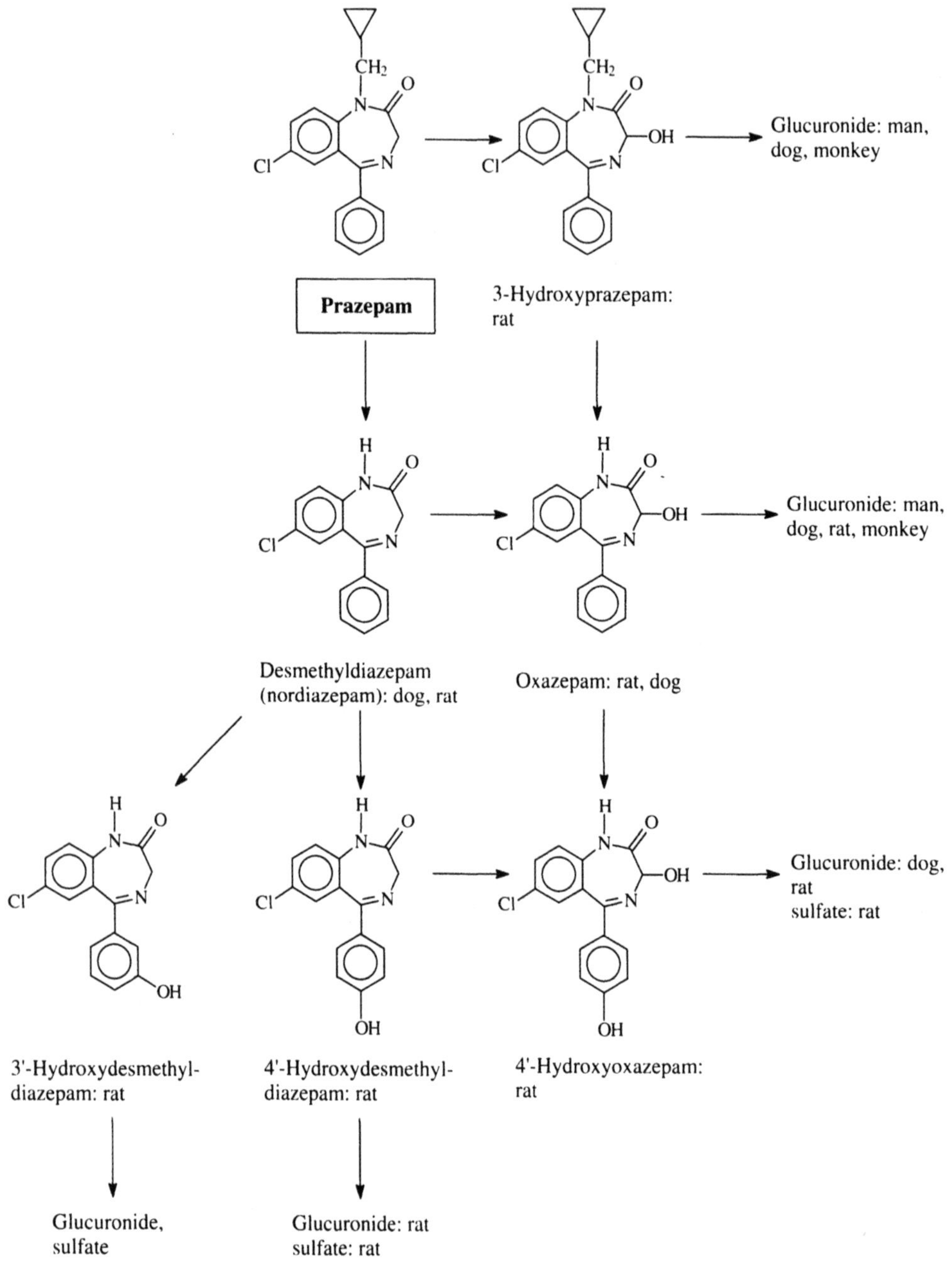

From Viau *et al.* (1973); Ishihama *et al.* (1978)

The plasma half-lives of [^{14}C]prazepam and of antipyrine were increased in male volunteers pretreated with unlabelled prazepam (0.4 mg/kg/day) for seven days (Vesell et al., 1972).

4.1.2 Experimental systems

Prazepam metabolism has been studied in rats, dogs and monkeys. Prazepam is well absorbed after oral dosing in rats, and is rapidly and extensively metabolized. In the rat, the plasma half-life of prazepam and its metabolites was 2.5 h (Viau et al., 1973). Nine identified metabolites in urine together accounted for only 50% of the dose of radio-isotope, while faecal excretion of radioisotope exceeded urinary excretion. The major pathway was N-dealkylation, and all identified metabolites were derived from N-des-methyldiazepam. Hydroxylation at the 4-position of the 5-phenyl ring (4′-hydroxylation) was extensive. Ishihama et al. (1978) additionally found substantial amounts of 3′-hydroxydesmethyldiazepam in urine and faeces. Both groups noted substantial amounts of unidentified polar metabolites. Metabolism in dogs was more similar to the pattern in humans. The major metabolite was oxazepam (excreted as the glucuronide), and smaller amounts of 3-hydroxyprazepam and 4′-hydroxyoxazepam (excreted as the glucuronides) were recovered (DiCarlo et al., 1969; DiCarlo & Viau, 1970). An even closer parallel to the human pattern was seen in cynomolgus monkeys, which excreted principally oxazepam and 3-hydroxyprazepam glucuronides, with only trace amounts of 4′-hydroxy-desmethyldiazepam, as the sulfate conjugate (Kabuto et al., 1978).

A preponderance of N-dealkylation over C_3-hydroxylation of prazepam was shown in metabolic studies using liver microsomes from Sprague-Dawley rats in vitro, pretreated with phenobarbital (Lu & Yang, 1989; Hooper et al., 1992). This was also shown for humans (Lu et al., 1991); these workers additionally showed that the 3-hydroxyprazepam was formed stereoselectively, with the 3R-enantiomer predominating in both rats and humans.

4.2 Toxic effects

4.2.1 Humans

(a) Acute toxicity

Prazepam has no significant effect on the cardiovascular system; however, respiratory depression may be observed following large doses or in sensitive individuals with chronic obstructive airway diseases (reviewed by Dollery et al., 1991). In a review of fatal poisoning attributed to benzodiazepines in the United Kingdom during the 1980s, only one lethal intoxication with prazepam was recorded (Serfaty & Masterton, 1993).

(b) Chronic toxicity

There is no evidence to suggest that prazepam causes any organ toxicity other than effects associated with its pharmacological action on the central nervous system (reviewed by Dollery et al., 1991).

4.2.2 *Experimental systems*

(a) *Acute toxicity*

Prazepam given intravenously to cats, dogs and rabbits caused convulsions at all doses (1–8 mg/kg bw) investigated. In contrast, oral administration of 3–36 mg/kg bw prazepam to mice suppressed convulsions induced by pentylenetetrazol, strychnine or electroshock with a similar potency to other benzodiazepines (Robichaud et al., 1970). Intravenous administration of prazepam to dogs at doses of up to 10 mg/kg did not induce significant autonomic or cardiovascular effects.

(b) *Subacute and chronic toxicity*

In male Sprague-Dawley rats, intraperitoneal administration of 100 mg/kg bw prazepam for four days resulted in increased levels of hepatic microsomal cytochrome P450 and increased activities of hepatic ethylmorphine N-demethylase and aniline hydroxylase (Vesell et al., 1972).

4.3 Reproductive and prenatal effects

4.3.1 *Humans*

No data were available to the Working Group

4.3.2 *Experimental systems*

Prazepam increased the incidence of congenital anomalies (mainly short tail and hydrops fetalis (subcutaneous oedema)) in rats. Body weights and organ weights of the offspring of rats treated orally with a daily dose of 100 mg/kg bw prazepam were decreased, but there was no adverse effect on behaviour, emotionality or learning ability of offspring (Kuriyama et al., 1978a; Ota et al., 1979a).

The fertility of male rats was suppressed by five weeks' treatment with 1000 mg/kg prazepam due to the retardation of spermatogenesis. Mating performance and fertility of female rats were inhibited by oral treatment with a daily dose of 1000 mg/kg prazepam, but recovered soon after discontinuation of treatment (Kuriyama et al., 1978b) and Ota et al. (1979a) found no adverse effect on the fertility of the offspring.

No increase in the occurrence of congenital abnormalities was observed in rabbits which received daily oral doses of 5, 12.5, 25 or 50 mg/kg bw on gestational days 6–18 (Ota et al., 1979b).

Chronic dietary administration of prazepam to breeding pairs of Swiss-Webster mice caused a significant decrease in mating performance and body weights at birth (Guerriero & Fox, 1976). Female mice which received prazepam prenatally had delay in the age of vaginal opening; however, the age of first oestrus was generally younger than that of controls due to disruption of normal hypothalamic-pituitary relations (Fox & Guerriero, 1978). Male mice which received prazepam prenatally and during early infancy exhibited enhanced performance of a Y-maze task as adults. The drug produced its greatest effects on learning measures when given prenatally (Fox et al., 1977).

4.4 Genetic and related effects (see also Table 3 for references and Appendices 1 and 2)

No chromosomal damage was observed in *Nigella damascena*. No increase in DNA single-strand breaks and/or alkali-labile sites was observed in the liver of rats given orally a single dose or multiple daily doses of prazepam.

Table 3. Genetic and related effects of prazepam

Test system	Result[a]		Dose[b] (LED/HID)	Reference
	Without exogenous metabolic system	With exogenous metabolic system		
PLC, *Nigella damascena*, chromosomal aberrations	–	NT	50	Moutschen et al. (1987)
DVA, DNA strand breaks, rat liver in vivo	–		325 po × 1	Carlo et al. (1989)
DVA, DNA strand breaks, rat liver in vivo	–		65 po × 15	Carlo et al. (1989)

[a] +, positive; (+), weak positive; –, negative; NT, not tested; ?, inconclusive
[b] LED, lowest effective dose; HID, highest ineffective dose; in-vitro tests, µg/mL; in-vivo tests, mg/kg bw/day

5. Summary of Data Reported and Evaluation

5.1 Exposure data

Prazepam is a benzodiazepine used since the late 1970s for treatment of anxiety.

5.2 Human carcinogenicity data

No data were available to the Working Group.

5.3 Animal carcinogenicity data

Prazepam was tested for carcinogenicity in one experiment in mice and in one experiment in rats by oral administration in the diet. No significant increase in the incidence of tumours was found.

5.4 Other relevant data

Prazepam is rapidly and extensively absorbed in humans, but its plasma concentrations are low and of short duration as a consequence of its rapid conversion to *N*-desmethyldiazepam and, to a lesser extent, 3-hydroxyprazepam. The elimination half-life is about 1 h.

Prazepam is extensively metabolized in rats, and the primary metabolite N-desmethyldiazepam is further converted to at least eight derivatives. Oxazepam is the major metabolite in dogs and monkeys.

There is no evidence to suggest that prazepam causes any organ toxicity other than effects associated with its pharmacological action on the central nervous system in humans or experimental animals.

There are no data on the teratogenicity of prazepam in humans. In one study, prazepam increased the incidence of short tail and hydrops fetalis (subcutaneous oedema) in rats. In a single study in the rabbit, it was not teratogenic.

The two available studies on genetic effects were negative.

5.5 Evaluation[1]

There is *inadequate evidence* in humans for the carcinogenicity of prazepam.

There is *inadequate evidence* in experimental animals for the carcinogenicity of prazepam.

Overall evaluation

Prazepam is *not classifiable as to its carcinogenicity to humans (Group 3)*.

6. References

Allen, M.D., Greenblatt, D.J., Harmatz, J.S. & Shader, R.I. (1979) Single-dose kinetics of prazepam, a precursor of desmethyldiazepam. *J. clin. Pharmacol.*, **19**, 445–450

Allen, M.D., Greenblatt, D.J., Harmatz, J.S. & Shader, R.I. (1980) Desmethyldiazepam kinetics in the elderly after oral prazepam. *Clin. Pharmacol. Ther.*, **28**, 196–202

Budavari, S., ed. (1995) *The Merck Index*, 12th Ed., Rahway, NJ, Merck & Co.

Carlo, P., Finollo, R., Ledda, A. & Brambilla, G. (1989) Absence of liver DNA fragmentation in rats treated with high oral doses of 32 benzodiazepine drugs. *Fundam. appl. Toxicol.*, **12**, 34–41

Chasseaud, L.F., Taylor, T. & Brodie, R.R. (1980) Prazepam metabolism in female subjects. *J. Pharm. Pharmacol.*, **32**, 652–653

DiCarlo, F.J., & Viau, J.-P. (1970) Prazepam metabolites in dog urine. *J. pharm. Sci.*, **59**, 322–325

DiCarlo, F.J., Crew, M.C., Melgar, M.D. & Haynes, L.J. (1969) Prazepam metabolism by dogs. *J. pharm. Sci.*, **58**, 960–962

DiCarlo, F.J., Viau, J.-P., Epps, J.E. & Haynes, L.J. (1970) Prazepam metabolism by man. *Clin. Pharmacol. Ther.*, **11**, 890–897

---

[1]For definition of the italicized terms, see Preamble, pp. 22–25.

Dollery, C., Boobis, A.R., Burley, D., Davies, D.M., Davies, D.S., Harrison, P.I., Orme, M.E., Park, B.K. & Goldberg, L.I. (1991) *Therapeutic Drugs, Prazepam*, Edinburgh, Churchill Livingstone, pp. P186–P189

El-Yazbi, F.A., Abdel-Hay, M.H. & Korany, M.A. (1986) Spectrophotometric determination of some 1,4-benzodiazepines by use of orthogonal polynomials. *Pharmazie*, **41**, 639–642

Farmindustria (1993) *Repertorio Farmaceutico Italiano* (Italian Pharmaceutical Directory), 7th Ed., Milan, Associazione Nazionale dell'Industria Farmaceutica, CEDOF S.P.A., pp. A-1212–A1213; A-1542–A-1543

Fox, K.A. & Guerriero, F.J. (1978) Effect of benzodiazepines on age of vaginal perforation and first estrus in mice. *Res. Commun. chem. Pathol. Pharmacol.*, **21**, 181–184

Fox, K.A., Abendschein, D.R. & Lahcen, R.B. (1977) Effects of benzodiazepines during gestation and infancy on Y-maze performance of mice. *Pharmacol. Res. Comm.*, **9**, 325–338

Gennaro, A.R., ed. (1995) *Remington: The Science and Practice of Pharmacy*, 19th Ed., Vol. II, Easton, PA, Mack Publishing Co., p. 1160

Greenblatt, D.J., Harmatz, J.S., Dorsey, C. & Shader, R.I. (1988) Comparative single-dose kinetics and dynamics of lorazepam, alprazolam, prazepam, and placebo. *Clin. Pharmacol. Ther.*, **44**, 326–334

Guerriero, F.J. & Fox, K.A. (1976) Benzodiazepines and reproduction of Swiss-Webster mice. *Res. Commun. chem. Pathol. Pharmacol.*, **13**, 601–610

Hollister, L.E., Müller-Oerlinghausen, B., Rickels, K. & Shader, R.I. (1993) Clinical uses of benzodiazepines. *J. clin. Psychopharmacol.*, **13** (Suppl. 1)

Hooper, W.D., Bruce, I. & Reilly, P.E.B. (1992) Comparative metabolism of clinically important precursors of N-desmethyldiazepam using phenobarbitone-pretreated rat liver microsomes. *Biochem. Pharmacol.*, **43**, 1377–1380

de la Iglesia, F.A., Barsoum, N., Gough, A., Mitchell, L., Martin, R.A., Di Fonzo, C. & McGuire, E.J. (1981) Carcinogenesis bioassay of prazepam (Verstran) in rats and mice. *Toxicol. appl. Pharmacol.*, **57**, 39–54

Ishihama, H., Kabuto, S., Kimata, H., Tamaki, T. & Yonemitsu, M. (1978) Studies on metabolism of prazepam. I. Metabolic fate of prazepam in rats. *Yakugaku Zasshi*, **98**, 720–736 (in Japanese)

Kabuto, S., Tamaki, T., Koide, T. & Ishihama, H. (1978) Studies on metabolism of prazepam. IV. Metabolic fate of prazepam in monkeys. *Yakugaku Zasshi*, **98**, 944–949 (in Japanese)

Köhler-Schmidt, H. & Bohn, G. (1983) Radioimmunoassay for determination of prazepam and its metabolites. *Forensic Sci. int.*, **22**, 243–248

Kuriyama, T., Nishigaki, K., Ota, T., Koga, T., Okubo, M. & Otani, G. (1978a) Safety studies of prazepam (K-373). (VI) Teratological study in rats. *Oyo Yakuri*, **15**, 797–811 (in Japanese)

Kuriyama, T., Ota, T., Nishigaki, K., Koga, T. & Otani, G. (1978b) Safety studies of prazepam (K-373). (VII). Study of fertility and general reproductive performance in rats. *Oyo Yakuri*, **15**, 813–828 (in Japanese)

Lensmeyer, G.L., Rajani, C. & Evenson, M.A. (1982) Liquid-chromatographic procedure for simultaneous analysis for eight benzodiazepines in serum. *Clin. Chem.*, **28**, 2274–2278

Lu, X.-L. & Yang, S.K. (1989) Metabolism of prazepam by rat liver microsomes: stereoselective formation and N-dealkylation of 3-hydroxyprazepam. *Mol. Pharmacol.*, **36**, 932–938

Lu, X.-L., Guengerich, F.P. & Yang, S.K. (1991) Stereoselective metabolism of prazepam and halazepam by human liver microsomes. *Drug Metab. Dispos.*, **19**, 637–642

Mañes, J., Civera, J., Font, G. & Bosch, F. (1987) Spectrophotometric determination of benzodiazepines in pharmaceuticals by ion pairing. *Cienc. ind. Farm.*, **6**, 333–338 (in Spanish)

Maurer, H. & Pfleger, K. (1987) Identification and differentiation of benzodiazepines and their metabolites in urine by computerized gas chromatography-mass spectrometry. *J. Chromatogr.*, **422**, 85–101

Medical Economics (1996) *PDR®: Physicians' Desk Reference*, 50th Ed., Montvale, NJ, Medical Economics Data Production Co., pp. 1721–1722

Moutschen, J., Gilot-Delhalle, J. & Moutschen-Dahmen, M. (1987) Clastogenic effects of benzodiazepines in a *Nigella damascena* seed test. *Environ. exp. Botany*, **27**, 227–231

Nau, H., Liddiard, C., Jesdinsky, D., Wittfoht, W. & Brendel, K. (1978) Quantitative analysis of prazepam and its metabolites by electron capture gas chromatography and selected ion monitoring: application to diaplacental passage and fetal hepatic metabolism in early human pregnancy. *J. Chromatogr.*, **146**, 227–239

Ota, T., Nishigaki, K., Kuriyama, T., Koga, T. & Otani, G. (1979a) Safety studies of prazepam (K-373). (9) Perinatal and postnatal studies in rats. *Oyo Yakuri*, **17**, 833–848 (in Japanese)

Ota, T., Okubo, M., Kuriyama, T., Koga, T. & Otani, G. (1979b) Safety studies of prazepam (K-373). (8) Teratological study in rabbits. *Oyo Yakuri*, **17**, 673–681 (in Japanese)

Parke-Davis (1996) *Prazepam*, Ann Arbor, MI

Peat, M.A. & Kopjak, L. (1979) Screening and quantitation of diazepam, flurazepam, chlordiazepoxide and their metabolites in blood and plasma by electron-capture gas chromatography and high-pressure liquid chromatography. *J. forensic Sci.*, **24**, 46–54

Prada, D., Vincente, J., Lorenzo, E., Blanco, M.H. & Hernández, L. (1988) Determination of 1,4-benzodiazepines by flow-injection analysis with spectrophotometric detection. *Quím. Analít. (Barcelona)*, **7**, 323–329 (in Spanish)

Quaglio, M.P. & Bellini, A.M. (1984) Simultaneous determination of maprotiline and some benzodiazepines in human plasma by gas chromatography. *Farmaco Ed. Prat.*, **39**, 431–437 (in Italian)

Reynolds, J.E.F., ed. (1993) *Martindale: The Extra Pharmacopoeia*, 30th Ed., London, The Pharmaceutical Press, pp. 611–612

Robichaud, R.C., Gylys, J.A., Sledge, K.L. & Hillyard, I.W. (1970) The pharmacology of prazepam, a new benzodiazepine derivative. *Arch. int. Pharmacodyn.*, **185**, 213–227

Serfaty, M. & Masterton, G. (1993) Fatal poisonings attributed to benzodiazepines in Britain during the 1980s. *Br. J. Psychiatr.*, **163**, 386–393

Smith, M.T., Evans, L.E.J., Eadie, M.J. & Tyrer, J.H. (1979) Pharmacokinetics of prazepam in man. *Eur. J. clin. Pharmacol.*, **16**, 141–147

Society of Japanese Pharmacopoeia (1992) *The Pharmacopoeia of Japan JP XII*, 12th Ed., Tokyo, pp. 462–464

United States National Library of Medicine (1996) *RTECS Database*, Bethesda, MD

United States Pharmacopeial Convention (1994) *The 1995 US Pharmacopeia*, 23rd Rev./*The National Formulary*, 18th Rev., Rockville, MD, pp. 1272–1274

Vesell, E.S., Passananti, G.T., Viau, J.-P., Epps, J.E. & DiCarlo, F.J. (1972) Effects of chronic prazepam administration on drug metabolism in man and rat. *Pharmacology*, **7**, 197–206

Viau, J.-P., Epps, J.E. & DiCarlo, F.J. (1973) Prazepam metabolism in the rat. *J. pharm. Sci.*, **62**, 641–645

Vidal (1995) *Dictionnaire* Vidal, 71st Ed., Paris, Editions du Vidal, pp. 876–877

RIPAZEPAM

1. Exposure Data

1.1 Chemical and physical data

1.1.1 *Nomenclature*

Chem. Abstr. Serv. Reg. No.: 26308-28-1

Chem. Abstr. Name: 1-Ethyl-4,6-dihydro-3-methyl-8-phenylpyrazolo[4,3-e][1,4]diazepin-5(1H)-one

IUPAC Systematic Name: 1-Ethyl-4,6-dihydro-3-methyl-8-phenylpyrazolo[4,3-e]-[1,4]diazepin-5(1H)-one

1.1.2 *Structural and molecular formulae and relative molecular mass*

$C_{15}H_{16}N_4O$ \hfill Relative molecular mass: 268.32

1.1.3 *Chemical and physical properties of the pure substance*

(a) *Description*: Pale-yellow crystalline solid (Fitzgerald *et al.*, 1984)

(b) *Melting-point*: 221–223 °C (DeWald *et al.*, 1973)

1.1.4 *Technical products and impurities*

One trade name of the chemical is available: Pyrazapon.

1.1.5 *Analysis*

No information on the analysis of ripazepam was available to the Working Group.

1.2 Production and use

1.2.1 Production

Ripazepam can be prepared by reacting 4-amino-1-ethyl-3-methylpyrazol-5-yl phenyl ketone and glycine ethyl ester hydrochloride in piperidine/pyridine solvent. The resulting intermediate is reacted with ammonium hydroxide in dichloromethane/ethyl acetate, and ripazepam is recrystallized from toluene (DeWald *et al.*, 1973).

1.2.2 Use

Ripazepam is a pyrazolodiazepine that demonstrated anxiolytic effects in pharmacological tests in animals, but was apparently never marketed for human use (Poschel *et al.*, 1974; Fitzgerald *et al.*, 1984).

1.3 Occurrence

Ripazepam is not known to occur as a natural product.

1.4 Regulations and guidelines

No information was available to the Working Group.

2. Studies of Cancer in Humans

No data were available to the Working Group.

3. Studies of Cancer in Experimental Animals

3.1 Oral administration

3.1.1 Mouse

Groups of 50 male and 50 female albino CD-1 mice, five to six weeks of age, were given 0, 15 or 150 mg/kg bw ripazepam (100% pure) in the diet for up to 78 weeks. The ripazepam concentration in the food was adjusted weekly for changes in body weight and food consumption. The ripazepam/diet mixtures were prepared freshly each week and offered *ad libitum*. In treated mice, body-weight gains exceeded those of controls at both doses in females and at 15 mg/kg bw in the males. Food consumption was similar in control and treated mice. From graphic presentations, there appeared to be a slight increase in mortality among high-dose males beginning at about week 40. Mortality rates were similar in all groups of female mice [statistics and exact numbers not given]. At 78 weeks, survival was 60–70% in all groups and all surviving animals were killed. Major organs [not specified] and visually apparent lesions were examined histologically. Data on the incidence of liver tumours are presented in Table 1 (Fitzgerald *et al.*, 1984).

Table 1. Incidence of benign and malignant hepatocellular tumours in mice and rats treated with ripazepam

Dose (mg/kg bw)	Mouse				Rat			
	Adenoma (neoplastic nodules)		Carcinoma		Adenoma (neoplastic nodules)		Carcinoma	
	Male	Female	Male	Female	Male	Female	Male	Female
0	10/50	5/50	0/50	0/50	5/50	4/50	0/50	0/50
15	15/50	2/50	0/50	0/50	4/50	6/50	0/50	0/50
150	33/50	11/50	1/50	0/50	9/50	6/50	1/50	2/50

From Fitzgerald *et al.* (1984)

3.1.2 *Rat*

Groups of 50 male and 50 female albino CD rats, five to six weeks of age, were given 0, 15 or 150 mg/kg bw ripazepam (100% pure) in the diet for up to 104 weeks. The ripazepam concentration in the food was adjusted weekly for changes in body weight and food consumption. The ripazepam/diet mixtures were prepared freshly each week and offered *ad libitum*. In treated rats, body-weight gains were depressed by 21% in male and by 36% in female rats given 150 mg/kg bw ripazepam. Food consumption was decreased slightly (7%) only in female rats at the 150-mg/kg dose. Mortality rates were similar in all groups. All surviving animals were killed at 104 weeks. Histological examinations were performed on major organs [not specified] and visually apparent lesions. An increase in centrilobular hypertrophy of hepatocytes, primarily at the 150-mg/kg bw dose level, was observed in treated rats. No significant increase in the incidence of tumours in treated groups was observed for either sex. Data on the incidence of liver tumours are presented in Table 1 (Fitzgerald *et al.*, 1984).

4. Other Data Relevant to an Evaluation of Carcinogenicity and its Mechanisms

No data were available to the Working Group.

5. Summary of Data Reported and Evaluation

5.1 Exposure data

Ripazepam is a pyrazolodiazepine with anxiolytic properties which has never been marketed for human use.

5.2 Human carcinogenicity data

No data were available to the Working Group.

5.3 Animal carcinogenicity data

Ripazepam was tested for carcinogenicity in one experiment in mice and in one experiment in rats by oral administration in the diet. An increased incidence of benign liver tumours was found in male mice. No increase in the incidence of tumours was found in female mice or in rats of either sex.

5.4 Other relevant data

No data were available to the Working Group on the metabolism, toxicity, reproductive or genetic and related effects of ripazepam.

5.5 Evaluation[1]

There is *inadequate evidence* in humans for the carcinogenicity of ripazepam.

There is *limited evidence* in experimental animals for the carcinogenicity of ripazepam.

Overall evaluation

Ripazepam is *not classifiable as to its carcinogenicity to humans (Group 3)*.

6. References

DeWald, H.A., Nordin, I.C., L'Italien, Y.J. & Parcell, R.F. (1973) Pyrazolodiazepines. 1,3- (and 2,3-) Dialkyl-4,6-dihydro-8-arylpyrazolo[4,3-*e*][1,4]diazepin-5-ones as antianxiety agents. *J. med. Chem.*, **16**, 1346–1354

Fitzgerald, J.E., de la Iglesia, F.A. & McGuire, E.J. (1984) Carcinogenicity studies in rodents with ripazepam, a minor tranquilizing agent. *Fundam. appl. Toxicol.*, **4**, 178–190

Poschel, B.P.H., McCarthy, D.A., Chen, G. & Ensor, C.R. (1974) Pyrazapon (CI-683): a new antianxiety agent. *Psychopharmacologia*, **35**, 257–271

---

[1]For definition of the italicized terms, see Preamble, pp. 22–25.

TEMAZEPAM

1. Exposure Data

1.1 Chemical and physical data

1.1.1 *Nomenclature*

Chem. Abstr. Serv. Reg. No.: 846-50-4

Chem. Abstr. Name: 7-Chloro-1,3-dihydro-3-hydroxy-1-methyl-5-phenyl-2H-1,4-benzodiazepin-2-one

IUPAC Systematic Name: 7-Chloro-1,3-dihydro-3-hydroxy-1-methyl-5-phenyl-2H-1,4-benzodiazepin-2-one

Synonyms: 3-Hydroxydiazepam; methyloxazepam; N-methyloxazepam; oxydiazepam

1.1.2 *Structural and molecular formulae and relative molecular mass*

$C_{16}H_{13}ClN_2O_2$ Relative molecular mass: 300.75

1.1.3 *Chemical and physical properties of the pure substance*

(a) *Description*: White crystals (Gennaro, 1995)

(b) *Melting-point*: 119–121 °C (Budavari, 1995)

(c) *Spectroscopy data*: Infrared spectroscopy data have been reported (British Pharmacopoeial Commission, 1993)

(d) *Solubility*: Very slightly soluble in water (< 1 in 10 000); sparingly soluble in ethanol (Dollery *et al.*, 1991; Gennaro, 1995); freely soluble in chloroform (British Pharmacopoeial Commission, 1993)

(e) *Dissociation constant*: pK_a, 1.6 (Gennaro, 1995)

1.1.4 Technical products and impurities

There are two enantiomeric forms of the temazepam structure (asymmetric at C_3), but temazepam in pharmaceutical preparations is invariably the racemic mixture (British Pharmacopoeial Commission, 1993).

Temazepam is available as 7.5-, 10-, 15-, 20- and 30-mg capsules, 10- and 20-mg tablets and an oral solution containing 10 mg/5 mL. Preparations also may contain benzyl alcohol, butylparaben, carboxymethylcellulose sodium, crospovidone (a crosslinked homopolymer of polyvinylpyrrolidone), edetate calcium disodium, gelatin, glycerol, lactose, magnesium stearate, mannitol, methylparaben, polyethylene glycol 400, propylparaben, silicon dioxide, sodium lauryl sulfate, sodium ethyl *para*-oxybenzoate, sodium propionate, sodium propyl *para*-oxybenzoate, sorbitol, synthetic red ferric oxide, titanium oxide, FD&C Blue 1 (Brilliant Blue FCF) or FD&C Red 3 (Erythrosine). Various capsule formulations of temazepam have been available (liquid, gel or powder formulations in hard or soft capsules), and differences in peak blood levels and half-life of temazepam among the various formulations have been noted (see Section 4.1 of this monograph) (Thomas, 1991; Farmindustria, 1993; Hingorani & Ainsworth, 1993; Reynolds, 1993; British Medical Association/Royal Pharmaceutical Society of Great Britain, 1994; Medical Economics, 1996)

A potential impurity limited by the requirements of the European Pharmacopoeia is 5-chloro-2-methylaminobenzophenone (Council of Europe, 1994). Another is the product of oxidation of the hydroxyl group of temazepam, the 2,3-dione (Fatmi & Hickson, 1988).

Trade names and designations of the chemical and its pharmaceutical preparations include: Crisonar; ER 115; Euhypnos; Euipnos; Gelthix; K 3917; Levanxene; Levanxol; Mabertin; Neodorm SP; Norkotral Tema; Normison; Perdorm; Planum; Pronervon; Razepam; Redupax Planpak; Remestan; Reposium; Restoril; Ro 5-5345; Signopam; Signopharm; Temaz; Temaze; Temazep; Temazin; Tenox; Tenso; Texapam; Veroqual; Wy 3917; Z-Pam.

1.1.5 Analysis

Several international pharmacopoeias specify potentiometric titration with perchloric acid or liquid chromatography as assays for purity of temazepam, and thin-layer and liquid chromatography for determining impurities and decomposition products, particularly 5-chloro-2-methylaminobenzophenone. The assay for temazepam in capsules applies liquid chromatography using a standard (British Pharmacopoeial Commission, 1993; Council of Europe, 1994; United States Pharmacopeial Convention, 1994). Other methods of analysis in pharmaceutical preparations include: fluorimetry (Walash *et al.*, 1994), polarography (Chan & Fogg, 1981), spectrophotometry (El-Brashy *et al.*, 1993), mass spectrometry (McCarley & Brodbelt, 1993) and high-performance liquid chromatography (Gordon *et al.*, 1986; Fatmi & Hickson, 1988).

Temazepam can be analysed in biological fluids and tissues by fluorimetry (Walash *et al.*, 1994), adsorptive stripping voltammetry (Zapardiel *et al.*, 1988), electron-capture gas chromatography (Divoll & Greenblatt, 1981; Löscher, 1982; Riva *et al.*, 1982), capillary gas chromatography (Beischlag & Inaba, 1992), gas chromatography–mass spectrometry (Maurer & Pfleger, 1987) and high-performance liquid chromatography (Ho et al., 1983; Komiskey et al., 1985; Patterson, 1986; Lau et al., 1987; Fernández et al., 1991; Kunsman et al., 1991; Chopineau et al., 1994).

1.2 Production and use

1.2.1 Production

Temazepam is prepared by acylating 2-(methylamino)-5-chlorobenzhydrol with chloroacetyl chloride. Heating the product with sodium iodide yields the iodoacetamido compound. Treatment of the iodoacetamido compound with hydroxylamine effects dehydration and dehydrohalogenation to form the benzodiazepine derivative, which rearranges to temazepam, with esterification when treated with acetic anhydride. Saponification liberates temazepam (Gennaro, 1995).

1.2.2 Use

Temazepam was first introduced in Europe in 1970 and in the United States of America in 1981 (Sternbach & Horst, 1982). During 1992–94, temazepam accounted for 40–45% of the United States pharmaceutical market for hypnotics (Sandoz Pharmaceuticals Corp., 1996).

Temazepam is a benzodiazepine hypnotic used in the short-term management of insomnia (see the monograph on diazepam, pp. 39–41, for a brief overview of the pharmacology of therapeutic action for this class of drugs). The usual oral dose for adults is 15 mg taken before retiring at night, although 7.5 mg may be sufficient for some patients and others may need 30 mg, or exceptionally up to 60 mg. Temazepam should be given at reduced dosages to elderly or debilitated patients: one half of the usual adult dose, or less, may be sufficient. For premedication before surgical or investigative procedures, the usual dose is 20–40 mg (Reynolds, 1993; Medical Economics, 1996).

Clinical uses of temazepam and other benzodiazepines have been reviewed (Hollister et al., 1993).

Comparative data on sales of temazepam in several countries are presented in Table 1. Overall, sales worldwide increased by approximately 7% from 1990 to 1995, and United States prescriptions increased by about 6% (see Table 2 in the monograph on diazepam, p. 43).

1.3 Occurrence

Temazepam is not known to occur as a natural product. It is a minor metabolite of diazepam in humans.

1.4 Regulations and guidelines

Temazepam is listed in the British, European, French and United States pharmacopoeias (Reynolds, 1993; British Pharmacopoeial Commission, 1993; Council of Europe, 1994; United States Pharmacopeial Convention, 1994; Vidal, 1995).

Table 1. Sales of temazepam in various countries[a] (no. of standard units[b], in thousands)

Country	1990	1995	Country	1990	1995
Africa			Europe		
South Africa	4 226	4 574	Belgium	2 480	1 577
North America			France	13 370	7 532
Canada	16 365	40 238	Germany	30 901	36 695
USA	177 054	200 677	Greece	2 394	2 111
South America			Italy	0	10 912
Venezuela	879	885	Netherlands	46 055	52 843
Asia			Portugal	4 426	4 378
Republic of Korea	15	16	Spain	2	0
Australia	80 984	79 864	Switzerland	2 312	2 109
			United Kingdom	324 041	311 519

[a] Data provided by IMS
[b] Standard dosage units, uncorrected for temazepam content

2. Studies of Cancer in Humans

No data were available to the Working Group (see the monograph on diazepam, pp. 44–54, for a discussion of benzodiazepines).

3. Studies of Cancer in Experimental Animals

3.1 Oral administration

3.1.1 *Mouse*

Groups of 100 male and 100 female Charles River CD-1 mice, five weeks of age, were given 0 (control), 10, 80 or 160 mg/kg bw temazepam (99% pure) per day in the diet for up to 78 weeks. The temazepam/diet mixtures were prepared freshly each week and offered *ad libitum*. Mice that died during the first 35 days were replaced. Body-weight gains tended to be slightly less than those of controls for both male and female treated mice throughout the study [exact details not given]. Food consumption was similar in control and treated mice. Mortality was increased in male mice receiving either

80 mg/kg bw (56% survival) or 160 mg/kg bw (47% survival) while the low-dose and control mice had survival greater than 80%. Among females, the mortality was generally similar in all groups (greater than 75% survival), with the mid- and high-dose groups tending to have slightly increased mortality. All surviving animals were killed at 78 weeks. Complete histological examinations were performed on 99–100 males per group and 100 females per group. Hepatic hyperplastic lesions occurred in 2% of control, 3% of low-dose, 3% of mid-dose and 10% of high-dose males, and in 0% of control, 0% of low-dose, 1% of mid-dose and 8% of high-dose female mice. No significant increase in the incidence of benign hepatocellular adenomas was observed for male or female mice. The incidence of hepatocellular adenomas was: males — control, 8/100; low-dose, 4/99; mid-dose, 2/100; and high-dose, 10/100; females — control, 0/100; low-dose, 1/100; mid-dose, 1/100; and high-dose, 4/100 (p = 0.056, Fisher exact test) [p = 0.014, trend test] (Robison *et al.*, 1984). [The Working Group noted that the study was terminated at 78 weeks.]

3.1.2 *Rat*

Groups of 90 male and 90 female Charles River weanling CD rats were given 0 (control), 10, 40 or 160 mg/kg bw temazepam (99% pure) per day in the diet for up to 104 weeks. The temazepam/diet mixtures were prepared freshly each week and offered *ad libitum*. Ten males and 10 females from each group were killed at weeks 27 and 53. In rats exposed to 160 mg/kg bw, body weights were less than those of controls for both males (except at weeks 13 and 26) and females. Food consumption was similar in control and treated rats. All treated males and low-dose females had higher mortality than the controls. The survival was satisfactory, with at least 24 animals remaining in each group. Complete histopathological examination, including visually apparent lesions, was performed. No significant increase in the incidence of tumours was observed in male or female rats. The incidence of hepatocellular carcinomas was: males — control, 10/90; low-dose, 9/90; mid-dose, 6/90; and high-dose, 10/90; females — control, 13/90; low-dose, 4/90; mid-dose, 10/90; and high-dose, 8/90. No liver adenoma was reported (Robison *et al.*, 1984).

3.2 Carcinogenicity of metabolites

See the monograph on oxazepam in this volume (pp. 119–123).

4. Other Data Relevant to an Evaluation of Carcinogenicity and its Mechanisms

4.1 Absorption, distribution, metabolism and excretion

4.1.1 *Humans*

Information on the absorption of temazepam is somewhat confused by the issue of differing formulations. Studies in the United States when the drug was first marketed in a hard gelatin capsule (1981) indicated relatively slow absorption, with maximal plasma concentrations attained about 2.5 h after dosing. This contrasted with data relating to the soft gelatin capsule, which became available earlier in Europe and gave peak plasma levels within 1.5 h. For example, after a 10-mg dose, Jochemsen et al. (1983) found peak plasma concentrations of 227 ± 92 ng/mL at 1.2 ± 0.9 h in Dutch subjects and Klem et al. (1986) found peak plasma concentrations of 306 ± 32 ng/mL at median 0.75 h in British geriatric patients given soft gelatin capsules. Fuccella et al. (1977) administered 20 mg temazepam in hard and soft capsules to male volunteers, and measured peak plasma concentrations of 668 ± 121 ng/mL and 892 ± 101 ng/mL at 1.44 ± 0.21 h and 0.83 ± 0.25 h, respectively. More recent data from the United States show that reformulation there achieved a product comparable with that marketed in Europe, and more appropriate for use as a hypnotic. In this study, the peak plasma concentration was 873 ± 43 ng/mL at 1.36 ± 0.15 h following a single 30-mg dose (Locniskar & Greenblatt, 1990). Controversy has also arisen in relation to the elimination half-life, but this study seems to confirm a mean value of 10 h. A sex difference was reported in another study (Divoll et al., 1981) in which, irrespective of age, the elimination half-life of temazepam was about 12 h in men and about 17 h in women. No such sex difference was seen in the much smaller study of Klem et al. (1986).

Schwarz (1979) reported that 80% of a 0.41-mg/kg bw dose was recovered in urine, while another 12% was recovered in faeces. The percentages of the dose excreted in urine were temazepam (1.5%), conjugated temazepam (72.5%), oxazepam (1.0%) and conjugated oxazepam (5.8%). Temazepam can cross the human placenta (Heel et al., 1981). Locniskar and Greenblatt (1990) found that direct conjugation of temazepam with glucuronic acid was a major pathway of metabolic clearance, and 39 ± 3% of the oral dose was eliminated in urine as the glucuronide; only 0.2% of the dose was recovered as temazepam. Oxazepam glucuronide accounted for a further 4.7% of the dose. Approximately 50% of the dose was not accounted for, possibly because of non-renal elimination or formation of unrecognized metabolites (see Figure 1).

4.1.2 *Experimental systems*

The disposition of temazepam has been studied in various animal species including mice, rats and dogs (Schwarz, 1979) (see Figure 1). Conjugation and N-demethylation were the major metabolic pathways in mice and dogs. In rats, excretion of temazepam was primarily in the faeces (78%), resulting from biliary excretion of metabolites (59%) rather than from incomplete absorption; only 15% was excreted in urine. Male Wistar rats excreted 85–90% of an intravenous dose of [^{14}C]temazepam in the bile within 8 h (Tse et al., 1983a) and about 85% of this material was reabsorbed to be re-excreted predominantly in the bile (Tse et al., 1983b). Mice and dogs excreted 37% in the urine and about 55% in the faeces. Temazepam can cross the placenta in rats and rabbits (Schwarz, 1979).

Expressed as percentages of the dose, the major urinary metabolites in mice were oxazepam conjugate(s) (23%), while in dogs approximately equal quantities of temazepam and oxazepam conjugates were excreted (15% and 16%, respectively). In rats, the major proportion in urine was unidentified metabolites (only about 1% of the dose was identified) (Schwarz, 1979). In metabolic studies using rat liver microsomes, it has been shown that CYP3A enzymes are involved in the C_3-hydroxylation of diazepam to yield temazepam, but not in the N-dealkylation of temazepam and diazepam (Reilly *et al.*, 1990).

Figure 1. Postulated metabolic pathways of temazepam

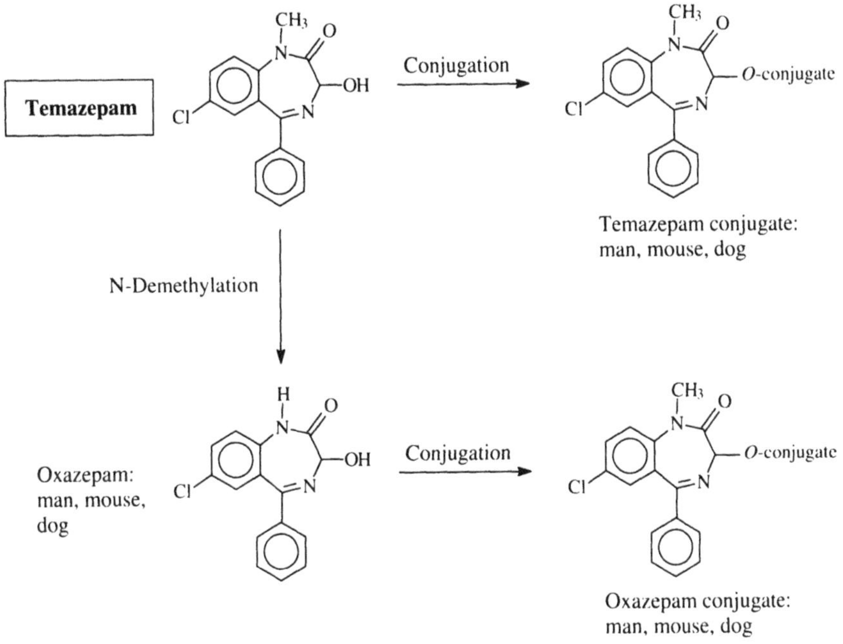

From Schwarz (1979)
Conjugate is glucuronide or sulfate

4.2 Toxic effects

4.2.1 Humans

(a) *Acute toxicity*

In a recent report on 573 lethal intoxications due to self-poisoning with temazepam alone or in combination in the United Kingdom during the 1980s, temazepam was found to be associated with a higher death rate per million prescriptions than any other benzodiazepine hypnotic drug except flurazepam (Serfaty & Masterton, 1993). In another study, temazepam was detected in post-mortem blood samples of 15 overdose deaths. In all cases, ethanol and additional drugs were identified, such as paracetamol, dextropropoxyphene, chlorpromazine and trifluoperazine. In 12 cases, the blood concentrations were well above the highest concentration found after therapeutic doses (750 μg/L) (Forrest *et al.*, 1986). Disulfiram has been reported to precipitate temazepam toxicity by increasing central nervous system depression (Hardman *et al.*, 1994). There are also several reports of deaths from pulmonary microembolisms after intravenous injection of temazepam from tablets by drug abusers. However, these are clearly not due to the compound itself but to other tablet constituents such as crospovidone (a plastic-like carrier material) which may cause pulmonary foreign-body reaction (Hingorani & Ainsworth, 1993).

(*b*) *Chronic toxicity*

In a post-marketing surveillance report, covering a period of three to five years, of 24 000 patients treated with 10–60 mg temazepam, approximately 10% of the patients experienced adverse effects. Gastrointestinal complaints, sleep disturbances, vertigo, headaches, weakness, lack of concentration, loss of equilibrium and falling were frequently reported. Severe adverse effects such as hypotension, blood dyscrasias and jaundice were reported only in single cases (reviewed by Dollery *et al.*, 1991).

4.2.2 *Experimental systems*

Toxicological tests lasting six months at doses up to 120 mg/kg bw per day in beagle dogs and rats did not show significant organ toxicity (Dollery *et al.*, 1991). In the study of Robison *et al.* (1984) described in Section 3.1.1, the increased mortality observed in the groups of male mice given 80 or 160 mg/kg bw per day was associated with an increased bite wound rate resulting from an apparently drug-related increase in fighting behaviour. There was no significant effect on food consumption, or organ or haematological toxicity in either rats or mice.

4.3 Reproductive and prenatal effects

4.3.1 *Humans*

Dusci *et al.* (1990) described the excretion of temazepam in plasma and breast milk from a lactating mother taking high-dose diazepam and oxazepam. The infant showed no overt physical or mental symptoms of benzodiazepine intoxication.

Kargas *et al.* (1985) reported a stillbirth at term of a female infant (3.82 kg) less than 8 h after maternal ingestion of therapeutic doses of diphenhydramine (50 mg) (Benadryl, an H1-receptor antagonist) and temazepam (30 mg); the authors suggested that a synergistic interaction of the drugs was the most likely cause of death (see Section 4.3.2).

4.3.2 *Experimental systems*

Kargas *et al.* (1985) treated 13 healthy pregnant New Zealand white rabbits on days 29 and 30 (parturition) of gestation with both diphenhydramine (15 mg/kg bw orally) and temazepam (10 mg/kg bw orally). Eighty-one per cent of the fetuses were stillborn or died shortly after birth, exhibiting marked irritability and seizures. In contrast, administration of diphenhydramine alone (up to 50 mg/kg bw) or temazepam alone (up to 80 mg/kg bw) did not increase mortality significantly.

4.4 Genetic and related effects

4.4.1 *Humans*

No data were available to the Working Group.

4.4.2 *Experimental systems* (see also Table 2 for references and Appendices 1 and 2)

No mitotic spindle abnormality was observed by electron microscopy in the marine flagellate, *Dunaliella bioculata*. No increase in DNA strand breaks and/or alkali-labile sites was observed in the liver of rats given a single or multiple daily doses of temazepam.

Table 2. Genetic and related effects of temazepam

Test system	Result^a		Dose^b (LED/HID)	Reference
	Without exogenous metabolic system	With exogenous metabolic system		
*, Mitotic abnormalities, protozoa	–	NT	30	Miernik *et al.* (1986)
DVA, DNA strand breaks, rat liver *in vivo*	–		300 po × 1	Carlo *et al.* (1989)
DVA, DNA strand breaks, rat liver *in vivo*	–		60 po × 15	Carlo *et al.* (1989)

*Not shown on profile

^{a} +, positive; (+), weak positive; –, negative; NT, not tested; ?, inconclusive

^{b} LED, lowest effective dose; HID, highest ineffective dose; in-vitro tests, µg/mL; in-vivo tests, mg/kg bw/day

5. Summary of Data Reported and Evaluation

5.1 Exposure data

Temazepam is a benzodiazepine prescribed widely since the 1970s for short-term management of insomnia. Temazepam is a minor metabolite of diazepam.

5.2 Human carcinogenicity data

No data were available to the Working Group.

5.3 Animal carcinogenicity data

Temazepam was tested for carcinogenicity in one experiment in mice and in one experiment in rats by oral administration in the diet. A slight increase in the incidence of liver adenomas was found in female mice.

5.4 Other relevant data

Temazepam is absorbed rapidly and completely in humans from appropriate oral formulations. It is eliminated mainly in urine as the glucuronide conjugate; oxazepam is a minor metabolite. The mean elimination half-life is about 10 h.

Conjugation and N-demethylation to oxazepam are the major metabolic pathways recognized in mice and dogs.

Chronic administration of pharmacological doses does not induce organ toxicity. Repeated-dose toxicity studies lasting up to six months did not reveal specific organ toxicity in dogs, rats or mice.

No data were available on teratogenic effects of temazepam.

Few data on genetic effects of temazepam were available. It did not produce DNA strand breaks in the livers of rats.

5.5 Evaluation[1]

There is *inadequate evidence* in humans for the carcinogenicity of temazepam.

There is *inadequate evidence* in experimental animals for the carcinogenicity of temazepam.

Overall evaluation

Temazepam is *not classifiable as to its carcinogenicity to humans (Group 3)*.

6. References

Beischlag, T.V. & Inaba, T. (1992) Determination of nonderivatized *para*-hydroxylated metabolites of diazepam in biological fluids with a GC megabore column system. *J. analyt. Toxicol.*, **16**, 236–239

British Medical Association/Royal Pharmaceutical Society of Great Britain (1994) *British National Formulary Number 27 (March 1994)*, London, p. 139

British Pharmacopoeial Commission (1993) *British Pharmacopoeia* 1993, Vols. I and II, London, Her Majesty' Stationery Office, pp. 652–653, 1121–1122

Budavari, S., ed. (1995) *The Merck Index*, 12th Ed., Rahway, NJ, Merck & Co.

---

[1]For definition of the italicized terms, see Preamble, pp. 22–25.

Carlo, P., Finollo, R., Ledda, A. & Brambella, G. (1989) Absence of liver DNA fragmentation in rats treated with high oral doses of 32 benzodiazepine drugs. *Fundam. appl. Toxicol.*, **12**, 34–41

Chan, H.K. & Fogg, A.G. (1981) Polarographic determination of temazepam in soft gelatin capsule formulations. *Analyst*, **106**, 768–775

Chopineau, J., Rivault, F., Sautou, V. & Sommier, M.F. (1994) Determination of temazepam and its active metabolite, oxazepam in plasma, urine and dialysate using solid-phase extraction followed by high-performance liquid chromatography. *J. liq. Chromatogr.*, **17**, 373–383

Council of Europe (1994) *European Pharmacopoeia*, 2nd Ed., Part II, 18th fasc., Sainte-Ruffine, France, Maisonneuve S.A., pp. 954-1–954-3

Divoll, M. & Greenblatt, D.J. (1981) Plasma concentrations of temazepam, a 3-hydroxybenzodiazepine, determined by electron-capture gas-liquid chromatography. *J. Chromatogr. biomed. Appl.*, **222**, 125–128

Divoll, M., Greenblatt, D.J., Harmatz, J.S. & Shader, R.I. (1981) Effect of age and gender on disposition of temazepam. *J. pharm. Sci.*, **70**, 1104–1107

Dollery, C., Boobis, A.R., Burley, D., Davies, D.M., Davies, D.S., Harrison, P.I., Orme, M.E., Park, B.K. & Goldberg, L.I. (1991) *Therapeutic Drugs: Temazepam*, Edinburgh, Churchill Livingstone, pp. T4–T8

Dusci, L.J., Good, S.M., Hall, R.W. & Ilett, K.F. (1990) Excretion of diazepam and its metabolites in human milk during withdrawal from combination high dose diazepam and oxazepam. *Br. J. clin. Pharmacol.*, **29**, 123–126

El-Brashy, A., Aly, F.A. & Belal, F. (1993) Determination of 1,4-benzodiazepines in drug dosage forms by difference spectrophotometry. *Mikrochim. Acta*, **110**, 55–60

Farmindustria (1993) *Repertorio Farmaceutico Italiano* (Italian Pharmaceutical Directory), 7th Ed., Milan, Associazione Nazionale dell'Industria Farmaceutica, CEDOF S.P.A., pp. A-552–A-553

Fatmi, A.A. & Hickson, E.A. (1988) Determination of temazepam and related compounds in capsules by high-performance liquid chromatography. *J. pharm. Sci.*, **77**, 87–89

Fernández, P., Hermida, I., Bermejo, A.M., López-Rivadulla, M., Cruz, A. & Concheiro, L. (1991) Simultaneous determination of diazepam and its metabolites in plasma by high-performance liquid chromatography. *J. liq. Chromatogr.*, **14**, 2587–2599

Forrest, A.R.W., Marsh, I., Bradshaw, C. & Braich, S.K. (1986) Fatal temazepam overdoses (Letter to the Editor). *Lancet*, **i**, 226

Fuccella, L.M., Bolcioni, G., Tamassia, V., Ferrario, L. & Tognoni, G. (1977) Human pharmacokinetics and bioavailability of temazepam administered in soft gelatin capsules. *Eur. J. clin. Pharmacol.*, **12**, 383–386

Gennaro, A.R., ed. (1995) *Remington: The Science and Practice of Pharmacy*, 19th Ed., Vol. II, Easton, PA, Mack Publishing Co., pp. 1160–1161

Gordon, S.M., Freeston, L.K. & Collins, A.J. (1986) Determination of temazepam and its major degradation products in soft gelatin capsules by isocratic reversed-phase high-performance liquid chromatography. *J. Chromatogr.*, **368**, 180–183

Hardman, M., Biniwale, A. & Clarke, C.E. (1994) Temazepam toxicity precipitated by disulfiram (Letter to the Editor). *Lancet*, **344**, 1231–1232

Heel, R.C., Brogden. R.N., Speight, T.M. & Avery, G.S. (1981) Temazepam: a review of its pharmacological properties and therapeutic efficacy as an hypnotic. *Drugs*, **21**, 321–340

Hingorani, A.D. & Ainsworth, R.W. (1993) Pulmonary microembolisation and temazepam (Letter to the Editor). *Br. med. J.*, **307**, 623–624

Ho, P.C., Triggs, E.J., Heazlewood, V. & Bourne, D.W.A. (1983) Determination of nitrazepam and temazepam in plasma by high-performance liquid chromatography. *Ther. Drug Monit.*, **5**, 303–307

Hollister, L.E., Müller-Oerlinghausen, B., Rickels, K. & Shader, R.I. (1993) Clinical uses of benzodiazepines. *J. clin. Psychopharmacol.*, **13** (Suppl. 1)

Jochemsen, R., van Boxtel, C.J., Hermans, J. & Breimer, D.D. (1983) Kinetics of five benzodiazepine hypnotics in healthy subjects. *Clin. Pharmacol. Ther.*, **34**, 42–47

Kargas, G.A., Kargas, S.A., Bruyere, H.J., Jr, Gilbert, E.F. & Opitz, J.M. (1985) Perinatal mortality due to interaction of diphenhydramine and temazepam (Letter to the Editor). *New Engl. J. Med.*, **313**, 1417–1418

Klem, K., Murray, G.R. & Laake, K. (1986) Pharmacokinetics of temazepam in geriatric patients. *Eur. J. clin. Pharmacol.*, **30**, 745–747

Komiskey, H.L., Rahman, A., Weisenburger, W.P., Hayton, W.L., Zobrist, R.H. & Silvius, W. (1985) Extraction, separation and detections of ^{14}C-diazepam and ^{14}C-metabolites from brain tissue of mature and old rats. *J. analyt. Toxicol.*, **9**, 131–133

Kunsman, G.W., Manno, J.E., Przekop, M.A., Manno, B.R., Llorens, K.A. & Kunsman, C.M. (1991) Determination of temazepam and temazepam glucuronide by reversed-phase high-performance liquid chromatography. *J. Chromatogr. biomed. Appl.*, **568**, 427–436

Lau, C.E., Dolan, S. & Tang, M. (1987) Microsample determination of diazepam and its three metabolites in serum by reversed-phase high-performance liquid chromatography. *J. Chromatogr. biomed. Appl.*, **416**, 212–218

Locniskar, A. & Greenblatt, D.J. (1990) Oxidative versus conjugative biotransformation of temazepam. *Biopharm. Drug Dispos.*, **11**, 499–506

Löscher, W. (1982) Rapid gas-chromatographic measurement of diazepam and its metabolites desmethyldiazepam, oxazepam and 3-hydroxydiazepam (temazepam) in small samples of plasma. *Ther. Drug Monit.*, **4**, 315–318

Maurer, H. & Pfleger, K. (1987) Identification and differentiation of benzodiazepines and their metabolites in urine by computerized gas chromatography-mass spectrometry. *J. Chromatogr.*, **422**, 85–101

McCarley, T.D. & Brodbelt, J. (1993) Structurally diagnostic ion-molecule reactions and collisionally activated dissociation of 1,4-benzodiazepines in a quadrupole ion trap mass spectrometer. *Analyt. Chem.*, **65**, 2380–2388

Medical Economics (1996) *PDR®: Physicians' Desk* Reference, 50th Ed., Montvale, NJ, Medical Economics Data Production Co., pp. 2284–2286

Miernik, A., Santa-Maria, A. & Marano, F. (1986) The antimitotic activities of some benzodiazepines. *Experientia*, **42**, 956–958

Patterson, S.E. (1986) Determination of temazepam in plasma and urine by high-performance liquid chromatography using disposable solid-phase extraction columns. *J. pharm. biomed. Analysis*, **4**, 271–274

Reilly, P.E.B., Thompson, D.A., Mason, S.R. & Hooper, W.D. (1990) Cytochrome P450IIIA enzymes in rat liver microsomes: involvement in C_3-hydroxylation of diazepam and nordazepam but not N-dealkylation of diazepam and temazepam. *Mol. Pharmacol.*, **37**, 767–774

Reynolds, J.E.F., ed. (1993) *Martindale: The Extra Pharmacopoeia*, 30th Ed., London, The Pharmaceutical Press, pp. 616–617

Riva, R., Albani, F. & Baruzzi, A. (1982) Determination of camazepam and its metabolite, temazepam, in man by gas-liquid chromatography with electron-capture detection. *Farm. Ed. Prat.*, **37**, 15–19

Robison, R.L., Van Ryzin, R.J., Stoll, R.E., Jensen, R.D. & Bagdon, R.E. (1984) Chronic toxicity/carcinogenicity study of temazepam in mice and rats. *Fundam. appl. Toxicol.*, **4**, 394–405

Sandoz Pharmaceuticals Corp. (1996) *Temazepam*, East Hanover, NJ, United States

Schwarz, H.J. (1979) Pharmacokinetics and metabolism of temazepam in man and several animal species. *Br. J. clin. Pharmacol.*, **8** (Suppl. 1), 23S–29S

Serfaty, M. & Masterton, G. (1993) Fatal poisonings attributed to benzodiazepines in Britain during the 1980s. *Br. J. Psychiatr.*, **163**, 386–393

Sternbach, L.H. & Horst, W.D. (1982) Psychopharmacological agents. In: Grayson, M. & Eckroth, D., eds, *Kirk-Othmer Encyclopedia of Chemical Technology*, 3rd Ed., Vol. 19, New York, John Wiley & Sons, pp. 342–379

Thomas, J., ed. (1991) *Prescription Products Guide 1991*, 20th Ed., Victoria, Australian Pharmaceutical Publishing Co., pp. 757–758, 1228–1229, 1605–1606

Tse, F.L.S., Ballard, F. & Jaffe, J.M. (1983a) Biliary excretion of [^{14}C]temazepam and its metabolites in the rat. *J. pharm. Sci.*, **72**, 311–312

Tse, F.L.S., Ballard, F., Jaffe, J.M. & Schwarz, H.J. (1983b) Enterohepatic circulation of radioactivity following an oral dose of [^{14}C]temazepam in the rat. *J. Pharm. Pharmacol.*, **35**, 225–228

United States Pharmacopeial Convention (1994) *The 1995 US Pharmacopeia*, 23rd Rev./*The National Formulary*, 18th Rev., Rockville, MD, pp. 1490–1491

Vidal (1995) *Dictionnaire Vidal*, 71st Ed., Paris, Editions du Vidal, pp. 1047–1048

Walash, M.I., Belal, F., Metwally, M.E. & Hefnawy, M.M. (1994) Selective fluorimetric method for the determination of some 1,4-benzodiazepine drugs containing a hydroxyl group at C-3. *J. pharm. biomed. Analysis*, **12**, 1417–1423

Zapardiel, A., Peréz Lopéz, J.A., Bermejo, E. & Hernández, L. (1988) Application of adsorptive stripping voltammetry to the determination of the psychoactive drug temazepam in urine. *Fresenius' Z. analyt. Chem.*, **330**, 707–710

PHENYTOIN

This substance was considered by previous working groups, in October 1976 (IARC, 1977) and March 1987 (IARC. 1987). Since that time, new data have become available, and these have been incorporated in the monograph and taken into consideration in the evaluation.

1. Exposure Data

1.1 Chemical and physical data

1.1.1 *Nomenclature*

Phenytoin

Chem. Abstr. Serv. Reg. No.: 57-41-0

Deleted CAS Reg. No.: 125-59-7

Chem. Abstr. Name: 5,5-Diphenyl-2,4-imidazolidinedione

IUPAC Systematic Name: 5,5-Diphenylhydantoin

Synonyms: Diphenylhydantoin; DPH

Phenytoin sodium

Chem. Abstr. Serv. Reg. No.: 630-93-3

Deleted CAS Reg. Nos: 143-75-9; 1421-15-4; 8017-52-5

Chem. Abstr. Name: 5,5-Diphenyl-2,4-imidazolidinedione, monosodium salt

IUPAC Systematic Name: 5,5-Diphenylhydantoin sodium salt

Synonyms: Diphenylhydantoin sodium; 5,5-diphenylhydantoin sodium; SDPH; sodium diphenylhydantoin; sodium 5,5-diphenylhydantoin; sodium diphenylhydantoinate; sodium 5,5-diphenyl-2,4-imidazolidinedione; sodium phenytoin; soluble phenytoin

1.1.2 *Structural and molecular formulae and relative molecular mass*

Phenytoin

$C_{15}H_{12}N_2O_2$ Relative molecular mass: 252.27

Phenytoin sodium

$C_{15}H_{11}N_2O_2 \cdot Na$ Relative molecular mass: 274.25

1.1.3 *Chemical and physical properties of the pure substances*

Phenytoin

(a) *Description*: White, odourless powder (Gennaro, 1995)
(b) *Melting-point*: 295–298 °C (Budavari, 1995)
(c) *Spectroscopy data*: Infrared, ultraviolet, nuclear magnetic resonance and mass spectral data have been reported (Philip et al., 1984).
(d) *Solubility*: Practically insoluble in water; soluble in acetone (1 g/30 mL), ethanol (1 g/60 mL) and alkali hydroxides (Budavari, 1995)
(e) *Dissociation constant*: pK_a = 8.06–8.33 (American Hospital Formulary Service, 1995)

Phenytoin sodium

(a) *Description*: White, odourless powder (Gennaro, 1995)
(b) *Spectroscopy data*: Infrared, ultraviolet, nuclear magnetic resonance and mass spectral data have been reported (Philip et al., 1984).
(c) *Solubility*: Soluble in water (approx. 1 g/66 mL) and ethanol (1 g/10.5 mL); insoluble in chloroform and diethyl ether (Budavari, 1995); freely soluble in warm propylene glycol (American Hospital Formulary Service, 1995)
(d) *Stability*: Easily dissociated by weak acids (including carbon dioxide absorbed on exposure to air) regenerating phenytoin; somewhat hygroscopic (Budavari, 1995)

1.1.4 *Technical products and impurities*

Both phenytoin and phenytoin sodium are used in pharmaceutical preparations worldwide, although phenytoin sodium is the more common form.

Phenytoin is available as 50-mg tablets which may also contain flavour, saccharin sodium, sucrose, talc, aluminium lake, D&C Yellow 10 (Quinoline Yellow) or FD&C Yellow 6 (Sunset Yellow FCF). It is also available as 30-, 100- and 125-mg/5 mL oral suspensions, with a maximal alcohol content not greater than 0.6%, and may contain anhydrous citric acid, carboxymethylcellulose, flavours, glycerin, magnesium aluminium silicate, polysorbate 40, sodium benzoate, sucrose, vanillin, D&C Red 33, FD&C Red 40 (Allura Red AC) or FD&C Yellow 6 (Thomas, 1991; British Medical Association/Royal Pharmaceutical Society of Great Britain, 1994; Medical Economics, 1996).

Phenytoin sodium is available as 25-, 30-, 50-, 100- and 300-mg capsules, 30- and 100-mg prompt- and extended-release capsules, and 50- and 100-mg coated tablets, which may also contain citric acid, colloidal silicon dioxide, gelatin, glyceryl monooleate, hydrogen peroxide, lactose, polyethylene glycol 200, sodium benzoate, sodium lauryl sulfate, sucrose, talc, titanium dioxide, FD&C Blue 1 (Brilliant Blue FCF), FD&C Red 3 (Erythrosine) or FD&C Yellow 6. It is also available as a 50-mg/mL injection solution in a vehicle containing 40% propylene glycol (0.4 g/mL) and 10% ethanol (0.1 g/mL) in water, adjusted to pH 12 with sodium hydroxide (Thomas, 1991; British Medical Association/Royal Pharmaceutical Society of Great Britain, 1994; American Hospital Formulary Service, 1995; Medical Economics, 1996).

Trade names for phenytoin and its pharmaceutical preparations include: Aleviatin; Denyl; Difhydan; Dihycon; Di-Hydan; Dihydantoin; Dilabid; Di-Lan; Dilantin; Dilantin-125; Dilantin Infatabs; Dilantin-30 Pediatric; Dintoina; Diphantoin; Diphedan; Diphentyn; Ekko; Enkefal; Epanutin; Epdantoin Simple; Epelin; Epiland; Epinat; Eptoin; Fenantoin; Hidantal; Hydantin; Hydantol; Lehydan; Lepitoin; Novophenytoin; Phenhydan; Phenhydantin; Sodanton; Tacosal; Zentropil.

Trade names for phenytoin sodium and its pharmaceutical preparations include: Alepsin; Aleviatin; Aleviatin sodium; Antisacer; Citrullamon; Danten; Dantoin; Denyl; Difenin; Difetoin; Difhydan; Dilantin; Di-Len; Dintoina; Diphantoine; Di-Phen; Diphenin; Diphenine; Diphenylan; Ditoin; Enkefal; Epanutin; Epdantoin Simple; Epelin; Epilan D; Epilantin; Epsolin; Eptoin; Hidantal; Hydantin; Hydantoinal; Idantoin; Minetoin; Muldis; Neosidantoina; Novodiphenyl; Om-Hydantoïne; Phenhydan; Pyorédol; Solantyl; Tacosal; Thilophenyt; Zentropil.

1.1.5 *Analysis*

Methods for the analysis of phenytoin have been reviewed (Glazko, 1982; Philip *et al.*, 1984; Burke & Thénot, 1985).

Several international pharmacopoeias specify liquid chromatography (LC) or titration with sodium hydroxide or sodium methoxide as the assay for purity of phenytoin, and LC, gas chromatography (GC) with flame ionization detection (FID) or thin-layer chromatography (TLC) for determining levels of benzil, benzophenone and other impurities and decomposition products. Assays for determining clarity and colour, acid or alkali, chloride, benzilic acid and heavy metals are also specified. The assay for phenytoin in powders, tablets and oral suspensions uses titration with sodium methoxide or sodium hydroxide or a gravimetric method following acidification and extraction (Society of Japanese Pharmacopoeia, 1992; British Pharmacopoeial Commission, 1993; United States Pharmacopeial Convention, 1994).

Several international pharmacopoeias specify LC or titration with sodium hydroxide as the assay for purity of phenytoin sodium, and LC, TLC or GC/FID for determining benzophenone levels and other impurities and decomposition products. Assays for determining clarity and colour, free phenytoin, water and heavy metals are also specified. The assay for phenytoin sodium in capsules, tablets and injectable solutions uses titration with tetrabutylammonium hydroxide, an LC method or a gravimetric method following acidification and extraction. Assays for determining bacterial endotoxins, clarity and colour, pH, alcohol and propylene glycol content, particulate matter and heavy metals for the injectable solution are also specified (Society of Japanese Pharmacopoeia, 1992; British Pharmacopoeial Commission, 1993; United States Pharmacopeial Convention, 1994).

Phenytoin and its metabolites can be analysed in biological fluids by spectrophotometry (colorimetry), radioimmunoassay, enzyme-mediated immunoassay techniques, differential pulse polarography, GC, GC–mass spectrometry and high-performance liquid chromatography (Glazko, 1982; Maya et al., 1992).

1.2 Production and use

1.2.1 Production

A method for preparing phenytoin sodium was first reported by Biltz in 1908 (Budavari, 1995).

Phenytoin and phenytoin sodium are prepared by treating benzaldehyde with sodium cyanide to form benzoin, which is oxidized to benzil with nitric acid or cupric sulfate. The benzil is then heated with urea in the presence of sodium ethoxide or isopropoxide, forming phenytoin sodium. Phenytoin sodium yields the base (phenytoin) on acidification of its aqueous solution (Gennaro, 1995).

In the United States of America, commercial production of phenytoin and phenytoin sodium was first reported in 1946 and 1938, respectively (United States Tariff Commission, 1939; 1948). Phenytoin (and/or its sodium salt) is currently available as a pharmaceutical in over 65 countries (Parke-Davis, 1995).

1.2.2 Use

Phenytoin is an anticonvulsant given orally (as phenytoin or phenytoin sodium) or by slow intravenous injection (as phenytoin sodium) in the treatment of epilepsy. Phenytoin exerts a stabilizing effect on excitable membranes of a variety of cells, including neurons and cardiac myocytes. It can decrease resting fluxes of sodium as well as sodium currents that flow during action potentials or chemically induced depolarizations (Jones & Wimbish, 1985). It is therefore used to control tonic-clonic (grand mal) and partial (focal) seizures; it has also been used for the prophylactic control of seizures developing during and after neurosurgery or following severe traumatic injury to the head. It is believed to stabilize rather than elevate the seizure threshold and to limit the spread of seizure activity. Phenytoin also has antiarrhythmic properties, which were discovered only in the 1950s (Goodman Gilman *et al.*, 1990; Reynolds, 1993).

The dose of phenytoin is typically adjusted to the needs of the individual patient to achieve adequate control of seizures, preferably with monitoring of plasma concentration; in many patients, control requires total plasma phenytoin concentrations of 10–20 µg/mL (40–80 µmol/L), but some are satisfactorily controlled at concentrations outside this range. A suggested initial oral dose of phenytoin or phenytoin sodium is 100 mg three times daily progressively increased with care to 600 mg daily if necessary; the suggested interval between increments ranges from about one week to about one month. Particular care is required at higher doses, where saturation of metabolism may mean that a small increment produces a large rise in plasma concentration. The usual maintenance dose is 300–400 mg daily (Reynolds, 1993).

A suggested initial dose for children is 5 mg/kg bw daily in two or three divided doses; a suggested maintenance dose is 4–8 mg/kg bw daily in divided doses. Young children may require a higher dose per kilogram body weight than adults, due to more rapid metabolism (Reynolds, 1993).

In the treatment of tonic-clonic status epilepticus, a benzodiazepine such as diazepam is usually given intravenously first, followed by intravenous administration of phenytoin sodium. For adults, a suggested dose of phenytoin sodium is 10–15 mg/kg bw, given by slow intravenous injection at a uniform rate of not more than 50 mg/min; thereafter maintenance doses of 100 mg are given orally or intravenously every 6–8 h. The suggested intravenous dose for children and neonates ranges from 10 to 20 mg/kg bw at a rate not exceeding 1–3 mg/kg bw/min (Reynolds, 1993).

Phenytoin sodium is absorbed only very slowly from an intramuscular site, and intramuscular administration is appropriate only in certain situations (e.g., prophylactic control of seizures during neurosurgery) (Reynolds, 1993; Medical Economics, 1996).

Phenytoin is also a class Ib antiarrhythmic agent (see Glossary, p. 447); it is used in the treatment of cardiac arrhythmias, particularly those associated with digitalis intoxication. The usual dose is 3.5–5 mg/kg bw administered by slow intravenous injection at a uniform rate of not more than 50 mg/min; this dose may be repeated once if necessary. Phenytoin has also been used in the treatment of trigeminal neuralgia refractory to carbamazepine or in patients intolerant of carbamazepine (Reynolds, 1993).

Comparative data on sales of phenytoin in several countries are shown in Table 1. Worldwide, sales decreased by approximately 8% from 1990 to 1995, while United States prescriptions increased by about 10% (see Table 2 in the monograph on diazepam, p. 43).

1.3 Occurrence

1.3.1 *Natural occurrence*

Phenytoin is not known to occur as a natural product.

1.3.2 *Occupational exposure*

In several hospital dispensaries in Japan, dust in the air and on surfaces was collected on several work days and analysed by microscopy, TLC and mass spectrometry. Drugs of several types, including phenytoin, were identified but exposure levels were not quantified (Ichiba *et al.*, 1984, 1986; Rikihisa *et al.*, 1984).

No quantitative data on occupational exposure levels were available to the Working Group.

Table 1. Sales of phenytoin in various countries[a] (no. of standard units[b], in thousands)

Country	1990	1995	Country	1990	1995
Africa			Australia	61 508	54 340
South Africa	10 175	9 290	Europe		
North America			Belgium	18 705	17 735
Canada	101 748	101 085	France	36 149	27 006
Mexico	103 204	96 439	Germany	91 567	77 451
United States	1 093 250	984 527	Greece	14 511	13 012
South America			Italy	46 206	39 557
Argentina	47 786	49 865	Netherlands	30 816	26 914
Brazil	131 010	98 831	Portugal	15 015	15 426
Colombia	29 063	27 253	Spain	75 760	77 944
Venezuela	15 570	19 655	Sweden	21 792	18 084
Asia			Switzerland	11 872	10 229
Japan	249 944	238 584	Turkey	24 125	44 232
Republic of Korea	6 146	5 439	United Kingdom	187 566	165 014

[a] Data provided by IMS
[b] Standard dosage units, uncorrected for phenytoin content

The National Occupational Exposure Survey conducted between 1981 and 1983 in the United States by the National Institute for Occupational Safety and Health indicated that approximately 23 400 and 11 850 employees were potentially occupationally exposed to phenytoin and phenytoin sodium, respectively. The estimate was based on a survey of United States companies and did not involve measurements of actual exposure (United States National Library of Medicine, 1996).

1.4 Regulations and guidelines

Phenytoin is listed in the following pharmacopoeias: Australian, British, Brazilian, Czech, French, German, Hungarian, International, Japanese, Mexican, Nordic, Romanian, Swiss, Turkish and United States (Reynolds, 1993; Vidal, 1995).

Phenytoin sodium is listed in the following pharmacopoeias: Australian, British, Brazilian, Chinese, Egyptian, European, French, German, Greek, Indian, International, Italian, Japanese, Mexican, Netherlands, Portuguese, Swiss, United States and former Yugoslavian (Reynolds, 1993; Vidal, 1995).

2. Studies of Cancer in Humans

2.1 Case reports

2.1.1 *Lymphomas and leukaemias*

In early years, numerous case reports described the occurrence of lymphomas and leukaemias in patients treated with phenytoin (IARC, 1977, 1987). Between 1962 and 1980, reports appeared of 79 cases of lymphoma worldwide in patients taking phenytoin, with or without other antiepileptic drugs (Scoville & White, 1981). Some difficulties were encountered in distinguishing benign lymph node changes from lymphoma; however, the hydantoin-induced lymph node reactions regress after drug withdrawal (see Section 4.2.1). Saltzstein and Ackerman (1959) introduced the term 'pseudolymphoma' for this phenomenon (Halevy & Feuerman, 1977). Some patients originally described as developing 'pseudolymphomas' following phenytoin (and in some cases also phenobarbital) treatment were later diagnosed with lymphoma (Gams *et al.*, 1968). In 1968, the term pseudo-pseudolymphoma was introduced by Gams *et al.* (1968) to underline the possibility that what is initially considered a non-malignant phenytoin reaction may, after long-term follow-up, turn out to be a true lymphoma (Scoville & White, 1981).

Most of the malignant lymphomas described in case reports were seen after long-term phenytoin therapy rather than early in therapy. An additional case appeared as an isolated malignant lymphoma of the jejunum (Rubinstein *et al.*, 1985).

2.1.2 *Childhood cancers*

Several case reports have suggested an association between childhood cancer and prenatal exposure to phenytoin. From 1976 to 1981, five cases of neuroblastoma were reported in infants and young children (up to five years of age) exposed *in utero* to phenytoin (Pendergrass & Hanson, 1976; Sherman & Roizen, 1976; Ramilo *et al.*, 1979; Allen *et al.*, 1980; Ehrenbard & Chaganti, 1981). These cases were also adversely affected by the fetal hydantoin syndrome (see Section 4.3.1(*b*)). After four cases had been described since 1976 in United States, Ehrenbard and Chaganti (1981) calculated that, within the United States, it should take 45 years for four to develop by chance. However, no more cases were reported until 1989 (Koren *et al.*, 1989). [The Working

Group noted that this may reflect a reporting bias, with clinicians lacking motivation to report additional cases of an 'established' phenomenon.] The last two cases (reported in 1989 and 1992) did not have major anomalies consistent with the fetal hydantoin syndrome (Koren *et al.*, 1989; Al-Shammri *et al.*, 1992).

Four cases of malignancies other than neuroblastoma in children exposed *in utero* to phenytoin have been reported (Blattner *et al.*, 1977; Taylor *et al.*, 1980; Jimenez *et al.*, 1981; Bostrom & Nesbit, 1983). In six of the 10 recorded cases of cancer associated with prenatal maternal phenytoin ingestion, the drug had not been given alone, but in combination with primidone or phenobarbital. Also, in some cases, there was evidence of alcohol abuse in the mother, which is associated with the fetal alcohol syndrome.

Koren *et al.* (1989) also examined 188 cases of childhood neuroblastoma diagnosed between January 1969 and October 1986 at the Hospital for Sick Children in Toronto, Canada. A review of medical records showed that none of the mothers or fathers had had epilepsy or been treated with phenytoin. In North America, the prevalence of epilepsy in the general population is 0.5%, and about half of all epileptic patients receive phenytoin. This serial cohort of 188 children indicates that, statistically, phenytoin cannot be incriminated in more than two cases of this series or in 1.5% of children with this malignancy in general.

2.2 Cohort studies

In a cohort study of members of the Kaiser Permanente Medical Care Program, described in the monograph on diazepam (pp. 44–45), phenytoin was used by 954 subjects (0.7%) (Selby *et al.*, 1989). Incidence of all cancers was marginally increased among phenytoin users (standard incidence ratio (SIR), 1.2 [95% confidence interval (CI), 0.9–1.5]; 61 cases), as were the incidences of brain cancer (SIR, 8.2 [95% CI, 3.3–17]; 7 deaths) and of oesophageal cancer (SIR, 5.0 [95% CI, 1.0–15]; 3 deaths). No other site showed a significant increase or decrease in cancer incidence. In an earlier study (Friedman, 1986), one case of multiple myeloma was reported in these subjects, with 0.6 expected. A case–control study of multiple myeloma in this population is described in Section 2.3.1.

Olsen *et al.* (1989) selected 8004 patients from all patients admitted for treatment of epilepsy to the Filadelfia treatment community in Denmark between 1933 and 1962 to compare cancer incidence with that in the general population. The patients had received powerful and prolonged treatment with anticonvulsants. During the 1940s, phenytoin became popular and was used alone (at daily doses of 100–400 mg) or in combination with phenobarbital. Time since hospitalization was used as a surrogate for cumulative drug exposure. To trace patients, the Central Population Register and mortality files were used (completeness of follow-up was > 90%). The follow-up lasted from 1943 to 1984. For each cancer site, expected numbers of cases were based on incidence rates in the general population by sex, five-year age group and calendar year. Tumour morphology and behaviour comparisons were made with population samples from Danish Cancer Registry records. For the 8004 patients (4246 men and 3758 women), the total person-years of follow-up amounted to 207 798 (average, 23.5 years). A total of 789 cancers (based on 7864 patients, excluding 140 patients known to have received Thorotrast) were reported, compared with 663.7 expected (relative risk (RR), 1.2; 95% CI, 1.1–1.3). Site-specific relative risks are presented in Table 2. Significant excesses were found for cancers of the lung and brain and central nervous system. Brain cancer risk was highest within one year after admission and declined markedly with time. No overall cancer risk was apparent after excluding the brain cancer cases (RR, 1.03). Nonsignificant risk elevations were also observed for cancers of the liver and biliary tract and for non-Hodgkin lymphoma. Significant deficits of urinary bladder cancer and melanoma were observed. [The Working Group noted that brain tumours may account for the seizure disorder and are unlikely to be due to exposure to the anticonvulsant treatment and, furthermore, that the excess of liver cancer may be due to unrecorded exposure to Thorotrast. The slight excess of lung cancer is difficult to interpret, because no information was available on smoking history.]

2.3 Case–control studies

2.3.1 *Multiple sites*

Four nested case–control studies based on the cohort of Olsen *et al.* (1989) were conducted to investigate the possible influence of anticonvulsant treatment on the risk of lung cancer and urinary bladder cancer (including cases of bladder papillomas), lymphoma and hepatobiliary cancer (Olsen *et al.*, 1993, 1995). The studies included 104 cases of lung cancer, 18 cases of urinary bladder cancer, 26 cases of primary liver cancer, 13 cases of biliary tract cancer, 15 cases of non-Hodgkin lymphoma and six cases of Hodgkin's disease. Cases were individually matched to controls on the basis of sex, year of birth (± 1 year) and survival time. The matching ratio was 2, except in the study of lymphoma, in which five controls were selected per case. Six percent of cases and 5% of controls were excluded because of missing medical records. Information about detailed drug use was abstracted from the medical records at the epilepsy centre. Cumulative doses were computed by assuming that treatment continued daily at the prescribed dose after each hospital discharge until the date of cancer diagnosis (or equivalent date for matched controls) or until the end of 1964, whichever occurred first. After the mid-1960s, many new anticonvulsants were released, and therefore no credible assumptions about continuation of previous treatment after discharge were possible for the years after 1964. The median cumulative dose of phenytoin was 750 g. Risk estimates were adjusted for other anticonvulsant treatments, but not for smoking. The prevalence of phenytoin use (alone or in combination with another drug) was around 50% among controls. Use of phenytoin was not associated with the risk for either lung (RR, 1.0; 95% CI, 0.6–1.7) or urinary bladder cancer (RR, 1.1; 95% CI, 0.4–3.5). Also, dose–response analyses revealed no consistent relationships between either lung cancer or bladder cancer and cumulative exposure to phenytoin. Data from a smoking survey among Danish epileptics indicated that the elevated risk in the cohort is probably attributable to confounding by smoking (Olsen *et al.*, 1993). Epileptic patients who had ever been given phenytoin had a slight, nonsignificantly increased risk for lymphoma

Table 2. Numbers of incident cancers occurring between 1943 and 1984 among patients hospitalized for epilepsy during 1933–62 at Filadelfia, Denmark, excluding 140 patients known to have received Thorotrast

Site	Observed	Observed/expected ratio (95% CI)
All malignant neoplasms	789	1.2 (1.1–1.3)
Buccal cavity and pharynx	18	1.2 (0.7–1.9)
Oesophagus	7	1.3 (0.5–2.8)
Stomach	33	1.0 (0.7–1.4)
Colon	48	1.1 (0.8–1.4)
Rectum	28	0.9 (0.6–1.2)
Liver (primary)	9	1.9 (0.9–3.6)
Liver (not otherwise specified)	2	0.8 (0.1–3.1)
Biliary tract	11	1.7 (0.9–3.1)
Pancreas	20	1.1 (0.7–1.7)
Larynx	10	1.6 (0.8–2.9)
Lung	106	1.4 (1.2–1.7)
Breast	80	1.0 (0.8–1.2)
Cervix uteri	32	0.8 (0.5–1.1)
Corpus uteri	19	1.0 (0.6–1.5)
Ovary	18	0.8 (0.5–1.3)
Prostate	19	0.8 (0.5–1.3)
Testis	13	1.6 (0.8–2.7)
Kidney	18	1.0 (0.6–1.6)
Bladder	18	0.6 (0.3–0.9)
Melanoma of skin	7	0.5 (0.2–1.0)
Other skin	60	1.0 (0.8–1.3)
Brain and central nervous system	118	5.7 (4.7–6.8)
Thyroid	4	1.2 (0.3–3.2)
Non-Hodgkin lymphoma	16	1.4 (0.8–2.3)
Hodgkin's disease	6	0.9 (0.3–2.1)
Multiple myeloma	3	0.5 (0.1–1.5)
Leukaemia	13[a]	0.8 (0.4–1.4)
Other specified sites	31	1.2 (0.8–1.8)
Secondary and unspecified sites	22[b]	1.9 (1.2–2.8)

From Olsen et al. (1989)

[a] Seven patients, chronic lymphocytic leukaemia; three, chronic myelogenous leukaemia; one, acute leukaemia; and two, leukaemia not otherwise specified

[b] Excluding liver

(RR, 1.6; 95% CI, 0.5–4.8). The risk was highest for the subgroup of non-Hodgkin lymphoma (RR, 1.8; 95% CI, 0.5–6.6). In this subgroup, patients who had received a cumulative dose of 750 g phenytoin or more had a nonsignificantly higher risk than patients who had been given less than 750 g (RR, 3.1; 95% CI, 0.6–15; versus RR, 1.0; 95% CI, 0.2–4.9). [The Working Group noted that the number of non-Hodgkin lymphoma patients in the study was very small.] The risk for hepatobiliary cancer was not increased among patients ever treated with phenytoin (RR, 1.2; 95% CI, 0.5–3.1) (Olsen et al., 1995).

2.3.2 Multiple myeloma

A case–control study was conducted to investigate (among other factors) the relationship between multiple myeloma and medicinal drugs, such as propoxyphene and phenytoin (Friedman, 1986). A total of 327 cases of multiple myeloma occurring during 1969–82 were identified among Kaiser Foundation Health Plan subscribers in northern California (United States) (96.6% based on pathological examination and 3.4% on strong clinical evidence). Controls (one per case) were selected from the Health Plan membership file of the same year as the case's year of first hospitalization for multiple myeloma, matched to the case by sex, year of birth, area of residence and, when feasible, race. No association was found between phenytoin use and multiple myeloma risk. [The Working Group noted that RR and 95% CI were not reported].

In the hospital-based, case–control study of multiple myeloma in whites in Baltimore area, MD, United States, in 1975–82, reported in the monograph on diazepam (p. 53), a nonsignificantly elevated risk was found for prior use of phenytoin (odds ratio, ∞; 95% CI, 0.6–∞; discordant pairs ratio: 3/0) (Linet et al., 1987). [The Working Group noted that the diagnostic categories for controls could have been associated with exposure to phenytoin. In addition, the greater number of proxy interviews for cases than for controls could not be adjusted for with phenytoin as the exposure.]

2.3.3 Hodgkin's disease

A case–control study was conducted to investigate a number of risk factors for Hodgkin's disease in Brazil (Kirchhoff et al., 1980). Cases were patients diagnosed from 1963 to 1976 at one hospital and were divided into three groups: private, self-paying patients; patients whose care was paid for by the national health insurance programme; and patients who were treated without charge. Out of a total of 546 patients, 70 patients of the last two groups were included in this study. A control group was made up of 128 siblings of the Hodgkin's disease patients. All of the patients and controls whose cooperation was solicited agreed to participate in the study. Exposure to phenytoin was assessed by asking whether the subjects had ever taken medicine for epilepsy, convulsions, fits or migraine headaches. The mean age of the cases was 27 years. For the sibling control group, the mean age was 22 years. Phenytoin had been used by 4% of the cases and 3% of the sibling controls. [The crude odds ratio for phenytoin use was 1.4; 95% CI, 0.3–6.4.] [The Working Group noted that the criteria for selection of cases were unclear.]

2.3.4 *Childhood cancer*

In a case–control study of 11 169 pairs of childhood cancer cases and matched controls in 1953–71 in the United Kingdom, use of drugs during pregnancy was assessed through hospital and general practitioners' records (Sanders & Draper, 1979). Phenytoin use was reported for mothers of 11 cases and 7 controls [crude odds ratio, 1.6; 95% CI, 0.6–4.0].

In a case–control study of incident cases of neuroblastoma diagnosed between 1970 and 1979 in the United States, drug use during pregnancy was investigated among mothers of 104 cases and 101 controls selected by telephone random digit dialling (Kramer *et al.*, 1987). No use of phenytoin during the index pregnancy was reported among mothers of cases or controls.

3. Studies of Cancer in Experimental Animals

3.1 Oral administration

3.1.1 *Mouse*

Groups of 48 female C57Bl, C3H/F or SJL/J mice, two to three months of age, were given 0 or 60 mg/kg bw phenytoin sodium (Dilantin) (pharmaceutical grade) in a liquid diet for 168 days. Of those surviving to 10 months, 3/24 treated C57Bl mice as well as 3/24 C3H/F mice developed thymic lymphosarcomas, whereas no pathological lesion was found in 48 controls [$p = 0.03$]. Of the treated SJL/J mice, 6/42 had generalized lymphomas during the fourth to eight months, but no lymphoma was seen in 48 controls after eight months [$p = 0.008$]. After the eighth month, 90% of the treated SJL/J mice developed reticulum-cell sarcomas which appeared 2–3 months earlier than in the controls (Krüger *et al.*, 1972).

Groups of 30 and 23 female C3H/Sn mice, 3.5 months of age, were given 0 or 2 mg/animal phenytoin sodium (Diphenin) (pharmaceutical grade) in 0.2 ml tap-water by gastric instillation five times per week for life. The life span of treated mice was significantly increased (mean: controls, 450 ± 19 days; treated, 558 ± 28 days; $p < 0.05$, Student's *t* test). The number of mice with mammary gland adenocarcinomas was significantly decreased (19/30 controls, 7/23 treated mice; $p < 0.05$, chi-square test); the numbers of mice with leukaemia were 5/30 controls and 2/23 treated mice; and the numbers of mice with polyps of the endometrium [not otherwise specified] were 4/30 controls and 0/23 treated mice (Dilman & Anisimov, 1980).

Groups of 50 male and 50 female B6C3F1 mice, six weeks old, were given 0, 60 or 120 mg/kg diet (ppm) phenytoin (purity, > 99%) in the diet for 78 weeks. The estimated mean total intake per mouse was 150 mg or 301 mg in males and 154 mg or 292 mg in females. The mice were kept for a further eight weeks, after which time all surviving animals were killed. Survival at week 86 was: males — 86% control, 72% low-dose and 82% high-dose; and females — 94% control, 88% low-dose and 86% high-dose. All major organs and visually apparent lesions were examined histologically. In male mice, the incidence of hepatocellular adenomas was decreased (19/46 control, 12/45 low-dose and 11/45 high-dose); that of hepatocellular carcinomas was 7/46 control, 8/45 low-dose and 5/45 high-dose. The decreased incidence of combined hepatocellular adenomas and carcinomas was statistically significant (26/46 control, 20/45 low-dose and 16/45 high-dose; $p < 0.05$, chi-square test). There was no significant difference in the incidence of tumours at other sites between treated and control males. No increase in tumours was seen in females (Maeda et al., 1988).

3.1.2 Rat

In a number of early carcinogenicity studies of phenytoin of limited duration, negative results were reported (Griswold et al., 1966, 1968; McDonald, 1969; Morris et al., 1969; Peraino et al., 1975). [The Working Group considered that these studies were inadequate for assessing carcinogenicity.]

Groups of 75 and 34 female rats [strain not specified], 3.5 months of age, were given 0 and 7.5 mg/rat phenytoin [purity not specified] in 5 mL tap-water by gastric instillation five times per week for life. Animals were killed when moribund. Neoplastic tissues were examined histologically. Mean life span was 681 ± 14 days in controls and 724 ± 36 days in treated animals. No treatment-related increase in tumour incidence was observed (Anisimov, 1980).

Groups of 50 male and 50 female Fischer 344/DuCrj rats, five weeks of age, were given 0, 250 or 500 (maximum tolerated dose) mg/kg diet (ppm) phenytoin (> 99% pure) in the diet for two years. After a further eight weeks, survival was greater than 60% in all groups, and all surviving rats were killed at that time. There was a dose-related decrease in mean body weight in treated females but not in males. All rats that died or were killed were autopsied. All lesions and most organs were examined histologically. There was no significant difference in tumour incidence between treated and control rats (Jang et al., 1987).

3.2 Perinatal and/or adult administration

3.2.1 Mouse

Groups of 60 female C57Bl/6N and 60 male C3H/HeN mice were exposed perinatally (F_0), as adults (B6C3F1 mice) (F_1) or both to various concentrations of phenytoin, as shown in Table 3. Four groups of 60 females aged 10–14 weeks were given 0, 21, 70 or 210 mg/kg diet (ppm) phenytoin (approximately 98% pure) in the diet for one week before breeding. After breeding with previously unexposed male mice, the females continued to receive the same diet throughout pregnancy and lactation. Weaning occurred on day 28 post-partum and dietary exposure of the pups continued at the same concentrations until they were approximately eight weeks of age. From eight weeks of age, groups of 60 male and 60 female pups were fed diets containing 0, 30, 100 or 300 ppm (males) and 0, 60, 200 or 600 ppm phenytoin (females), respectively, for up to two years (perinatal/adult exposure). The highest dose was set on the basis of body weight changes in prechronic studies. Additional groups of 60 male and 60 female adults, 10–14 weeks of age, were given diets containing 0, 100 or 300 ppm and 0, 200 or 600 ppm

Table 3. Incidence of hepatocellular adenoma or carcinoma in mice exposed to phenytoin in the diet

Concentration (ppm)		Liver tumour incidence		
F_0	F_1	Adenoma	Carcinoma[a]	Adenoma or carcinoma[a]
Males				
Adult exposure groups				
0	0[b]	19/50	13/50	29/50
0	100	19/49	15/49	29/49
0	300	22/49	7/49	26/49
Perinatal/adult exposure group				
21	30	16/50[c]	13/50[c]	25/50[c]
70	100	20/50	18/50	31/50
210	100	23/49	18/49	35/49
210	300	31/50[c,d]	20/50	41/50[c,d]
Perinatal exposure group				
210	0	23/50	14/50	33/50
Females				
Adult exposure groups				
0	0[b]	5/48	0/48	5/48
0	200	13/49[d]	1/49	14/49[d]
0	600	22/50[e]	12/50[e]	30/50[e]
Perinatal/adult exposure groups				
21	60	11/50[c]	4/50	13/50[c,d]
70	200	25/50[c,f]	3/50	26/50[c,f]
210	200	12/50	4/50	16/50[c,f]
210	600	26/50[c,f]	10/50[b,c]	34/50[c,f]
Perinatal exposure group				
210	0	11/49	1/49	12/49[g]

From United States National Toxicology Program (1993)

[a] For adult exposure: carcinoma is hepatoblastoma or hepatocellular carcinoma

[b] Historical control rates at the laboratory: males — 167/410 (40%; range, 17–68%); females — 56/416 (13%; range, 3–26%) (Chhabra et al., 1993)

[c] From Chhabra et al. (1993)

[d] Significantly different ($p < 0.05$) from the 0:0 group (logistic regression analysis)

[e] Significantly different ($p < 0.001$) from the 0:0 group (logistic regression analysis)

[f] Significantly different ($p \leq 0.01$) from the 0:0 group (logistic regression analysis)

[g] Not significantly different ($p = 0.055$) from the 0:0 group (logistic regression analysis)

phenytoin for two years. After nine months of phenytoin administration, 10 animals from each group were killed. Surviving animals were killed at the end of the two-year study period. Survival at that time was similar in control (males, 78%; females, 72%) and treated groups (66–88%). Incidences of hepatocellular tumours are summarized in Table 3. In male mice, perinatal exposure alone did not increase the incidence of liver tumours. However, there was a significant $F_0 : F_1$ interaction, which reflected the enhancing effects of combined 210 ppm perinatal treatment and 300 ppm adult treatment on the incidences of liver neoplasms. In female mice, both adult exposures and perinatal plus adult exposure resulted in increased incidence of liver tumours (United States National Toxicology Program, 1993).

3.2.2 Rat

Groups of 60 female and 60 male Fischer 344/N rats were exposed perinatally (F_0), as adults (F_1) or both to various concentrations of phenytoin, as shown in Table 4. Four groups of 60 females aged 10–12 weeks were given 0, 63, 210 or 630 mg/kg diet (ppm) phenytoin (approximately 98% pure) in the diet for one week before breeding. After breeding with previously unexposed male rats, the females continued to receive the same diet throughout pregnancy and lactation. Weaning occurred on day 28 post-partum and dietary exposure of pups continued at the same concentrations until they were approximately eight weeks of age. From eight weeks of age, groups of 60 male and 60 female pups were fed diets containing 0, 240, 800 or 2400 ppm phenytoin for up to two years (perinatal/adult exposure). The highest dose was set on the basis of body weight changes in prechronic studies. Additional groups of 60 male and 60 female adults, 10–12 weeks of age, were given diets containing 0, 800 or 2400 ppm phenytoin for two years. After nine months of phenytoin administration, 10 animals from each group were killed. Surviving animals were killed at the end of the two-year study period. Survival at that time was similar in control (males, 52%; females, 62%) and treated groups (44–76%). Incidences of hepatocellular tumours (adenoma and carcinoma combined) are summarized in Table 4. In male rats, the incidence of liver tumours was slightly increased in the high-dose perinatal/adult treatment group ($p < 0.05$, logistic regression analysis) (US National Toxicology Program, 1993).

3.3 Intraperitoneal administration

Mouse: A group of 50 male and female random-bred albino mice, weighing 18–20 g [age not specified], was given 0.6 mg/animal phenytoin as phenytoin sodium [purity not specified] suspended in water or in saline daily by intraperitoneal injection over a 66-day period (total of 57 injections; 34.2 mg/animal). No weight gain was observed and 10 animals died during this period. The remaining 40 animals were observed for nine months. A group of 50 untreated controls was observed for 11 months. Ten treated mice developed tumours, comprising four thymic and two mesenteric lymphomas and four leukaemias. The leukaemias were found between 60 and 142 days and the lymphomas between 100 and 255 days. In controls, one thymic lymphoma and one lung adenoma were observed (Juhász et al., 1968).

Table 4. Incidence of hepatocellular adenoma and carcinoma combined in rats exposed to phenytoin in the diet

Concentration (ppm)		Liver tumour incidence	
F_0	F_1	Male	Female
Adult exposure groups			
0	0[a]	0/50	0/50
0	800	2/50 (1 carcinoma)	1/50
0	2400	4/50	1/50
Perinatal/adult exposure groups			
63	240	3/49 (1 carcinoma)	0/50
210	800	2/49	1/50
630	800	1/49	0/50
630	2400	5/49[b]	0/50
Perinatal exposure group			
630	0	1/50	0/49

From United States National Toxicology Program (1993)
[a] Historical control rates at the laboratory: males — 6/302 (2%; range 0–10%); females — 0/300 (Chhabra et al., 1993)
[b] Significantly different ($p < 0.05$) from the 0:0 group (logistic regression analysis) (Chhabra et al., 1993)

3.4 Administration with known carcinogens

Mouse: In a short-term assay based upon lung adenoma induction in mice, three groups of SWR inbred mice [age and sex not specified] were given 0.5 mg/g bw urethane [purity not specified] in water as a single intraperitoneal injection. Two groups also received seven daily subcutaneous injections either of 0.5 mg/animal phenytoin [purity and solvent not specified] or of the solvent only before and after the administration of urethane, while one group received no further treatment. Twelve weeks after the injection of urethane, all animals were killed and their lungs were examined macroscopically for the presence of adenomas. The incidence of lung adenomas was 100% in the urethane-treated controls (15 mice) and in animals treated with urethane plus solvent (15 mice) and was 85.7% in animals treated with urethane plus phenytoin (14 mice). The number of adenomas per mouse was reduced in the phenytoin-treated group (mean ± SE : 4.5 ± 0.6, 4.7 ± 0.6 and 2.9 ± 0.6 ($p < 0.025$, Student's t test) in the three groups, respectively) (Levo, 1974).

Groups of 25 male D2B6F1 mice, five weeks of age, were given 0 or 90 mg/kg bw *N*-nitrosodiethylamine (NDEA; 99% pure) in tricaprylin as a single intraperitoneal injection. Two weeks later, the mice were given 0, 125, 250 or 500 mg/kg diet (ppm) phenytoin [purity not specified] in the diet. Ten mice from each group were killed at 30 weeks of age, at which time the incidence of hepatocellular lesions (foci) in NDEA-treated mice was 2 (lesions)/10, 4 (eosinophilic foci)/10, 0/10 and 10 (lesions)/10 ($p < 0.01$, Mann-Whitney U test) in the groups treated with 0 (control), 125, 250 and 500 ppm phenytoin, respectively. Three NDEA-treated mice receiving 500 ppm phenytoin developed hepatocellular adenomas. Control mice and mice given only phenytoin displayed no hepatocellular lesions at 30 weeks. All surviving mice were killed at 60 weeks of age. Selected portions of liver lobe (two sections per lobe), all liver lesions and lesions in other organs were examined histologically. Survival was not affected by phenytoin in NDEA-treated or vehicle-treated mice. Phenytoin enhanced the hepatocarcinogenesis initiated by NDEA at week 60 (see Table 5). No significant difference in either incidence or multiplicity of lung adenomas was observed between the groups (Diwan et al., 1993).

Table 5. Effect of phenytoin on hepatocellular carcinogenesis initiated by *N*-nitrosodiethylamine (NDEA) in mice

Treatment groups	No. of mice with tumours/total no. at risk (%)[a]	No. of tumours per tumour-bearing mouse (mean ± SD)		
		Adenomas	Carcinomas	Hepato-blastomas
NDEA	9/15 (60)	1.8 ± 0.8	0	0
NDEA/125 ppm phenytoin	10/14 (71)	2.6 ± 1.3	0	0
NDEA/250 ppm phenytoin	10/13 (77)	4.4 ± 3.3[b]	0	0
NDEA/500 ppm phenytoin	15/15 (100)[b]	11.6 ± 5.6[c]	2.3 ± 2.2	1.4 ± 0.5
Vehicle/250 ppm phenytoin	1/15 (7)	1 ± 0	0	0
Vehicle/500 ppm phenytoin	1/15 (7)	1 ± 0	0	0
Vehicle	0/15	0	0	0

From Diwan et al. (1993)
[a] Animals with severe post-mortem changes were not included
[b] Statistically significant compared with NDEA group ($p < 0.05$, Fisher's exact test)
[c] Statistically significant compared with NDEA group ($p < 0.001$, Fisher's exact test)

4. Other Data Relevant to an Evaluation of Carcinogenicity and its Mechansms

4.1 Absorption, distribution, metabolism and excretion

4.1.1 *Humans*

Phenytoin is well absorbed following oral dosing with well formulated pharmaceutical preparations (capsules, tablets, suspensions); absorption occurs predominantly in the duodenum, from which the absorption rate is limited by its dissolution in intestinal fluids (solubility approximately 100 μg/mL) and plasma (75 μg/mL). Peak plasma concentrations are usually reached within 4–8 h. The drug is widely distributed in the body (volume of distribution averages about 0.8 L/kg), readily crosses the blood–brain barrier and is bound extensively (~90%) to plasma protein, predominantly albumin (Treiman & Woodbury, 1995). Phenytoin is metabolized extensively (Figure 1), principally to 5-(4'-hydroxyphenyl)-5-phenylhydantoin (*para*-HPPH), which is excreted as the glucuronide conjugate in the urine, typically accounting for 67–88% of the dose. This is formed via the well known epoxide-diol pathway, like the 5-(3',4'-dihydrodiol), which is also found in urine, representing some 7–11% of the dose (Browne & LeDuc, 1995). The arene oxide, which is the primary metabolite on this pathway, has never been isolated but its occurrence is inferred. This class of metabolic intermediates has attracted considerable attention because of their possible role in the mechanisms of toxicity, mutagenicity and teratogenicity (see Section 4.3.3) (Van Dyke *et al.*, 1991; Finnell *et al.*, 1992). In addition to the two major excretion products mentioned, a number of minor metabolites including the 3',4'-catechol, the corresponding 3'-*O*-methylcatechol, a bis-(4-hydroxyphenyl) derivative and the *N*-glucuronide of phenytoin have been identified. These never account for more than trace quantities of a phenytoin dose in humans. The *meta*-isomer of HPPH (namely the 5-(3'-hydroxyphenyl) derivative) has been reported (Browne & LeDuc, 1995), but this may be an analytical artefact. Early workers also reported the identification of two ring-opened products, diphenylhydantoic acid and α-aminodiphenylacetic acid, as minor metabolites. Since phenytoin is prochiral, any metabolic change in one of the phenyl substituents will give rise to chiral derivatives. In humans, the *para*-HPPH excreted in urine is predominantly the *S*-enantiomer (the $S:R$ ratio is typically about 3 : 1) (Poupaert *et al.*, 1975; Maguire *et al.*, 1980; Browne & LeDuc, 1995).

There has recently been considerable study of the cytochrome P450 isoforms responsible for the hydroxylation of phenytoin. Doecke *et al.* (1990) suggested that isoforms of the CYP2C subfamily were responsible for phenytoin metabolism in rabbits and humans, and recent work by Veronese *et al.* (1993) strongly suggests that CYP2C9/10 isoforms are responsible for most of the *para*-HPPH formation in humans.

Phenytoin displays non-linear elimination pharmacokinetics which are adequately described by a model based on the Michaelis–Menten equation (Browne & LeDuc, 1995). One consequence of this non-linearity is that the apparent elimination half-life varies with plasma concentration. Strictly speaking, it is inappropriate to refer to a 'half-life', but in practical terms a mean value of around 22 h is a useful guide. It seems clear that the non-linearity in the elimination of phenytoin results from saturation of the enzyme(s) responsible for the formation of the arene oxide metabolite.

Phenytoin crosses the placenta (Mirkin, 1971). Similar concentrations have been measured in maternal and umbilical cord plasma at delivery, indicating an equilibrium state after long-term administration (Nau *et al.*, 1982). Neonatal elimination of placentally transferred phenytoin was very slow on post-partum days 1 and 2, increased markedly on post-partum day 3 and was complete by post-partum day 5. Phenytoin levels are low in breast milk obtained from epileptic mothers (Mirkin, 1971). The maternal serum level falls during the second and third trimesters of pregnancy (Eadie *et al.*, 1977; Nau *et al.*, 1982). Free and total plasma levels of phenytoin were determined

Figure 1. Postulated metabolic pathways of phenytoin

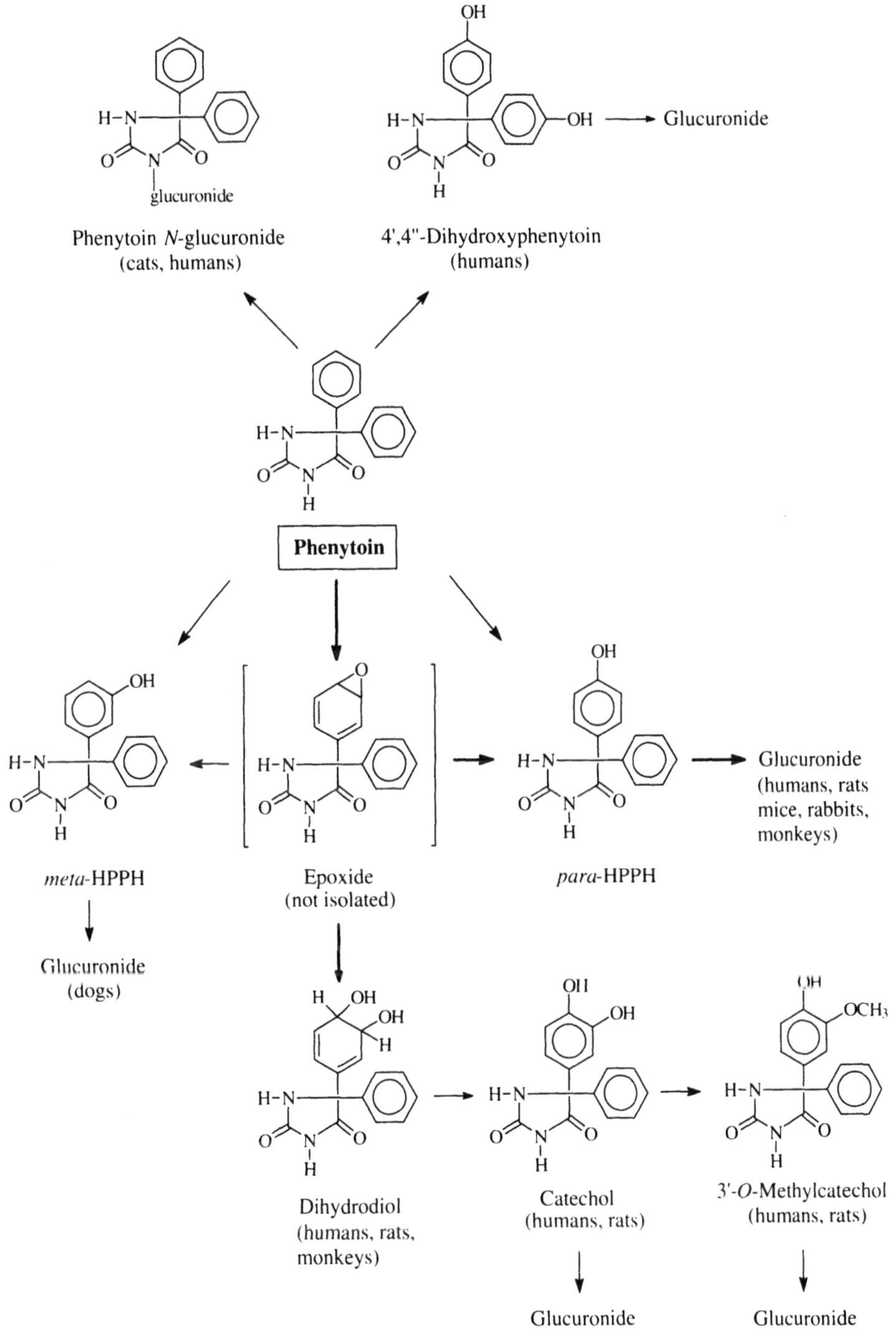

From Browne & Leduc (1995)

in a prospective study of 29 pregnant women receiving phenytoin monotherapy. Total clearance of plasma phenytoin increased from the first trimester and a less pronounced, but significant, increase was observed for clearance of free phenytoin during the third trimester (Tomson *et al.*, 1994). In a study of 10 epileptic women, the proportion of the phenytoin dose excreted as *para*-HPPH tended to rise during pregnancy and overall the increased excretion of *para*-HPPH appeared sufficient to account for the elimination of the entire increase in the daily dose of phenytoin required during pregnancy. Excretion of unmetabolized phenytoin and certain of its minor metabolites appeared essentially unaltered. Thus pregnancy does not enhance uniformly the various pathways of phenytoin metabolism (Eadie *et al.*, 1992). The plasma level of phenytoin returns to normal values during the post-partum period (Lander *et al.*, 1977).

4.1.2 *Experimental systems*

para-HPPH glucuronide appears to be the major metabolite in all species studied (e.g., rats, mice, rabbits, monkeys) except dogs, in which the major excretion product is the glucuronide of *meta*-HPPH (Atkinson *et al.*, 1970), and cats, in which the *N*-glucuronide of phenytoin predominates (Hassell *et al.*, 1984). All of the major metabolites found in humans have been identified in most of the animal species studied, although there are some interspecies differences in the relative quantities and in the extent of conjugation (Browne & LeDuc, 1995).

A single intragastric dose of phenytoin to pregnant Sprague-Dawley rats was transferred to the fetuses and was concentrated more in the kidney than in the liver, in contrast to the situation in adult rats (Gabler & Falace, 1970). Transplacental transport has been documented in mice (Waddell & Mirkin, 1972; Stevens & Harbison, 1974), rats (Mirkin, 1971; Stevens & Harbison, 1974), Syrian hamsters (Stevens & Harbison, 1974), goats (Shoeman *et al.*, 1972) and rhesus monkeys (Gabler & Hubbard, 1972).

Studies with CYP2C3 purified from rabbit liver have shown that this enzyme plays a major role in the 4'-hydroxylation of phenytoin, and further suggested than an orthologue to this enzyme was in part responsible for this metabolic reaction in humans (Doecke *et al.*, 1990). The hydroperoxidase component of prostaglandin synthetase, as well as thyroid peroxidase and other peroxidases, can bioactivate phenytoin to a reactive free radical intermediate, which may have toxicological relevance (Kubow & Wells, 1989). Whether this free radical or the arene oxide intermediate is the principal mediator of toxic effects remains unclear.

4.2 Toxic effects

4.2.1 *Humans*

(a) *Acute toxicity*

Death from acute phenytoin overdosage in humans is very uncommon (reviewed by Dollery *et al.*, 1991). Intravenous administration of high doses of phenytoin (e.g., in the emergency treatment of cardiac arrhythmias or status epilepticus) may induce severe cardiac arrhythmias and hypotension as well as central and peripheral nervous system toxicity. Nystagmus, ataxia, diplopia, dysarthria, vertigo and other cerebellar-vestibular effects are common symptoms of phenytoin intoxication; acute oral overdosage has been reported to cause irreversible cerebellar atrophy (Earnest et al., 1983; Masur et al., 1989, 1990; Reynolds, 1993). Since phenytoin has a narrow therapeutic range and patients respond with considerable interindividual variability, intoxications are frequently iatrogenic or due to inappropriate self-adjustment of doses (Manon-Espaillat et al., 1991).

Phenytoin is a potent inducer of certain hepatic cytochrome P450 activities, increasing the clearance of antipyrine, dicoumarol, primidone, carbamazepine, prednisolone, dexamethasone and other glucocorticoids (Nation et al., 1990a,b; Dollery et al., 1991).

(b) *Chronic toxicity*

(i) *Effects on the nervous system*

Chronic phenytoin intake may induce a variety of adverse effects on the nervous system, including drowsiness, nystagmus, ataxia, blurred vision and diplopia; in the past when patients were treated with very high doses for many years, intellectual dulling and depression of mood were frequently reported (reviewed by Dollery et al., 1991).

Although central and peripheral nervous system toxicity is the most consistent effect of acute phenytoin overdosage, the chronic effects of phenytoin on the nervous system are a subject of debate, since it remains unclear if they can be attributed solely to the drug or if and to what extent they result from recurrent seizures. The most severe histopathological feature associated with chronic phenytoin administration is development of cerebellar atrophy. However, literature on neuropathology from before the introduction of phenytoin documents that convulsions are associated with cerebellar atrophy. The molecular mechanism of phenytoin damage to the cerebellum has not been elucidated and the causal role of phenytoin in the induction of cerebellar atrophy cannot be considered as proven (Ghatak et al., 1976; Rapport & Shaw, 1977; McLain, et al., 1980; Hammond & Wilder, 1983; Ney et al., 1994).

A rare, albeit well documented complication of phenytoin administration is the induction of dyskinesias consisting mainly of generalized choreoathetosis with or without orofacial symptoms. Phenytoin has been shown to interfere with the dopaminergic system; however, the precise mechanism remains to be elucidated (Harrison et al., 1993).

(ii) *Gingival overgrowth*

Phenytoin-induced gingival overgrowth was first reported in 1939 (Kimball, 1939); later studies revealed extremely high incidences of up to 50% of gingival hyperplasia in patients medicated with phenytoin (Hassell, 1981). However, these high incidences were based mainly on investigations carried out in hospital patients usually taking several anticonvulsant drugs because they experienced complications with the control of their epilepsy (Angelopoulos, 1975). A recent community-based study of patients in general medical practice revealed a 13% incidence of phenytoin-induced, clinically significant gingival overgrowth (Thomason et al., 1992).

Gingival overgrowth can commence within three months after initiation of phenytoin therapy and is most rapid in the first year of medication. Early signs often arise as diffuse swelling of the interdental papillae; in severe cases, the overgrowth may induce impairment of speech and eating (Thomason et al., 1992; Seymour, 1993). There is no strict dose–effect relationship. Polypharmacy significantly increases the prevalence of gingival overgrowth, especially co-medication with sodium valproate, phenobarbital and carbamazepine, which can result in alterations in phenytoin kinetics (Maguire et al., 1986). The overgrowth of tissue appears to involve altered collagen metabolism, which in rare cases and after many years of treatment may result in facial coarsening (Ohta et al., 1995), mainly manifested as broadening of the lips and nose. Rodents and other small mammals do not appear to be susceptible to phenytoin-induced gingival overgrowth, but this side-effect can be reproduced in the monkey *Macaca arctoides* (Staple et al., 1977) and cats (Hassell et al., 1982; Thomason et al., 1992).

Studies on the mechanisms underlying phenytoin-induced gingival hyperplasia show that fibroblasts derived from patients with phenytoin-associated gingival hyperplasia synthesize a higher amount of total protein and collagen and have higher proliferation rates compared with control cells or with cells from patients with idiopathic gingival fibromatosis (Hou, 1993). Phenytoin inhibits calcium transport and, since gingival hyperplasia is also induced by nifedipine and other calcium-channel blockers, it has been suggested that interference with calcium transport may be involved in the gingival overgrowth (Fujii et al., 1994).

(iii) *Folic acid deficiency*

Patients taking phenytoin may exhibit folic acid deficiency (Mallek & Nakamoto, 1981; Reynolds, 1993). In addition to increasing the risk for developing megaloblastic anaemia, folic acid deficiency has been implicated in the development of gingival hyperplasia by impairing maturation of the gingival epithelium, thus rendering the underlying connective tissue more susceptible to inflammation and increased proliferation.

(iv) *Hypersensitivity reactions — effects on the immune system*

Phenytoin has been associated with numerous cutaneous hypersensitivity reactions. Morbilliform rash arises in 2–5% of patients and in rare cases more severe reactions may be observed, such as toxic epidermal necrolysis (Stevens–Johnson syndrome) or lupus erythematosus. The skin reactions may be accompanied by lymphadenopathy, eosinophilia, fever, diverse haematological disorders (leukocytosis, leukopenia, thrombocytopenia) and systemic organ manifestations such as hepatitis or nephritis (Reynolds, 1993). This hypersensitivity syndrome complex, referred to as the phenytoin hypersensitivity syndrome, usually appears early (e.g., two to four weeks) after initiation of treatment, and does not exhibit a dose–response relationship (Delattre et al., 1988; Braddock et al., 1992).

In some patients exhibiting the triad of skin reactions, fever and lymphadenopathy, biopsy specimens of enlarged lymph nodes display a broad spectrum of histopathological changes, ranging from benign hyperplasia to malignant-appearing cells (Saltzstein & Ackerman, 1959; Hyman & Sommers, 1966; Anthony, 1970). The possible effects of phenytoin on the lymphatic tissue can be categorized into four groups, although some symptoms may overlap: benign lymphoid hyperplasia, pseudolymphoma, pseudo-pseudolymphoma and malignant lymphoma (see Section 2.1.1) (Harris *et al.*, 1992).

Lymphoid hyperplasia and pseudolymphoma are clinically indistinguishable; however, histological examination reveals normal lymph node structure in the hyperplasia group, while loss of normal lymph node architecture, focal necrosis and infiltration with eosinophils are seen in the pseudolymphoma group. Development of pseudolymphoma has been reported in a few hundred patients receiving normal doses of phenytoin (100 mg daily) and, in view of the many hundreds of thousands of treated patients, can be considered as a rare, albeit severe, side-effect (see Section 2.1.1). The clinical symptoms develop within an average of three weeks, five days to three months after initiation of therapy. In addition to high spiking fever and intensely pruritic maculopapular rash (sometimes with pustulation progressing to exfoliative erythroderma), marked localized or generalized enlargement of lymph nodes is observed. Myalgia and arthralgia as well as hepatitis and in rare cases splenomegaly and histological skin features suggestive of mycosis fungoides have also been reported in some patients. The symptoms resolve in most cases after withdrawal of the drug and recurrence is usually observed upon readministration (Gams *et al.*, 1968; Rosenthal *et al.*, 1982; Cooke *et al.*, 1988; Rijlaarsdam *et al.*, 1991; Singer *et al.*, 1993).

(v) *Endocrine effects*

A variety of endocrine effects have been associated with chronic phenytoin administration. Osteomalacia with hypocalcaemia (Dollery *et al.*, 1991) and elevated alkaline phosphatase activity may arise from altered vitamin D metabolism, inhibition of intestinal absorption of calcium and reduced concentrations of vitamin K, which is important for normal calcium metabolism in the bone (Keith *et al.*, 1983; Kumar *et al.*, 1993). Hyperglycaemia and glucosuria appear to be due to inhibition of insulin secretion (Dollery *et al.*, 1991).

Long-term administration of phenytoin affects blood thyroid hormone levels in a specific manner. Phenytoin reduces the plasma concentration of total thyroxine (T_4) as well as that of free T_4, while there are reports of variable effects upon the concentrations of other thyroid and related hormones. Deda *et al.* (1992) reported that, in addition to T_4, there were reductions in total triiodothyronine (T_3), free T_3 and reverse T_3 levels in phenytoin-treated epileptic children. Similar effects on T_3 and reverse T_3 were found in adults in one study (Yeo *et al.*, 1978), while in another study on adults, T_3 and thyrotropin were within normal ranges (Larkin *et al.*, 1989). In a number of studies, the T_4 and T_3 reductions were accompanied by unaltered thyroid stimulating hormone (TSH) levels (see Schröder-Van der Elst & Van der Heide, 1990). Patients appear to be clinically euthyroid, but experimental studies do not indicate whether phenytoin acts as a thyroid hormone agonist or antagonist. Although much emphasis has been placed on the role of occupancy by phenytoin of binding sites on the circulating thyroxine-binding globulin, the experimental evidence does not support impairment of hormone-binding capacity in the observed side-effects (Yeo *et al.*, 1978; Larkin *et al.*, 1989; Deda *et al.*, 1992).

4.2.2 *Experimental systems*

(a) *Acute toxicity*

The nervous system is the major target of acute phenytoin toxicity in experimental animals. Seizures may be induced after single intraperitoneal administration of 75 mg/kg bw phenytoin in seven-day-old rats, while doses of about 200 mg/kg bw are required in 18-day-old rats. Lethal doses after single intraperitoneal administration are in the range of 1000 mg/kg bw phenytoin (Mareš *et al.*, 1987).

Treatment of mice with phenytoin (150 mg/kg intraperitoneally for three days) induced a 33–43% increase in hepatic cytochrome P450 content compared with controls (Kim *et al.*, 1993). Analysis of the specific enzymes by immunoblot quantification and by metabolic activities revealed a several-fold increase in CYP2B and hexobarbital hydroxylase activities. In contrast, phenytoin treatment did not raise CYP1A activity in mice.

(b) *Subacute and chronic toxicity*

Groups of 10 male and 10 female B6C3F1 mice 7–9 weeks old were given phenytoin in the diet at concentrations between 0 and 1200 mg/kg diet (ppm) for 13 weeks. Nine males and all females exposed to 1200 ppm died before the end of the study and all treated animals showed depressed body-weight gain, although food consumption was not significantly lower than that of the controls. Dose-dependent centrilobular hypertrophy was observed in animals exposed to doses of 300 ppm or more (United States National Toxicology Program, 1993). In another 13-week study, B6C3F1 mice were given 60–4000 ppm phenytoin in the diet. Most mice receiving 1000 ppm or more phenytoin died before the end of the study. Weight gain impairment and focal necrosis of liver cells were observed in the groups receiving 500 and 250 ppm, while no sign of toxicity was observed in animals given 120 ppm (Maeda *et al.*, 1988).

Groups of 10 male and 10 female Fischer 344/N rats, 7–9 weeks old, were given phenytoin in the diet at concentrations between 0 and 4800 mg/kg diet (ppm) for 13 weeks. Mean body-weight gains were significantly lower in the 2400-ppm and 4800-ppm males and females. There was no clinical sign of toxicity and no gross lesion of any organ related to chemical exposure. Chemical-related microscopic lesions were limited to mild centrilobular hypertrophy in the liver of the 4800-ppm group, which was slightly more prominent in males than in females (United States National Toxicology Program, 1993). Similar impairment in body weight-gain and histopathological changes in the liver were reported in another 13-week study in Fischer 344/N rats given phenytoin at concentrations of 1000 and 2000 ppm in the diet, while no change was induced with concentrations of 120–500 ppm. In addition, the relative weights of the liver and spleen in females and of the liver and kidney in males were increased by 1000 and 2000 ppm phenytoin. Increases were measured in alkaline phosphatase activity and in levels of triglyceride and total protein in males and in total cholesterol, total protein and blood urea nitrogen in females (Jang *et al.*, 1987).

(i) *Effects on the liver*

In male D2B6F1 mice given diets containing 250 or 500 mg/kg diet (ppm) phenytoin, hepatic CYP2B-mediated benzyloxyresorufin *O*-dealkylase activity was induced 30-fold and 43-fold after 30 weeks and 41-fold and 57-fold after 60 weeks, respectively. Male B6C3F1 mice given 125, 250, 500 or 1000 ppm phenytoin for 14 days showed significant increases in liver weights at all but the lowest dose and in hepatic CYP2B-mediated benzyloxyresorufin *O*-dealkylase activity at all doses relative to controls (Diwan *et al.*, 1993).

(ii) *Effects on the nervous system*

The chronic effects of phenytoin on the peripheral nervous system were investigated in female Sprague-Dawley rats given 300 mg/kg bw phenytoin per day orally for 180 days. A time-dependent slowing of sensory and motor conduction velocity was observed, and animals with impaired motor conduction velocity also had histopathological changes in the myelinated fibres of the sciatic nerve (Moglia *et al.*, 1981). In male Wister rats, a single intraperitoneal dose of 150 mg/kg bw phenytoin induced a complete blockage of muscle action potential in the dorsal segmental muscles of the tail evoked by electric stimulation of the caudal nerve and a 40% decrease in the Na^+,K^+-ATPase activity of the sciatic nerve compared with control values (Raya *et al.*, 1992).

Exposure of immortalized mouse hippocampal neurons to 1–100 µM phenytoin (concentrations spanning the human therapeutic serum levels and the concentrations in the human brain) impaired the formation of normal neuronal processes by preventing the assembly of several cytoskeletal constituents such as actin, tubulin, neurofilament, tau protein and MAP 5; these constituents accumulated within membrane blebs or cytoplasmic condensations instead of forming normally organized processes. However, at these concentrations, no reduction in the overall cell protein synthesis was seen, an effect observed with concentrations above 200 µM (Bahn *et al.*, 1993).

In addition to its established anticonvulsive activity, phenytoin has been reported to have beneficial effects on the nervous system in other situations. Six-day-old Wistar rats were given 50 mg/kg bw phenytoin (a dose known to give anticonvulsive activity in rats) intraperitoneally, 1 h before induction of brain hypoxia by ligation of the left carotid artery. This dose markedly reduced hypoxic-ischaemic infarction in the cerebral cortex and in the striatum assessed histopathologically 72 h later. This protective effect was not observed when phenytoin was administered immediately after the hypoxia. The authors proposed attenuation of hypoxia-induced release of glutamate (an excitatory amino acid) as a mechanism for this neuroprotective action of phenytoin (Hayakawa *et al.*, 1994). In albino rats of the Wistar-derived Sabra strain, systemically (1–10 mg into the left carotid artery) or topically (0.1–1 mM) applied phenytoin on the neuroma surface suppressed spontaneous ectopic discharge in sciatic nerve neuromas without blocking impulse conductance. Since phenytoin is known to provide effective relief in some kinds of human neuralgia, the authors suggested that the clinical analgesic action of phenytoin may involve direct suppression of ectopic impulses generated in the region of nerve damage (Yaari & Devor, 1985).

(iii) *Effects on the immune system*

Oral administration of phenytoin (25, 50 or 100 mg/kg bw per day for seven days) to BALB/c mice significantly depressed both humoral and cellular immune responses compared with control animals, as assessed by the enumeration of direct and indirect splenic plaque-forming cells and the delayed-type hypersensitivity reaction against sheep red blood cells. Furthermore, spleen cells and lymphocytes obtained from mice treated with 100 mg/kg bw phenytoin suppressed the physiological responses of normal cells in these systems. These immunosuppressing effects were observed in spite of the fact that phenytoin induced a rise in spleen cellularity in the treated mice (Andrade-Mena *et al.*, 1994). Similar results concerning the effects of phenytoin on the murine immune system were also obtained in previous studies in mice (de Souza Queiroz & Mullen, 1980; Margaretten & Warren, 1987).

Lorand *et al.* (1976) assessed morphological changes in lymphoid organs induced by administration of phenytoin (10 or 50 mg/kg bw) to female Wistar rats for two to four months. The morphological changes indicated blockage of cellular differentiation in the thymus; in the lymph nodes, depletion of T lymphocytes together with an increase in plasma cells implied a functional disturbance of the lymphoreticular system. Atypical cells or other morphological features potentially indicative of lymphoma production were not found in this study. Experimental results relating to lymphoma induction are described in Section 3.1.1.

(iv) *Endocrine effects*

Dietary administration of phenytoin to male Wistar rats (50 mg/kg bw for 8 or 20 days) resulted in 20–30% reductions in the serum concentrations of thyroxine (T_4) and triiodothyronine (T_3) but no change in TSH (Schröder-Van der Elst & Van der Heide, 1990; Cageao *et al.*, 1992). At the same doses, the pituitary deiodination of T_4 to T_3 was significantly increased and this increase in the conversion rate is known to inhibit the feedback response of TSH. The observations in rats are consistent with the clinical findings (see Section 4.2.1).

(v) *Bone effects*

Long-term treatment of epileptic patients with phenytoin has been associated with increased thickness mainly of craniofacial bones. This side-effect has been observed in Sprague-Dawley rats given 5 mg/kg bw per day phenytoin for 36 days by intraperitoneal injection, in which increased histomorphometric (osteoblast number, bone mineral apposition rate) and biochemical parameters (skeletal alkaline phosphatase activity, osteocalcin concentration in the serum) of bone formation were measured. Simultaneous administration of sodium fluoride (50 mg/L (ppm)) in drinking water for 36 days acted in collaboration to stimulate bone formation and to increase bone volume (Ohta *et al.*, 1995).

(vi) *Effects on cell proliferation*

Phenytoin is commonly used in brain tumour patients with epileptic seizures. Although phenytoin cannot be considered as a cytostatic drug, it has been reported to inhibit microtubule polymerization (MacKinney et al., 1978), and it enhances the cytotoxicity of vincristine, a prototype microtubule inhibitor, in multidrug-resistant human glioma cell lines (Ganapathi et al., 1993).

4.3 Reproductive and prenatal effects

4.3.1 *Humans*

Four kinds of effects and consequences of phenytoin treatment can be differentiated.

(*a*) Reproductive effects concerning germ cells, sexual hormones and sexual activity;

(*b*) Structural abnormalities, i.e. classical teratogenic effects, when used mainly in the first trimester of gestation;

(*c*) Short-term functional alterations, manifested postnatally and related mainly to treatment in the perinatal period;

(*d*) Long-term developmental (including behavioural) effects, in general connected with use in the second and third trimesters of gestation.

(*a*) *Reproductive effects*

Swanson et al. (1978) found phenytoin in the semen at a concentration of 0.2 relative to plasma. A diminution of sperm production in epileptic males is due to a decrease in free testosterone level (Cramer & Jones, 1991). This phenomenon results from an increased prolactin level (Aminoff et al., 1984; Laxer et al., 1985) caused by seizures which can inhibit gonadotrophin-releasing hormone secretion from the hypothalamus that in turn inhibits follicle-stimulating hormone (FSH) and luteinizing hormone (LH) production. Taneja et al. (1994) compared the effect of phenytoin on semen with data from untreated epileptic and healthy males. A smaller volume of seminal fluid, and lower spermatozoal concentration and total sperm count were seen in untreated epileptics and phenytoin-treated patients compared with the healthy males, but no difference was evident between the two patient groups. The number of morphologically abnormal sperm was greater in untreated patients than in phenytoin-treated or control subjects.

Male patients treated with phenytoin commonly complain of diminished libido and impotence (Toone et al., 1983). Hyposexuality may be the result of altered levels of pituitary hormones, sex hormone-binding globulin and free testosterone (Mattson & Cramer, 1985; Macphee et al., 1988). Phenytoin decreases free testosterone levels by induction of aromatase and sex hormone-binding globulin synthetase, enhancing conversion of free testosterone to oestradiol. Oestradiol exerts a potent inhibitory influence on LH secretion and it may have a major role in negative feedback in men as well as women. Suppression of LH secretion results in hypogonadotropic hypogonadism, which accounts for reproductive and sexual dysfunction among men with epilepsy (Herzog et al., 1991). The higher level of oestrogen during pregnancy can lower the seizure threshold (Mattson & Cramer, 1985).

(b) Congenital abnormalities

The maternal metabolism of phenytoin during pregnancy is discussed in Section 4.1.1.

In Europe, about 0.4% of pregnant women have epilepsy (Czeizel *et al.*, 1992). During epileptic convulsive attacks there may be breathing disorders up to apnoea and alterations in cardiac output that, in pregnancy, may effect fetal well-being, especially in the case of frequent attacks (Yerby, 1991). About 40% of women have increased frequency of seizures, mainly due to the decreased serum level of phenytoin, particularly in the first trimester, in parallel with hyperemesis gravidarum, during labour (Schmidt *et al.*, 1983) or if the fetus is male (Dansky & Finnel, 1991). Pregnant epileptic women therefore need higher doses of anticonvulsant treatment. The risk of stillbirth, microcephaly and mental retardation is doubled in the offspring of women with seizures during pregnancy (Nelson & Ellenberg, 1982).

Meadow (1968) reported five cases of congenital malformation in the offspring of epileptic women treated with phenytoin. Subsequently, a total of 32 children born to mothers who took anticonvulsants, including phenytoin, throughout pregnancy were found to have a similar constellation of abnormalities including cleft lip and palate, and cardiovascular and skeletal (limb, skull, face) abnormalities (Meadow, 1970). Subsequent case reports of epileptic women treated during pregnancy with phenytoin and phenobarbital have described affected infants with similar abnormalities (IARC, 1977).

In the early 1970s, nearly all analytical epidemiological studies indicated a 2–3-fold greater risk for congenital abnormalities after phenytoin treatment in the first trimester of gestation (IARC, 1977). However, the risk is five- to six-fold higher for the fetal hydantoin syndrome (Hanson & Smith, 1975; Hanson, 1976). The most characteristic symptom of this syndrome is hypoplasia of the nails and distal phalanges, which occurs in up to 18% of the exposed fetuses (Barr *et al.*, 1974; Hill *et al.*, 1974). Distal digital and nail hypoplasia has been documented through radiographic hand analyses in about 30% of exposed children (Kelly, 1984). Other abnormalities include cleft lip and palate or unusual face (hypoplasia of the mid-face, broad depressed nasal bridge, short upturned nose, mild hypertelorism, inner epicanthal folds, ptosis of the eyelid), microcephaly and congenital cardiovascular malformations. Mild to moderate mental retardation and prenatal-onset growth retardation may also occur. Hanson *et al.* (1976) concluded that as many as 11% of exposed fetuses develop the fetal hydantoin syndrome. However, there is no obvious borderline between lesser manifestations of this syndrome and normal babies. Thus, at present there is evidence for the teratogenicity of phenytoin ingested at 100–800 mg/day during the first trimester of gestation (Adams *et al.*, 1990).

Gaily *et al.* (1988) reported that several minor anomalies previously regarded as symptoms of fetal hydantoin syndrome were genetically linked to epilepsy. Only hypertelorism and digital hypoplasia were specifically associated with phenytoin exposure.

Most studies in which epileptic mothers taking phenytoin alone (namely those receiving monotherapy) were identified indicated a significantly higher rate of fetal hydantoin syndrome compared with untreated non-epileptic women (Lowe, 1973; Fedrick, 1973; Bertollini *et al.*, 1987; Kaneko *et al.*, 1992). It is difficult to calculate the specific teratogenic risk of phenytoin as the drug is frequently given with other anticonvulsants (polytherapy) and because maternal epilepsy itself is teratogenic. The teratogenic risk of polytherapy has consistently been found to be higher than that of monotherapy. For example, Kaneko et al. (1988, 1992) found that the overall rate of congenital abnormalities was 6.2–6.5% in children born to epileptic women with monotherapy, while the rate was 13.5–15.6% after polytherapy.

The teratogenicity of phenytoin afflicts only some exposed fetuses, possibly due to genetic variation in susceptibility. Strickler et al. (1985) demonstrated a genetic defect in the detoxification of arene oxide metabolites of phenytoin, which may increase the risk for fetal hydantoin syndrome. Buehler et al. (1990) assessed epoxide hydrolase levels in cultures of both fetal fibroblasts and amniocytes and found a deficiency of the enzyme in fetuses at high risk for fetal hydantoin syndrome. In a prospective study of 19 pregnancies monitored by amniocentesis, an adverse outcome was predicted for four fetuses on the basis of low epoxide hydrolase activity (< 30% of the standard). In all four cases, the mother was receiving phenytoin monotherapy and, after birth, the infants had clinical findings compatible with the fetal hydantoin syndrome. The fetuses with enzyme activity above 30% of the standard after use of the same doses of phenytoin were not considered to be at risk and all 15 neonates lacked any characteristic features of the fetal hydantoin syndrome.

Data on congenital abnormality rates among babies born to women with epilepsy but without anticonvulsant therapy are contradictory (Speidel & Meadow, 1972; Monson et al., 1973; Lowe, 1973; Shapiro et al., 1976; Czeizel et al., 1992). A summary of 12 prospective studies (Kaneko & Kondó, 1995) showed that the overall rate of congenital abnormalities was 11.1% (122/1099), 5.7% (6/105) and 4.8% (4081/85 361) in children born to epileptic women treated with anticonvulsants during pregnancy, to epileptic women without anticonvulsant therapy and to non-epileptic control women, respectively.

(c) Short-term functional alterations

Clinical manifestations of withdrawal syndrome including hyperirritability, tremor, seizures, vomiting, poor suckling and sleep disturbances may occur shortly after birth in infants exposed to phenytoin during pregnancy (Watson & Spellacy, 1971; Koch et al., 1985). These symptoms do not affect psychomotor development (Hirano et al., 1984).

In newborns exposed to phenytoin during pregnancy, a tendency to bleeding may develop during the first day of life due to decreased levels of vitamin K-dependent clotting factors, despite normal levels in the mother (Bleyer & Skinner, 1976). Haemorrhage secondary to thrombocytopenia may also be caused occasionally by phenytoin (Page et al., 1982).

(d) Long-term developmental effects

Developmental and behavioural neurotoxicity in humans has been studied (Hirano et al., 1984; Adams et al., 1990). The prospective study of Scolnik et al. (1994) indicated a mean global IQ in children of mothers treated with phenytoin during pregnancy 10 points lower (95% CI, 4.9–15.8) than that of matched controls, and specific weakness in performance of non-verbal tasks. The deficits were unrelated to seizure activity, but correlated with serum levels of phenytoin. However, behavioural dysfunction was generally limited to global measures of intellectual function. [The Working Group noted that the studies were limited by the short study period, which in general did not extend past infancy.]

4.3.2 Experimental systems

In rabbits (as in humans), Swanson *et al.* (1978) found phenytoin in the semen at a concentration of 0.2 relative to plasma. A single intragastric dose of phenytoin to pregnant Sprague-Dawley rats was transferred to the fetuses and was concentrated more in the kidney than in the liver, in contrast to the situation in adult rats (Gabler & Falace, 1970). Transplacental transport has been documented in mice, rats, hamsters, goats and monkeys (see Section 4.1.2).

A/Jax mice were treated with 12.5, 25 or 50 mg/kg bw phenytoin sodium by subcutaneous injection at various times from days 9 to 15 of pregnancy; the highest dose produced cleft palates in 26–43% of the offspring (Massey, 1966). Similar treatment with 50 mg/kg bw phenytoin sodium on days 7–9 or 11–13 of gestation induced significant increases in the incidence of cleft palates in the offspring of Swiss-Webster (15%) and A/J mice (31%) (Gibson & Becker, 1968). The teratogenicity of phenytoin has been confirmed in other experiments in mice (Elshove, 1969; Harbison & Becker, 1969; Marsh & Fraser 1973; Sullivan & McElhatton, 1975), rats (Harbison & Becker, 1972; Mercier-Parot & Tuchman-Duplessis, 1974) and rabbits (McClain & Langhoff, 1980). In a mouse model, it has been shown that phenytoin, and not epileptic disease state nor seizure frequency, was associated with congenital abnormalities (Finnel, 1981; Finnel *et al.*, 1989). The major metabolite of phenytoin, *para*-HPPH, and diphenylhydantoic acid and α-aminodiphenylacetic acid were less teratogenic *in vivo* in mice than phenytoin itself (Harbison & Becker, 1974).

Phenytoin (100 mg/kg bw) administered by gastric instillation on gestational days 9, 11 and 13 to Sprague-Dawley rats interfered with sexual dimorphism in cranofacial pattern (Zengel *et al.*, 1989).

Groups of 10 female Fischer 344/N rats and C57Bl/6N mice were given phenytoin in the diet for two weeks before breeding and throughout gestation and lactation (United States National Toxicology Program, 1993). The concentrations were 0, 80, 240, 800 and 2400 mg/kg diet (ppm) for the rats and 0, 20, 60, 200 and 600 mg/kg diet (ppm) for the mice. The females were mated with unexposed males. Four pregnant rats only from each group were killed on gestational day 18 and their uterine contents assessed. The remaining rats and all of the mice were permitted to litter and rear their pups until lactational day 28, after which the pups were weaned and continued to be exposed to the experimental diets for another four weeks. None of the sperm-positive rats given the 2400-ppm diet and none of the mice given 600 ppm delivered any litters. In offspring of the group of rats given 800 ppm phenytoin, there was increased postnatal death. No gross external malformation was observed among rat fetuses or rat or mouse pups surviving to term in any dose group. No gross or histological lesion was found in the rats exposed to 800 ppm or in any of the groups of mice during the four weeks following weaning.

No obvious teratogenic effects (major defects) were seen in monkeys (rhesus macaque, *Macaca mulata*, Wilson, 1974; Hendrie *et al.*, 1990; *Macaca fascicularis*, Phillips & Lockard, 1985, 1989, 1990, 1993), but there was an increased risk for hyperexcitability.

Phenytoin produces multiple behavioural dysfunctions in rat offspring at subteratogenic and non-growth-retarding doses. Elmazar and Sullivan (1981) found an impairment of motor function, primarily of gross motor coordination. Mullenix *et al.* (1983) reported an increase in the activity level of males but not of females. Exposure to phenytoin *in utero* caused a permanent alteration in the hypothalamic-pituitary-thyroid axis in rats (Theodoropoulos *et al.*, 1990). Significant learning and memory deficits, delayed auditory startle, increased locomotor activity and an extremely abnormal spontaneous circling behaviour have been reported (Vorhees, 1983, 1987a,b; Minck *et al.*, 1989; Vorhees & Minck, 1989; Vorhees *et al.*, 1989; Adams *et al.*, 1990). These dysfunctions were dose-dependent and exposure period-dependent in offspring of treated rats. Pizzi and Jersey (1992) found lower birth weight, later lower body weight and a significant increase in locomotor activity.

4.3.3 *Possible mechanisms of prenatal effects of phenytoin*

Various mechanisms have been suggested for the origin of phenytoin-induced cleft palate and other congenital abnormalities.

Genetic susceptibility

The genetic basis of susceptibility to the fetal hydantoin syndrome became clear from the difference in the incidence and pattern of defects in three inbred mouse strains (Finnel & Chernoff, 1984a,b). It was possible to characterize 'fast' and 'slow' metabolizers among several inbred strains of mice, but there was no correlation between the rate of metabolism and the sensitivity to the teratogenic effect of phenytoin (Atlas *et al.*, 1980). The available human data (Strickler *et al.*, 1985; Buehler *et al.*, 1990) were discussed in Section 4.3.1.

Reactive intermediates

Phenytoin is a potent inducer of liver microsomal oxidation in humans (Conney, 1969). The human fetus has hepatic and extrahepatic monooxygenase systems which may catalyse the formation of epoxide (Pelkonen & Kärki, 1975) and has hepatic and extrahepatic enzymes (e.g. glutathione *S*-transferase, epoxide hydrolase) that metabolize epoxides (Pacifici *et al.*, 1981; Pacifici & Rane, 1983). In human fetal liver, sulfhydryl groups and glutathione are also present which react with metabolites of phenytoin (Rollins *et al.*, 1981). Martz *et al.* (1977) demonstrated the binding of an oxidized metabolite of phenytoin to cellular macromolecules (trichloroacetic acid-precipitable material) in mouse fetuses and showed that this binding was associated with an increased teratogenic potential of phenytoin. These findings suggest that an intermediary metabolite such as an arene oxide may be the causative agent in the teratogenic effect. Phenytoin enhances epoxide metabolism in cultured fetal hepatocytes (Rane & Peng,

1985) and may also induce the metabolism of its own epoxide. Thus, the balance between the enzyme activities that catalyse the formation and the elimination of epoxides could be a determinant of the risk for developmental abnormalities.

Human evidence to support a role for an epoxide intermediate in phenytoin-induced teratogenesis was presented by Strickler *et al.* (1985), who found that increased toxicity of murine microsome-generated phenytoin metabolites to the lymphocytes of 24 children exposed to phenytoin throughout gestation was highly correlated with major birth defects. Each of the 14 children with a 'positive' assay had a parent whose lymphocytes also scored 'positive'. However, no association was found with the presence of minor anomalies, which seem to be independent, mainly familial traits, a conclusion also reached by Gaily *et al.* (1988), who found that only hypertelorism and digital hypoplasia were associated with phenytoin exposure. Thus, a genetic defect of detoxification of arene oxide metabolites of phenytoin may increase the risk for or can select fetuses having abnormalities. This hypothesis was supported by the study of Buehler *et al.* (1990) described in Section 4.3.1, who found that epoxide hydrolase activity in amniocytes of fetuses with fetal hydantoin syndrome was significantly lower than that in fetuses without this syndrome.

The arene oxide of phenytoin can be formed through cytochrome P450-mediated oxidation and yields the dihydrodiol metabolite, 5-(3,4-dihydroxy-1,5-cyclohexadien-1-yl-5-phenylhydantoin), in a reaction catalysed by the enzyme epoxide hydrolase (Chang *et al.*, 1970) and possibly direct or indirect interactions with glutathione (Harbison, 1978; Pantarotto *et al.*, 1982; Wong *et al.*, 1989). Substitution of hydrogen by deuterium at the *para* position of one of the phenyl rings, which favours arene oxide formation, causes an increase in the teratogenic effect of phenytoin (Lambotte-Vandepaer *et al.*, 1989). Embryonic peroxidase-catalysed bioactivation of phenytoin and glutathione-dependent detoxifying and cytoprotective pathways are critical determinants of phenytoin teratogenicity (Miranda *et al.*, 1994). When the rate of bioactivation exceeds the detoxifying capacity of the organism, the electrophilic centre of the arene oxide is capable of binding covalently to nucleophilic sites found in fetal macromolecules, such as nucleic acid (Jerina & Daly, 1974), and such irreversible binding at the critical periods of development may explain the teratogenic effect of phenytoin. Finnel *et al.* (1993, 1994) reduced the teratogenic effect of phenytoin in mice by co-administration of stiripentol, a potent inhibitor of cytochrome P450 enzymes. This suggests that cytochrome P450 oxidation products may be the primary teratogenic agent(s) in phenytoin-induced teratogenesis.

Besides an arene oxide, free radicals may also be reactive intermediates generated by cytochromes P450 and/or prostaglandin synthetase (Kubow & Wells, 1986; Wells *et al.*, 1989). Increased oxygen consumption and free radical intermediates were detected during bioactivation of phenytoin by prostaglandin synthetase *in vitro* (Kubow & Wells, 1989). Phenytoin embryopathy was enhanced by concurrent treatment with 12-*O*-tetradecanoylphorbol 13-acetate, which activates phospholipase A_2, leading to release of membrane-bound arachidonic acid and enhanced prostaglandin biosynthesis (Wells & Vo, 1989). Furthermore, administration to CD-1 mice of phenytoin together with acetylsalicylic acid (an irreversible inhibitor of prostaglandin synthetase), caffeic acid (an antioxidant) or α-phenyl-N-tert-butylnitrone (a free radical spin-trapping agent) led to 50%, 71% and 82% reductions in the rate of phenytoin-caused cleft palate, respectively (Wells et al., 1989). These results indicated that prostaglandin synthetase contributes to the enzymatic bioactivation of phenytoin to a teratogenic free radical intermediate. Phenytoin teratogenicity in mice was also reduced by the antioxidant vitamin E (Sanyal & Wells, 1993) and by dietary *n*–3 fatty acids (Kubow, 1992) via inhibition of embryonic prostaglandin synthetase. Liu and Wells (1994) showed that peroxidase-catalysed bioactivation of phenytoin may initiate oxidative damage to lipids and proteins in embryonic tissues.

It has been suggested that phenytoin and glucocorticoids disrupt normal palatal development by the same or a very similar mechanism (Fritz, 1976; McDevitt et al., 1981). Phenytoin treatment of A/J mice increased endogenous maternal corticosterone concentrations for approximately 48 h after dosing (Hansen et al., 1988). Thus, Hansen et al. (1992) hypothesized that phenytoin causes clefting through the glucocorticoid-mediated effect; however, it appeared that phenytoin is capable of producing clefts in the absence of endogenous maternal corticosterone. Involvement of glucocorticoids or of interaction between phenytoin and the glucocorticoid receptor (Sonawane & Goldman, 1981; Katsumata et al., 1982; Hansen & Hodes, 1983; Gupta et al., 1985; Katsumata et al., 1985; Hansen, 1991) has not been ruled out. Binding of phenytoin to the glucocorticoid receptor could stimulate the release of a protein that can inhibit the phospholipase A_2-mediated release from membrane phospholipids of arachidonic acid, a precursor in the synthesis of leukotrienes, thromboxanes and prostaglandins (Kay et al., 1988). In experimental systems, addition of arachidonic acid decreased the incidence of phenytoin-induced abnormalities, suggesting that phenytoin somehow caused a deficiency of arachidonic acid (Kay et al., 1990). However, a significant amount of work remains to be done to examine the involvement of the arachidonic acid cascade in phenytoin-induced teratogenicity *in vivo*.

In conclusion, the bulk of experimental data and some human evidence suggests some role for reactive intermediates in phenytoin-induced teratogenicity. These observations may also contribute to the understanding of the effect of phenytoin on the central nervous system (Kempermann et al., 1994).

Effect on folate metabolism

Phenytoin alters the metabolism of folate (Malpas et al., 1966; Reynolds, 1973). This water-soluble B vitamin is required for DNA synthesis (it provides one-carbon units for the de-novo synthesis of guanine, adenine and thymine) and plays an important role in the methylation cycle in supplying the methyl group (Czeizel, 1995). Folate deficiency is seen in epileptics, mainly in pregnant epileptic women (Hiilesmaa et al., 1983; Dansky et al., 1987), although there is an increased demand for folate during pregnancy.

In experimental systems, conflicting results have been obtained when phenytoin and folate were given concurrently. Folic acid had no effect on the rate of abnormalities produced by phenytoin treatment in mice (Marsh & Fraser, 1973; Mercier-Parot & Tuchmann-Duplessis, 1974). Although folic acid was initially said to decrease the rate of cleft palate (Marsh & Fraser, 1973), this was not confirmed in subsequent reports (Schardein et al., 1973; Sullivan & McElhatton, 1975). The embryonic concentration of folate decreased after intraperitoneal administration of phenytoin (Netzloff et al., 1979), but not after dietary supplementation (Hansen & Billings, 1985), and further intervention studies (e.g., Chatot et al., 1984; Zhu & Zhou, 1989) have also given contradictory results. Nevertheless, phenytoin and/or its arene oxide metabolite can decrease the activity of hepatic 5,10-methylenetetrahydrofolate reductase (Billings, 1984) and, consequently, may affect S-adenosylmethionine synthesis, which is central to methyl group transfer reactions. Neither folate absorption (Nelson et al., 1983) nor folate catabolism (Guest et al., 1983) is adversely affected by phenytoin. Data from human randomized double-blind intervention studies suggest that a high dose (4 mg) of folic acid alone can reduce the recurrence (MRC Vitamin Study Research Group, 1991) and a low dose (0.8 mg) of folic acid-containing multivitamins can prevent the first occurrence of neural-tube defects (Czeizel & Dudás, 1992) and some other major congenital abnormalities (Czeizel, 1993), including oral clefts. This is supported by a case–control study (Shaw et al., 1995).

Fetal hypoxia

The experimental studies of Danielson et al. (1992) and Danielsson et al. (1992) indicated that phenytoin exerts its teratogenic effects by inducing fetal hypoxia, leading to vascular disruption and necrosis of existing and developing structures.

4.4 Genetic and related effects (see also Table 6 for references and Appendices 1 and 2)

4.4.1 *Humans*

Bone-marrow cells from epileptic patients treated with phenytoin were analysed in two studies. Alving et al. (1977) found no evidence of either chromosomal damage or induction of hyperploidy in 10 adult patients (four women and six men), aged 19–49 years (mean, 33 years), treated for 4–20 years; in none of the patients did the serum level of phenytoin exceed 20 mg/L during the last year of treatment. The controls in this study were bone-marrow aspirates and peripheral blood samples from 10 patients without haematological disorders who had not received treatment with ionizing radiation or cytostatic drugs. The bone-marrow smears from five of the patients were also studied for the presence of micronuclei: a doubling of the number of erythroblasts with micronuclei was observed, but the difference was not statistically significant. Knuutila et al. (1977) reported on a series of 22 patients with epilepsy (12 women and 10 men), aged 4–47 years (mean, 21 years); the effective serum concentrations of phenytoin varied between 4 and 113 µmol/L [1 and 29 mg/L]. The results of the study were compared with those from a simultaneously conducted study of 20 healthy persons (11 women and nine men), aged 23–37 years (mean, 27 years): none had taken medicines and none of the women contraceptive pills for at least half a year before the study (Knuutila et al., 1976). The mean frequency of all chromosomal structural changes among the patients was 0.5%

Table 6. Genetic and related effects of phenytoin or its sodium salt

Test system	Result[a] Without exogenous metabolic system	Result[a] With exogenous metabolic system	Dose[b] (LED/HID)	Reference
PRB, SOS repair test (chromo-test)	–	NT	6300	Brams et al. (1987)
SA0, Salmonella typhimurium TA100, reverse mutation	–	–	385	Sezzano et al. (1982)
SA0, Salmonella typhimurium TA100, reverse mutation	–	–	323	Haworth et al. (1983)
SA0, Salmonella typhimurium TA100, reverse mutation	–	–	185	Léonard et al. (1984)
SA0, Salmonella typhimurium TA100, reverse mutation	–	–	370	Brams et al. (1987)
SA3, Salmonella typhimurium TA1530, reverse mutation	–	–	185	Léonard et al. (1984)
SA5, Salmonella typhimurium TA1535, reverse mutation	–	–	385	Sezzano et al. (1982)
SA5, Salmonella typhimurium TA1535, reverse mutation	–	–	323	Haworth et al. (1983)
SA7, Salmonella typhimurium TA1537, reverse mutation	–	–	385	Sezzano et al. (1982)
SA7, Salmonella typhimurium TA1537, reverse mutation	–	–	323	Haworth et al. (1983)
SA7, Salmonella typhimurium TA1537, reverse mutation	–	–	185	Léonard et al. (1984)
SA8, Salmonella typhimurium TA1538, reverse mutation	–	(+)	100	Sezzano et al. (1982)
SA8, Salmonella typhimurium TA1538, reverse mutation	–	–	370	Léonard et al. (1984)
SA9, Salmonella typhimurium TA98, reverse mutation	–	–	385	Sezzano et al. (1982)
SA9, Salmonella typhimurium TA98, reverse mutation	–	–	323	Haworth et al. (1983)
SA9, Salmonella typhimurium TA98, reverse mutation	–	–	370	Léonard et al. (1984)
SA9, Salmonella typhimurium TA98, reverse mutation	–	–	370	Brams et al. (1987)
SAS, Salmonella typhimurium TA97, reverse mutation	–	–	185	Léonard et al. (1984)
SAS, Salmonella typhimurium TA97, reverse mutation	–	–	370	Brams et al. (1987)
DMX, Drosophila melanogaster, sex-linked recessive lethal mutation	–		100 inj.	Woodruff et al. (1985)
DMX, Drosophila melanogaster, sex-linked recessive lethal mutation	–		5000 feed	Woodruff et al. (1985)
GCO, Gene mutation, Chinese hamster ovary cells, hprt locus, in vitro	?	?	800	Oberly et al. (1993)
G5T, Gene mutation, mouse lymphoma L5178Y cells, tk locus, in vitro	–	–	400	Oberly et al. (1993)
SIC, Sister chromatid exchange, Chinese hamster ovary cells in vitro	–		300	Riedel & Obe (1984)
SIA, Sister chromatid exchange, Wg 3h cells in vitro	0	+	75	Tan et al. (1985) (abstract)

Table 6 (contd)

Test system	Result[a] Without exogenous metabolic system	Result[a] With exogenous metabolic system	Dose[b] (LED/HID)	Reference
CIC, Chromosomal aberrations, Chinese hamster ovary cells in vitro	–	–	300	Riedel & Obe (1984)
CIC, Chromosomal aberrations, Chinese hamster ovary cells in vitro	–	–	300	Kindig et al. (1992)
CIM, Chromosomal aberrations, mouse primary embryonic fibroblasts in vitro	–	NT	200	de Oliveira & Machado-Santelli (1987)
AIA, Aneuploidy, mouse primary embryonic fibroblasts in vitro (hyperdiploidy)	+	NT	200	de Oliveira & Machado-Santelli (1987)
T7S, Cell transformation, SA7/Syrian hamster embryo cells in vitro	+	NT	50	Hatch et al. (1986)
SHL, Sister chromatid exchange, human lymphocytes in vitro	+	NT	15	Maurya & Goyle (1985)
CHL, Chromosomal aberrations, human lymphocytes in vitro	–	NT	70	Bishun et al. (1975)
CHL, Chromosomal aberrations, human lymphocytes in vitro	–	NT	100	Alving et al. (1976)
CHL, Chromosomal aberrations, human lymphocytes in vitro	–	NT	500	Léonard et al. (1984)
CHL, Chromosomal aberrations, human lymphocytes in vitro	+	NT	54	Ramadevi et al. (1984)
CHL, Chromosomal aberrations, human lymphocytes in vitro	+	NT	10	García Sagredo (1988)
CIH, Chromosomal aberrations, human amnion cells in vitro	–	NT	200	de Oliveira & Machado-Santelli (1987)
AIH, Aneuploidy, human lymphocytes in vitro (hyperdiploidy and polyploidy)	–	NT	70	Bishun et al. (1975)
AIH, Aneuploidy, human lymphocytes in vitro (hyperdiploidy)	–	NT	100	Alving et al. (1976)
AIH, Aneuploidy, human amnion cells in vitro (hyperdiploidy)	+	NT	200	de Oliveira & Machado-Santelli (1987)
TVI, Transformation of mouse peritoneal macrophages treated in vivo, scored in vitro	+		50 ip × 1	Massa et al. (1990)
TVI, Cell transformation, human fibroblasts treated in vivo, scored in vitro	+		NG	Dhanwada et al. (1992)
MVM, Micronucleus test, mouse (Swiss) bone marrow in vivo	+		100 po × 2	Das et al. (1983)

Table 6 (contd)

Test system	Result[a]		Dose[b] (LED/HID)	Reference
	Without exogenous metabolic system	With exogenous metabolic system		
MVM, Micronucleus test, mouse (BALB/c) bone marrow *in vivo*	+		0.5 iv × 1	Montes de Oca-Luna *et al.* (1984)
MVM, Micronucleus test, mouse (Swiss CD-1) liver *in utero*	(+)[c]		100 ip × 1	Barcellona *et al.* (1987)
MVM, Micronucleus test, mouse (Swiss CD-1) bone marrow *in vivo*	−		100 ip × 1	Barcellona *et al.* (1987)
MVM, Micronucleus test, mouse (CD-1) bone marrow *in vivo*	−		40 ip × 2	Kindig *et al.* (1992)
MVM, Micronucleus test, mouse (BALB/c) bone marrow *in vivo*	−		20 iv × 1	McFee *et al.* (1992)
MVM, Micronucleus test, mouse (B6C3F1) tone marrow *in vivo*	−		70 ip × 3	McFee *et al.* (1992)
MVM, Micronucleus test, mouse (B6C3F1) peripheral blood erythrocytes *in vivo*	−		70 ip × 3	McFee *et al.* (1992)
SVA, Sister chromatid exchange, mouse (ICR) bone marrow *in vivo*	−		80 ip × 1	Sharma *et al.* (1985)
SVA, Sister chromatid exchange, mouse (ICR) liver *in utero*	(+)		80 ip × 1	Sharma *et al.* (1985)
SVA, Sister chromatid exchange, mouse (B6C3F1) bone marrow *in vivo*	−		250 ip × 1	McFee *et al.* (1992)
SVA, Sister chromatid exchange, female mouse (CD-1) bone marrow *in vivo*	−		40 ip × 1	Kindig *et al.* (1992)
SVA, Sister chromatid exchange, mouse (ICR) liver *in utero*	−		40 ip × 2	Kindig *et al.* (1992)
CBA, Chromosomal aberrations, rat (Lister) bone-marrow cells *in vivo*	−		50 × 3	Alving *et al.* (1976)
CBA, Chromosomal aberrations, mouse (BALB/c) bone marrow *in vivo*	−		0.48 po 3d/wk 2 m	de Oliveira *et al.* (1987)
CBA, Chromosomal aberrations, mouse (BALB/c) bone marrow *in vivo*	−		100 ip × 3	de Oliveira *et al.* (1987)
CBA, Chromosomal aberrations, mouse (B6C3F1) bone marrow *in vivo*	−		500 ip × 1	McFee *et al.* (1992)
DLM, Dominant lethal test, mouse *in vivo*	+		145 ip × 1	Epstein *et al.* (1972)
AVA, Aneuploidy, rat (Lister) bone-marrow *in vivo* (hyperdiploidy)	−		50 × 3	Alving *et al.* (1976)
AVA, Aneuploidy, mouse (BALB/c) bone marrow *in vivo*	−		0.48 po 3d/wk 2 m	de Oliveira *et al.* (1987)

Table 6 (contd)

Test system	Result[a] Without exogenous metabolic system	With exogenous metabolic system	Dose[b] (LED/HID)	Reference
AVA, Aneuploidy, mouse (BALB/c) bone marrow in vivo	+		50 ip × 3	de Oliveira et al. (1987)
SLH, Sister chromatid exchange, human lymphocytes in vivo	+		NG	Habedank et al. (1982)
SLH, Sister chromatid exchange, human lymphocytes in vivo	–		NG	Sinués et al. (1982)
SLH, Sister chromatid exchange, human lymphocytes in vivo	+		NG	Schaumann et al. (1985)
SLH, Sister chromatid exchange, human lymphocytes in vivo	–		NG	Tan et al. (1985) (abstract)
SLH, Sister chromatid exchange, human lymphocytes in vivo	–		NG	Schaumann et al. (1989)
SLH, Sister chromatid exchange, human lymphocytes in vivo	–		270[d] daily > 1 yr	Flejter et al. (1989)
SLH, Sister chromatid exchange, human lymphocytes in vivo	+		NG	Taneja et al. (1992)
MVH, Micronucleus test, human lymphocytes in vivo	–		6 daily > 6 mo	Hashem & Shawki (1976)
MVH, Micronucleus test, human bone-marrow cells in vivo	–		NG	Alving et al. (1977)
CBH, Chromosomal aberrations, human bone-marrow cells in vivo	–		NG	Alving et al. (1977)
CBH, Chromosomal aberrations, human bone-marrow cells in vivo	–		NG	Knuutila et al. (1977)
CLH, Chromosomal aberrations, human lymphocytes in vivo	+		6 daily > 6 mo	Hashem & Shawki (1976)
CLH, Chromosomal aberrations, human lymphocytes in vivo	–		NG	Alving et al. (1977)
CLH, Chromosomal aberrations, human lymphocytes in vivo	–		6 daily > 8 mo	Esser et al. (1981)
CLH, Chromosomal aberrations, human lymphocytes in vivo	–		NG	Tan et al. (1985) (abstract)
CLH, Chromosomal aberrations, human lymphocytes in vivo	–		270[d] daily > 1 yr	Flejter et al. (1989)

Table 6 (contd)

Test system	Result[a]		Dose[b] (LED/HID)	Reference
	Without exogenous metabolic system	With exogenous metabolic system		
AVH, Polyploidy, human lymphocytes in vivo	+		6 daily > 6 mo	Hashem & Shawki (1976)
AVH, Aneuploidy, human bone-marrow cells in vivo	–		NG	Alving et al. (1977)
AVH, Aneuploidy, human lymphocytes in vivo	–		NG	Alving et al. (1977)
AVH, Aneuploidy, human bone-marrow cells in vivo	–		NG	Knuutila et al. (1976)
*, Inhibition of tubulin polymerization in vitro	–	0	2520	Léonard et al. (1984)
ICR, Inhibition of gap-junctional intercellular communication, Chinese hamster (V79) cells in vitro	+	0	23	Welsch & Stedman (1984)
ICR, Inhibition of gap-junctional intercellular communication, Chinese hamster (V79) cells in vitro	+[c]	0	60	Jone et al. (1985)
SPM, Sperm morphology, mouse (Swiss) in vivo	+		10 po × 5	Ramaniah et al. (1980)
*, Increase in c-sis expression	+		10	Dill et al. (1993)

* Not shown on profile

[a] +, positive; (+), weak positive; –, negative; NT, not tested; ?, inconclusive

[b] LED, lowest effective dose; HID, highest ineffective dose; in-vitro tests, μg/mL; in-vivo tests, mg/kg bw/day; NG, dose not given

[c] Pretreatment with epoxide hydrolase inhibitor 1,2-epoxy-3,3,3-trichloropropane (100 mg/kg bw sc) increased genotoxicity

[d] Average daily dose from 10 patients

[e] Combination treatment with phenobarbital enhanced the effect of phenytoin

(range, 0–5.4%), compared with 0.4% (0–2%) in controls. No increase in polyploidy or hyperdiploidy (except one cell in two patients) was found.

Many studies have been conducted on possible cytogenetic effects induced by phenytoin in lymphocytes (and two in bone marrow) of children and adult patients affected by grand mal or petit mal seizure. Almost all of the adequately conducted studies had negative findings for micronucleus frequencies (2/2 studies), chromosomal aberrations (5/6 studies) and aneuploidy (2/2 studies). The only positive finding was that of Hashem and Showki (1976) for chromosomal aberrations and polyploidy. Their study subjects were 21 epileptic patients aged 3–12 years (11 boys and 10 girls) treated for grand mal epilepsy with the sodium salt of phenytoin at a dose of 3–6 mg/kg bw per day for durations ranging between six months and five years; serum levels were not reported. The control group comprised 25 subjects (3–15 years); 10 were epileptics and 15 were normal subjects aged 3–14 years (nine boys and six girls). There was no difference between epileptics not receiving any treatment and normal controls, but a significant increase was seen in gaps, chromatid breaks, chromosome pulverization, polynuclei and polyploidy in treated epileptics relative to untreated epileptics or normal controls. In normal controls, the percentages of cells with single chromatid breaks and polyploidy, were 2.5 ± 0.25 and 0.2, respectively; neither fragmentation/pulverization nor gaps were observed. In untreated epileptic patients, the percentages of cells with single chromatid breaks and polyploidy were 3.0 ± 0.2 and 0.3, respectively. In treated patients, the corresponding frequencies were 6.8 ± 0.87 and 2.8 ± 0.35; induction of gaps ($5.2 \pm 0.31\%$) and isochromatid breaks ($5.6 \pm 0.21\%$), as well as fragmentation/pulverization ($1.8 \pm 0.67\%$), was observed.

Results on sister chromatid exchange (SCE) in lymphocytes are contradictory. Habedank et al. (1982) were the first to describe increased SCE in lymphocyte cultures of nine children (6–16 years of age) suffering from epilepsy and therefore treated with phenytoin monotherapy for 6–60 months; serum levels of phenytoin were rather uniform (40–80 µM) [10–20 mg/L]. Their average SCE rate (10.03 ± 1.31 per metaphase) clearly exceeded that of a control group of healthy children (6.49 ± 0.46 per metaphase). Schaumann et al. (1985) also found significantly increased frequencies of SCE in lymphocyte cultures of 12 adult male epileptic patients (37.25 ± 2.26 years of age; 12.28 ± 0.69 SCE/metaphase) on long-term monotherapy (1.3–14 years) compared with 12 controls matched for age and smoking (37.08 ± 2.21 years of age; 7.81 ± 0.44 SCE/metaphase); the serum levels of the patients were consistently within the therapeutic range of 10–20 mg/L (with exception of two patients with subtherapeutic levels). More recently, an extensive study (Taneja et al., 1992) compared SCE frequencies in 29 phenytoin-treated epileptics (8.29 ± 2.67 SCE/metaphase in 22 men; 7.52 ± 2.92 SCE/metaphase in seven women), 32 untreated epileptics (8.44 ± 2.40 SCE/metaphase in 16 men; 9.76 ± 2.73 SCE/metaphase in 16 women) and 32 normal healthy controls (5.0 ± 1.13 SCE/metaphase in 16 men; 4.95 ± 1.08 SCE/metaphase in 16 women). Age ranged from 16 to 41 years (20.9 ± 7.8 years) in the patients and from 16 to 38 (24.5 ± 5.5 years) in the controls, but no information was available on smoking habits. The authors concluded that SCE frequencies were similar in untreated patients and in patients receiving phenytoin monotherapy, but that both groups had significantly increased frequencies compared with controls. No correlation of SCE frequency with sex or duration of therapy was observed. None of the subjects in this study were heavy smokers or on any drugs. The disease itself might therefore be responsible for inducing genetic damage. [The Working Group noted that the distribution of smokers in the groups was not presented.]

In contrast with these results, Schaumann et al. (1989) undertook a larger, better controlled study than that published in 1985 and observed no increase in SCE frequency in lymphocytes of treated patients. Sixteen adult male patients with epilepsy receiving long-term phenytoin monotherapy (serum level, 3–20 mg/L; age, 38.8 ± 2.4 years) were matched with 16 healthy controls (age, 38.9 ± 2.4 years) for sex, age and smoking habits. Statistical analysis did not reveal any significant difference between rates of SCE in phenytoin-treated persons (5.52 ± 0.25 per metaphase) and controls (5.78 ± 0.29 per metaphase). These data agree with those from three other studies, one published as an abstract (Tan et al., 1985), on 12 adult epileptics and two more extensive studies. Sinués et al. (1982) analysed the lymphocytes of 64 epileptic adults (6.84 ± 1.18 per metaphase) and 30 controls taking no medication (6.66 ± 1.15 per metaphase); no information was reported on age, smoking habits or serum levels of phenytoin. Flejter et al. (1989) compared a mixed population of five epileptic children and four adults [6.10 ± 1.93 per metaphase] with 10 control adults aged 23–52 years and taking no medication (6.83 ± 1.65 per metaphase). The blood levels of phenytoin ranged from 2.7 to 22.0 mg/L.

4.4.2 Experimental systems

In bacteria, all gene mutation tests performed without exogenous metabolic systems were negative, while one of these studies was positive in the presence of an exogenous metabolic activation system.

No sex-linked recessive lethal mutations were observed in Drosophila melanogaster after phenytoin was injected or fed to the adults.

No mutation was induced at the tk locus in mouse lymphoma L5178Y cells; the results concerning the hprt locus in Chinese hamster ovary cells are unclear.

There was no evidence for the induction of SCE in one study on Chinese hamster cells in vitro, but one abstract reported positive effects in Wg 3h cells in the presence of an exogenous metabolic system. Chromosomal aberrations were not found in Chinese hamster ovary cells or in mouse primary embryonic fibroblasts. Aneuploidy induction, mitotic delay and abnormal chromosome/spindle segregation were observed in one study of primary embryonic fibroblasts in vitro (de Oliveira & Machado-Santelli, 1987).

Cell transformation was induced in one study with Syrian hamster embryo cells. Gap-junctional intercellular communication in Chinese hamster lung V79 cells was inhibited by phenytoin treatment.

In cultured human lymphocytes, SCE was observed in a single study and chromosomal aberrations were increased in two of five studies. In one of these, there was an increase in hyperdiploidy, but without a dose–response relationship, while the results of two others were negative for both aneuploidy and polyploidy. Mitotic delay and abnormal chromosome/spindle segregation have also been reported in human lymphocyte or amnion cell cultures (Maurya & Goyle, 1985; de Oliveira & Machado-Santelli, 1987).

The frequency of cell transformation was enhanced *in vitro* in hyperplastic gingival tissue derived from one patient treated with phenytoin and in murine peritoneal macrophages in a host-mediated assay.

Micronuclei were induced in two of six studies performed *in vivo* in mouse bone marrow but not in single studies in mouse liver and circulating erythrocytes. Inhibition of epoxide hydrolase by subcutaneous injection of mice on day 13 of gestation with 1,2-epoxy-3,3,3-trichloropropane (TCPO) (100 mg/kg) 1 h before intraperitoneal injection of phenytoin increased the frequency of micronuclei in liver cells of the fetal mice (TCPO control, 0.23 ± 0.120 versus TCPO + phenytoin, 1.05 ± 0.658) over that observed with phenytoin, but without TCPO treatment (control, 0.23 ± 0.116 versus phenytoin, 0.43 ± 0.206) (Barcellona *et al.* 1987). There is no evidence for the induction of either SCE or chromosomal aberrations in adult mouse in bone marrow *in vivo* or in mouse liver *in utero*. Increased frequencies of aneuploidy were observed in mouse bone marrow after three intraperitoneal injections of 50 mg/kg bw phenytoin, but not after two months oral dosing with 0.48 mg/mouse/day three days per week; no increased hyperploidy was reported with the former protocol in rat bone marrow. Phenytoin administered to male mice induced dominant lethal effects and sperm-head morphological abnormalities.

5-(4'-Hydroxyphenyl)-5-phenylhydantoin (para-HPPH)

This metabolite of diphenylhydantoin was reported to slightly increase mutations in *S. typhimurium* in the presence of S9 in one study (Sezzano *et al.*, 1982), but not in another in which higher dose levels were used (Léonard *et al.*, 1984).

Following intraperitoneal treatment of pregnant mice, micronuclei were not induced in the bone-marrow cells of the adults or in the liver cells of the fetuses (Barcellona *et al.*, 1987).

5. Summary of Data Reported and Evaluation

5.1 Exposure data

Phenytoin, often administered as its sodium salt, has been widely used since the 1930s as an anticonvulsant in the treatment of epilepsy and, to a lesser extent and more recently, in the treatment of certain cardiac arrhythmias.

5.2 Human carcinogenicity data

Many case reports have suggested that there may be a relationship between lymphomas and anticonvulsants, especially phenytoin. In a cohort study in Denmark of epileptic patients exposed to anticonvulsants, including phenytoin, there was an increase in overall cancer risk, attributable to an excess of brain and lung cancer. Nevertheless, brain tumours probably caused the seizure disorder; an evaluation of brain tumour risk over time showed that these tumours were unlikely to be drug-related.

Nested case–control studies based on the Danish cohort investigated in detail the influence of several treatments with anticonvulsants on the risk of cancers of the lung, bladder and liver and non-Hodgkin lymphoma. Anticonvulsant treatment with phenytoin was not associated with lung, bladder or liver cancer. There was an elevated risk for non-Hodgkin lymphoma associated with phenytoin use, but this was not significant.

Two case–control studies investigated the relationship between multiple myeloma and the use of phenytoin, among many other factors. One found no association between phenytoin use and at risk for multiple myeloma risk. The other study found a nonsignificantly elevated risk associated with the use of phenytoin. The power of both studies to assess an effect of phenytoin was low.

5.3 Animal carcinogenicity data

Phenytoin was tested for carcinogenicity by oral administration in three experiments in mice and in two experiments in rats. It was also tested by perinatal/adult exposure in one study in mice and rats and by intraperitoneal administration in one study in mice.

In one experiment in three strains of female mice, oral administration of the sodium salt of phenytoin was reported to increase the incidence of lymphomas. Oral administration to female mice in another study decreased the incidence of mammary gland adenocarcinomas, leukaemias and polyps of the endometrium; in a further study, the incidence of hepatocellular tumours was reduced in males. Oral administration to rats did not increase the incidence of tumours in two studies.

In the experiment using combinations of adult and perinatal exposure, adult exposure resulted in a dose-dependent increase in the incidence of hepatocellular tumours in female mice. Perinatal treatment followed by adult exposure increased the incidence of hepatocellular tumours in both male and female mice and slightly in male rats.

Following intraperitoneal injection of phenytoin into mice, leukaemias and lymphomas were observed.

In one experiment in mice, phenytoin increased the incidence of hepatocellular tumours induced by N-nitrosodiethylamine. In a mouse lung adenoma assay, phenytoin decreased the multiplicity of lung adenomas induced by urethane.

5.4 Other relevant data

Phenytoin is well absorbed in humans. It is eliminated mainly as the glucuronide of the major metabolite, 5-(4'-hydroxyphenyl)-5-phenylhydantoin, which typically accounts for 67–88% of the dose in urine. Several other metabolites are known. The elimination kinetics are non-linear, but an apparent mean half-life of 22 h is a useful guide.

5-(4'-Hydroxyphenyl)-5-phenylhydantoin is the main metabolite in all animal species except dogs (5-(3'-hydroxyphenyl)-5-phenylhydantoin) and cats (the N-glucuronide).

Acute phenytoin intoxication in humans presents usually with cerebellar-vestibular effects such as nystagmus, ataxia, diplopia, vertigo and dysarthria. Chronic administration of phenytoin at therapeutic doses may rarely induce various adverse health effects such as symptoms associated with impairment of the nervous system described above.

Gingival overgrowth, sometimes together with increased thickness of the craniofacial bones as well as folic acid deficiency and development of megaloblastic anaemia, are well established adverse effects of the drug. Phenytoin has also been associated with various forms of cutaneous hypersensitivity reactions, sometimes accompanied by lymphadenopathy and benign lymphoid hyperplasia. In rare cases, the histological architecture of the lymph nodes is lost (pseudolymphoma). Phenytoin may also induce a variety of endocrine effects such as reduction of thyroxine concentrations, hypocalcaemia, osteomalacia and hyperglycaemia.

The nervous system appears to be the major target of acute and chronic phenytoin toxicity in experimental animals. In addition, repeated administration of phenytoin induces increased liver and kidney weights, centrilobular hepatic hypertrophy and diverse immunosuppressive effects. Phenytoin may reduce thyroxine concentrations and increase bone thickness in rodents, but gingival hyperplasia has been observed only in cats and monkeys and not in rodents.

Phenytoin is an inducer of certain hepatic cytochrome P450 activities in humans and mice.

There is evidence for the teratogenicity of phenytoin in humans ingesting 100–800 mg per day during the first trimester of gestation. Phenytoin is teratogenic in mice and rats. Animal and a few human studies suggest that neurobehavioural deficits occur at doses which produce no dysmorphic effect.

Phenytoin induced mutations in *Salmonella typhimurium* in the presence of a metabolic activation system in one study.

No mutagenic effect was observed in *Drosophila* or in mammalian cells *in vitro* in the absence of an exogenous metabolic system. Aneuploidy was induced in one study in primary mouse embryonic fibroblasts *in vitro*. Cell transformation was induced in Syrian hamster embryo. A single study showed increased clone sizes of murine macrophages in a host-mediated assay. Phenytoin inhibited gap-junctional intercellular communication.

In human lymphocytes *in vitro*, sister chromatid exchanges were induced in one study and chromosomal aberrations were induced in two of five studies. Aneuploidy was observed in human amnion cells but not in lymphocytes.

Phenytoin induced micronuclei in three of five studies in rodents *in vivo*. Aneuploidy, in one of two studies, aberrant sperm morphology and dominant lethal mutations were induced, but not sister chromatid exchange or chromosomal aberrations.

In general, studies of human lymphocytes *in vivo* showed no induction of micronuclei, chromosomal aberrations or aneuploidy but an increase of polyploidy was found in one study and of sister chromatid exchange frequencies in three of seven studies. Neither chromosomal aberrations nor aneuploidy were induced in human bone marrow.

The metabolite 5-(4'-hydroxyphenyl)-5-phenylhydantoin was mutagenic in *Salmonella typhimurium* in the presence of a metabolic activation system; it did not induce micronuclei in mouse bone marrow *in vivo*.

Mechanistic considerations

Evidence is available to support the conclusion that phenytoin induces liver tumours in mice by a promoting mechanism. The increase in liver weight, centrilobular hypertrophy and pattern of cytochrome P450 induction are similar to those observed with other non-genotoxic mouse liver tumour promoters such as phenobarbital. In addition, the inhibition of cell–cell communication by phenytoin *in vitro* supports the role of promotion in mouse carcinogenesis.

The metabolic activation of phenytoin to a reactive intermediate has been proposed to account for the teratogenicity and possible genotoxicity of phenytoin. One possible intermediate is an arene oxide, that is hypothesized to result in binding to cellular macromolecules. However, this possibility has not been evaluated definitively, and studies of potential DNA damage in mouse liver or hepatocytes have not been reported.

The mechanism of induction of aneuploidy by phenytoin *in vitro* is unclear, as is its relationship to carcinogenicity in mouse liver.

5.5 Evaluation[1]

There is *inadequate evidence* in humans for the carcinogenicity of phenytoin.

There is *sufficient evidence* in experimental animals for the carcinogenicity of phenytoin.

Overall evaluation

Phenytoin is *possibly carcinogenic to humans (Group 2B)*.

6. References

Adams, J., Vorhees, C.V. & Middaugh, L.D. (1990) Developmental neurotoxicity of anticonvulsants: human and animal evidence on phenytoin. *Neurotoxicol. Teratol.*, **12**, 203–214

Allen, R.W., Jr, Ogden, B., Bentley, F.L. & Jung, A.L. (1980) Fetal hydantoin syndrome, neuroblastoma and hemorrhagic disease in a neonate. *J. Am. med. Assoc.*, **244**, 1464–1465

Al-Shammri, S., Guberman, A. & Hsu, E. (1992) Neuroblastoma and fetal exposure to phenytoin in a child without dysmorphic features. *Can. J. neurol. Sci.*, **19**, 243–245

Alving, J., Jensen, M.K. & Meyer, H. (1976) Diphenylhydantoin and chromosome morphology in man and rat: a negative report. *Mutat. Res.*, **40**, 173–176

Alving, J., Jensen, M.K. & Meyer, H. (1977) Chromosome studies of bone marrow cells and peripheral blood lymphocytes from diphenylhydantoin-treated patients. *Mutat. Res.*, **48**, 361–366

American Hospital Formulary Service (1995) *AHFS Drug Information* 95, Bethesda, MD, American Society of Health-System Pharmacists, pp. 1441–1444

---

[1] For definition of the italicized terms, see Preamble, pp. 22–25.

Aminoff, M.J., Simon, R.P. & Wiedemann, E. (1984) The hormonal responses to generalized tonic-clonic seizures. *Brain*, **107**, 569–578

Anderson, R.C. (1976) Cardiac defects in children of mothers receiving anticonvulsant therapy during pregnancy. *J. Pediatr.*, **89**, 318–319

Andrade-Mena, C.E., Sardo-Olmedo, J.A.J. & Ramirez-Lizardo, E.J. (1994) Effects of phenytoin administration on murine immune function. *J. Neuroimmunol.*, **50**, 3–7

Angelopoulos, A.P. (1975) A clinicopathological review: diphenylhydantoin gingival hyperplasia: 2. Aetiology, pathogenesis, differential diagnosis and treatment. *J. Can. dent. Assoc.*, **5**, 275–277

Anisimov, V.N. (1980) Effect of buformin and diphenylhydantoin on the life span, oestrous function and spontaneous tumours incidence in rats. *Vopr. Onkol.*, **26**, 42–48 (in Russian)

Anthony, J.J. (1970) Malignant lymphoma associated with hydantoin drugs. *Arch. Neurol.*, **22**, 450–454

Atkinson, A.J, Jr, MacGee, J., Strong, J., Garteiz, D. & Gaffney, T.E. (1970) Identification of 5-*meta*-hydroxyphenyl-5-phenylhydantoin as a metabolite of diphenylhydantoin. *Biochem. Pharmacol.*, **19**, 2483–2491

Atlas, S.A., Zweier, J.L. & Nebert, D.W. (1980) Genetic differences in phenytoin pharmacokinetics. In vivo clearance and in vitro metabolism among inbred strains of mice. *Dev. Pharmacol. Ther.*, **1**, 281–304

Bahn, S., Ganter, U., Bauer, J., Otten, U. & Volk, B. (1993) Influence of phenytoin on cytoskeletal organization and cell viability of immortalized mouse hippocampal neurons. *Brain Res.*, **615**, 160–169

Barcellona, P.S., Barale, R., Campana, A., Zucconi, D., Rossi, V. & Caranti, S. (1987) Correlations between embryotoxic and genotoxic effects of phenytoin in mice. *Teratog. Carcinog. Mutag.*, **7**, 159–168

Barr, M., Jr, Poznanski, A.K. & Schmickel, R.D. (1974) Digital hypoplasia and anticonvulsants during gestation: a teratogenic syndrome? *J. Pediatr.*, **84**, 254–256

Bertollini, R., Kallen, B., Mastroiacova, P. & Robert, A. (1987) Anticonvulsant drugs in monotherapy. Effect on the fetus. *Eur. J. Epidemiol.*, **3**, 164–171

Billings, R.E. (1984) Decreased hepatic 5,10-methylenetetrahydrofolate reductase activity in mice after chronic phenytoin treatment. *Mol. Pharmacol.*, **25**, 459–466

Bishun, N.P., Smith, N.S. & Williams, D.C. (1975) Chromosomes and anticonvulsant drugs. *Mutat. Res.*, **28**, 141–143

Blattner, W.A., Henson, D.E., Young, R.C. & Fraumeni, J.F., Jr (1977) Malignant mesenchymoma and birth defects. Prenatal exposure to phenytoin. *J. Am. med. Assoc.*, **238**, 334–335

Bleyer, W.A. & Skinner, A.L. (1976) Fatal neonatal hemorrhage after maternal anticonvulsant therapy. *J. Am. med. Assoc.*, **235**, 626–627

Bostrom, B. & Nesbit, M.E., Jr (1983) Hodgkin disease in a child with fetal alcohol-hydantoin syndrome. *J. Pediatr.*, **103**, 760–762

Braddock, S.W., Harrington, D. & Vose, J. (1992) Generalized nodular cutaneous pseudolymphoma associated with phenytoin therapy. Use of T-cell receptor gene rearrangement in diagnosis and clinical review of cutaneous reactions to phenytoin. *J. Am. Acad. Dermatol.*, **27**, 337–340

Brams, A., Buchet, J.P., Crutzen-Fayt, M.C., de Meester, C., Lauwerys, R. & Léonard, A. (1987) Comparative study, with 40 chemicals, of the efficiency of the *Salmonella* assay and the SOS chromotest (kit procedure). *Toxicol. Lett.*, **38**, 123–133

British Medical Association/Royal Pharmaceutical Society of Great Britain (1994) *British National Formulary Number 27 (March 1994)*, London, pp. 189–190, 193–194

British Pharmacopoeial Commission (1993) *British Pharmacopoeia* 1993, Vols. I & II, London, Her Majesty's Stationery Office, pp. 511–512, 1056–1058

Browne, T.R. & LeDuc, B. (1995) Phenytoin: chemistry and biotransformation. In: Levy, R.H., Mattson, R.H. & Meldrum, B.S., eds, *Antiepileptic Drugs*, 4th Ed., New York, Raven Press, pp. 283–300

Budavari, S., ed. (1995) *The Merck Index*, 12th Ed., Rahway, NJ, Merck & Co.

Buehler, B.A., Delimont, D., van Waes, M. & Finnell, R.H. (1990) Prenatal prediction of risk of the fetal hydantoin syndrome. *New Engl. J. Med.*, **322**, 1567–1572

Burke, J.T. & Thénot, J.P. (1985) Determination of antiepileptic drugs. *J. Chromatogr.*, **340**, 199–241

Cageao, L.F., Ceppi, J.A., Boado, R.J. & Zaninovich, A.A. (1992) Diphenylhydantoin stimulates the intrapituitary conversion of thyroxine to triiodothyronine in the rat. *Neuroendocrinology*, **56**, 453–458

Chang, T., Savory, A. & Glazko, A.J. (1970) A new metabolite of 5,5-diphenylhydantoin (dilantin). *Biochem. biophys. Res. Comm.*, **38**, 444–449

Chatot, C.L., Klein, N.W., Clapper, M.L., Resor, S.R., Singer, W.D., Russman, B.S., Holmes, G.L., Mattson, R.H. & Cramer, J.A. (1984) Human serum teratogenicity studied by rat embryo culture: epilepsy, anticonvulsant drugs, and nutrition. *Epilepsia*, **25**, 205–216

Chhabra, R.S., Bucher, J.R., Haseman, J.K., Elwell, M.R., Kurtz, P.J. & Carlton, B.D. (1993) Comparative carcinogenicity of 5,5-diphenylhydantoin with or without perinatal exposure in rats and mice. *Fundam. appl. Toxicol.*, **21**, 174–186

Conney, A.H. (1969) Microsomal enzyme induction by drugs. *Pharmacol. Phys.*, **3**, 1–6

Cooke, L.E., Hardin, T.C. & Hendrickson, D.J. (1988) Phenytoin-induced pseudolymphoma with mycosis fungoides manifestations. *Clin Pharmacol.*, **7**, 153–157

Cramer, J.A. & Jones, E.E. (1991) Reproductive function in epilepsy. *Epilepsia*, **32** (Suppl. 6), S19–S26

Czeizel, A.E. (1993) Prevention of congenital abnormalities by periconceptional multivitamin supplementation. *Br. med. J.*, **306**, 1645–1648

Czeizel, A.E. (1995) Folic acid in the prevention of neural tube defect. *J. Pediatr. Gastroenterol. Nutr.*, **20**, 4–16

Czeizel, A.E. & Dudás, I. (1992) Prevention of the first occurrence of neural-tube defects by periconceptional vitamin supplementation. *New Engl. J. Med.*, **327**, 1832–1835

Czeizel, A.E., Bod, M. & Halász, P. (1992) Evaluation of anticonvulsant drugs during pregnancy in a population-based Hungarian study. *Eur. J. Epidemiol.*, **8**, 122–127

Dabee, V., Hart, A.G. & Hurley, R.M. (1975) Teratogenic effects of diphenylhydantoin. *Can. med. Assoc. J.*, **112**, 75–76

Danielson, M.K., Danielsson, B.R.G., Marchner, H., Lundin, M., Rundqvist, E. & Reiland, S. (1992) Histopathological and hemodynamic studies supporting hypoxia and vascular disruption as explanation to phenytoin teratogenicity. *Teratology*, **46**, 485–497

Danielsson, B.R.G., Danielson, M.K., Rundqvist, E. & Reiland, S. (1992) Identical phalangeal defects induced by phenytoin and nifedipine suggest fetal hypoxia and vascular disruption behind phenytoin teratogenicity. *Teratology*, **45**, 247–258

Dansky, L.V. & Finnel, R.H. (1991) Parental epilepsy, anticonvulsant drugs, and reproductive outcome: epidemiologic and experimental findings spanning three decades. II. Human studies. *Reprod. Toxicol.*, **5**, 301–335

Dansky, L.V., Andermann, E., Rosenblatt, D., Sherwin, A.L. & Andermann, F. (1987) Anticonvulsants, folate levels, and pregnancy outcome: a prospective study. *Ann. Neurol.*, **21**, 176–182

Das, U.N., Devi, G.R., Rao, K.P., Nandan, S.D. & Rao, M.S. (1983) Prevention and/or reversibility of genetic damage induced by phenytoin in the bone marrow cells of mice by colchicine: possible relevance to prostaglandin involvement. *IRCS med. Sci.*, **11**, 122–123

Deda, G., Akinci, A., Teziç, T. & Karagöl, U. (1992) Effects of anticonvulsant drugs on thyroid hormones in epileptic children. *Turk. J. Pediatr.*, **34**, 239–244

DeLattre, J.-Y., Safai, B. & Posner, J.B. (1988) Erythema multiforme and Stevens-Johnson syndrome in patients receiving cranial irradiation and phenytoin. *Neurology*, **38**, 194–198

Dhanwada, K.R., Veerisetty, V., Zhu, F., Razzaque, A., Thompson, K.D. & Jones, C. (1992) Characterization of primary human fibroblasts transformed by human papilloma virus type 16 and herpes simplex virus type 2 DNA sequences. *J. gen. Virol.*, **73**, 791–799

Dill, R.E., Miller, E.K., Weil, T., Lesley, S., Farmer, G.R. & Iacopino, A.M. (1993) Phenytoin increases gene expression for platelet-derived growth factor B chain in macrophages and monocytes. *J. Periodontol.*, **64**, 169–173

Dilman, V.M. & Anisimov, V.N. (1980) Effect of treatment with phenformin, diphenylhydantoin or L-dopa on life span and tumour incidence in C3H/Sn mice. *Gerontology*, **26**, 241–246

Diwan, B.A., Hennemen, J.R., Nims, R.W. & Rice, J.M. (1993) Tumor promotion by an anticonvulsant agent, phenytoin, in mouse liver: correlation with CYP2B induction. *Carcinogenesis*, **14**, 2227–2231

Doecke, C.J., Sansom, L.N. & McManus, M.E. (1990) Phenytoin 4-hydroxylation by rabbit liver P450IIC3 and identification of orthologs in human liver microsomes. *Biochem. biophys. Res. Commun.*, **166**, 860–866

Dollery, C., Boobis, A.R., Burley, D., Davies, D.M., Davies, D.S., Harrison, P.I., Orme, M.E., Park, B.K. & Goldberg, L.I. (1991) *Therapeutic Drugs: Phenytoin (sodium)*, Edinburgh, Churchill Livingstone, pp. P93–P98

Eadie, M.J., Lander, C.M. & Tyrer, J.H. (1977) Plasma drug level monitoring in pregnancy. *Clin. Pharmacokinet.*, **2**, 427–436

Eadie, M.J., McKinnon, G.E., Dickinson, R.G., Hooper, W.D. & Lander, C.M. (1992) Phenytoin metabolism during pregnancy. *Eur. J. clin. Pharmacol.*, **43**, 389–392

Earnest, M.P., Marx, J.A. & Drury, L.R. (1983) Complications of intravenous phenytoin for acute treatment of seizures. Recommendations for usage. *J. Am. med. Assoc.*, **249**, 762–765

Ehrenbard, L.T. & Chaganti, R.S.K. (1981) Cancer in the fetal hydantoin syndrome (Letter to the Editor). *Lancet*, **ii**, 97

Elmazar, M.M.A. & Sullivan, F.M. (1981) Effect of prenatal phenytoin administration on postnatal development of the rat: a behavioral teratology study. *Teratology*, **24**, 115–124

Elshove, J. (1969) Cleft palate in the offspring of female mice treated with phenytoin (Letter to the Editor). *Lancet*, **ii**, 1074

Epstein, S.S., Arnold, E., Andrea, J., Bass, W. & Bishop, Y. (1972) Detection of chemical mutagens by the dominant lethal assay in the mouse. *Toxicol. appl. Pharmacol.*, **23**, 288–325

Esser, K.J., Kotlarek, F., Habedank, M., Mühler, U. & Mühler, E. (1981) Chromosomal investigations in epileptic children during long-term therapy with phenytoin or primidone. *Hum. Genet.*, **56**, 345–348

Fedrick, J. (1973) Epilepsy and pregnancy: a report from the Oxford Record Linkage Study. *Br. med. J.*, **ii**, 442–448

Finnel, R.H. (1981) Phenytoin-induced teratogenesis: a mouse model. *Science*, **211**, 483–484

Finnel, R.H. & Chernoff, G.F. (1984a) Editorial comment: Genetic background: the elusive component in the fetal hydantoin syndrome. *Am. J. med. Genet.*, **19**, 459–462

Finnel, R.H. & Chernoff, G.F. (1984b) Variable pattern of malformation in the mouse fetal hydantoin syndrome. *Am. J. med. Genet.*, **19**, 463–471

Finnel, R.H., Abbott, L.C. & Taylor, S.M. (1989) The fetal hydantoin syndrome: answers from a mouse model. *Reprod. Toxicol.*, **3**, 127–133

Finnell, R.H., Buehler, B.A., Kerr, B.M., Ager, P.L. & Levy, R.H. (1992) Clinical and experimental studies linking oxidative metabolism to phenytoin-induced teratogenesis. *Neurology*, **42** (Suppl. 5), 25–31

Finnel, R.H., Van Waes, M., Musselman, A., Kerr, B.M. & Levy, R.H. (1993) Differences in the patterns of phenytoin-induced malformations following stiripentol coadministration in three inbred mouse strains. *Reprod. Toxicol.*, **7**, 439–448

Finnel, R.H., Kerr, B.M., Van Waes, M., Stewart, R.L. & Levy, R.H. (1994) Protection from phenytoin-induced congenital malformations by coadministration of the antiepileptic drug striripentol in a mouse model. *Epilepsia*, **35**, 141–148

Flejter, W.L., Astemborski, J.A., Hassel, T.M. & Cohen, M.M. (1989) Cytogenetic effects of phenytoin and/or carbamazepine on human peripheral leukocytes. *Epilepsia*, **30**, 374–379

Friedman, G.D. (1986) Multiple myeloma: relation to propoxyphene and other drugs, radiation and occupation. *Int. J. Epidemiol.*, **15**, 424–426

Fritz, H. (1976) The effect of cortisone on the teratogenic action of acetylsalicylic acid and diphenylhydantoin in the mouse. *Experientia*, **32**, 721–722

Fujii, A., Matsumoto, H., Nakao, S., Teshigawara, H. & Akimoto, Y. (1994) Effect of calcium-channel blockers on cell proliferation, DNA synthesis and collagen synthesis of cultured gingival fibroblasts derived from human nifedipine responders and non-responders. *Arch. oral Biol.*, **39**, 99–104

Gabler, W.L. & Falace, D. (1970) The distribution and metabolism of dilantin in non-pregnant, pregnant and fetal rats. *Arch. int. Pharmacodyn.*, **184**, 45–58

Gabler, W.L. & Hubbard, G.L. (1972) The distribution of 5,5-diphenylhydantoin (DPH) and its metabolites in maternal and fetal rhesus monkey tissues. *Arch. int. Pharmacodyn.*, **200**, 222–230

Gabrys, K., Medras, E., Kowalski, P. & Gola, A. (1983) Malignant lymphoma in the course of antiepileptic therapy. *Polsk. Tyg. Lek.*, **38**, 505–507 (in Polish)

Gaily, E., Granström, M.-L., Hiilesmaa, V. & Bardy, M. (1988) Minor anomalies in the offspring of epileptic mothers. *J. Pediatr.*, **112**, 520–529

Gams, R.A., Neal, J.A. & Conrad, F.G. (1968) Hydantoin-induced pseudo-pseudolymphoma. *Ann. intern. Med.*, **69**, 557–568

Ganapathi, R., Hercbergs, A., Grabowski, D. & Ford, J. (1993) Selective enhancement of vincristine cytotoxicity in multidrug-resistant tumor cells by dilantin (phenytoin). *Cancer Res.*, **53**, 3262–3265

García Sagredo, J.M. (1988) Effect of anticonvulsants on human chromosomes. 2. In vitro studies. *Mutat. Res.*, **204**, 623–626

Gennaro, A.R., ed. (1995) *Remington: The Science and Practice of Pharmacy*, 19th Ed., Vol. II, Easton, PA, Mack Publishing Co., pp. 1177–1178

Ghatak, N.R., Santoso, R.A. & McKinney, W.M. (1976) Cerebellar degeneration following long-term phenytoin therapy. *Neurology*, **26**, 818–820

Gibson, J.E. & Becker, B.A. (1968) Teratogenic effects of diphenylhydantoin in Swiss-Webster and A/J mice. *Proc. Soc. exp. Biol. Med.*, **128**, 905–909

Glazko, A.J. (1982) Phenytoin: chemistry and methods of determination. In: Woodbury, D.M., Penry, J.K. & Pippenger, C.E., eds, *Antiepileptic Drugs*, New York, Raven Press, pp. 177–189

Goodman Gilman, A., Rall, T.W., Nils, A.S. & Taylor, P., eds (1990) *Goodman and Gilman's. The Pharmacological Basis of Therapeutics*, 8th Ed., New York, Pergamon, pp. 439–443; 857–861

Griswold, D.P., Jr, Casey, A.E., Weisburger, E.K., Weisburger, J.H. & Schabel, F.M., Jr (1966) On the carcinogenicity of a single intragastric dose of hydrocarbons, nitrosamines, aromatic amines, dyes, coumarins and miscellaneous chemicals in female Sprague-Dawley rats. *Cancer Res.*, **26**, 619–625

Griswold, D.P., Jr, Casey, A.E., Weisburger, E.K. & Weisburger, J.H. (1968) The carcinogenicity of multiple intragastric doses of aromatic and heterocyclic nitro or amino derivatives in young female Sprague-Dawley rats. *Cancer Res.*, **28**, 924–933

Guest, A.E., Saleh, A.M., Pheasant, A.E. & Blair, J.A. (1983) Effects of phenobarbitone and phenytoin on folate catabolism in the rat. *Biochem. Pharmacol.*, **32**, 3179–3182

Gupta, C., Katsumata, M. & Goldman, A.S. (1985) H-2 histocompatibility region influences the inhibition of arachidonic acid cascade by dexamethasone and phenytoin in mouse embryonic palates. *J. craniofac. Genet. dev. Biol.*, **9**, 277–285

Habedank, M., Esser, K.-J., Brüll, D., Kotlarek, F. & Stumpf, C. (1982) Increased sister chromatid exchanges in epileptic children during long-term therapy with phenytoin. *Hum. Genet.*, **61**, 71–72

Halery, S. & Feuerman, E.J. (1977) Pseudolymphoma syndrome. *Dermatologica*, **155**, 321–327

Hammond, E.J. & Wilder, B.J. (1983) Immunofluorescent evidence for a specific binding site for phenytoin in the cerebellum. *Epilepsia*, **24**, 269–274

Hansen, D.K. (1991) The embryotoxicity of phenytoin: an update on possible mechanisms. *Proc. Soc. exp. Biol. Med.*, **197**, 361–368

Hansen, D.K. & Billings, R.E. (1985) Phenytoin teratogenicity and effects on embryonic and maternal folate metabolism. *Teratology*, **31**, 363–371

Hansen, D.K. & Hodes, M.E. (1983) Comparative teratogenicity of phenytoin among several inbred strains of mice. *Teratology*, **28**, 175–179

Hansen, D.K., Holson, R.R., Sullivan, P.A. & Grafton, T.F. (1988) Alterations in maternal plasma corticosterone levels following treatment with phenytoin. *Toxicol. appl. Pharmacol.*, **96**, 24–32

Hansen, D.K., Branham, W.S., Sheehan, D.M. & Holson, R.R. (1992) Embryotoxicity of phenytoin in adrenalectomized CD-1 mice. *Proc. Soc. exp. Biol. Med.*, **199**, 501–508

Hanson, J.W. (1976) Fetal hydantoin syndrome. *Teratology*, **13**, 185–187

Hanson, J.W. & Smith, D.W. (1975) The fetal hydantoin syndrome. *J. Pediatr.*, **87**, 285–290

Hanson, J.W., Myrianthopoulos, N.C., Sedgwick Harvey, M.A. & Smith, D.W. (1976) Risks to the offspring of women treated with hydantoin anticonvulsants, with emphasis on the fetal hydantoin syndrome. *J. Pediatr.*, **89**, 662–668

Harbison, R.D. (1978) Chemical-biological reactions common to teratogenesis and mutagenesis. *Environ. Health Perspectives*, **29**, 87–100

Harbison, R.D. & Becker, B.A. (1969) Relation of dosage and time of administration of diphenylhydantoin to its teratogenic effect in mice. *Teratology*, **2**, 305–311

Harbison, R.D. & Becker, B.A. (1972) Diphenylhydantoin teratogenicity in rats. *Toxicol. appl. Pharmacol.*, **22**, 193–200

Harbison, R.D. & Becker, B.A. (1974) Comparative embryotoxicity of diphenylhydantoin and some of its metabolites in mice. *Teratology*, **10**, 237–242

Harris, D.W.S., Ostlere, L., Buckley, C., Whittaker, S., Sweny, P. & Rustin, M.H.A. (1992) Phenytoin-induced pseudolymphoma. A report of a case and review of the literature. *Br. J. Dermatol.*, **127**, 403–406

Harrison, M.B., Lyons, G.R. & Landow, E.R. (1993) Phenytoin and dyskinesias: a report of two cases and review of the literature. *Movement Disorders*, **8**, 19–27

Hashem, N. & Shawki, R. (1976) Cultured peripheral lymphocytes: one biologic indicator of potential drug hazard. *Afr. J. Med. med. Sci.*, **5**, 155–163

Hassell, T.M. (1981) *Epilepsy and the Oral Manifestation of Phenytoin Therapy*, Basel, Karger, pp. 116–202

Hassell, T.M., Roebuck, S., Page, R.C. & Wray, S.H. (1982) Quantitative histopathologic assessment of developing phenytoin-induced gingival overgrowth in the cat. *J. clin. Periodontol.*, **9**, 365–372

Hassell, T.M., Maguire, J.H., Cooper, C.G. & Johnson, P.T. (1984) Phenytoin metabolism in the cat after long-term oral administration. *Epilepsia*, **25**, 556–563

Hatch, G.G., Anderson, T.M., Lubet, R.A., Kouri, R.E., Putman, D.L., Cameron, J.W., Nims, R.W., Most, B., Spalding, J.W., Tennant, R.W. & Schechtman, L.M. (1986) Chemical enhancement of SA7 virus transformation of hamster embryo cells: evaluation of interlaboratory testing of diverse chemicals. *Environ. Mutag.*, **8**, 515–513

Haworth, S., Lawlor, T., Mortelmans, K., Speck, W. & Zeiger, E. (1983) *Salmonella* mutagenicity test results for 250 chemicals. *Environ. mol. Mutagen.*, **5** (Suppl. 1), 3–142

Hayakawa, T., Hamada, Y., Maihara, T., Hattori, H. & Mikawa, H. (1994) Phenytoin reduces neonatal hypoxic-ischemic brain damage in rats. *Life Sci.*, **54**, 387–392

Hendrie, T.A., Rowland, J.R., Binkerd, P.E. & Hendricks, A.G. (1990) Developmental toxicity and pharmacokinetics of phenytoin in the rhesus macaque: an interspecies comparison. *Reprod. Toxicol.*, **4**, 257–266

Herzog, A.G., Levesque, L.A., Drislane, F.W., Ronthal, M. & Schomer, D.L. (1991) Phenytoin-induced elevation of serum estradiol and reproductive dysfunction in men with epilepsy. *Epilepsia*, **32**, 550–553

Hiilesmaa, V.K., Teramo, K., Granström, M.-L. & Bardy, A.H. (1983) Serum folate concentrations during pregnancy in women with epilepsy: relation to antiepileptic drug concentrations, number of seizures, and fetal outcome. *Br. med. J.*, **287**, 577–579

Hill, R.M., Verniaud, W.M., Horning, M.G., McCulley, L.B. & Morgan, N.F. (1974) Infants exposed *in utero* to antiepileptic drugs: a prospective study. *Am. J. Dis. Child.*, **127**, 645–653

Hirano, T., Kaneko, S. & Fujioka, K. (1984) Prospective study on psychomotor development in the offspring of epileptic mother: risk factors for developmental retardation. *Ann. Rep. pharmacopsychiat. Res. Found.*, **15**, 282–291

Hou, L.-T. (1993) Synthesis of collagen and fibronectin in fibroblasts derived from healthy and hyperplastic gingivae. *J. Formos. med. Assoc.*, **92**, 367–372

Hyman, G.A. & Sommers, S.C. (1966) The development of Hodgkin's disease and lymphoma during anticonvulsant therapy. *Blood*, **28**, 416–427

IARC (1977) *IARC Monographs on the Evaluation of Carcinogenic Risk of Chemicals to Man*, Vol. 13, *Some Miscellaneous Pharmaceutical Substances*, Lyon, pp. 201–225

IARC (1987) *IARC Monographs on the Evaluation of Carcinogenic Risks to Humans*, Suppl. 7, *Overall Evaluations of Carcinogenicity: An Update of* IARC Monographs *Volumes 1 to 42*, Lyon, pp. 319–321

Ichiba, M., Kanazawa, H., Kobo, M., Takenobu, S., Taguchi, S., Senga, K. & Tamura, Z. (1984) Analysis of drugs in fallen dust in a dispensary using thin-layer chromatography and chemical ionization mass spectrometry. *Yakuzaigaku*, **44**, 231–238 (in Japanese)

Ichiba, M., Kanazawa, H., Shimizu, N., Kobo, M., Senga, K. & Tamura, Z. (1986) Identification of drugs with optical, fluorescence and polarizing microscopes: drugs in fallen and floating dust in a dispensary. *Bunseki Kagaku*, **35**, 157–160 (in Japanese)

Isobe, T., Horimatsu, T., Fujita, T., Miyazaki, K. & Sugiyama, T. (1980) Adult T-cell lymphoma following diphenylhydantoin therapy. *Acta haematol. jpn.*, **43**, 711–714

Jang, J.J., Takahashi, M., Furukawa, F., Toyoda, K., Hasegawa, R., Sato, H. & Hayashi, Y. (1987) Long-term in vivo carcinogenicity study of phenytoin (5,5-diphenylhydantoin) in F344 rats. *Food chem. Toxicol.*, **25**, 697–702

Jerina, D.M. & Daly, J.W. (1974) Arene oxides: a new aspect of drug metabolism. *Science*, **185**, 573–582

Jimenez, J.F., Brown, R.E., Seibert, R.W., Seibert, J.J. & Char, F. (1981) Melanotic neuroectodermal tumor of infancy and fetal hydantoin syndrome. *Am. J. pediatr. Hemat./Oncol.*, **3**, 9–15

Jone, C.M., Erickson, L.M., Trosko, J.E., Netzloff, M.L. & Cheng, C.-C. (1985) Inhibition of metabolic cooperation by the anticonvulsants, diphenylhydantoin and phenobarbital. *Teratog. Carcinog. Mutag.*, **5**, 379–391

Jones, G.L. & Wimbish, G.H. (1985) Hydantoins. In: Frey, H.-H. & Janz, D., eds, *Handbook of Experimental Pharmacology*, Vol. 74, *Anti-epileptic Drugs*, Berlin, Springer-Verlag, pp. 351–419

Juhász, J., Baló, J. & Szende, B. (1968) Experimental tumours developing upon the effect of diphenylhydantoin treatment. *Magyar Onkol.*, **12**, 39–44 (in Hungarian)

Kaneko, S. & Kondo, T. (1995) Antiepileptic agents and birth defects. Incidence, mechanisms and prevention. *CNS Drugs*, **3**, 41–55

Kaneko, S., Otani, K., Fukushima, Y., Ogawa, Y., Nomura, Y., Ono, T., Nakane, Y., Teranishi, T. & Goto, M. (1988) Teratogenicity of antiepileptic drugs: analysis of possible risk factors. *Epilepsia*, **29**, 459–467

Kaneko, S., Otani, K., Kondo, T., Fukushima, Y., Nakamura, Y., Ogawa, Y., Kan, R., Takeda, A., Nakane, Y. & Teranishi, T. (1992) Malformation in infants of mothers with epilepsy receiving antiepileptic drugs. *Neurology*, **42** (Suppl. 5), 68–74

Katsumata, M., Gupta, C., Baker, M.K., Sussdorf, C.E. & Goldman, A.S. (1982) Diphenylhydantoin: an alternative ligand of a glucocorticoid receptor affecting prostaglandin generation in A/J mice. *Science*, **218**, 1313–1315

Katsumata, M., Gupta, C. & Goldman, A.S. (1985) Glucocorticoid receptor IB: mediator of antiinflammatory and teratogenic functions of both glucocorticoids and phenytoin. *Arch. Biochem. Biophys.*, **243**, 385–395

Kay, E.D., Goldman, A.S. & Daniel, J.C. (1988) Arachidonic acid reversal of phenytoin-induced neural tube and craniofacial defects *in vitro* in mice. *J. craniofac. Genet. dev. Biol.*, **8**, 179–186

Kay, E.D., Goldman, A.S. & Daniel, J.C. (1990) Common biochemical pathway of dysmorphogenesis in murine embryos: use of the glucocorticoid pathway by phenytoin. *Teratog. Carcinog. Mutag.*, **10**, 31–39

Keith, D.A., Gundberg, C.M., Japour, A., Aronoff, J., Alvarez, N. & Gallop, P.M. (1983) Vitamin K-dependent proteins and anticonvulsant medication. *Clin. Pharmacol. Ther.*, **34**, 529–532

Kelly, T.E. (1984) Teratogenicity of anticonvulsant drugs. III. Radiographic hand analysis of children exposed *in utero* to diphenylhydantoin. *Am. J. med. Genet.*, **19**, 445–450

Kempermann, G., Knoth, R., Gebicke-Haerter, P.J., Stolz, B.-J. & Volk, B. (1994) Cytochrome P450 in rat astrocytes *in vivo* and *in vitro*: intracellular localization and induction by phenytoin. *J. Neurosci. Res.*, **39**, 576–588

Kim, N.D., Yoo, J.K., Won, S.M., Park, S.S. & Gelboin, H.V. (1993) Phenytoin induction of cytochrome P4502B in mice: effects on hexobarbital hydroxylase activity. *Xenobiotica*, **23**, 217–225

Kimball, O.P. (1939) The treatment of epilepsy with sodium diphenylhydantoinate. *J. Am. med. Assoc.*, **112**, 1244–1246

Kindig, D., Garriott, M.L., Parton, J.W., Brunny, J.D. & Beyers, J.E. (1992) Diphenylhydantoin is not genotoxic in a battery of short-term cytogenetic assays. *Teratog. Carcinog. Mutag.*, **12**, 43–50

Kirchhoff, L.V., Evans, A.S., McClelland, K.E., Carvalho, R.P.S. & Pannuti, C.S. (1980) A case–control study of Hodgkin's disease in Brazil. I. Epidemiological aspects. *Am. J. Epidemiol.*, **112**, 595–608

Knuutila, S., Simell, O., Lipponen, P. & Saarinen, I. (1976) Bone-marrow chromosomes in healthy subjects. *Hereditas*, **82**, 29–35

Knuutila, S., Siimes, M., Simell, O., Tammisto, P. & Weber, T. (1977) Long-term use of phenytoin: effects on bone-marrow chromosomes in man. *Mutat. Res.*, **43**, 309–312

Koch, S., Göpfert-Geyer, E., Häuser, I., Hartmann, A., Jakob, S., Jäger-Roman, E., Nau, H., Rating, D. & Helge, H. (1985) Neonatal behaviour disturbance in infants of epileptic women treated during pregnancy. *Prof. clin. biol. Res.*, **163B**, 453–461

Koren, G., Demitrakoudis, D., Weksberg, R., Rieder, M., Shear, N.H., Sonely, M., Shandling, B. & Spielberg, S.P. (1989) Neuroblastoma after prenatal exposure to phenytoin: cause and effect? *Teratology*, **40**, 157–162

Kramer, S., Ward, E., Meadows, A.T. & Malone, K.E. (1987) Medical and drug risk factors associated with neuroblastoma: a case–control study. *J. natl Cancer Inst.*, **78**, 797–804

Krüger, G., Harris, D. & Sussman, E. (1972) Effect of dilantin in mice. II. Lymphoreticular tissue atypia and neoplasia after chronic exposure. *Z. Krebsforsch.*, **78**, 290–302

Kubow, S. (1992) Inhibition of phenytoin bioactivation and teratogenicity by dietary n-3 fatty acids in mice. *Lipids*, **27**, 721–728

Kubow, S. & Wells, P.G. (1986) In vitro evidence for prostaglandin synthetase-catalysed bioactivation of phenytoin to a free radical intermediate (Abstract no. 23). *Pharmacologist*, **28**, 195

Kubow, S. & Wells, P.G. (1989) In vitro bioactivation of phenytoin to a reactive free radical intermediate by prostaglandin synthetase, horseradish peroxidase, and thyroid peroxidase. *Mol. Pharmacol.*, **35**, 504–511

Kumar, N., Khwaja, G.A., Gupta, M. & Sharma, S. (1993) Antiepileptic drug induced osteomalacic myopathy with hyperparathyroidism and nephrolithiasis. *J. Assoc. Phys. India*, **41**, 748–749

Lambotte-Vandepaer, M., Brams, A., Crutzen-Fayt, M.C., Duverger-Van Bogaert, M., Dumont, P. & Léonard, A. (1989) Comparison of teratogenic properties in mice, strain BALB-c by diphenylhydantoin and ^{3}H-diphenylhydantoin. *C.R. Soc. Biol.*, **183**, 358–361 (in French)

Lander, C.M., Edwards, V.E., Eadie, M.J. & Tyrer, J.H. (1977) Plasma anticonvulsant concentrations during pregnancy. *Neurology*, **27**, 128–131

Larkin, J.G., Macphee, G.J.A., Beastall, G.H. & Brodie, M.J. (1989) Thyroid hormone concentrations in epileptic patients. *Eur. J. clin. Pharmacol.*, **36**, 213–216

Laxer, K.D., Mullooly, J.P. & Howell, B. (1985) Prolactin changes after seizures classified by EEG monitoring. *Neurology*, **35**, 31–35

Léonard, A., de Meester, C., Fabry, L., de Saint-Georges, L. & Dumont, P. (1984) Lack of mutagenicity of diphenylhydantoin in in vitro short-term tests. *Mutat. Res.*, **137**, 79–88

Levo, Y. (1974) The protective effect of hydantoin treatment on carcinogenesis. *Naunyn-Schmiedeberg's Arch. Pharmacol.*, **285**, 29–30

Li, F.P., Willard, D.R., Goodman, R. & Vawter, G. (1975) Malignant lymphoma after diphenylhydantoin (dilantin) therapy. *Cancer*, **36**, 1359–1362

Linet, M.S., Harlow, S.D. & McLaughlin, J.K. (1987) A case–control study of multiple myeloma in whites: chronic antigenic stimulation, occupation, and drug use. *Cancer Res.*, **47**, 2978–2981

Liu, L. & Wells, P.G. (1994) In vivo phenytoin-initiated oxidative damage to proteins and lipids in murine maternal hepatic and embryonic tissue organelles: potential molecular targets of chemical teratogenesis. *Toxicol. appl. Pharmacol.*, **125**, 247–255

Lorand, I.G.H., Hadler, W.A. & Prigenzi, L.S. (1976) Morphological changes in the lymphoid organs induced by diphenylhydantoin sodium (DPH). *Virchows Arch. A. Pathol. Anat. Histol.*, **372**, 81–88

Lowe, C.R. (1973) Congenital malformations among infants born to epileptic women. *Lancet*, **i**, 9–10

MacKinney, A.A., Vyas, R.S. & Walker, D. (1978) Hydantoin drugs inhibit polymerization of pure microtubular protein. *J. Pharmacol. exp. Ther.*, **204**, 189–202

Macphee, G.J.A., Larkin, J.G., Butler, E., Beastall, G.H. & Brodie, M.J. (1988) Circulating hormones and pituitary responsiveness in young epileptic men receiving long-term antiepileptic medication. *Epilepsia*, **29**, 468–475

Maeda, T., Sano, N., Togei, K., Shibata, M., Izumi, K. & Otsuka, H. (1988) Lack of carcinogenicity of phenytoin in (C57Bl/6 × C3H)F$_1$ mice. *J. Toxicol. environ. Health*, **24**, 111–119

Maguire, J.H., Butler, T.C. & Dudley, K.H. (1980) Absolute configurations of the dihydrodiol metabolites of 5,5-diphenylhydantoin (phenytoin) from rat, dog, and human urine. *Drug Metab. Dispos.*, **8**, 325–331

Maguire, J.H., Greenwood, R.S., Lewis, D.V. & Hassell, T.M. (1986) Phenytoin-induced gingival overgrowth incidence is dependent upon co-medication. *J. dent. Res.*, **65**, 249

Mallek, H.M. & Nakamoto, T. (1981) Dilantin and folic acid status. Clinical implications for the periodontist. *J. Periodontol.*, **14**, 255–259

Malpas, J.S., Spray, G.H. & Witts, L.J. (1966) Serum folic-acid and vitamin-B$_{12}$ levels in anticonvulsant therapy. *Br. med. J.*, **i**, 955–957

Manon-Espaillat, R., Burnstine, T.H., Remler, B., Reed, R.C. & Osorio, I. (1991) Antiepileptic drug intoxication: factors and their significance. *Epilepsy*, **32**, 96–100

Mareš, P., Lišková-Bernášková, K. & Mudrochová, M. (1987) Convulsant action of diphenylhydantoin overdose in young rats. *Act. Nerv. Sup. (Praha)*, **29**, 30–35

Margaretten, N.C. & Warren, R.T. (1987) Effect of phenytoin on antibody production: use of a murine model. *Epilepsia*, **28**, 77–80

Marsh, L. & Fraser, F.C. (1973) Studies on dilantin-induced cleft palate in mice (Abstract). *Teratology*, **7**, A-23

Martz, F., Failinger, C., III & Bake, D.A. (1977) Phenytoin teratogenesis: correlation between embryopathic effect and covalent binding of putative arene oxide metabolite in gestational tissue. *Pharmacol. exp. Ther.*, **203**, 231–239

Massa, T., Gerber, T., Pfaffenholz, V., Chandra, A., Schlatterer, A. & Chandra, P. (1990) A host-mediated in vivo/in vitro assay with peritoneal murine macrophages for the detection of carcinogenic chemicals. *J. Cancer Res. clin. Oncol.*, **116**, 357–364

Massey, K.M. (1966) Teratogenic effects of dyphenylhydantoin sodium. *J. oral Ther. Pharmacol.*, **2**, 380–385

Masur, H., Elger, C.E., Ludolph, A.C. & Galanski, M. (1989) Cerebellar atrophy following acute intoxication with phenytoin. *Neurology*, **39**, 432–433

Masur, H., Fahrendorf, G., Oberwittler, C. & Reuther, G. (1990) Cerebellar atrophy following acute intoxication with phenytoin. *Neurology*, **40**, 1800

Mattson, R.H. & Cramer, J.A. (1985) Epilepsy, sex hormones and antiepileptic drugs. *Epilepsia*, **26** (Suppl.), S40–S51

Maurya, A.K. & Goyle, S. (1985) Mutagenic potential of anticonvulsant diphenylhydantoin (DPH) on human lymphocytes *in vitro*. *Meth. Find exp. clin. Pharmacol.*, **7**, 109–112

Maya, M.T., Farinha, A.R., Lucas, A.M. & Morais, J.A. (1992) Sensitive method for the determination of phenytoin in plasma, and phenytoin and 5-(4-hydroxyphenyl)-5-phenylhydantoin in urine by high-performance liquid chromatography. *J. pharm. biomed. Analysis*, **10**, 1001–1006

McClain, R.M. & Langhoff, L. (1980) Teratogenicity of diphenylhydantoin in the New Zealand white rabbit. *Teratology*, **21**, 371–379

McDevitt, J.M., Gautieri, R.F. & Mann, D.E., Jr (1981) Comparative teratogenicity of cortisone and phenytoin in mice. *J. pharm. Sci.*, **70**, 631–634

McDonald, D.F. (1969) Lack of effect of diphenylhydantoin ingestion on vesical transitional epithelium in the rat. *J. surg. Oncol.*, **1**, 77–79

McFee, A.F., Tice, R.R. & Shelby, M.D. (1992) In vivo cytogenetic activity of diphenylhydantoin in mice. *Mutat. Res.*, **278**, 61–68

McLain, L.W., Jr, Martin, J.T. & Allen, J.H. (1980) Cerebellar degeneration due to chronic phenytoin therapy. *Ann. Neurol.*, **7**, 18–23

Meadow, S.R. (1968) Anticonvulsant drugs and congenital abnormalities (Letter to the Editor). *Lancet*, **ii**, 1296

Meadow, S.R. (1970) Congenital abnormalities and anticonvulsant drugs. *Proc. roy. Soc. Med.*, **63**, 48–49

Medical Economics (1996) *PDR®: Physicians' Desk Reference*, 50th Ed., Montvale, NJ, Medical Economics Data Production Co., pp. 1906–1913

Mercier-Parot, L. & Tuchmann-Duplessis, H. (1974) The dysmorphogenic potential of phenytoin: experimental observations. *Drugs*, **8**, 340–353

Minck, D.R., Erway, L.C. & Vorhees, C.V. (1989) Preliminary findings of a reduction of otoconia in the inner ear of adult rats prenatally exposed to phenytoin. *Neurotoxicol. Teratol.*, **11**, 307–311

Miranda, A.F., Wiley, M.J. & Wells, P.G. (1994) Evidence for embryonic peroxidase-catalyzed bioactivation and glutathione-dependent cytoprotection in phenytoin teratogenicity. Modulation by eicosatetraynoic acid and buthionine sulfoximine in murine embryo culture. *Toxicol. appl. Pharmacol.*, **124**, 230–241

Mirkin, B.L. (1971) Diphenylhydantoin: placental transport, fetal localisation, neonatal metabolism, and possible teratogenic effects. *J. Pediatr.*, **78**, 329–337

Moglia, A., Tartara, A., Arrigo, A., Poggi, P., Scelsi, M. & Scelsi, R. (1981) Chronic treatment with phenytoin in rats: effects on peripheral nervous system. *Farm. Sci.*, **36**, 419–424

Monson, R.R., Rosenberg, L., Hartz, S.C., Shapiro, S., Heinonen, O.P. & Slone, D. (1973) Diphenylhydantoin and selected congenital malformations. *New Engl. J. Med.*, **289**, 1049–1052

Montes de Oca-Luna, R., Leal-Garza, C.H., Baca-Sevilla, S. & Garza-Chapa, R. (1984) The effect of diphenylhydantoin on the frequency of micronuclei in bone-marrow polychromatic erythrocytes of mice. *Mutat. Res.*, **141**, 183–187

Morris, J.E., Price, J.M., Lalich, J.J. & Stein, R.J. (1969) The carcinogenic activity of some 5-nitrofuran derivatives in the rat. *Cancer Res.*, **29**, 2145–2156

MRC Vitamin Study Research Group (1991) Prevention of neural tube defects. Results of the Medical Research Council Vitamin Study. *Lancet*, **338**, 131–137

Mullenix, P., Tassinari, M.S. & Keith, D.A. (1983) Behavioral outcome after prenatal exposure to phenytoin in rats. *Teratology*, **27**, 149–157

Nation, R.L., Evans, A.M. & Milne, R.W. (1990a) Pharmacokinetic drug interactions with phenytoin (Part I). *Clin. Pharmacokinet.*, **18**, 37–60

Nation, R.L., Evans, A.M. & Milne, R.W. (1990b) Pharmacokinetic drug interactions with phenytoin (Part II). *Clin. Pharmacokinet.*, **18**, 131–150

Nau, H., Kuhnz, W., Egger, H.-J., Rating, D. & Helge, H. (1982) Anticonvulsants during pregnancy and lactation. Transplacental, maternal and neonatal pharmacokinetics. *Clin. Pharmacokinet.*, **7**, 508–543

Nelson, K.B. & Ellenberg, J.H. (1982) Maternal seizure disorder, outcome of pregnancy, and neurological abnormalities in the children. *Neurology*, **32**, 1247–1254

Nelson, E.W., Crick, W.F., Cerda, J.J., Wilder, B.J. & Streiff, R.R. (1983) The effect of diphenylhydantoin (phenytoin) on the sequential stages of intestinal folate absorption. *Drug. Nutr. Interact.*, **2**, 47–56

Netzloff, M.L., Streiff, R.R., Frias, J.L. & Rennert, O.M. (1979) Folate antagonism following teratogenic exposure to diphenylhydantoin. *Teratology*, **19**, 45–50

Ney, G.C., Lantos, G., Barr, W.B. & Schaul, N. (1994) Cerebellar atrophy in patients with long-term phenytoin exposure and epilepsy. *Arch. Neurol.*, **51**, 767–771

Oberly, T.J., Michaelis, K.C., Rexroat, M.A., Bewsey, B.J. & Garriott, M.L. (1993) A comparison of the CHO/HGPRT$^+$ and the L5178Y/TK$^{+/-}$ mutation assays using suspension treatment and soft agar cloning: results for 10 chemicals. *Cell Biol. Toxicol.*, **9**, 243–257

Ohta, T., Wergedal, J.E., Matsuyama, T., Baylink, D.J. & Lau, K.-H.W. (1995) Phenytoin and fluoride act in concert to stimulate bone formation and to increase bone volume in adult male rats. *Calcif. Tissue int.*, **56**, 390–397

de Oliveira, A.R. & Machado-Santelli, G.M. (1987) Diphenylhydantoin and mitotic spindle abnormalities in cultured mouse and human cells. *Mutat. Res.*, **187**, 91–97

de Oliveira, A.R., Mori, L. & Machado-Santelli, G.M. (1987) Diphenylhydantoin effects in Balb/c mouse bone marrow cells: cytogenetic aspects (Short communication). *Rev. Brasil. Genet.*, **10**, 127–134

Olsen, J.H., Boice, J.D., Jr, Jensen, J.P.A. & Fraumeni, J.F., Jr (1989) Cancer among epileptic patients exposed to anticonvulsant drugs. *J. natl Cancer Inst.*, **81**, 803–808

Olsen, J.H., Wallin, H., Boice, J.D., Jr, Rask, K., Schulgen, G. & Fraumeni, J.F., Jr (1993) Phenobarbital, drug metabolism, and human cancer. *Cancer Epidemiol. Biomarkers Prev.*, **2**, 449–452

Olsen, J.H., Schulgen, G., Boice, J.D., Jr., Whysner, J., Travis, L.B., Williams, G.M., Johnson, F.B. & McGee, J.O'D. (1995) Antiepileptic treatment and risk for hepatobiliary cancer and malignant lymphoma. *Cancer Res.*, **55**, 294–297

Pacifici, G.M. & Rane, A. (1983) Epoxide hydrolase in human fetal liver. *Pharmacology*, **26**, 241–248

Pacifici, G.M., Norlin, A. & Rane, A. (1981) Glutathione S-transferase in human fetal liver. *Biochem. Pharmacol.*, **30**, 3367–3371

Page, T.E., Hoyme, H.E., Markarian, M. & Jones, K.L. (1982) Neonatal haemorrhage secondary to thrombocytopenia: an occasional effect of prenatal hydantoin exposure. *Birth Defect. orig. Art. Ser.*, **18**, 47–50

Pantarotto, C., Arboix, M., Sezzano, P. & Abbruzi, R. (1982) Studies of 5,5-diphenylhydantoin irreversible blinding to rat liver microsomal proteins. *Biochem. Pharmacol.*, **31**, 1501–1507

Parke-Davis (1995) *Phenytoin*, Morris Plains, NJ, USA

Pelkonen, O. & Kärki, N.T. (1975) Epoxidation of xenobiotics in the human fetus and placenta: a possible mechanism of transplacental drug-induced injuries. *Biochem. Pharmacol.*, **24**, 1445–1448

Pendergrass, T.W. & Hanson, J.W. (1976) Fetal hydantoin syndrome and neuroblastoma (Letter to the Editor). *Lancet*, **ii**, 150

Peraino, C., Fry, R.J.M., Staffeldt, E. & Christopher, J.P. (1975) Comparative enhancing effects of phenobarbital, amobarbital, diphenylhydantoin and dichlorodiphenyltrichloroethane on 2-acetylaminofluorene-induced hepatic tumorigenesis in the rat. *Cancer Res.*, **35**, 2884–2890

Philip, J., Holcomb, I.J. & Fusari, S.A. (1984) Phenytoin. In: Florey, K., ed., *Analytical Profiles of Drug Substances*, Vol. 13, New York, Academic Press, pp. 417–445

Phillips, N.K. & Lockard, J.S. (1985) A gestational monkey model: effects of phenytoin versus seizures on neonatal outcome. *Epilepsia*, **26**, 697–703

Phillips, N.K. & Lockard, J.S. (1989) Stiripentol, phenytoin, valproate and pregnancy in monkey (Abstract). *Epilepsia*, **30**, 666

Phillips, N.K. & Lockard, J.S. (1990) Object permanence development in monkey infants prenatally exposed to phenytoin or stiripentol (Abstract). *Epilepsia*, **31**, 600

Phillips, N.K. & Lockard, J.S. (1993) Phenytoin and/or stiripentol in pregnancy: infant monkey hyperexcitability. *Epilepsia*, **34**, 1117–1122

Pizzi, W.J. & Jersey, R.M. (1992) Effects of prenatal diphenylhydantoin treatment on reproductive outcome, development, and behavior in rats. *Neurotoxicol. Teratol.*, **14**, 111–117

Poupaert, J.H., Cavalier, R., Claesen, M.H. & Dumont, P.A. (1975) Absolute configuration of the major metabolite of 5,5-diphenylhydantoin, 5-(4'-hydroxyphenyl)-5-phenylhydantoin. *J. med. Chem.*, **18**, 1268–1271

Ramadevi, G., Das, U.N., Rao, K.P. & Rao, M.S. (1984) Prostaglandins and mutagenesis: modification of phenytoin induced genetic damage by prostaglandins in lymphocyte cultures. *Prostaglandins Leukotrienes Med.*, **15**, 109–113

Ramaniah, T.V., Nandan, S.D., Rao, K.P. & Rao, M.S. (1980) Mutagenicity of phenytoin in the male germ cells of Swiss mice. *IRCS med. Sci.*, **8**, 853

Ramilo, J. & Harris, V.J. (1979) Neuroblastoma in a child with the hydantoin and fetal alcohol syndrome. The radiographic features. *Br. J. Radiol.*, **52**, 993–995

Rane, A. & Peng, D. (1985) Phenytoin enhances epoxide metabolism in human fetal liver culture. *Drug Metab. Dispos.*, **13**, 382–385

Rapport, R.L., II. & Shaw, C.-M. (1977) Phenytoin-related cerebellar degeneration without seizures. *Ann. Neurol.*, **2**, 437–439

Raya, A., Gallego, J., Hermenegildo, C., Puertas, F.J., Romero, F.J., Felipo, V., Miñana, M.D., Grisolía, S. & Romá, J. (1992) Prevention of the acute neurotoxic effects of phenytoin on rat peripheral nerve by H7, an inhibitor of protein kinase C. *Toxicology*, **75**, 249–256

Reynolds, E.H. (1973) Anticonvulsants, folic acid, and epilepsy. *Lancet*, **i**, 1376–1378

Reynolds, J.E.F., ed. (1993) *Martindale: The Extra Pharmacopoeia*, 30th Ed., London, The Pharmaceutical Press, pp. 304–309

Riedel, L. & Obe, G. (1984) Mutagenicity of antiepileptic drugs. II. Phenytoin, primidone and phenobarbital. *Mutat. Res.*, **138**, 71–74

Rijlaarsdam, U., Scheffer, E., Meijer, C.J.L.M., Kruyswijk, M.R.J. & Willemze, R. (1991) Mycosis fungoides-like lesions associated with phenytoin and carbamazepine therapy. *J. Am. Acad. Dermatol.*, **24**, 216–220

Rikihisa, T., Takeda, Y., Nakata, K.-I. & Kanakubo, Y. (1984) Composition of fallen dust in a dispensing room. *Yakuzaigaku*, **44**, 169–174 (in Japanese)

Rollins, D., Larsson, A., Steen, B., Krishnaswamy, K., Hagenfeldt, L., Moldéns, P. & Rane, A. (1981) Glutathione and gamma-glutamyl cycle enzymes in fetal liver. *J. Pharmacol. exp. Ther.*, **217**, 697–700

Rosenthal, C.J., Noguera, C.A., Coppola, A. & Kapelner, S.N. (1982) Pseudolymphoma with mycosis fungoides manifestations, hyperresponsiveness to diphenylhydantoin, and lymphocyte disregulation. *Cancer*, **49**, 2305–2314

Rubinstein, I., Langevitz, P. & Shibi, G. (1985) Isolated malignant lymphoma of the jejunum and long-term diphenylhydantoin therapy. *Oncology*, **42**, 104–106

Saltzstein, S.L. & Ackerman, L.V. (1959) Lymphadenopathy induced by anticonvulsant drugs and mimicking clinically and pathologically malignant lymphomas. *Cancer*, **12**, 164–182

Sanders, B.M. & Draper, G.J. (1979) Childhood cancer and drugs in pregnancy. *Br. med. J.*, **i**, 717–719

Sanyal, S. & Wells, P.G. (1993) Reduction in phenytoin teratogenicity by pretreatment with the antioxidant D-α-tocopherol acetate (vitamin E) in CD-1 mice (Abstract no. 950). *Toxicologist*, **13**, 252

Schardein, J.L., Dresner, A.J., Hentz, D.L., Petrere, J.A., Fitzgerald, J.E. & Kurtz, S.M. (1973) The modifying effect of folinic acid on diphenylhydantoin-induced teratogenicity in mice. *Toxicol. appl. Pharmacol.*, **24**, 150–158

Schaumann, B.A., Johnson, S.B., Wang, N. & Van Brunt, S. (1985) Sister chromatid exchanges in adult epileptic patients on phenytoin therapy. *Environ. Mutag.*, **7**, 711–714

Schaumann, B.A., Winge, V.B. & Garry, V.F. (1989) Lack of sister chromatid exchange induction in phenytoin-treated patients with epilepsy. *Epilepsia*, **30**, 240–245

Schmidt, D., Canger, A., Avanzini, G., Battino, D., Cusi, C., Beck-Mannagetta, G., Koch, S., Rating, D. & Janz, D. (1983) Changes in seizure frequency in pregnant epileptic women. *J. Neurol. Neurosurg. Psychiat.*, **46**, 751–755

Schöder-Van der Elst, J.P. & Van der Heide, D. (1990) Effects of 5,5'-diphenylhydantoin on thyroxine and 3,5,3'-triiodothyronine concentrations in several tissues of the rat. *Endocrinology*, **126**, 186–191

Schreiber, M.M. & McGregor, J.G. (1968) Pseudolymphoma syndrome, a sensitivity to anticonvulsant drugs. *Arch. Dermatol.*, **97**, 297–300

Scolnik, D., Mulman, D., Rovet, J., Gladstone, D., Czuchta, D., Gardner, H.A., Gladstone, R., Ashby, P., Weksberg, R., Einarson, T. & Koren, G. (1994) Neurodevelopment of children exposed *in utero* to phenytoin and carbamazepine monotherapy. *J. Am. med. Assoc.*, **271**, 767–770

Scoville, B. & White, B.G. (1981) Carcinogenicity of hydantoins: history, data, hypotheses, and public policy. In: Dam, M., Gram, L. & Penry, J.K., eds, *Advances in Epileptology: XIIth Epilepsy International Symposium*, New York, Raven Press, pp. 589–596

Selby, J.V., Friedman, G.D. & Fireman, B.H. (1989) Screening prescription drugs for possible carcinogenicity: eleven to fifteen years of follow-up. *Cancer Res.*, **49**, 5736–5747

Seymour, R.A. (1993) Drug-induced gingival overgrowth. *Adverse Drug React. Toxicol. Rev.*, **12**, 215–232

Sezzano, P., Raimondi, A., Arboix, M. & Pantarotto, C. (1982) Mutagenicity of diphenylhydantoin and some of its metabolites towards *Salmonella typhimurium* strains. *Mutat. Res.*, **103**, 219–228

Shapiro, S., Hartz, S.C., Siskind, V., Mitchell, A.A., Slone, D., Rosenberg, L., Monson, R.R., Heinonen, O.P., Idänpään-Heikkilä, J., Härö, S. & Saxén, L. (1976) Anticonvulsants and parental epilepsy in the development of birth defects. *Lancet*, **i**, 272–275

Sharma, R.K., Jacobson-Kram, D., Lemmon, M., Bakke, J,. Galperin, I. & Blazak, W.F. (1985) Sister-chromatic exchange and cell replication kinetics in fetal and maternal cells after treatment with chemical teratogens. *Mutat. Res.*, **158**, 217–231

Shaw, G.M., Lammer, E.J., Wasserman, G.R., O'Malley, C.D. & Tolarevo, M.M. (1995) Risks of orofacial clefts in children born to women using multivitamins containing folic acid periconceptionally. *Lancet*, **345**, 393–396

Sherman, S. & Roizen, N. (1976) Fetal hydantoin syndrome and neuroblastoma. *Lancet*, **ii**, 517

Shoeman, D.W., Kauffman, R.E., Azarnoff, D.L. & Boulos, B.M. (1972) Placental transfer of diphenylhydantoin in the goat. *Biochem. Pharmacol.*, **21**, 1237–1243

Singer, J., Schmid, C., Souhami, R. & Isaacson, P.G. (1993) Bone marrow involvement in phenytoin induced 'pseudolymphoma'. *Clin. Oncol.*, **5**, 397–398

Sinués, B,. Martínez, P., Tamparillas, M. & Bartolomé, M. (1982) Cytogenetic study of the treatment with phenytoin using SCE. *Arch. Farmacol. Toxicol.*, **8**, 165–170 (in Spanish)

Society of Japanese Pharmacopoeia (1992) *The Pharmacopoeia of Japan JP XII*, 12th Ed., Tokyo, pp. 451–453

Sonawane, B.R. & Goldman, A.S. (1981) Susceptibility of mice to phenytoin-induced cleft palate correlated with inhibition of fetal palatal RNA and protein synthesis. *Proc. Soc. exp. biol. Med.*, **168**, 175–179

de Souza Queiroz, M.L. & Mullen, P.W. (1980) The effects of phenytoin, 5-(*para*-hydroxyphenyl)-5-phenylhydantoin and valproic acid on humoral immunity in mice (Abstract no. 31). *Int. J. Immunopharmacol.*, **2**, 224–225

Speidel, B.D. & Meadow, S.R. (1972) Maternal epilepsy and abnormalities of the fetus and newborn. *Lancet*, **ii**, 839–843

Staple, P.H., Reed, M.J. & Mashimo, P.A. (1977) Diphenylhydantoin gingival hyperplasia in *Macaca arctoides*: a new human model. *J. Periodontol.*, **48**, 325–336

Stevens, M.W. & Harbison, R.D. (1974) Placental transfer of diphenylhydantoin: effects of species, gestational age and route of administration. *Teratology*, **9**, 317–326

Strickler, S.M., Dansky, L.V., Miller, M.A., Seni, M.-H., Andermann, E. & Spielberg, S.P. (1985) Genetic predisposition to phenytoin-induced birth defects. *Lancet*, **ii**, 746–749

Sullivan, F.M. & McElhatton, P.R. (1975) Teratogenic activity of the antiepileptic drugs phenobarbital, phenytoin and primidone in mice. *Toxicol. appl. Pharmacol.*, **34**, 271–282

Swanson, B.N., Leger, R.M., Gordon, W.P., Lynn, R.K. & Gerber, N. (1978) Excretion of phenytoin into semen of rabbits and man. Comparison with plasma levels. *Drug. Metab. Dispos.*, **6**, 70–74

Tan, Y.-D., Qiu, X.-F. & Xie, J.-R. (1985) Diphenylhydantoin: clinical investigation and cytogenetic research on mammalian cells *in vitro* (Abstract). *Environ. Mutag.*, **7**, 35

Taneja, N., Jain, S., Maheswari, M.C., Tandon, J.K. & Kucheria, K. (1992) Induction of sister chromatid exchanges in phenytoin treated and untreated patients with epilepsy. *Indian J. med. Res.*, **96**, 302–305

Taneja, N., Kucheria, K., Jain, S. & Maheshwari, M.C. (1994) Effect of phenytoin on semen. *Epilepsia*, **35**, 136–140

Taylor, W.F., Myers, M. & Taylor, W.R. (1980) Extrarenal Wilm's tumour in an infant exposed to intrauterine phenytoin (Letter to the Editor). *Lancet*, **ii**, 481–482

Theodoropoulos, T.J., Pappolla, M.A., Goussis, O.S., Zolman, J.C. & Benson, D.M. (1990) Permanent alterations in the hypothalamic-pituitary-thyroid axis in the rat following phenytoin exposure in utero. *Horm. Metab. Res.*, **22**, 521–523

Thomas, J., ed. (1991) *Prescription Products Guide 1991*, 20th Ed., Victoria, Australian Pharmaceutical Publishing Co., pp. 652–653

Thomason, J.M., Seymour, R.A. & Rawlins, M.D. (1992) Incidence and severity of phenytoin-induced gingival overgrowth in epileptic patients in general medical practice. *Community Dent. oral Epidemiol.*, **20**, 288–291

Tomson, T., Lindbom, U., Ekqvist, B. & Sundqvist, A. (1994) Disposition of carbamazepine and phenytoin in pregnancy. *Epilepsia*, **35**, 131–135

Toone, B.K., Wheeler, M., Nanjee, M., Fenwick, P. & Grant, P. (1983) Sex hormones, sexual activity and plasma anticonvulsant levels in male epileptics. *J. Neurol. Neurosurg. Psychiat.*, **46**, 824–826

Treiman, D.M. & Woodbury, D.M. (1995) Phenytoin: absorption, distribution, and excretion. In: Levy, R.H., Mattson, R.H. & Meldrum, B.S., eds, *Antiepileptic Drugs*, 4th Ed., New York, Raven Press, pp. 301–314

United States National Library of Medicine (1996) *RTECS Database*, Bethesda, MD

United States National Toxicology Program (1993) *Toxicology and Carcinogenesis Studies of 5,5-Diphenylhydantoin (Phenytoin) (CAS No. 57-41-0) in F344/N Rats and B6C3F1 Mice (Feed Studies)* (Technical Report Series 404; NIH Publication no. 94-2859), Research Triangle Park, NC

United States Pharmacopeial Convention (1994) *The 1995 US Pharmacopeia*, 23rd Rev./*The National Formulary*, 18th Rev., Rockville, MD, pp. 1216–1221

United States Tariff Commission (1939) *Synthetic Organic Chemicals, US Production and Sales, 1938*, Report No. 136, Second Series, Washington DC, US Government Printing Office, p. 103

United States Tariff Commission (1948) *Synthetic Organic Chemicals, US Production and Sales, 1946*, Report No. 159, Second Series, Washington DC, US Government Printing Office, p. 103

Van Dyke, D.C., Berg, M.J. & Olson, C.H. (1991) Differences in phenytoin biotransformation and susceptibility to congenital malformations: a review. *Drug Intell. clin. Pharm.*, **25**, 987–992

Veronese, M.E., Doecke, C.J., Mackenzie, P.I., McManus, M.E., Miners, J.O., Rees, D.L.P., Gasser, R., Meyer, U.A. & Birkett, D.J. (1993) Site-directed mutation studies of human liver cytochrome *P*-450 isoenzymes in the CYP2C subfamily. *Biochem. J.*, **289**, 533–538

Vidal (1995) *Dictionnaire Vidal*, 71st Ed., Paris, Editions du Vidal, pp. 449–450, 1247

Vorhees, C.V. (1983) Fetal anticonvulsant syndrome in rats: dose- and period-response relationships of prenatal diphenylhydantoin, trimethadione and phenobarbital exposure on the structural and functional development of the offspring. *J. Pharmacol. exp. Ther.*, **227**, 274–287

Vorhees, C.V. (1987a) Fetal hydantoin syndrome in rats: dose-effect relationship of prenatal phenytoin on postnatal development and behavior. *Teratology*, **35**, 287–303

Vorhees, C.V. (1987b) Maze learning in rats: a comparison of performance in two water mazes in progeny prenatally exposed to different doses of phenytoin. *Neurotoxicol. Teratol.*, **9**, 235–241

Vorhees, C.V. & Minck, D.R. (1989) Long-term effects of prenatal phenytoin exposure on offspring behavior in rats. *Neurotoxicol. Teratol.*, **11**, 295–305

Vorhees, C.V., Weisenburger, W.P. & Minck, D.R. (1989) An analysis of factors influencing water maze learning in rats: effects of escape assistance, task complexity, and path order using prenatal exposure to phenytoin as a positive control (Abstract no. BTS41). *Teratology*, **39**, 513

Waddell, W.J. & Mirkin, B.L. (1972) Distribution and metabolism of diphenylhydantoin-^{14}C in fetal and maternal tissues of the pregnant mouse. *Biochem. Pharmacol.*, **21**, 547–552

Watson, J.D. & Spellacy, W.N. (1971) Neonatal effects of maternal treatment with the anticonvulsant drug diphenylhydantoin. *Obstet. Gynec.*, **37**, 881–885

Wells, P.G. & Vo, H.P.N. (1989) Effect of the tumor promoter 12-*O*-tetradecanoylphorbol-13 acetate on phenytoin-induced embryopathy in mice. *Toxicol. appl. Pharmacol.*, **97**, 398–405

Wells, P.G., Zubovits, J.T., Wong, S.T., Molinari, L.M. & Ali, S. (1989) Modulation of phenytoin teratogenicity and embryonic covalent binding by acetylsalicylic acid, caffeic acid, and α-phenyl-*N*-t-butylnitrone: implications for bioactivation by prostaglandin synthetase. *Toxicol. appl. Pharmacol.*, **97**, 192–202

Welsch, F. & Stedman, D.D. (1984) Inhibition of metabolic cooperation between Chinese hamster V79 cells by structurally diverse teratogens. *Teratog. Carcinog. Mutag.*, **4**, 285–301

Willington, S.E., Zajac, W., McGregor, D.B. & Combes, R.D. (1989) Methods and criteria for assessing the V79 metabolic cooperation assay (Abstract no. 36). *Mutat. Res.*, **216**, 283

Wilson, J.G. (1974) Teratologic causation in man and its evaluation in non-human primates. In: Motulsky, A.G., Lenz, W. & Ebling, F.J.G., eds, *Birth Defects*, Amsterdam, Excerpta Medica, pp. 191–203

Wong, M., Helston, L.M.J. & Wells, P.G. (1989) Enhancement of murine phenytoin teratogenicity by the gamma-glutamylcysteine synthetase inhibitor L-buthionine-(S,R)-sulfoximine and by the glutathione depletor diethyl maleate. *Teratology*, **40**, 127–141

Woodruff, R.C., Mason, J.M., Valencia, R. & Zimmering, S. (1985) Chemical mutagenesis testing in *Drosophila*. V. Results of 53 coded compounds tested for the National Toxicology Program. *Environ. Mutag.*, **7**, 677–702

Yaari, Y. & Devor, M. (1985) Phenytoin suppresses spontaneous ectopic discharge in rat sciatic nerve neuromas. *Neurosci. Lett.*, **58**, 117–122

Yeo, P.P.B., Bates, D., Howe, J.G., Ratcliffe, W.A., Schardt, C.W., Heath, A. & Evered, D.C. (1978) Anticonvulsants and thyroid function. *Br. med. J.*, **i**, 1581–1583

Yerby, M.S. (1991) Pregnancy and epilepsy. *Epilepsia*, **32** (Suppl. 6), S51–S59

Zengel, A.E., Keith, D.A. & Tassinari, M.S. (1989) Prenatal exposure to phenytoin and its effect on postnatal growth and craniofacial proportion in the rat. *J. craniofac. Genet. dev. Biol.*, **9**, 147–160

Zhu, M.-X. & Zhou, S.-S. (1989) Reduction of the teratogenic effects of phenytoin by folic acid and a mixture of folic acid, vitamins, and amino acids: a preliminary trial. *Epilepsia*, **30**, 246–251

ANTI-OESTROGENIC COMPOUNDS

DROLOXIFENE

1. Exposure Data

1.1 Chemical and physical data

1.1.1 *Nomenclature*

Droloxifene

Chem. Abstr. Serv. Reg. No.: 82413-20-5

Chem. Abstr. Name: (*E*)-3-(1-(4-(2-(Dimethylamino)ethoxy)phenyl)-2-phenyl-1-butenyl)phenol

IUPAC Systematic Name: (*E*)-α-[*para*-[2-(Dimethylamino)ethoxy]phenyl]-α′-ethyl-3-stilbenol

Synonyms: (*E*)-1-(4′-(2-Dimethylaminoethoxy)phenyl)-1-(3-hydroxyphenyl)-2-phenylbut-1-ene; *trans*-1-(4-β-dimethylaminoethoxyphenyl)-1-(3-hydroxyphenyl)-2-phenylbut-1-ene; 3-hydroxytamoxifen

Droloxifene citrate

Chem. Abstr. Serv. Reg. No.: 97752-20-0

Chem. Abstr. Name: (*E*)-3-(1-(4-(2-(Dimethylamino)ethoxy)phenyl)-2-phenyl-1-butenyl)phenol, 2-hydroxy-1,2,3-propanetricarboxylate (1:1)

IUPAC Systematic Name: (*E*)-α-[*para*-[2-(Dimethylamino)ethoxy]phenyl]-α′-ethyl-3-stilbenol citrate

Synonyms: (*E*)-1-(4′-(2-Dimethylaminoethoxy)phenyl)-1-(3-hydroxyphenyl)-2-phenylbut-1-ene citrate; *trans*-1-(4-β-dimethylaminoethoxyphenyl)-1-(3-hydroxyphenyl)-2-phenylbut-1-ene citrate; 3-hydroxytamoxifen citrate

1.1.2 *Structural and molecular formulae and relative molecular mass*

Droloxifene

$C_{26}H_{29}NO_2$ Relative molecular mass: 387.52

Droloxifene citrate

$C_{26}H_{29}NO_2 \cdot C_6H_8O_7$ Relative molecular mass: 579.65

1.1.3 *Chemical and physical properties of the pure substances*

From Budavari (1995); Pfizer (1996)

Droloxifene

(a) *Description*: Colourless crystals

(b) *Melting-point*: 160–163 °C

Droloxifene citrate

(a) *Description*: Off-white, crystalline powder

(b) *Melting-point*: 142 °C

(c) *Solubility*: Slightly soluble in water (0.078 mg/mL (unbuffered, pH 3.4)); soluble in methanol; sparingly soluble in ethanol; insoluble in chloroform

(d) *Stability*: Stable in aqueous solutions at pHs 3–7 at temperatures up to 50 °C

1.1.4 *Technical products and impurities*

In its pharmaceutical preparations, droloxifene is normally formulated as the citrate salt.

Trade names and designations of droloxifene citrate and its pharmaceutical preparation include: *E*-Droloxifene; FK 435; K 060; K 060E; K 21.060E.

1.1.5 *Analysis*

Droloxifene and its metabolites can be analysed in biological fluids by high-performance liquid chromatography (Lien *et al.*, 1995).

1.2 Production and use

1.2.1 *Production*

Droloxifene can be prepared by the reaction of 3-(tetrahydropyran-2-yloxy)phenyl bromide with magnesium or *n*-butyllithium followed by addition of the resulting reagent to 1-[4-[2-(dimethylamino)ethoxy]phenyl]-2-phenylbutan-1-one. Acid-catalysed dehydration of the resulting tertiary alcohol gives a mixture of droloxifene and its Z-isomer, which can be separated by chromatography and recrystallization (Ruenitz et al., 1982; Foster et al., 1985).

1.2.2 Use

Droloxifene (a phenolic analogue of tamoxifen) is a new non-steroidal antioestrogenic drug which has a high affinity for oestrogen receptors (see Glossary, p. 448) (Roos et al., 1983), a low oestrogenic to antioestrogenic activity ratio (Löser et al., 1985) and rapid pharmacokinetics (Grill & Pollow, 1991).

Phase I and II trials (see Glossary, p. 449) of droloxifene in postmenopausal women with metastatic breast cancer in various countries (Breitbach et al., 1987; Stamm et al., 1987) have shown that the drug has very little short-term toxicity (Bellmunt & Solé, 1991; Deschênes 1991; Miller et al., 1991; Bruning, 1992; Haarstad et al., 1992; Rauschning & Pritchard, 1994). Response (see Glossary, p. 449) rates and durations are similar, within the limits of cross-study comparison, to those seen with tamoxifen. Doses of up to 300 mg daily seem to be well tolerated (Buzdar et al., 1993). A large multicentre phase III trial (see Glossary, p. 449) comparing droloxifene (40 mg) with tamoxifen (20 mg) is in progress in Europe, North and South America, South Africa and India (Pfizer, 1996). Droloxifene has not yet been tested for use in adjuvant therapy.

1.3 Occurrence

Droloxifene is not known to occur as a natural product.

1.4 Regulations and guidelines

Droloxifene is not registered for use as a pharmaceutical in any country (Pfizer, 1996).

2. Studies of Cancer in Humans

No report of carcinogenicity or preventive activity of droloxifene in humans has been published.

3. Studies of Cancer in Experimental Animals

3.1 Oral administration

Rat: In a study that also included tamoxifen, groups of 49–50 male and 50 female Sprague-Dawley rats, 4–5 weeks old, after 13 weeks of adaptation, were given 0 (control), 4, 12, 36 or 90 mg/kg bw droloxifene citrate (> 99.1% pure) by gastric instillation daily for 24 months. No increase in the incidence of liver tumours was reported (Dahme & Rattel, 1994; Hasmann et al., 1994). [The Working Group noted the inadequate information on dose selection and inadequate reporting.]

3.2 Administration with known carcinogens

3.2.1 Mouse

Groups of five or six male and female BALB/c/Bln mice, 8–12 weeks of age, were given intraperitoneal injections of diluted serum from leukaemic mice infected with the Rauscher murine leukaemia virus. Starting one day later, mice were given intraperitoneal injections of 0.5, 1.0 or 2 mg per animal droloxifene citrate [purity not specified] in dimethyl sulfoxide three times a week for 1–2 weeks. The mice were killed when moribund and spleens were weighed as an index of leukaemic disease. Compared to the controls, the spleen weights of the droloxifene-treated animals were about 70%, 60% and 45% in the low-, mid- and high-dose groups, respectively (Sydow & Wunderlich, 1994).

3.2.2 Rat

Three groups of 10 female Sprague-Dawley rats, seven weeks of age, were given 20 mg per animal 7,12-dimethylbenz[a]anthracene in sesame oil orally; starting one day later, two of the groups were given 1.0 or 10.0 mg/kg bw droloxifene citrate [purity not specified] in methylcellulose orally for seven days, while the third group received no further treatment. At 20 weeks, mammary tumours were found in 8/9 controls, 7/9 low-dose droloxifene citrate-treated rats and 3/10 ($p < 0.05$) high-dose droloxifene citrate-treated rats (Kawamura et al., 1991).

Two groups of 21 and 20 female Sprague-Dawley rats, 50 days of age, were given 50 mg/kg bw N-methyl-N-nitrosourea as a single intravenous injection. When at least one mammary tumour reached a diameter of 10 mm, the animals were given 6 or 12 mg/kg bw droloxifene citrate [purity not specified] in Tween 80/distilled water by gastric instillation on five and three days a week, respectively, for four weeks. A control group of 50 female rats received N-methyl-N-nitrosourea alone. At 207 days, the multiplicity of mammary tumours was 1.1 in controls, 1.1 in low-dose droloxifene citrate-treated rats and 1.4 in high-dose droloxifene citrate-treated rats (Winterfeld et al., 1992).

4. Other Data Relevant to an Evaluation of Carcinogenicity and its Mechanisms

4.1 Absorption, distribution, metabolism and excretion

4.1.1 Humans

Droloxifene is rapidly and completely absorbed from the intestinal tract. Results from a phase II clinical trial (Kvinnsland, 1991) in postmenopausal women with metastatic breast cancer treated with droloxifene at 20 mg (34 patients), 40 mg (43 patients) or 100 mg (71 patients) once daily for up to one year showed that, with the 20-mg dose, peak plasma concentrations were reached after 2–4 h and the terminal half-life was 24 h. The mean plasma levels at steady-state concentration were about 15, 30 and 80 ng/mL with the 20-, 40- and 100-mg doses, respectively. These results are consistent with the plasma levels of 81 ng/mL droloxifene, 1 ng/mL 4-methoxydroloxifene and 6 ng/mL N-desmethyldroloxifene measured in a breast cancer patient following a single oral dose of 100 mg droloxifene (Lien *et al.*, 1995).

In humans, droloxifene is rapidly metabolized to droloxifene glucuronide, N-desmethyldroloxifene and 4-methoxydroloxifene (Löser *et al.*, 1989; Hasmann *et al.*, 1994) (see Figure 1). Consequently, accumulation of droloxifene or its metabolites, if it occurs, is slight.

4.1.2 *Experimental systems*

In rats and mice, droloxifene is metabolized to droloxifene glucuronide, N-desmethyldroloxifene, 4-methoxydroloxifene, 3-methoxy-4-hydroxytamoxifen (4-hydroxydroloxifene) and droloxifene N-oxide. The proportion of 3-methoxy-4-hydroxytamoxifen formed is much higher in mice (> 40%) than in rats (< 20%) (Hasmann *et al.*, 1994).

White *et al.* (1993) showed that droloxifene (0.12 mmol/kg bw per day for four days) administered by gastric instillation to rats had little or no effect on the metabolism of ethoxy-, benzyloxy- or pentoxyresorufin.

4.2 Toxic effects

4.2.1 *Humans*

Results from the phase II clinical trial described in Section 4.1.1 showed dose-related decreases in luteinizing hormone and follicle-stimulating hormone levels. A rise in sex hormone-binding globulin level was found (particularly at doses of 40 and 100 mg). These changes were all observed during the first three months of therapy (Kvinnsland, 1991). When droloxifene was administered to 369 postmenopausal women with advanced breast cancer in a dose-finding phase II trial at levels of 20, 40 or 100 mg/day, common side-effects included hot flushes (32%, 32%, 29%), lassitude (28%, 23%, 26%) and nausea (22%, 24%, 29%) in the 20-mg, 40-mg and 100-mg dose groups, respectively. In 1200 patients who received 20, 40, 100 or more than 100 mg doses, signs of serious toxicity were infrequent, but pulmonary embolism in two patients and superficial venous thrombosis of the leg in one patient receiving 20 mg-doses were observed. In patients receiving 100-mg doses, these effects were observed in four and eight patients, respectively, and among those receiving more than 100 mg, they were each observed in one patient (Rauschning & Pritchard, 1994).

4.2.2 *Experimental systems*

Groups of 25 male or 25 female rats were given 1, 10 or 100 mg/kg bw droloxifene orally for four weeks. Droloxifene was tolerated at all doses, with no sign of systemic toxicity. A substance-related increase in the weight of the male and female sexual organs was found; this and histological changes in these organs can be explained by the antioestrogenic effect of droloxifene (Löser *et al.*, 1986).

Figure 1. Postulated metabolic pathways of droloxifene

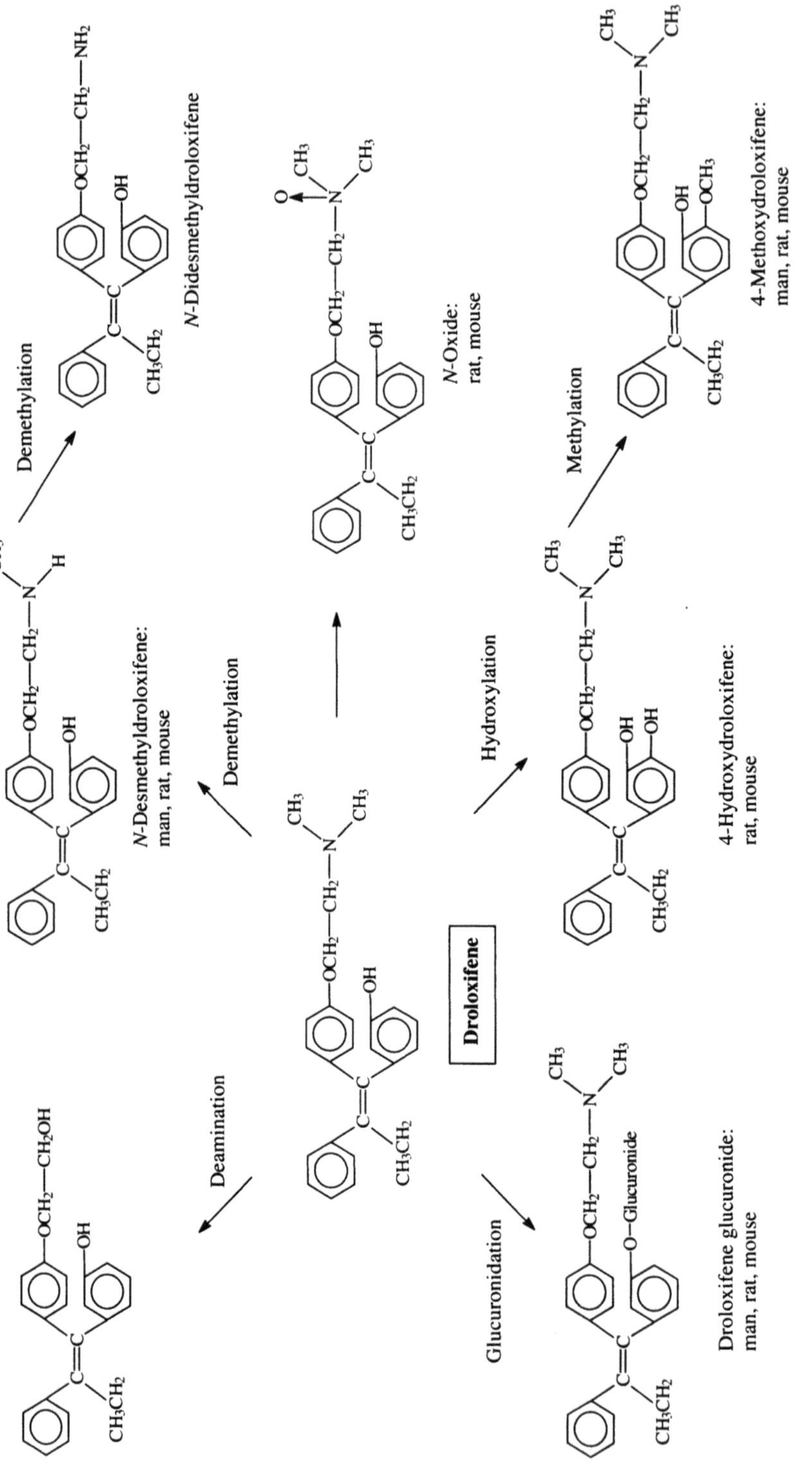

From Grill and Pollow (1991)

Groups of 25 male and 25 female Sprague-Dawley rats, four to five weeks old, after 13 weeks of adaptation, were given 0, 2, 20 or 200 mg/kg bw droloxifene citrate (purity, > 99.1%) per day by gastric instillation in 0.25% agar suspension (volume 10 mg/mL) for six months [body weights, survival not reported.] Six weeks after the end of the treatment period, animals were killed and complete necropsy and histology were carried out but only liver histology was reported. No preneoplastic or neoplastic liver change was found at either dose level (Dahme & Rattel, 1994).

Droloxifene and its major metabolite, N-desmethyldroloxifene, exhibit high binding affinity to the oestrogen receptor in the oestrogen receptor-positive human breast cancer cell line MCF-7. The affinity of droloxifene for the oestrogen receptor was more than 60-fold higher than that of tamoxifen and the IC_{50} value of droloxifene for displacement of 17β-oestradiol from the receptor was approximately 1×10^{-8} M (maximal blood concentration, $1-4 \times 10^{-7}$ M) (Hasmann et al., 1994).

Droloxifene inhibits lipid peroxidation in microsomal and liposomal membranes, but to a lower extent than 17β-oestradiol. The inhibition of lipid peroxidation by droloxifene may result from membrane stabilization that could be associated in cancer cells with decreased membrane fluidity, that might antagonize cell division (Wiseman et al., 1992).

Other effects of droloxifene in rats include prevention of increased bone turnover and bone loss and reduced total serum cholesterol (Chen et al., 1995a,b; Ke et al., 1995a,b).

4.3 Reproductive and developmental effects

No data were available to the Working Group.

4.4 Genetic and related effects (see also Table 1 for references and Appendices 1 and 2)

Droloxifene did not cause significant morphological transformation of Syrian hamster embryo cells.

DNA adducts were not detected by ^{32}P-postlabelling in the livers of female Fischer 344 rats given 0.12 mmol/kg bw droloxifene per day by gastric instillation for four days (White et al., 1992).

5. Summary of Data Reported and Evaluation

5.1 Exposure data

Droloxifene is a phenolic analogue of tamoxifen which is undergoing clinical trials for the treatment of metastatic breast cancer, but is not yet registered in any country.

5.2 Human carcinogenicity data

No data were available to the Working Group.

Table 1. Genetic and related effects of droloxifene

Test system	Result[a]		Dose[b] (LED/HID)	Reference
	Without exogenous metabolic system	With exogenous metabolic system		
TCS, Cell transformation, Syrian hamster embryo cells, clonal assay	–	NT	3.9	Metzler & Schiffmann (1991)
BVD, Binding (covalent) to DNA, Fischer 344/N rat liver in vivo (^{32}P-postlabelling)	–		47 po × 4	White et al. (1992)

[a] +, positive; (+), weak positive; –, negative; NT, not tested; ?, inconclusive

[b] LED, lowest effective dose; HID, highest ineffective dose; in-vitro tests, μg/mL; in-vivo tests, mg/kg bw/day

5.3 Animal carcinogenicity data

Droloxifene was tested for carcinogenicity by oral administration in one study in rats. No increase in the incidence of tumours was reported.

Droloxifene was studied in two experiments in rats for its modulation of chemically induced mammary tumours. In one study with 7,12-dimethylbenz[a]anthracene, inhibition of mammary tumours was observed, while in another study with N-methyl-N-nitrosourea, there was no effect or a slight increase in the incidence of mammary tumours.

5.4 Other relevant data

Droloxifene is well absorbed in humans after oral doses. It undergoes both oxidative metabolism and direct glucuronidation, and the elimination half-life is about 24 h. Metabolites were identified in rats and mice that were not found in humans.

Toxic effects were infrequent in a phase II trial in postmenopausal women with metastatic breast cancer. Short- (four weeks) and longer- (six months) term toxicity studies in rats at doses of up to 200 mg/kg bw showed biochemical changes but little toxicity.

Droloxifene did not induce cell transformation *in vitro* or form DNA adducts in rat liver *in vivo*.

5.5 Evaluation[1]

There is *inadequate evidence* in humans for the carcinogenicity of droloxifene.

There is *inadequate evidence* in experimental animals for the carcinogenicity of droloxifene.

Overall evaluation

Droloxifene is *not classifiable as to its carcinogenicity to humans (Group 3)*.

6. References

Bellmunt, J. & Solé, L. (1991) European early phase II dose-finding study of droloxifene in advanced breast cancer. *Am. J. clin. Oncol. Cancer clin. Trials,* **14** (Suppl. 2), S36–S39

Breitbach, G.P., Moous, V., Bastert, G., Kreienberg, R., Muset, M.J. & Staab, H.J. (1987) Droloxifene: efficacy and endocrine effects in treatment of metastatic breast cancer. *J. Steroid Biochem.*, **28** (Suppl.), 1095

Bruning, P.F. (1992) Droloxifene, a new anti-oestrogen in postmenopausal advanced breast cancer: preliminary results of a double-blind dose-finding phase II trial. *Eur. J. Cancer*, **28A**, 1404–1407

Budavari, S., ed. (1995) *The Merck Index*, 12th Ed., Rahway, NJ, Merck & Co.

Buzdar, A.U., Kau, S., Hortobagyi, G.N., Theriault, R.L., Booser, D., Holmes, F.A., Walters, R. & Krakoff, I.H. (1993) Phase I trial of droloxifene in patients with metastatic breast cancer. *Cancer Chemother. Pharmacol.*, **33**, 313–316

Chen, H.K., Ke, H.Z., Jee, W.S.S., Ma, Y.F., Pirie, C.M., Simmons, H.A. & Thompson, D.D. (1995a) Droloxifene prevents ovariectomy-induced bone loss in tibiae and femora of aged female rats: a dual energy X-ray absorptiometric and histomorphometric study. *J. Bone miner. Res.*, **10**, 1256–1262

Chen, H.K., Ke, H.Z., Lin, C.H., Ma, Y.F., Qi, H., Crawford, D.T., Pirie, C.M., Simmons, H.A., Jee, W.S.S. & Thompson, D.D. (1995b) Droloxifene inhibits cortical bone turnover associated with estrogen deficiency in rats. *Bone*, **17**, 175S–179S

Dahme, E. & Rattel, B. (1994) Droloxifene induces, in contrast to tamoxifen, no liver tumour in the rat. *Onkologie*, **17** (Suppl. 1), 6–16 (in German)

Deschênes, L. (1991) Droloxifene, a new antiestrogen, in advanced breast cancer. A double-blind dose-finding study. *Am. J. clin. Oncol. Cancer clin. Trials*, **14** (Suppl. 2), S52–S55

Foster, A.B., Jarman, M., Leung, O.-T., McCague, R., Leclercq, G. & Devleeschouwer, N. (1985) Hydroxy derivatives of tamoxifen. *J. med. Chem.*, **28**, 1491–1497

Grill, H.J. & Pollow, K. (1991) Pharmacokinetics of droloxifene and its metabolites in breast cancer patients. *Am. J. clin. Oncol. Cancer clin. Trials*, **14** (Suppl. 2), S21–S29

---

[1]For definition of the italicized terms, see Preamble, pp. 22–25.

Haarstad, H., Gundersen, S., Wist, E., Raabe, N., Mella, O. & Kvinnsland, S. (1992) Droloxifene — a new anti-estrogen. A phase II study in advanced breast cancer. *Acta oncol.*, **31**, 425–428

Hasmann, M., Rattel, B. & Löser, R. (1994) Preclinical data for droloxifene. *Cancer Lett.*, **84**, 101–116

Kawamura, I., Mizota, T., Kondo, N., Shimomura, K. & Kohsaka, M. (1991) Antitumor effects of droloxifene, a new antiestrogen drug, against 7,12-dimethylbenz(*a*)anthracene-induced mammary tumors in rats. *Jpn. J. Pharmacol.*, **57**, 215–224

Ke, H.Z., Chen, H.K., Qi, H., Pirie, C.M., Simmons, H.A., Ma, Y.F., Jee, W.S.S. & Thompson, D.D. (1995a) Effects of droloxifene on prevention of cancellous bone loss and bone turnover in the axial skeleton of aged, ovariectomized rats. *Bone*, **17**, 491–496

Ke, H.Z., Simmons, H.A., Pirie, C.M., Crawford, D.T. & Thompson, D.D. (1995b) Droloxifene, a new estrogen antagonist/agonist prevents bone loss in ovariectomised rats. *Endocrinology*, **136**, 2435–2441

Kvinnsland, S. (1991) Droloxifen, a new antioestrogen. Hormonal influences in postmenopausal breast cancer patients. *Am. J. clin. Oncol. Cancer clin. Trials*, **14** (Suppl. 2), S46–S51

Lien, E.A., Anker, G., Lønning, P.E. & Ueland, P.M. (1995) Determination of droloxifene and two metabolites in serum by high-pressure liquid chromatography. *Therap. Drug Monit.*, **17**, 259–265

Löser, R., Seibel, K., Roos, W. & Eppenberger, U. (1985) In vivo and in vitro antiestrogenic action of 3-hydroxytamoxifen, tamoxifen and 4-hydroxytamoxifen. *Eur. J. Cancer clin. Oncol.*, **21**, 985–990

Löser, R., Seibel, K., Liehn, H.D. & Staub, H.-J. (1986) Pharmacology and toxicology of the antiestrogen droloxifene. *Contr. Oncol.*, **23**, 64–72

Löser, R., Hasmann, M., Seibel, K., Jank, P. & Eppenberger, U (1989) Pharmacological activity of the metabolites of the antiestrogen droloxifene (Abstract no. 89). *Breast Cancer Res. Treat.*, **14**, 155

Metzler, M. & Schiffmann, D. (1991) Structural requirements for the in vitro transformation of Syrian hamster embryo cells by stilbene estrogens and triphenylethylene-type antiestrogens. *Am. J. clin. Oncol. Cancer clin. Trials*, **14** (Suppl. 2), S30–S35

Miller, A.B., Hoogstraten, B., Staquet, M. & Winkler, A. (1981) Reporting results of cancer treatment. *Cancer*, **47**, 207–214

Pfizer (1996) *Droloxifene*, Groton, CT, United States

Rauschning, W. & Pritchard, K.I. (1994) Droloxifene: a new antiestrogen: its role in metastatic breast cancer. *Breast Cancer Res. Treat.*, **31**, 83–94

Roos, W., Oeze, L., Löser, R. & Eppenberger, U. (1983) Antiestrogenic action of 3-hydroxytamoxifen in the human breast cancer cell line MCF-7. *J. natl Cancer Inst.*, **71**, 55–59

Ruenitz, P.C., Bagley, J.R. & Mokler, C.M. (1982) Estrogenic and antiestrogenic activitiy of monophenolic analogues of tamoxifen, (Z)-2-[*p*-(1,2-diphenyl-1-butenyl)phenoxy]-*N*,*N*-dimethylethylamine. *J. med. Chem.*, **25**, 1056–1060

Stamm, H., Roth, R., Almendral, A. Staab, H.J. & Heil, M. (1987) Tolerance and efficacy of the antiestrogen droloxifene in patients with advanced breast cancer. *J. Steroid Biochem.*, **28** (Suppl.), 1085

Sydow, G. & Wunderlich, V. (1994) Effects of tamoxifen, droloxifene and 17β-estradiol on Rauscher mouse leukemogenesis. *Cancer Lett.*, **82**, 89–94

White, I.N.H., de Matteis, F., Davies, A., Smith, L.L., Crofton-Sleigh, C., Venitt, S., Hewer, A. & Phillips, D.H. (1992) Genotoxic potential of tamoxifen and analogues in female Fischer F344/n rats, DBA/2 and C57Bl/6 mice and in human MCL-5 cells. *Carcinogenesis*, **13**, 2197–2203

White, I.N.H., Davies, A., Smith, L.L., Dawson, S. & de Matteis, F. (1993) Induction of CYP2B1 and 3A1, and associated monooxygenase activities by tamoxifen and certain analogues in the livers of female rats and mice. *Biochem. Pharmacol.*, **45**, 21–30

Winterfield, G., Hauff, P., Görlich, M., Arnold, W., Fichtner, I. & Staab, H.J. (1992) Investigations of droloxifene and other hormone manipulations on *N*-nitrosomethylurea-induced rat mammary tumours. 1. Influence on tumour growth. *J. Cancer Res. clin. Oncol.*, **119**, 91–96

Wiseman, H., Smith, C., Halliwell, B., Cannon, M., Arnstein, M.R.V. & Lennard, M.S. (1992) Droloxifene (3-hydroxytamoxifen) has membrane antioxidant ability: potential relevance to its mechanism of therapeutic action in breast cancer. *Cancer Lett.*, **66**, 61–68

TAMOXIFEN

1. Exposure Data

1.1 Chemical and physical data

1.1.1 *Nomenclature*

Tamoxifen

Chem. Abstr. Serv. Reg. No.: 10540-29-1

Chem. Abstr. Name: (Z)-2-[4-(1,2-Diphenyl-1-butenyl)phenoxy]-*N,N*-dimethylethanamine

IUPAC Systematic Name: (Z)-2-[*para*-(1,2-Diphenyl-1-butenyl)phenoxy]-*N,N*-dimethylethylamine

Synonyms: 1-*para*-β-Dimethylaminoethoxyphenyl-*trans*-1,2-diphenylbut-1-ene; (Z)-2-[4-(1,2-diphenylbut-1-enyl)phenoxy]ethyldimethylamine

Tamoxifen citrate

Chem. Abstr. Serv. Reg. No.: 54965-24-1

Chem. Abstr. Name: (Z)-2-[4-(1,2-Diphenyl-1-butenyl)phenoxy]-*N,N*-dimethylethanamine, 2-hydroxy-1,2,3-propanetricarboxylate (1:1)

IUPAC Systematic Name: (Z)-2-[*para*-(1,2-Diphenyl-1-butenyl)phenoxy]-*N,N*-dimethylethylamine citrate (1:1)

Synonyms: Tamoxifen citrate; Z-tamoxifen citrate

1.1.2 *Structural and molecular formulae and relative molecular mass*

$C_{26}H_{29}NO$ Relative molecular mass: 371.52

$C_{26}H_{29}NO.C_6H_8O_7$ Relative molecular mass: 563.65

1.1.3 *Chemical and physical properties of the pure substances*

From Budavari (1995), unless otherwise specified

Tamoxifen

(a) *Description*: White crystals

(b) *Melting-point*: 96–98 °C

Tamoxifen citrate

(a) *Description*: Fine, white, odourless crystalline powder

(b) *Melting-point*: 140–142 °C

(c) *Spectroscopy data*: Infrared spectral data have been reported (British Pharmacopoeial Commission, 1993).

(d) *Solubility*: Slightly soluble in water; soluble in acetone, ethanol and methanol

(e) *Stability*: Hygroscopic at high relative humidities; sensitive to ultraviolet light

(f) *Dissociation constant*: $pK_a = 8.85$ (Medical Economics, 1996)

1.1.4 *Technical products and impurities*

Tamoxifen in pharmaceutical formulations is invariably present as its citrate salt. Tamoxifen citrate is available as 15.2-, 30.4- and 45.6-mg (equivalent to 10, 20 and 30 mg tamoxifen base) tablets which also may contain carboxymethylcellulose calcium, croscarmellose sodium (type A) [a polymer of carboxymethylcellulose sodium], gelatin, hydroxypropyl methylcellulose 2.910, lactose, Macrogel 300, magnesium stearate, mannitol, polyvinylpyrrolidone (povidone), sodium carboxymethylstarch, corn starch or titanium oxide (Thomas, 1991; Farmindustria, 1993; Reynolds, 1993; British Medical Association/Royal Pharmaceutical Society of Great Britain, 1994; Medical Economics, 1996).

The impurities limited by the requirements of the European Pharmacopoeia include: (*E*)-2-[4-(1,2-diphenylbut-1-enyl)phenoxy]ethyldimethylamine (the *E*-isomer of tamoxifen); 2-[4-(1-hydroxy-1,2-diphenylbutyl)phenoxy]ethyldimethylamine; 2-[4-(1,2-diphenylvinyl)phenoxy]ethyldimethylamine; 2-[4-(1,2-diphenylprop-1-enyl)phenoxy]dimethylamine; 2-[2-(1,2-diphenylbut-1-enyl)phenoxy]ethyldimethylamine; (*Z*)-2-[4-(1,2-diphenylbut-1-enyl)phenoxy]ethylmethylamine; and 1-(4-dimethylaminoethoxyphenyl)-2-phenylbutan-1-one (Council of Europe, 1995). The United States of America and

British pharmacopoeias limit the *E*-isomer content to not more than 0.3% and 1%, respectively (British Pharmacopoeial Commission, 1993; United States Pharmacopeial Convention, 1994).

Trade names and designations for tamoxifen citrate and its pharmaceutical preparations include: Apo-Tamox; Citofen; Dignotamoxi; Duratamoxifen 5; Emblon; ICI-46 474; Jenoxifen; Kessar; Ledertam; Noltam; Nolvadex; Nourytam; Novofen; Oestrifen; Oncotam; Retaxim; Tafoxen; Tam; Tamaxin; Tamifen; Tamofen; Tamone; Tamoplex; Tamoxasta; Tamox-Gry; Tamoxigenat; Tamox-Puren; Taxfeno; Terimon; Valodex; Zemide; Zitazonium.

1.1.5 *Analysis*

Several international pharmacopoeias specify potentiometric titration with perchloric acid as the assay for purity of tamoxifen citrate, and liquid chromatography (LC) or gas chromatography with flame ionization detection for determining levels of the *E*-isomer and other impurities and decomposition products. The assays specified for tamoxifen citrate in tablets use LC and ultraviolet/visible absorption spectroscopy with standards. An assay for heavy metal impurities is also specified (British Pharmacopoeial Commission, 1993; United States Pharmacopeial Convention, 1994; Council of Europe, 1995).

Tamoxifen and its metabolites can be analysed in biological fluids and tissues by thin-layer chromatography (Furr & Jordan, 1984), gas chromatography–mass spectrometry (MS) (Furr & Jordan, 1984) and high-performance liquid chromatography with ultraviolet, fluorimetric or electrochemical detection (Chamart *et al.*, 1989; Berthou & Dréano, 1993; Lim *et al.*, 1993; Fried & Wainer, 1994).

1.2 Production and use

1.2.1 *Production*

Tamoxifen is prepared by reacting 4-β-dimethylaminoethoxy-α-ethyldesoxybenzoin with phenylmagnesium bromide or phenyl lithium to form 1-(4-β-dimethylaminoethoxyphenyl)-1,2-diphenylbutanol, which on dehydration yields a mixture of tamoxifen and its *E*-isomer that may be separated with petroleum ether. Tamoxifen is converted to the 1:1 citrate for pharmaceutical use (Gennaro, 1995).

Worldwide production of tamoxifen citrate has increased from approximately 7.0 tonnes in 1989 to 8.5 tonnes in 1991, 10.1 tonnes in 1993 and 10.3 tonnes in 1995.

1.2.2 *Use*

Tamoxifen was first synthesized by Bedford and Richardson in the United Kingdom (Bedford & Richardson, 1966). It was shown to be an anti-fertility agent in rats (Harper & Walpole, 1967a,b), but was soon found to induce ovulation in women and to have either oestrogenic or antioestrogenic effects, depending on species specificity and tissue and receptor status (Harper & Walpole, 1966, 1967a). The earliest clinical studies were carried out in postmenopausal women with advanced breast cancer in Manchester,

United Kingdom (Cole *et al.*, 1971). It was soon appreciated that tamoxifen was a successful palliative therapy for advanced breast cancer, yielding response (see Glossary, p. 449) rates similar to those seen with other endocrine approaches while producing few side-effects (Ward 1973; O'Halloran & Maddock, 1974). It was approved for use as a pharmaceutical in the United Kingdom in 1973 (Jordan, 1988). By 1978, it was being widely adopted as first-line endocrine therapy for postmenopausal women with advanced disease, particularly after it was shown to be as effective as, and less toxic than, diethylstilboestrol, the previous standard in that setting (Ingle *et al.*, 1981). It was tested in premenopausal women for therapy of metastatic breast cancer from the late 1970s (Manni *et al.*, 1979; Pritchard *et al.*, 1980; Planting *et al.*, 1985; Buchanan *et al.*, 1986; Ingle *et al.*, 1986; Sawka *et al.*, 1986) and shown to be 20–30% effective, but it has probably been far less widely used in this younger group, with chemotherapy or ovarian ablation remaining the more usual approaches (Sunderland & Osborne, 1991; Early Breast Cancer Trialists' Collaboration Group, 1992).

Since the early 1980s, tamoxifen has been widely accepted as first-line endocrine therapy for metastatic disease in postmenopausal women (Ingle, 1984). Most postmenopausal women who develop metastatic disease will at some point undergo at least one attempt at endocrine therapy, either as a palliative treatment or as first-line therapy for metastatic disease. Even those women who respond to tamoxifen for metastatic disease generally receive it for, on average, only 9–12 months (Muss, 1992).

In the mid- to late 1970s, many investigators became interested in using tamoxifen as adjuvant therapy in women at high risk for recurrence of breast cancer following surgery, because of the equivalence of this approach to other endocrine therapies and the drug's extremely low short-term toxicity profile. Several large trials of adjuvant tamoxifen therapy in mostly postmenopausal, axillary node-positive women demonstrated a small but statistically significant improvement (about 25%) in both recurrence-free and overall survival in these patient groups (Nolvadex Adjuvant Trial Organisation, 1983; Ribeiro & Swindell, 1985). Although the relative merits of tamoxifen and chemotherapy for use in this setting were widely debated, particularly between the United Kingdom and the United States, the final results from the Oxford Overview (Early Breast Cancer Trialists' Collaborative Group, 1988) convinced clinicians on both sides of the Atlantic of the benefit of tamoxifen not only in this patient group but in others as well (Breast Cancer Chemotherapy Consensus Conference, 1985; Glick *et al.*, 1992).

From the early days of trials of adjuvant tamoxifen therapy, British clinicians in particular favoured the use of tamoxifen in node-negative (lower-risk) and premenopausal women as well as in postmenopausal, node-positive women. Several large trials soon supported the use of tamoxifen in this setting and showed that it improved overall and recurrence-free survival (Breast Cancer Trials Committee, 1987; Fisher *et al.*, 1989a,b).

From the early days of these trials, dose and dosage varied from one country to another. In the United States and the United Kingdom, 20 mg daily given for one to two years was the early norm (Nolvadex Adjuvant Trial Organisation, 1983; Fisher *et al.*, 1986; Nolvadex Adjuvant Trial Organisation, 1988), while in continental Europe doses of 30–40 mg daily for one to two years were more usual (Fornander et al., 1991; Mouridsen et al., 1988; Rutqvist et al., 1992; Rutqvist & Mattsson, 1993; Rutqvist et al., 1995). The wide variety of dosing is clear from the summary tables of the Early Breast Cancer Trialists' Collaborative Group (1988, 1992). In addition, data from rat models suggested that longer tamoxifen treatment would be advantageous (Jordan, 1978; Jordan et al., 1979, 1980) and trials examining two versus five years, five versus ten years and two or five years versus indefinite tamoxifen were undertaken. From the mid-1980s to the mid-1990s, tamoxifen therapy of five years or longer was used increasingly in many countries. Further, with reports of its effectiveness in node-negative women, the use of tamoxifen spread widely, to the point where it was sometimes used to treat even very small (< 1 cm) invasive carcinomas and carcinomas *in situ* for which it had never been tested in randomized trials. Trials of its use for very small invasive cancers and carcinoma *in situ* are now in progress: National Surgical Adjuvant Breast and Bowel Project, B21, B24.

Tamoxifen has been the adjuvant therapy of choice for postmenopausal, node-positive women and oestrogen receptor-positive or progesterone receptor-positive (see Glossary, p. 448) since the mid-1980s and for postmenopausal, node-negative and oestrogen receptor-positive or progesterone receptor-positive women since the early 1990s. It is also used in many cases in postmenopausal receptor-negative women and in premenopausal women with low-risk (node-negative) receptor-positive disease (Glick et al., 1992; National Institutes of Health Consensus Development Panel, 1992; Goldhirsch et al., 1995). In both pre- and postmenopausal women, it is also often given concurrently with or following chemotherapy as a type of adjuvant maintenance (Glick et al., 1992; Tormey et al., 1993; Goldhirsch et al., 1995). Thus, a high proportion (40–60%) of all women who undergo potentially curative surgery for breast cancer now receive adjuvant tamoxifen therapy for a period of some two to five years.

Most breast cancer patients with metastatic disease receive, at some time in the course of their treatment, cytotoxic chemotherapy as well as tamoxifen and often other hormonal therapies. Similarly, many women, particularly in the postmenopausal, axillary node-positive subset, receive cytotoxic chemotherapy as well as tamoxifen as part of their adjuvant therapy. Again, the Early Breast Cancer Trialists' Collaborative Group (1988, 1992) summary tables document the use of these drugs, which are mainly cyclophosphamide, methotrexate and 5-fluorouracil-based combinations, but also include other cytotoxic agents such as melphalan and adriamycin, many of which are documented carcinogens in their own right (see IARC, 1987a). There are nevertheless many randomized trials of tamoxifen adjuvant therapy versus no therapy, particularly in postmenopausal axillary node-positive and pre- and postmenopausal node-negative subjects, from which information relating to tamoxifen exposure without accompanying cytotoxic agents can be obtained (Early Breast Cancer Trialists' Collaborative Group, 1992).

Tamoxifen has also been commonly used, without surgery, as a primary therapy for breast cancer in elderly women who are considered poor candidates for surgery (Akhtar et al., 1991), although two randomized studies have suggested that surgical removal of the primary tumour plus tamoxifen treatment is preferable, leading to fewer problems with local recurrence (Bates et al., 1991; Mustacchi et al., 1994).

In the mid-1980s, because of its known cytostatic action and because of the reduction in new contralateral breast cancers observed in many clinical trials of tamoxifen (Breast Cancer Chemotherapy Consensus Conference, 1985; Nolvadex Adjuvant Trial Organisation, 1988; Early Breast Cancer Trialists' Collaborative Group, 1992), considerable interest arose in using tamoxifen as a preventive agent. At least three large trials are in progress in Italy (hysterectomized women), North America and the United Kingdom (Powles *et al.*, 1990; National Surgical Adjuvant Breast and Bowel Project, 1992; Redmond *et al.*, 1993; Vanchieri, 1993; Costa *et al.*, 1996). The subjects are women believed to be at high risk for developing breast cancer. These so-called high-risk women include those at a risk as low as that of the average 60-year-old in at least one trial (National Surgical Adjuvant Breast and Bowel Project, 1992). Although the practice is discouraged by most investigators, it is known that some women are currently prescribed tamoxifen as a preventive agent outside of study, in various high-risk situations (such as women with lobular carcinoma *in situ* or a family history of breast cancer).

Tamoxifen has been widely adopted as the appropriate first-line therapy for hormone-responsive male breast cancer and is also used frequently as adjuvant therapy for men with oestrogen receptor- or progesterone receptor-positive breast cancer, in spite of the lack of any large randomized trials in this relatively small group of patients (Jaiyesimi *et al.*, 1992).

Tamoxifen, at doses similar to those used in breast cancer treatment, has given response rates of 20–30% in several phase II trials in women with advanced endometrial cancer (Quinn & Campbell, 1989; Barakat & Hoskins, 1994; Lentz, 1994) and has been accepted as a second-line endocrine therapy for unresectable or recurrent endometrial cancer (Swenerton *et al.*, 1984).

There have also been studies, but probably not wide use, of tamoxifen treatment for a variety of other malignancies, including hepatocellular carcinoma (Martínez Cerezo *et al.*, 1994), carcinoma of the stomach (Harrison *et al.*, 1989), renal-cell carcinoma (Yagoda *et al.*, 1995), melanoma (McClay & McClay, 1994), adenocarcinoma of the pancreas (Taylor *et al.*, 1993; Wong & Chan, 1993), carcinoma of the cervix (Vargas Roig *et al.*, 1993), carcinoma of the ovary (Hatch *et al.*, 1991), glioblastoma multiforme (Baltuch *et al.*, 1993), carcinoma of the biliary tract (West *et al.*, 1990), desmoid tumours (Brooks *et al.*, 1992) and meningiomas (Goodwin *et al.*, 1993). In addition, tamoxifen has been suggested to be useful in treating certain non-malignant conditions including retroperitoneal fibrosis, the POEMS syndrome (a multi-system syndrome consisting of polyneuropathy, organomegaly, endocrinopathy, serum M-band and skin changes) (Enevoldson & Harding, 1992), oligoospermia in men with incomplete androgen sensitivity (Gooren, 1989), idiopathic oligozoospermia (Sterzik *et al.*, 1993), pulmonary lymphangioleiomyomatosis (Kitaichi *et al.*, 1995), rectal polyps in patients with Gardner's syndrome (Parry *et al.*, 1993), Peyronie's disease (Ralph *et al.*, 1992), autoimmune progesterone dermatitis (Stephens *et al.*, 1989), menstrual migraine (O'Dea & Davis, 1990) and painful idiopathic gynaecomastia (McDermott *et al.*, 1990). It has also been shown to have anti-candidal activity (Beggs, 1993).

Tamoxifen has also been suggested to be useful as an adjuvant to cancer chemotherapy of various types, in that it displays synergy with drugs such as cisplatin (McClay et al., 1993). Tamoxifen has also been shown to cause apoptotic effects which appear to be independent of the oestrogen receptor status of the cells affected (Perry et al., 1985).

Interest has focused more recently on positive effects of tamoxifen on cardiovascular lipid profiles (Bruning et al., 1988; Love et al., 1990, 1991; Shewmon et al., 1994; Thangaraju et al., 1994; Grey et al., 1995a; Guetta et al., 1995; Gylling et al., 1995; Kenny et al., 1995), on cardiovascular events (Rutqvist & Mattsson, 1993) and cardiovascular deaths (McDonald & Stewart, 1991) and on bone density (Love et al., 1988; Wolter et al., 1988; Kristensen et al., 1994; Love et al., 1994a; Wright et al., 1994; Grey et al., 1995b; Kenny et al., 1995; Leslie et al., 1995). These apparently positive effects have made the drug even more attractive for long-term use in early breast cancer and as a preventive agent. Some authors have even hypothesized that it may have more beneficial preventive effects on mortality and morbidity from causes other than breast cancer, at least for women over 60 (Gray, 1993).

Thus, tamoxifen has become very widely used around the world. It is estimated that there have been over 7 million patient-years of treatment with tamoxifen since it was first approved in 1973. Tamoxifen is now registered for use in 97 countries. Most women and men with metastatic breast cancer receive it at some time in their therapy, and 40–60% of women may receive it as adjuvant therapy, in some instances for five years or longer. It is being increasingly tested as a preventive agent against the development of breast cancer. Studies are in progress to examine potential effects of its long-term use on risks for cardiovascular disease and osteoporosis.

1.3 Occurrence

Tamoxifen is not known to occur as a natural product.

The National Occupational Exposure Survey conducted between 1981 and 1983 in the United States by the National Institute for Occupational Safety and Health indicated that approximately 350 and 2100 employees were potentially occupationally exposed to tamoxifen and tamoxifen citrate, respectively. The estimate was based on a survey of companies and did not involve measurements of actual exposure (United States National Library of Medicine, 1996).

1.4 Regulations and guidelines

Tamoxifen citrate is listed in the following pharmacopoeias: British, French, Greek and United States (Reynolds, 1993; Vidal, 1995).

2. Studies of Cancer in Humans

Introduction

In this section, epidemiological evidence is considered with regard to the occurrence of second primary cancers after the use of tamoxifen (invariably as tamoxifen citrate) for the treatment of breast cancer. These data include descriptive studies of single cases and case series, case–control studies, cohort studies and randomized clinical trials. Data on the use of tamoxifen in healthy women are currently very limited.

2.1 Endometrial cancer

2.1.1 *Case reports*

Following an initial report by Killackey *et al.* (1985) of three cases of endometrial cancer in women who received tamoxifen for breast cancer, a large number of case reports have been published. Those available to the Working Group are summarized in Table 1. One hundred and two cases of endometrial cancer were reported in 32 case reports, ranging from isolated cases to series of up to 20 cases. The reports concern 72 adenocarcinomas, including 8 mucinous, 3 clear-cell adenocarcinomas and 1 serous papillary adenocarcinoma, 14 Müllerian mixed tumours, 1 stromal sarcoma and 13 carcinomas not otherwise specified. [The Working Group noted that rare histological types of endometrial cancer are over-represented in these reports.]

2.1.2 *Case series*

Two groups of case series were available to the Working Group. The first comprises series of cases of endometrial cancer following breast cancer, among whom tamoxifen use was assessed (Table 2). In one of these series, 15 of 53 cases had received tamoxifen, and more of these had high-grade tumours (poorly differentiated endometrial carcinomas) (67%) than in the group not treated with tamoxifen (24%; $p = 0.03$) (Magriples *et al.*, 1993). In another series of 73 cases, of whom 23 had received tamoxifen, the proportion of high-grade tumours was 23% in tamoxifen-treated patients and 19% in non-treated patients. The disease stage (according to the current International Federation of Gynecology and Obstetrics (FIGO) criteria) in this series did not differ between tamoxifen-treated and untreated cases (Barakat *et al.*, 1994). The second group comprises series of cases of breast cancer treated with tamoxifen, among whom the development of endometrial cancer was assessed (Table 3).

2.1.3 *Case–control studies*

The case–control studies considered by the Working Group were those which compared tamoxifen use in women with breast cancer who did (cases) or did not (controls) subsequently develop endometrial cancer. A fundamental requirement for these controls is that they, like the cases, were at risk for developing endometrial cancer (namely, that they had an intact uterus). The failure to consider the hysterectomy status

Table 1. Case reports of gynaecological cancers in patients receiving tamoxifen for breast cancer

Reference, country	No. of cases	Dose (mg/day)	Duration (years)	Latency (years)	Additional therapy[a]	Endometrial cancers[b]	Other cancers, when specified	Histological grade[c]	Tumour stage[d]
Killackey et al. (1985) United States	3 (1 premenopausal)	all, 20	all, <2	all, <2	2 cases, chemo	2 adenocarcinomas 1 carcinoma (NOS)	—	2G1, 1G2	all, I
Atlante et al. (1990) Italy	4	2 cases, 40 2 cases, 60	3 cases, 2–5 1 case, >5	3 cases, 3–5 1 case, >5	3 cases, chemo 1 case, radio	4 adenocarcinomas	—	1G1, 2G2, 1G3	all, I
Dauplat et al. (1990) France	2	1 case, 30 1 case, 20	1 case, <2 1 case, 2	1 case, <2 1 case, 2–5	NS	1 adenocarcinoma 1 adenoacanthoma	—	G1 NS	NS
Malfetano (1990) United States	7	all, 40	2 cases, <2 5 cases, 2–4	1 case, <2 5 cases, 2–5 1 case, >5	3 cases, chemo	7 carcinomas (NOS)	—	2G1, 3G2, 2G3	6 cases, I 1 case, NS
Mathew et al. (1990) United States	5	3 cases, 20 2 cases, NG	2 cases, 2–5 3 cases, >5	2 cases, 2–5 3 cases, >5	NS	3 adenocarcinomas 2 carcinomas (NOS)	—	2G1 3NS	1 case, I 4 cases, NS
Rodier et al. (1990) France	1	40	<2	<2	Radio	Adenocarcinoma	—	G1	II
Lang-Avérous et al. (1991) Germany	3	10–30	2–5	2–5	NS	3 adenocarcinomas (2 mucinous)	—	2G1, 1G2	NS
Rasmussen & Nielsen (1991) Denmark	2	both, 30	both, >5	both, >5	both, radio	2 adenocarcinomas	—	1G2, 1G3	1 case, IV 1 case, II
Spinelli et al. (1991) Italy	3 (premenopausal)	all, 40	1 case, <2 1 case, 2–5 1 case, >5	1 case, <2 1 case, 2–5 1 case, >5	2 cases, chemo	3 adenocarcinomas	—	2G1, 1G3	all, I
Bocklage et al. (1992) United States	1	20	<2	<2	Radio and chemo	Müllerian mixed tumour	—	G3	I

Table 1 (contd)

Reference, country	No. of cases	Dose (mg/day)	Duration (years)	Latency (years)	Additional therapy[a]	Endometrial cancers[b]	Other cancers, when specified	Histological grade[c]	Tumour stage[d]
Deprest et al. (1992) Belgium	1	40	> 5	> 5	Chemo	Serous papillary adenocarcinoma	–	G3	III
Le Bouëdec & Dauplat (1992) France	4	2 cases, 20; 2 cases, 30	2 cases, < 2; 2 cases, 2–3	2 cases, < 2; 2 cases, 2–5	1 radio, 1 chemo; 2 radio + chemo	3 adenocarcinomas; 1 adenoacanthoma	–	3G1; G2	All, I
Mignotte et al. (1992) France	20	all, 20	14 cases, 2–5; 6 cases, > 5	1 case, 2–5; 1 case, 2; 2 cases, < 2	13 chemo	8 in situ adenocarcinomas; 10 invasive adenocarcinomas; 2 Müllerian mixed tumours	–	16 G1; 2 G2; 2 NS	8 cases, 0; 10 cases, I; 1 case, II; 1 case, III
Segna et al. (1992) United States	11	2 cases, 10; 9 cases, 20	2 cases, < 2; 8 cases, 2–5; 1 case, > 5	NG	–	11 adenocarcinomas	–	5G1; 4G2; 2G3	All, I
Altaras et al. (1993) Israël	1	20	> 5	> 5	Radio	Müllerian mixed tumour	–	G3	I
Clarke (1993) United States	1	20	> 5	> 5	0	Müllerian mixed tumour	–	G3	I
McAuliffe (1993) Ireland	5	NG	NG	NG	NG	3 carcinomas (NOS); 1 Müllerian mixed tumour; 1 papillary adenocarcinoma	–	3G3; 2 NS	NS
Palacios et al. (1993) Spain	1	20	> 5	> 5	Radio	Adenocarcinoma	–	G2	I

Table 1 (contd)

Reference, country	No. of cases	Dose (mg/day)	Duration (years)	Latency (years)	Additional therapy[a]	Endometrial cancers[b]	Other cancers, when specified	Histological grade[c]	Tumour stage[d]
Seoud et al. (1993) United States	5	20	2 cases, < 2 3 cases, > 2	NG	NS	3 adenocarcinomas 1 Müllerian mixed tumour	1 fallopian tube adenocarcinoma	3G2 NS	2 cases, I 1 case, III III
Bardi et al. (1994) Italy	1	30	> 2	2–5	Chemo	None	Endometrioid carcinoma in pelvic endometriosis	G1	–
Cohen et al. (1994) Israël	1	20	1	< 2	None	None	Ovarian endometrioid carcinoma	G2	I
Gherman et al. (1994) United States	1	20	< 2	2	Radio	None	Ovarian granulosa cell tumour	NS	I
Krause & Gerber (1994) Germany	1	30	~ 2	~ 2	NS	Adenocarcinoma	–	G1	NS
Lanza et al. (1994) Italy	2	1 case, 20 1 case, 40	1 case, 5 1 case, > 5	1 case, 5 1 case, > 5	Chemo	2 adenocarcinomas	–	1G1, 1G3	1 case, II 1 case, III
Sonnendecker et al. (1994) South Africa	1	20	2	2	Radio	None	Fallopian tube adenocarcinoma *in situ*	G1	0
Beer et al. (1995) United Kingdom	1	20	5	5	None	1 adenocarcinoma + 1 stromal sarcoma in the same patient	–	G1 NS	Both, I

Table 1 (contd)

Reference, country	No. of cases	Dose (mg/day)	Duration (years)	Latency (years)	Additional therapy[a]	Endometrial cancers[b]	Other cancers, when specified	Histological grade[c]	Tumour stage[d]
Dallenbach-Hellweg & Hahn (1995) Germany	10	1 case, 10 2 cases, 20 7 cases, 30	2 cases, <2 5 cases, 2–5 2 cases, >5 1 case, NG	NS	NS	3 clear-cell adenocarcinomas 6 mucinous adenocarcinomas 1 papillary adenocarcinoma of endometrioid type	–	1G1, 9G2	All, I
Evans et al. (1995) United Kingdom	6	NG	1 case, 3 5 cases, >5	NG	NS	6 Müllerian mixed tumours	–	NS	NS
Gillett (1995) Australia	1	20	4.5	>5	NS	None	1 leiomyosarcoma of myometrium uteri	–	I
Jose et al. (1995) India	1	20	>5	>5	Radio	Adenocarcinoma	–	G1	I
LiVolsi et al. (1995) United States	1	20	1	1	Radio	–	Papillary mucinous endocervical adenocarcinoma	G1	I
Sasco et al. (1995) France	1	20	<5	>5	Radio	Müllerian mixed tumour	–	NS	II

[a] Chemo, chemotherapy; radio, radiotherapy
[b] NOS, not otherwise specified; NS, not specified; NG, not given
[c] Histological classification: G1, grade 1, well differentiated; G2, grade 2, moderately differentiated; G3, grade 3, poorly differentiated
[d] FIGO stages [International Federation of Gynecology and Obstetrics]: 0, carcinoma in situ; I, tumour confined to corpus; II, tumour invades cervix but does not enter beyond uterus; III, local and/or regional spread; IV, distant metastasis or/and tumour invades bladder mucosa and/or bowel mucosa.

Table 2. Use of tamoxifen among endometrial cancer case series following breast cancer

Reference	Country (period)	No. of endometrial cancer cases	No. (%) of tamoxifen users	Dose (mg/day)	Duration (years)[a]	Comments
Hardell (1988a)	Sweden (1959–88)	23	11 (48)	40	1–9	Series also included in the case–control study, p. 267. In tamoxifen users, 6 cases also had pelvic radiotherapy for ovarian ablation and 2 cases also had adjuvant chemotherapy; the tumours of the corpus uteri were: 9 carcinomas, 1 carcinosarcoma, 1 anaplastic cancer.
Magriples et al. (1993)	USA (1980–90)	53	15 (28) (5 deaths)[b]	40	0.2–10 (4.2)	Higher-grade tumours in tamoxifen users (67% versus 24%). The endometrial cancers were: 9 endometrioid carcinomas, 3 papillary serous carcinomas, 1 clear-cell carcinoma, 2 Müllerian mixed tumours; 3 cases had also adjuvant chemotherapy and 1 case pelvic radiotherapy for ovarian ablation. One premenopausal woman among the 53 cases.
Barakat et al. (1994)	USA (1980–92)	73	23 (32) (5 deaths)[b]	20	1–10.5 (4.5)	No difference in stage between tamoxifen-treated and untreated patients. In tamoxifen users, 17 had adenocarcinoma of the corpus uteri, 1 had a papillary serous carcinoma, 5 had Müllerian mixed tumours; 5 cases received adjuvant chemotherapy; some cases received radiotherapy.
Silva et al. (1994)	USA (NA)	72	15 (20) (1 death)[b]	20	0.2–5.5 (2)	In tamoxifen users, the tumours of the uterine corpus were: 3 endometrial carcinomas, 4 clear-cell carcinomas, 5 serous carcinomas, 1 Müllerian mixed tumour, 2 leiomyosarcomas. 2/15 also received premarin.

NA, not available
[a] Mean or median in parentheses
[b] Number of deaths from endometrial cancer

Table 3. Case series of endometrial cancer among breast cancer patients treated with tamoxifen

Reference	Country (period)	No. of tamoxifen users[a]	Dose (mg/day)	Duration (years)[b]	No. (%) of endometrial cancer cases	Comments
De Muylder et al. (1991)	Belgium (NA)	46 (23 LRT, 15 CT)	NA	0.5–3	2 (4)	Both adenocarcinomas were of grade 3 and stage I; 12 premenopausal women
Samelis et al. (1992)	Greece (NA)	243	20–40	2–13 (4)	1 (0.5)	Six other cancers found (2 ovarian); 64 pre-menopausal women
Lahti et al. (1993)	Finland (1991)	51 (1 CT, 48 LRT)	20–40	0.5–8 (2.5)	1 (2)	One adenocarcinoma of grade 1
Uziely et al. (1993)	Israel (1990–92)	95	20	1–7 (2)	3 (3)	All endometrial cancers have been found in women with > 1 year tamoxifen therapy.
Gibson et al. (1994)	USA (1986–93)	72	NA	2	6 (8)	Six adenocarcinomas

NA, not available
[a] Patients had also local radiotherapy (LRT) and chemotherapy (CT)
[b] Mean or median in parenthesis

of controls may invalidate a case–control study of endometrial cancer. Other issues to be considered include factors which either may be determinants of risk for endometrial cancer (age, nulliparity, obesity, diabetes, hypertension, age at menopause and use of unopposed oestrogen therapy) or may influence the likelihood of tamoxifen prescription (calendar year of breast cancer diagnosis, menopausal status, and stage and oestrogen receptor status of the breast cancer). Determinants of risk for endometrial cancer are confounding factors in the studies discussed below only to the extent that they influence the likelihood of tamoxifen prescription. As in any case–control study, information and selection bias may also pertain. Finally, the possibility that endometrial cancer was diagnosed preferentially in women who had received tamoxifen constitutes a potential bias that is considered in greater detail in the introductory remarks to cohort studies and randomized trials (Sections 2.1.4 and 2.1.5).

Hardell (1988a) described a case series from a Swedish registry, covering 32 cases of endometrial cancer diagnosed at least one year after breast cancer. He then examined the same group in a case–control study (Hardell, 1988b), including 23 of these cases compared to 92 age- and breast cancer-matched controls. Eleven cases (48%) compared with 18 controls (20%) had received tamoxifen at 40 mg/day and nine (39%) cases compared with 10 (11%) controls had received pelvic irradiation. The odds ratio for patients receiving both treatments was 7.1 (95% confidence interval (CI), 2.3–22.1) compared to neither treatment, that for tamoxifen alone was 2.6 (95% CI, 0.7–9.6) and that for pelvic irradiation alone was 4.7 (95% CI, 0.8–27.3). [The Working Group noted that the presence of an intact uterus was not confirmed in the controls.]

van Leeuwen *et al.* (1994) conducted a large case–control study in the Netherlands in which 98 cases of endometrial cancer diagnosed at least three months following breast cancer were matched by age and date of diagnosis of breast cancer with 285 controls with breast cancer who survived with an intact uterus at least up to the time of diagnosis of endometrial cancer of the cases. Twenty-three cases and 58 controls had had treatment with tamoxifen. The relative risk associated with any use of tamoxifen was 1.3 (95% CI, 0.7–2.4). Statistically significant trends with duration and cumulative dose were found ($p < 0.05$ for both). The odds ratio for women who had taken tamoxifen for more than two years was 2.3 (95% CI, 0.9–5.9). Most women were treated with doses of 40 mg/day (59%), 17% received 30 mg/day and 23%, ≤ 20 mg/day. The duration–response trends were similar with daily doses of 40 mg or 30 mg and less. No difference in stage or histology between the exposed and unexposed cases was found. [The Working Group noted that the statistical power to detect differences in risk associated with different dose intensities of tamoxifen was low.]

Cook *et al.* (1995) conducted a case–control study involving women under the age of 85 years registered in the Washington State Cancer Registry with a diagnosis of breast cancer between 1978 and 1990, who subsequently developed endometrial cancer at least six months after breast cancer. These were matched with controls without second primary cancer by age, year of breast cancer diagnosis and stage of cancer. Controls had to have an intact uterus and to have survived at least up to the time of diagnosis of endometrial cancer of their matched cases. Thirty-four endometrial cancer patients and 64 matched controls were analysed. All but two cases were postmenopausal. Tamoxifen use [mainly 20 mg/day] was more common in the controls (31% versus 26%). After adjustment for cytotoxic chemotherapy and duration of oestrogen replacement therapy, the matched odds ratio for any use was 0.6 (95% CI, 0.2–1.9). The mean duration of use was 14 months for cases and 21 months for controls. The odds ratio for more than one year's use was 0.2 (95% CI, 0.1–1.0) based on three cases and 16 controls. [The Working Group noted the inability of this study to address risks associated with long-term use of tamoxifen.]

Sasco *et al.* (1996) conducted a case–control study in Lyon and Dijon, France. Forty-three cases of endometrial cancer occurring at least one year after the diagnosis of breast cancer were matched with 177 controls for age, region, year of diagnosis of breast cancer, intact uterus and survival with breast cancer. The median dose was 20 mg/day; the median duration of treatment was greater in cases (63 months) than in controls (37 months); and tamoxifen was used in 67% of cases and 60% of controls (odds ratio, 1.4; 95% CI, 0.6–3.5). Information on duration of use was missing for 21% of exposed cases and 45% of exposed controls. The risk appeared to increase with duration of use, with a relative risk of 3.5 (95% CI, 0.9–12.7) for more than five years of use. [The Working Group noted that a difference in the percentages of cases and controls with unknown duration of treatment could have exaggerated the estimate of the effect of duration.]

2.1.4 *Cohort studies*

Detection bias may pertain to both cohort studies and randomized clinical trials, since tamoxifen is known to increase the frequency of symptoms such as vaginal bleeding or discharge which may lead to gynaecological evaluation. In addition, tamoxifen is known to induce benign gynaecological changes such as endometrial hyperplasia and polyps. Other changes include poorly defined thickening of the endometrium that may be revealed by ultrasound examination. Growth of leiomyomata may occur and provide a further opportunity for the diagnosis of endometrial cancer.

The longer survival of tamoxifen-treated patients may lead to greater duration of follow-up in which second cancers may occur. The appropriate methods of statistical analysis in this context are life table analysis or analysis of rates based on person-years at risk.

In an abstract, Champion *et al.* (1991) reported a breast cancer registry-based series from northern Alberta, Canada. Between 1953 and 1988, a total of 1874 women had taken tamoxifen, 20 mg/day for 22, 36 and 39 months and 8201 had not. Thirty-one women developed uterine cancer, three (two sarcomas and one adenocarcinoma) in the tamoxifen group and 28 in the other group. [The Working Group noted that no adjustment for period of diagnosis was made in this study and the results therefore could not be interpreted.]

Robinson *et al.* (1995) reviewed 586 eligible breast cancer patients without a previous hysterectomy in a medical centre series from Texas, United States. Of 108 patients who received tamoxifen (20 mg/day for at least one year), four developed endometrial adenocarcinoma and, of 478 breast cancer patients who did not receive tamoxifen, four developed endometrial cancer [odds ratio, 4.6; 95% CI, 1.3–16.0]. After adjustment for hypertension and diabetes mellitus, the odds ratio for development of endometrial cancer after tamoxifen use was 15.2 (95% CI, 2.8–84.4). [The Working Group noted the imprecision of the estimates and the difference between the crude and adjusted odds ratios, that the results were not adjusted for follow-up time and that the presence of an intact uterus during follow-up was not controlled for.]

Curtis et al. (1996) examined the effect of tamoxifen on risk for endometrial cancer in 87 323 women with breast cancer reported to the SEER (Surveillance, Epidemiology and End Results) Program in the United States. All women included in this study were diagnosed with early-stage (localized or regional) breast cancer between 1980 and 1992, were aged at least 50 years at diagnosis and had not been given chemotherapy as an initial treatment. For 14 358 women defined as the study group, the SEER database indicated that they had received hormonal therapy (which for over 90% was tamoxifen treatment). After a mean follow-up of [4.4] years, 73 cancers of the uterine corpus were observed, resulting in a standardized incidence ratio (SIR) (based on SEER incidence rates) of 2.0 (95% CI, 1.6–2.6). The SIR for women not known to have received hormones was significantly lower (1.2; 95% CI, 1.1–1.4). The differences in risk for endometrial cancer between hormone-treated women and women with no/unknown hormone treatment status were greater in five-year survivors (SIRs of 3.6 and 1.2, respectively). There was little difference in the severity of grade or stage of cancer of the uterine corpus according to initial therapy: in hormone-treated patients, 59% of the uterine cancers which developed were grade 1 or 2, 25% were grade 3 or 4 and for 16% the grade was unknown (versus 63%, 21% and 16% in no/unknown hormone treatment). The stage distribution was: localized, 78%; regional, 12%; distant, 4%; unknown, 6% (versus 76%, 11%, 8% and 5%, respectively). [The Working Group noted that no information on hysterectomy status was available and that misclassification of hormonal treatment in the study may have led to an underestimation of the difference in risk for cancer of the uterine corpus between the two groups.]

2.1.5 Randomized clinical trials (see Table 4)

The design of randomized trials is such that they allow both known and unknown confounding factors to be distributed randomly between treatment groups. Therefore, these studies offer the best evidence regarding tamoxifen and the occurrence of second cancers. However, assessment of the risk for endometrial cancer was not the principal aim of the trials considered by the Working Group. None of the trials included procedures which would assure complete reporting of second primary tumours. Even in the trials (such as those in Scandinavia) that ascertained second primary tumours after linkage of the trial data to a population-based cancer registry, complete ascertainment of such tumours cannot be assumed, as second primary tumours are not reported systematically to cancer registries. However, there is no reason to believe that the reporting of such tumours would be biased by being related to tamoxifen therapy. Other biases which are relevant to randomized clinical trials are the same as those already discussed for cohort studies.

Table 4. Endometrial cancers in patients treated for breast cancer: summary results of randomized clinical trials of adjuvant use of tamoxifen

Reference, country	No. of patients and treatment[a]		Dose of tamoxifen (mg/day)	Duration (years)	Median follow-up (years)	No. of endometrial cancers	Odds ratio (95% CI)
Pritchard et al. (1987) (updated by Nayfield et al., 1991) Canada	198	Tamoxifen	20	2	5.8	0	—
	202	Observation				1	
NATO (1988) (updated by Nayfield et al., 1991) United States	564	Tamoxifen	20	2	5.5	0	—
	567	Observation				0	
Palshof (1988) Denmark	164	Tamoxifen (52 postmenopausal)	30	2	9	2	—
	153	Placebo (52 postmenopausal)				0	
Castiglione et al. (1990) Several countries	167	Tamoxifen + prednisone	20	1	8	0	—
	153	Observation				0	
Andersson et al. (1992) Denmark	864	Tamoxifen + LRT	30	0.9	8	7	3.3 (0.6–31[b])
	846	LRT				2	
Ribeiro & Swindell (1992a) United Kingdom	199	Premenopausal, tamoxifen	20	1	13	0	—
	174	Premenopausal, pelvic irradiation for ovary ablation				0	
	282	Postmenopausal, tamoxifen	20	1	max. 13	1	[1.0 (0.1–16)]
	306	Postmenopausal, observation				1	
Rydén et al. (1992) South Sweden	244	Tamoxifen	30	1	9	5	[2.4 (0.5–12)] LRT-tamoxifen versus LRT
	239	Tamoxifen + LRT				4	
	236	LRT				2 (1 death[c])	
Stewart (1992) as updated in Nayfield et al. (1991) Scotland	661	Tamoxifen	20	≥ 5	4–10	4	[2.0 (0.4–11)]
	651	Observation				2	

Table 4 (contd)

Reference, country	No. of patients and treatment[a]		Dose of tamoxifen (mg/day)	Duration (years)	Median follow-up (years)	No. of endometrial cancers	Odds ratio (95% CI)
Cummings et al. (1993) United States	85	Tamoxifen	20	2	10	1	[1.0 (0.1–15)]
	83	Placebo				1	
Boccardo et al. (1994a) Italy	168	Tamoxifen	30	5	≥5	0	—
	171	Tamoxifen + Chemotherapy					
		77 premenopausal				0	
		94 postmenopausal				1	
	165	Chemotherapy				0	
Fisher et al. (1994)[d] Canada, United States	1419	Tamoxifen	20	5	8	15 (4 deaths[c,e])	7.5 (1.7–32.7)
	1424	Placebo				2 (Both received tamoxifen)	
Kedar et al. (1994) United Kingdom	61	Tamoxifen	20	NG	2	0	—
	50	Placebo				0	
Rivkin et al. (1994) United States	295	Tamoxifen	20	1	6.5	2	—
	303	Tamoxifen + Chemotherapy				3	—
	300	Chemotherapy				0	
Rutqvist et al. (1995) Stockholm, Sweden	1372	Tamoxifen	40	2 or 5	9	23[c] (4 deaths[c])	5.6 (1.9–16.2)
	1357	Observation				4	

NG, not given; LRT, local radiotherapy
[a] Observation: patients receiving no adjuvant therapy
[b] The upper 95% confidence limit reported by Andersson et al. (1992) is probably overestimated.
[c] Death from endometrial cancer
[d] Fisher et al. (1994) in a non-randomized population reported 8 cancers of the endometrium (7 endometrioid cancers) in 1220 registered breast cancer patients given tamoxifen for breast cancer
[e] One did not receive tamoxifen

In a trial in Canada (Pritchard *et al.*, 1987, updated by Nayfield *et al.*, 1991), no case of endometrial cancer was found among 198 breast cancer patients treated with 20 mg/day tamoxifen for two years, but one occurred among 202 patients receiving no adjuvant therapy for breast cancer.

In a trial in the United States of tamoxifen therapy (20 mg/day) for two years for treatment of early breast cancer in women ≤ 75 years old versus no treatment, the NATO (Nolvadex Adjuvant Trial Organization) (1988) reported no case of endometrial cancer in 564 tamoxifen patients or in 567 patients receiving no further treatment following mastectomy during 1977–81 and followed up for eight years.

In a trial carried out in Denmark during 1975–78 with follow-up until 1988 of tamoxifen therapy (30 mg/day) for two years in women who were admitted for breast tumour (stage I, II and III), Palshof (1988) reported two endometrial cancers in 52 tamoxifen-treated postmenopausal patients (< 70 years old) and none in 52 patients in the placebo group. In premenopausal women, no case was found in either 112 tamoxifen-treated patients or 101 placebo patients.

In the IBCSG (International Breast Cancer Study Group) trial of tamoxifen (20 mg/day) plus low-dose prednisone (7.5 mg/day) therapy for one year, no endometrial cancer was observed in either 167 treated patients aged 66–80 years with operable breast cancer or 153 women randomized to observation (Castiglione *et al.*, 1990). Subjects were entered into this trial during 1978–81 and were followed up for a median observation time of eight years.

A Danish study (Andersson *et al.*, 1992) reported seven cases of endometrial cancer among 864 postmenopausal patients receiving radiotherapy and 30 mg tamoxifen for 48 weeks compared with two cases among 846 patients receiving radiotherapy alone. Eleven cases were reported among a third group of 1828 untreated, 'low-risk' patients. SIRs for endometrial cancer were computed from the incidence rates of the female Danish population. [The most valid comparison was between women with and without tamoxifen treatment in the radiotherapy group.] The SIRs for endometrial cancer were 1.9 (95% CI, 0.8–3.9) for patients who received radiotherapy and tamoxifen and 0.6 (95% CI, 0.1–2.1) for patients who received radiotherapy without tamoxifen (ratio of the SIRs, 3.3 (95% CI, 0.6–31).

After a maximal follow-up of 13 years, Ribeiro and Swindell (1992) reported one case of endometrial cancer among 282 postmenopausal patients ≤ 70 years old treated with tamoxifen (20 mg/day) for one year and one endometrial cancer among 306 untreated patients. There was no case of endometrial cancer among 199 premenopausal patients randomized to tamoxifen treatment or 174 patients randomized to irradiation-induced menopause.

In a trial in postmenopausal women, < 71 years old, in Sweden, of radiotherapy alone (236 patients), radiotherapy plus tamoxifen (30 mg/day) for one year (239 patients) or the same tamoxifen regimen alone (244 patients), two, four and five cancers of the corpus uteri were reported, respectively (Rydén *et al.* 1992). One endometrial cancer death was reported in the group receiving radiotherapy only. The median follow-up period was nine years.

In a Scottish trial of tamoxifen treatment (20 mg/day) for five or more years, Stewart and Knight (1989) found three uterine sarcomas in 539 tamoxifen-treated postmenopausal patients and two endometrial cancers in 531 untreated patients. In a subsequent set of 374 adjuvant tamoxifen-treated patients and 373 untreated patients, one endometrial cancer was observed in each group (Stewart, 1992). In another report of the same trial (Nayfield et al., 1991), four cases of endometrial cancer were reported among 661 tamoxifen-treated patients and two cases among 651 untreated patients.

The ECOG (Eastern Cooperation Oncology Group) in the United States open to accrual during 1978–82 (Cummings et al., 1993) found one case of endometrial cancer among 85 treated patients 65–84 years old (20 mg/day tamoxifen for two years) and another case among 83 placebo patients.

In a trial of the Cooperative Group for Chemohormonal Therapy of Early Breast Cancer (GROCTA) in Italy comparing tamoxifen (30 mg/day) for five years with six cycles of cyclophosphamide + methotrexate + 5-fluorouracil followed by four cycles of epidoxorubicin or a combination of the two, no case of endometrial cancer was seen among the 168 patients randomized to tamoxifen alone or among the 165 patients randomized to chemotherapy. One case was observed among 94 postmenopausal women who received both treatments. Women were 35–65 years old (Boccardo et al., 1994a).

In a large placebo-controlled trial, the National Surgical Adjuvant Breast and Bowel Project in Canada and the United States in 1982–88, Fisher et al. (1994) reported 15 cases of endometrial cancer among women with invasive breast cancer randomized to tamoxifen (20 mg/day) for five years compared with two cases among the placebo group. It was known at randomization that the proportion of women with hysterectomy was similar in the two groups. Both of the placebo patients with endometrial cancer had received tamoxifen for breast cancer relapse. One of the 15 patients who developed endometrial cancer was allocated to tamoxifen but never received it. One of the 15 endometrial cancers after review was found not to be a cancer. The annual hazard rate in the treated group was 1.6/1000 compared to 0.2/1000 in the placebo group. The latter rate was below that of the general population, from which about seven cancers would have been expected. The relative risk estimates were 7.5 (95% CI, 1.7–32.7) using the placebo control group and 2.2 [95% CI, 1.2–2.9] using population rates. The histological characteristics and grades of endometrial cancer were similar to those in patients who had not been treated with tamoxifen; 9/15 were grade 1 and 11 were stage I. Four patients allocated to tamoxifen died of endometrial cancer (among whom one never received the treatment). [The Working Group noted that the most valid comparison was between the group allocated to tamoxifen and the placebo control group. The rates used for calculating the expected numbers were from the United States SEER Program, whereas seven of the 12 major contributing centres were from Canada, where the rates for endometrial cancer are lower than in the United States.]

Kedar et al. (1994) in the United Kingdom recruited a randomized cohort of healthy postmenopausal women with a family history of breast cancer into groups given tamoxifen (20 mg/day) (61) or placebo (50) [duration of treatment not specified]. Fifty-five of the treated women had detectable serum levels of tamoxifen. No endometrial cancer was found in either group (median follow-up period, two years). [The Working Group noted the small numbers and short follow-up period.]

The SWOG (Southwest Oncology Group) in the United States (Rivkin *et al.*, 1994) reported two cases of endometrial cancer among 295 postmenopausal patients treated with tamoxifen alone, three cases among 303 patients given tamoxifen and chemotherapy and none among 300 patients given chemotherapy alone during 1979–89.

Fornander *et al.* (1989) and Rutqvist *et al.* (1995) reported a study of endometrial cancer in the trial of treatment of postmenopausal women < 71 years old with tamoxifen (40 mg/day) for two or five years. 'Low-risk' patients (1774) and 'high-risk' patients (955) were randomized to tamoxifen or no tamoxifen; 678 of the 'high-risk' patients were also randomized to receive either radiotherapy or chemotherapy. Of the patients who received tamoxifen for two years, 809 were re-randomized to stop treatment or receive an additional three years of tamoxifen therapy. After a median follow-up time of nine years, 23 (one refused to take tamoxifen) endometrial cancers were found in 1372 patients randomized to tamoxifen versus four in 1357 untreated women (RR, 5.6; 95% CI, 1.9–16.2). Other corpus uteri cancers were reported: one in the tamoxifen-allocated group and three in the untreated group. A joint analysis of three Scandinavian trials (in Stockholm, Denmark (Andersson *et al.*, 1992) and the south Sweden (Rydén *et al.*, 1992)) presented in the same paper also showed a significant increase in the risk for endometrial cancer in tamoxifen-allocated patients (RR, 4.1; 95% CI, 1.9–8.9). Fornander *et al.* (1993) provided further details of 22 of the cases in the Stockholm trial, 17 of whom had actually received tamoxifen (out of 19 patients assigned to receive it). All cases were grade 1 or grade 2, and all but three were stage I. Endometrial cancer developed less than two years from the beginning of tamoxifen treatment in five of the 17 treated cases and after five years in four cases. Nine cases had received radiotherapy and two others had received chemotherapy. There were three deaths from endometrial cancer among the 17 cases receiving tamoxifen.

2.2 Breast cancer

2.2.1 *Case–control study*

Cook *et al.* (1995) conducted the only case–control study that considered contralateral breast cancer. A total of 188 (18 receiving tamoxifen) < 85-year-old cases in Washington State, United States, were matched to 328 (58 receiving tamoxifen) controls without second primary cancer as described in Section 2.1.3. A 50% reduction in new breast tumours was observed for any use of tamoxifen (matched odds ratio, 0.5; 95% CI, 0.3–0.9) and an increased protection in women who used tamoxifen for more than one year (matched odds ratio, 0.4; 95% CI, 0.2–0.9). Odd ratios for any use of tamoxifen were somewhat larger in premenopausal than in postmenopausal women (0.7 versus 0.4), but were similar in pre- and postmenopausal women who used tamoxifen for more than one year (0.3 versus 0.4).

2.2.2 Cohort study

In the study by Curtis *et al.* (1996) (described in Section 2.1.4) of 87 323 breast cancer patients reported to the United States SEER Program, tamoxifen-treated patients had an SIR for contralateral breast cancer of 1.1 (95% CI, 1.0–1.3), compared with an SIR of 1.6 (95% CI, 1.5–1.7) for patients not known to have received tamoxifen. This represents a significant reduction [of approximately 30%] in the risk for contralateral breast cancer in tamoxifen-treated patients.

2.2.3 Randomized clinical trials

Results of trials of contralateral breast cancer following tamoxifen treatment are summarized in Table 5.

In Canada, Pritchard *et al.* (1987) (updated by Nayfield *et al.*, 1991) found no difference in the risk of contralateral breast cancer: 3 cases in 198 tamoxifen-treated patients and 3 cases in 202 untreated patients.

In a trial of tamoxifen (20 mg/day) for two years versus no treatment, the NATO (Nolvadex Adjuvant Trial Organization) (1988) and Nayfield *et al.* (1991) reported 15 contralateral tumours in 564 tamoxifen-treated patients and 17 in 567 untreated patients.

A Danish study (Andersson *et al.*, 1992) reported 8 cases of contralateral breast cancer occurring at least one year after the first primary cancer among 864 patients receiving radiotherapy and tamoxifen (30 mg/day) for 48 weeks compared with 10 cases among 846 patients receiving radiotherapy alone. A third group of 1828 untreated, 'low-risk' patients [with longer survival] experienced 10 cases in this period.

Baum *et al.* (1992), of the Cancer Research Campaign Breast Cancer Trials Group in the United Kingdom, in a 2 × 2 trial of 20 mg/day tamoxifen or perioperative cyclophosphamide found no overall effect of tamoxifen on contralateral breast tumours (RR, 0.9; 95% CI, 0.5–1.5). However, a reduction was seen in postmenopausal women (RR, 0.5; 95% CI, 0.2–1.1), but not in premenopausal women (RR, 1.4; 95% CI, 0.6–3.3).

After a maximal 13 years of follow-up, Ribeiro and Swindell (1992) reported seven cases of contralateral breast cancer in 282 postmenopausal patients treated with tamoxifen (20 mg/day) for one year and nine in 306 untreated patients.

In a trial in southern Sweden of radiotherapy alone (236 patients), radiotherapy plus tamoxifen (30 mg/day) for one year (239 patients) or the same tamoxifen regimen alone (244 patients), 15, 11 and 9 contralateral breast cancers were reported, respectively (Rydén *et al.*, 1992).

In a Scottish trial of tamoxifen (20 mg/day) treatment for five or more years, Stewart (1992) found seven contralateral breast cancers in 374 tamoxifen-treated patients and 20 in 373 untreated patients.

The ECOG (Eastern Cooperative Oncology Group) group (Cummings *et al.*, 1993) found one case of contralateral breast cancer among 85 patients treated with tamoxifen (20 mg/day) for two years and five among 83 untreated patients.

In a trial of the Cooperative Group for Chemohormonal Therapy of Early Breast Cancer (GROCTA) in Italy comparing tamoxifen (30 mg/day) for five years against

Table 5. Contralateral breast cancers: summary results of randomized clinical trials of adjuvant use of tamoxifen

Reference, country	No. of patients and treatment		Dose of tamoxifen (mg/day)	Duration (years)	Median follow-up (years)	No. of contralateral breast cancers	Odds ratio (95% CI)
Pritchard et al. (1987) (updated by Nayfield, 1991) Canada	198 202	Tamoxifen Observation	20	2	5.8	3 3	[1.0 (0.2–5.0)]
NATO (1988) (updated by Nayfield et al., 1991) United States	564 567	Tamoxifen Observation	20	2	5.5	15 17	[0.9 (0.4–1.8)]
Palshof (1988) Denmark	164 153	Tamoxifen Placebo	30	2	9	3 4	[0.7 (0.2–3.1)]
Castiglione et al. (1990) Several countries	167 153	Tamoxifen + prednisone Observation	20	1	8	1 4	[0.2 (0.03–2.0)]
Andersson et al. (1992) Denmark	864 846	Tamoxifen + LRT LRT	30	0.9	8	8 10	[0.8 (0.3–2.0)]
Ribeiro & Swindell (1992a) United Kingdom	199 174	Pre-menopausal Tamoxifen Pelvic irradiation	20	1	Max. 13	3 2	[1.3 (0.2–7.6)]
	282 306	Post-menopausal Tamoxifen Observation	20	1	Max. 13	7 9	[0.8 (0.3–2.2)]

Table 5 (contd)

Reference, country	No. of patients and treatment		Dose of tamoxifen (mg/day)	Duration (years)	Median follow-up (years)	No. of contralateral breast cancers	Odds ratio (95% CI)
Rydén et al. (1992) Southern Sweden	244	Tamoxifen	30	1	9	9	[0.6 (0.3–1.3)]
	239	Tamoxifen + LRT				11	[0.7 (0.3–1.5)]
	236	LRT				15	
Stewart (1992) Scotland	374	Tamoxifen	20	≥ 5	4–10	7	[0.3 (0.1–0.8)]
	373	Observation				20	
Cummings et al. (1993) United States	85	Tamoxifen	20	2	10	1	[0.2 (0.02–1.6)]
	83	Placebo				5	
Boccardo et al. (1994a) Italy	168	Tamoxifen	30	5	≥ 5	0	—
	171	Tamoxifen + Chemotherapy				1	
	165	Chemotherapy				4	[0.2 (0.03–2.1)]
Fisher et al. (1994) Canada, United States	1419	Tamoxifen	20	5	8	30	[0.6 (0.4–1.0)]
	1424	Placebo				49	
Rutqvist et al. (1995) Stockholm, Sweden	1372	Tamoxifen	40	2	9	40	0.6 (0.4–0.9)
	1357	Observation				66	

LRT, localized radiation therapy

chemotherapy or a combination of the two, four contralateral breast tumours were seen in the 165 patients randomized to chemotherapy, one contralateral tumour in the 171 patients who received both treatments and none in the 168 patients who received tamoxifen alone (Boccardo et al., 1994a).

In a placebo-controlled trial of tamoxifen (20 mg/day) for five years, Fisher et al. (1994) found 30 primary contralateral tumours in 1419 patients who received tamoxifen in the first five years of follow-up compared with 49 cases among 1424 patients receiving placebo. The reduction in incidence rate was 42%.

In a Swedish trial of treatment with tamoxifen (40 mg/day) for two or five years, Rutqvist et al. (1995) reported 40 contralateral tumours in 1372 women in the tamoxifen group and 66 in 1357 untreated patients. The risk ratio was 0.6 (95% CI, 0.4–0.9).

All of the studies mentioned above, and many other randomized trials, were included in an overview of data available up to 1990 on the occurrence of contralateral breast cancer in women allocated to tamoxifen treatment in trials (EBCTCG (Early Breast Cancer Trialists' Collaborative Group), 1992). In contrast to the analyses in some of the original reports, the life table method of analysis was used in this overview. Based on the occurrence of 122 contralateral breast cancers in 9128 tamoxifen-allocated women and 184 breast cancers in 9135 control patients, a 39% reduction in risk for contralateral breast cancer was observed ($p < 0.00001$). The effects were greater in trials using longer duration of tamoxifen treatment (reductions of risk were 26% for less than two years of tamoxifen treatment, 37% for two years of treatment and 53% for more than two years of treatment), although this was not statistically significant.

2.3 Liver cancer

2.3.1 Case report

Johnstone et al. (1991) reported a single case of primary hepatocellular carcinoma in a woman who had received 20 mg tamoxifen daily and chemotherapy. The tumour developed six months after treatment began.

2.3.2 Cohort studies

There is probably some under-reporting of primary liver cancer in follow-up studies of breast cancer patients, because of confusion of these tumours with metastases from the breast.

Mühlemann et al. (1994) examined the incidence of hepatocellular cancer from 1974 to 1989 in white women aged 50 years or more with breast cancer in the United States and found no evidence of an increase after the introduction of tamoxifen in 1977.

Curtis et al. (1996) reported on liver cancer risk in 87 323 breast cancer patients reported to the United States SEER Program (see Section 2.1.4). In tamoxifen-treated patients, three cases of liver cancer were observed (SIR, 1.1; 95% CI, 0.2–3.2) and, in the larger group of patients not known to have received tamoxifen, eight cases were seen (SIR, 0.4; 95% CI, 0.2–0.7). [The Working Group noted that the low SIR for liver cancer in patients not known to have received tamoxifen may indicate underascertainment of liver cancers following breast cancer.]

2.3.2 *Randomized clinical trials*

In the Swedish trial (see p. 274), Rutqvist *et al.* (1995) reported three cases of hepatobiliary (two liver) cancer among subjects randomized to tamoxifen (40 mg/day) for two or five years and one case among untreated patients. Two of the three cases had been treated for 20 and 46 months, respectively (Rutqvist, 1993). Verification of the exposure was not reported for the third case.

The Danish study by Andersson *et al.* (1991) (see p. 271) reported one case of hepatobiliary cancer among 864 treated breast cancer patients (30 mg/day tamoxifen for 48 weeks + radiotherapy) and two cases among 846 radiation-treated breast cancer patients.

A study from southern Sweden (Rydén *et al.* 1992) reported two cases of hepatobiliary cancer among 244 patients who had received tamoxifen (30 mg/day) for one year, no case among 239 patients who had received tamoxifen plus radiotherapy and no case among 236 patients treated with radiotherapy alone.

No case of liver cancer was reported among 1419 tamoxifen-treated (20 mg/day for 5 years) patients and 1424 controls in the NSABP (National Surgical Adjuvant Breast and Bowel Project) B-14 trial (Fisher *et al.*, 1994).

2.4 Other cancers

2.4.1 *Case reports*

Reports exist of one case of papillary mucinous endocervical adenocarcinoma, one in-situ and one invasive fallopian tube adenocarcinoma, one endometrioid carcinoma of the pelvic endometrium, one endometrioid carcinoma, one granulosa cell tumour of the ovary and one leiomyosarcoma of the myometrium uteri among women treated with tamoxifen (see Table 1).

2.4.2 *Case–control study*

Cook *et al.* (1995) reported on a population-based study of ovarian, endometrial and contralateral breast cancers following tamoxifen therapy of breast cancer patients. The results for endometrium and breast cancer have been reported above (pp. 267–268 and 274). For ovarian cancer, 34 cases (6 given tamoxifen) were compared with 89 controls who did not develop a second primary cancer, of whom 18 were given tamoxifen (matched odds ratio, 0.6; 95% CI, 0.2–1.8).

2.4.3 *Cohort studies*

Curtis *et al.* (1996) reported the risks for various second cancers in 87 323 breast cancer patients reported to the United States SEER Program (see p. 269). Between patients who had initial tamoxifen treatment and those not known to have received such treatment, there was no difference in the risks for ovarian cancer, digestive tract cancers or cancers at various other sites (other than endometrial cancer and contralateral breast cancer). The observed/expected ratios for all digestive system cancers combined were 1.0 (95% CI, 0.9–1.2) in tamoxifen-treated women and 0.9 (95% CI, 0.9–1.0) in women not known to have received tamoxifen treatment.

2.4.3 Randomized clinical trials

Two reports of randomized trials have been published which address the risks for second cancers other than those of the endometrium, breast and liver.

In a large trial (see p. 273), Fisher et al. (1994) found no significant difference between women allocated to tamoxifen and women allocated to placebo in the risk for second cancers of the colon, rectum, ovary or other sites.

In a joint analysis of three Scandinavian trials (see p. 274), Rutqvist et al. (1995) reported an excess risk for gastrointestinal cancer in tamoxifen-allocated women compared with those in untreated groups (RR, 1.9; 95% CI, 1.2–2.9). The relative risk for colorectal cancer was 1.9 (95% CI, 1.1–3.3) and that for stomach cancer was 3.2 (95% CI, 0.9–11.7). For other sites, no difference was observed between tamoxifen-allocated patients and untreated patients. [In view of the number of comparisons made, these results should be interpreted with caution.]

3. Studies of Cancer in Experimental Animals

In the studies reviewed here, the usual form of tamoxifen citrate will be referred to as tamoxifen.

3.1 Oral administration

3.1.1 Mouse

In a study reported in a monograph, groups of 25 male and 25 female Alderley Park Strain 1 mice [age unspecified] were given 0 (control), 5 or 50 mg/kg bw tamoxifen [purity not specified] per day by gastric instillation for three months. The mice were then maintained for 12 months on a diet containing tamoxifen at concentrations to provide 0, 5 or 50 mg/kg bw tamoxifen, after which the experiment was terminated because of skeletal abnormalities in many of the exposed mice. Numbers surviving at 15 months were 16/25 control, 11/25 low-dose and 17/25 high-dose males and 15/25 control, 17/25 low-dose and 12/25 high-dose females. In males, interstitial cell tumours of the testes were found in 0/25 control, 2/25 low-dose and 21/25 high-dose animals. In females, granulosa-cell adenomas of the ovary were found in 0/25 control, 9/25 low-dose and 9/25 high-dose animals. Two other studies at lower doses were briefly described (Tucker et al., 1984). [The Working Group noted that the descriptions of these lower-dose studies did not provide sufficient information for evaluation.]

3.1.2 *Rat*

Groups of 51 male and 52 female Alderley Park Wistar-derived rats, five weeks of age, were given 5, 20 or 35 mg/kg bw tamoxifen [purity not specified] per day by gastric instillation in 0.5% hydroxypropyl methylcellulose for two years. A control group of 102 male and 104 female rats was given the vehicle alone. Moribund animals and those surviving to the end of the exposure period were killed and subjected to necropsy; all major tissues were examined histologically. Growth was reduced (by about 30% in females and 40% in males) in all tamoxifen-treated groups compared with controls. Survival was reduced in the groups given the two higher doses but increased in those given the lower dose. The reduced survival was attributed to early deaths from liver tumours and resulted in termination of the study at 87 weeks for the mid-dose group and at 71 weeks for the high-dose group. Hepatocellular adenomas occurred in 1/102 control, 8/51 low-dose, 11/51 mid-dose and 8/51 high-dose males and in 1/104 control, 2/52 low-dose, 6/52 mid-dose and 9/52 high-dose females ($p < 0.0001$ for trend). Hepatocellular carcinomas were found in 1/102 control, 8/51 low-dose, 34/51 mid-dose and 34/51 high-dose males and in 0/104 control, 6/52 low-dose, 37/52 mid-dose and 37/52 high-dose females [$p < 0.001$]. Hepato/cholangiocellular carcinomas were found in 0/102 control, 0/51 low-dose, 2/51 mid-dose and 5/51 high-dose males and in 0/104 control, 0/52 low-dose, 4/52 mid-dose and 5/52 high-dose females ($p < 0.0001$ for trend). No increase in the incidence of tumours was observed at any other site. Significant decreases in tumour incidence were observed in the pituitary and parathyroid glands of males and in the pituitary and mammary glands of females (see Table 6) (Greaves *et al.*, 1993). [The Working Group noted that part of the reduction in tumour rates may have been related to decreased body-weight gain.]

In a study that also evaluated toremifene, groups of 57, 84 and 75 female Sprague-Dawley [Crl:CD(BR)] rats, approximately six weeks of age, were given 0, 11.3 and 22.6 mg/kg bw tamoxifen (99% pure) per day by gastric instillation in 0.5% carboxymethylcellulose on seven days per week for up to 12 months followed by a three-month recovery period. Nine rats from each group were killed at three and six months. At 12 months, 18 control, 36 low-dose and 24 high-dose rats were killed. The experiment was terminated at 15 months. All rats, including those found dead or moribund, were subjected to necropsy; organs examined histopathologically included liver, ovaries, uterus, mammary gland, adrenal glands, kidneys, tail bone, sternum, brain and pituitary. Weight gain in both groups receiving tamoxifen was less than that in controls. In the group killed at 15 months, uterine weights were significantly reduced in both high- and low-dose treated groups. A significant increase in the incidence of hepatocellular carcinomas occurred in both treated groups, compared with controls. At 12 months, the incidence of hepatocellular carcinomas was 0/18 control, 16/36 low-dose and 24/24 high-dose animals ($p < 0.001$); that at 15 months was 0/13, 13/21 and 8/9, respectively ($p < 0.001$). The incidence of hyperplasia in the mammary gland and the incidence of pituitary adenomas were decreased in tamoxifen-treated animals (Hard *et al.*, 1993). [The Working Group noted the small numbers of animals, that the exposure was for one year and that the study was terminated at 15 months.]

Table 6. Incidence (%) of tumours in Alderley Park Wistar-derived rats exposed to tamoxifen

Tumour	Dose (mg/kg bw per day)			
	0	5	20	35
Females				
Mammary adenocarcinomas[a]	9	0	0	0
Pituitary adenomas[b]	73	0	0	0
Liver adenomas[b]	1	4	12	17
Liver carcinomas[b]	0	12	71	71
Males				
Pituitary adenomas[c]	14	2	0	0
Parathyroid gland adenomas[d]	10	0	0	0
Liver adenomas[b]	1	16	22	16
Liver carcinomas[b]	1	16	67	67

From Greaves et al. (1993)
[a] $p < 0.02$, trend test
[b] $p < 0.0001$, trend test
[c] $p = 0.009$, trend test
[d] $p = 0.003$, trend test

In a study that also included toremifene, groups of 20 female Sprague-Dawley rats, six weeks of age, were given 0, 11.3 or 45 (maximum tolerated dose, MTD) mg/kg bw tamoxifen (purity > 99%) in carboxymethylcellulose per day by gastric instillation on seven days per week for up to one year. Five animals from each group were killed after 26 weeks and 52 weeks of treatment; all surviving rats were killed 65 weeks after the beginning of treatment. Weight gain was reduced in both tamoxifen-treated groups. No tumour was found in animals killed at 26 weeks. At 52 weeks, the incidences of hepatocellular carcinomas were 0/5 control, 0/5 low-dose and 3/5 high-dose animals; those at 65 weeks were 0/8, 0/8 and 5/6, respectively. Histopathological findings in tissues other than the liver were not reported (Hirsimäki et al., 1993). [The Working Group noted the small numbers of animals, that the exposure was for one year and that the study was terminated at 65 weeks.]

Groups of 55–57 female Sprague-Dawley [Crl:CD(BR) Charles River] rats, six weeks of age, were given 0, 2.8, 11.3 or 45.2 mg/kg bw tamoxifen [purity not specified] per day by gastric instillation in 0.5% carboxymethylcellulose on seven days per week for up to 12 months, followed by a three-month recovery period. Mortality was 5.3% in control, 9.0% in low-dose, 1.7% in mid-dose and 40% in high-dose animals. All tamoxifen-treated animals had weight gain depression and some developed alopecia. Among the seven high-dose rats examined at six months, five had adenomas and two had carcinomas. At 12 months of exposure, the incidences of hepatic adenomas were 5/10 mid-dose and 2/4 high-dose rats. The incidence of liver carcinomas in these groups was 1/10 and 3/4, respectively. During the three months of recovery, the occurrence of carcinomas in the mid-dose group increased to 5/11. No liver tumour was seen in control or low-dose groups (Williams *et al.*, 1993). [The Working Group noted that exposure was for only one year and that the study was terminated at 15 months.]

In a study that included toremifene, groups of five female Sprague-Dawley rats, six weeks of age, were given 0, 11.3 or 45 (MTD) mg/kg bw tamoxifen (purity > 99%) per day by gastric instillation in 0.5% carboxymethylcellulose seven days per week for 12 months. Groups were killed at 12 months or after a further 13 weeks of recovery. The incidence of liver tumours (hepatocellular carcinomas) at 12 months was 0/5 control, 0/5 low-dose and 4/5 high-dose animals; that at 65 weeks was 0/5, 0/5 and 5/5, respectively (Ahotupa *et al.*, 1994). [The Working Group noted the small number of animals and that the exposure was for only one year.]

In a study that also included droloxifene, groups of 50 male and 50 female rats [strain and age not specified] were given to 0 (control), placebo [not specified] or 36 mg/kg bw tamoxifen [purity not specified] in the diet for 24 months. The incidences of hepatocellular carcinomas were: males — control, 0/50; placebo, 0/50; tamoxifen, 49/50; females — control, 0/50; placebo, 0/50; tamoxifen, 50/50 (Hasmann *et al.*, 1994). [The Working Group noted the lack of experimental detail.]

Groups of 10 female Fischer (344/Tox), Wistar (LAC-P) and Lewis (LEW Oka) rats, six weeks of age, were fed either basal diet or diets containing 420 mg/kg diet (ppm) tamoxifen (purity > 98%) until 50% mortality was reached, at which time all surviving animals were killed. In groups of five rats killed after 90 days of exposure, the incidence of hepatocellular altered foci was increased in the Wistar and Lewis animals (Table 7). In rats killed at 180 days, no liver tumour was present in controls, while, in treated rats, the incidence was 3/5 in Wistar, 1/5 in Lewis and 0/5 in Fischer rats. By 11 months, 50% of the tamoxifen-treated Wistar and Lewis rats developed palpable liver nodules or were in ill health and these animals were killed. In the Wistar and Lewis rats killed at or before 11 months, all 10 had multiple liver tumours of which one or more was a carcinoma. In Fischer rats, 50% mortality was reached at 20 months and the remaining animals were killed at this time. All 10 rats exhibited at least one hepatocellular carcinoma (Carthew *et al.*, 1995a).

In a compilation of three experiments also including toremifene, reported in the proceedings of a meeting, groups of 109, 25 or 104 female Sprague-Dawley rats [age not specified] were given tamoxifen (> 99% pure) at 0, 11.3 or 45.0 mg/kg bw per day 7 days per week, for 20, 26 or 52 weeks with recovery periods of 12 or 13 weeks. In the high-dose group, squamous-cell metaplasia of the endometrium was found in 10 rats, dysplasia with metaplasia in three and squamous-cell carcinoma in two. The carcinomas were found after 20 or 26 weeks of dosing and a recovery period of 12–13 weeks. Among control or low-dose animals, no lesion of the uterus was reported (Mäntylä *et al.*, 1995, 1996). [The Working Group noted the lack of study details.]

Table 7. Hepatocellular altered foci in tamoxifen-exposed rats at 90 days of treatment

Strain	Exposure	Foci per cm^2
Wistar	None	1.5 ± 0.4
	Tamoxifen	14.0 ± 2.2^a
Lewis	None	0.9 ± 0.3
	Tamoxifen	3.8 ± 1.0^a
Fischer	None	1.0 ± 0.6
	Tamoxifen	1.5 ± 0.6

From Carthew *et al.* (1995a)
$^a p < 0.05$

As part of a tumour-promotion study in which toremifene was also included, groups of 14–22 female Sprague-Dawley rats, weighing 130 ± 10 g [age not specified], were subjected to partial hepatectomy and two weeks later were exposed to tamoxifen [purity not specified] in the diet at concentrations of 0 (control), 250 or 500 mg/kg diet (ppm) for up to 18 months. Both exposures to tamoxifen suppressed body-weight gain. In animals killed at six months, uterine weights were reduced. At this time, increases were found in both the number and volume of hepatocellular altered foci identified by staining for γ-glutamyl transpeptidase. Incidences of hepatic neoplastic nodules were not increased. In the remaining animals killed at 18 months, hepatocellular carcinomas were found in 0/22 controls, 1/15 low-dose and 8/15 high-dose rats (Dragan *et al.*, 1995).

3.2 Subcutaneous administration

3.2.1 *Mouse*

In a study using a strain of mouse with a high incidence of mammary tumours, groups of female C3H/OUJ mice, received a subcutaneous implantation of a silastic capsule containing 28 mg tamoxifen (release, 125 μg/day for at least six months) [purity not specified] on the back at two weeks (11 mice) or at five weeks (15 mice) after a pregnancy/weaning cycle (3.5 months of age). A control group of 11 mice received implantations of a placebo silastic capsule at the start of the experiment. After 15 months, the percentage of mice with mammary tumours was 100% in the controls, about 20% in the group exposed to tamoxifen at two weeks and about 50% in the group exposed to tamoxifen at five weeks (Jordan *et al.*, 1990). [The Working Group noted that only the uterus and mammary glands were examined and only macroscopically.]

In a study using a strain of mouse with a high incidence of mammary tumours, two groups of 30 female C3H/OUJ mice, 2.5 months of age, were ovariectomized and two further groups of 30 females were left intact. Two weeks later, one ovariectomized and one intact group received an implantation of a silastic capsule containing 28 mg tamoxifen (release, approximately 125 μg/day for six months) [purity not specified]. The capsules were replaced every six months up to 17 months of treatment. Mice were observed up to 27 months of age. In the intact controls, the mammary tumour incidence was 100% by about 20 months of age. This was reduced to about 20% by tamoxifen. In ovariectomized mice, the incidence of mammary tumours was 50%, which was reduced to about 20% by tamoxifen. In a further experiment, four groups of 20 female C3H/OUJ mice, three months old, received a tamoxifen capsule implant for three, six or 12 months (capsule replaced at six months in this group). The incidence of mammary tumours in controls was 100% by 17 months, whereas all tamoxifen-treated groups had an incidence of about 25% (Jordan et al., 1991). [The Working Group noted that only the mammary gland was examined and only macroscopically.]

3.2.2 Rat

As part of a tumour-promotion study, groups of 10 female Sprague-Dawley rats, weighing 125–175 g [age not specified], were subjected to partial hepatectomy and, one week later, received subcutaneous implants of time-release tablets providing 0 or 50 µg/day tamoxifen. At four months, the body weights of treated rats were significantly lower than those of controls. The livers were examined for γ-glutamyl transpeptidase-positive altered hepatocellular foci. Controls had 0.07 ± 0.08 foci/cm^2, whereas tamoxifen-exposed rats had 1.11 ± 0.25 foci/cm^2 (Yager et al., 1986).

3.3 Administration with known carcinogens

3.3.1 Mouse

Groups of 25–70 female Swiss mice, six to eight weeks of age, were ovariectomized or left intact and were divided into seven groups, one of which was left untreated; the others received a beeswax-impregnated thread inserted into the canal of the uterine cervix; subcutaneous injection of olive oil thrice weekly; an intracervical insertion of thread impregnated with 3-methylcholanthrene (MCA); an MCA-impregnated thread plus subcutaneous injections of 50 µg/kg bw tamoxifen in olive oil three times per week; a beeswax thread plus tamoxifen; or tamoxifen alone. The experiment lasted for at least 393 days. Vaginocervical smears were taken to monitor cervical dysplasia and carcinoma. In intact mice, the incidence of cervical carcinoma in mice exposed to MCA was $60 \pm 8.2\%$, while, in mice receiving MCA and tamoxifen, it was $30 \pm 6.8\%$. No other intact mouse developed a carcinoma. In ovariectomized mice, the incidence of cervical carcinoma in the MCA-treated group was $62 \pm 7.2\%$ and that in the mice also receiving tamoxifen was $27 \pm 6.7\%$. No other ovariectomized mouse developed a carcinoma (Sengupta et al., 1991).

Groups of four to six male and female BALB/c/Bln mice, 8–12 weeks of age, were given intraperitoneal injections of diluted serum from leukaemic mice infected with the Rauscher murine leukaemia virus. Starting one day later, mice were given intraperitoneal injections of 0.2, 0.5 or 1 mg/animal tamoxifen [purity not specified] in dimethyl sulfoxide three times a week for three weeks (total doses, 1.6, 4 and 8 mg). At the end of treatment, the mice were killed and spleens were weighed as an index of leukaemic disease. Compared to the controls, the spleen weights of the tamoxifen-treated animals were about 60%, 45% and 20% in the low-, mid- and high-dose groups, respectively, indicative of reduced leukaemic activity (Sydow & Wunderlich, 1994).

3.3.2 Rat

A group of 36 male Fischer rats, approximately three months of age, was given a single gastric instillation of 100 mg/kg bw N-nitrosodiethylamine (NDEA), then fed a diet containing 200 mg/kg diet (ppm) 2-acetylaminofluorene (2-AAF) [duration not specified] and underwent partial hepatectomy. Six weeks after cessation of 2-AAF treatment, one group of 17 rats was maintained with no further treatment. The remaining rats were divided into three groups of seven, five and five animals that were given subcutaneous injections of 0.25, 1.0 and 2.5 mg/animal tamoxifen [purity not specified] in peanut oil twice a week. The experiment was terminated at 10 months. From graphic presentations, the incidence of liver malignancy [not further specified] was about 75% in controls and 10% in the low-dose, 25% in the mid-dose and 35% in the high-dose tamoxifen-treated groups (Mishkin *et al.*, 1985).

Groups of 7–15 female Sprague-Dawley rats, 50 ± 2 days of age, were given 12 mg 7,12-dimethylbenz[*a*]anthracene (DMBA) per animal as a single gastric instillation in sesame oil. After six weeks, when mammary tumours had reached about 1 cm in diameter, groups were treated with 0, 1.0, 3.0 or 7.5 mg/kg bw tamoxifen (> 98% pure) per day by gastric instillation for at least five weeks. The numbers of new tumours per animal were 3.0 ± 2.6 in controls and 2.0 ± 0.6 in low-dose, 2.1 ± 1.4 in mid-dose and 0.3 ± 0.5 in high-dose tamoxifen-treated groups (Kangas *et al.*, 1986) [The Working Group noted the small numbers of animals.]

Groups of 10 female Sprague-Dawley rats, weighing 125–175 g [age not specified], were given 25 mg/kg bw NDEA by intraperitoneal injection 24 h after partial hepatectomy (Yager & Shi, 1991). One week later, the animals received implants of a time-release tablet containing quantities of tamoxifen to give a daily release of 15 or 50 µg or no tamoxifen. At four months, liver samples were examined for γ-glutamyl transpeptidase-positive altered hepatocellular foci. The body weights of treated rats were substantially lower than those of controls. The incidence of altered foci per cm^2 was 0.9 ± 0.3 in controls, 7.1 ± 1.9 in low-dose and 4.9 ± 1.0 in high-dose tamoxifen-treated rats (Yager *et al.*, 1986).

Male Sprague-Dawley rats, eight weeks of age, were given 200 mg/kg bw NDEA by intraperitoneal injection and were allocated to four groups two weeks later: four rats were fed olive oil in the diet; 12 rats were fed 1 mg/animal tamoxifen (analytical grade) in the diet daily; eight rats were fed 0.5 mg/animal diethylstilboestrol (DES) in olive oil in the diet daily; and 11 rats were fed both DES and tamoxifen. At eight months, the incidence of altered foci in the liver was quantified using γ-glutamyl transpeptidase as a marker. The numbers of foci per cm^2 [derived from graphic presentations] were about 10 in the NDEA-treated rats, about 20 in the NDEA/tamoxifen-treated rats, about 16 in the NDEA/DES-treated rats and about 22 in the NDEA/DES/tamoxifen-treated rats. The lesions in the NDEA/tamoxifen-treated group were larger than those in the group given

NDEA alone, whereas, when tamoxifen was given with NDEA/DES, the lesions were smaller than with NDEA/DES alone (Kohigashi et al., 1988).

Groups of 20 female Sprague-Dawley rats, 50 days of age, were given 20 mg/animal DMBA in peanut oil by gastric instillation. Twenty-eight days later, one group was treated with 200 μg/animal tamoxifen per day by gastric instillation, the other one with peanut oil. At 100 days after DMBA administration, 75% of the rats given DMBA alone had developed mammary tumours, whereas, in the group also receiving tamoxifen, less than 20% had tumours. Cessation of tamoxifen treatment after four months led to the development of mammary tumours, so that by 4.5 months about 70% of animals had tumours (Robinson et al., 1988).

Groups of 12 female Sprague-Dawley rats, weighing 140–160 g [age not specified], and 12 female Fischer 344 rats, weighing 120–140 g [age not specified], were allocated to one of two protocols. To evaluate initiating activity, groups of Sprague-Dawley rats either remained untreated as controls or were fed diets containing 10 mg/kg diet (ppm) ethinyloestradiol, 400 ppm tamoxifen or ethinyloestradiol plus tamoxifen for six weeks. After seven days, all rats underwent partial hepatectomy and, on day 49 after a one-week recovery phase on basal diet, were fed a diet containing 200 ppm 2-AAF for two weeks; at the midpoint, they were given 1 mL [1.6 mg]/kg bw carbon tetrachloride by gastric instillation in corn oil. In order to evaluate promoting activity, groups of 12 Sprague-Dawley and 12 Fischer 344 rats were fed a diet containing 200 ppm 2-AAF for two weeks and, on day 7, were given 1 mL/kg bw carbon tetrachloride by gastric instillation in corn oil. On day 21, after a one-week recovery period, these groups were maintained as untreated controls or were fed diets containing 10 ppm ethinyloestradiol, 400 ppm tamoxifen or ethinyloestradiol plus tamoxifen for six weeks; on day 28 animals were subjected to partial hepatectomy. All treated rats showed reduced weight gain. Liver samples were examined for γ-glutamyl transpeptidase-positive altered hepatocellular foci. After the initiation protocol, the numbers of foci per cm^2 were 15.6 ± 6.5 in controls, 67.4 ± 10 in tamoxifen-treated rats, 68.2 ± 13.9 in ethinyloestradiol-treated rats and 140.7 ± 21.2 in ethinyloestradiol/tamoxifen-treated rats. In the promotion protocol, the numbers per cm^2 were 25.9 ± 6.9, 72.0 ± 13.0, 56 ± 10.4 and 98.5 ± 18.4 in the respective groups (Ghia & Mereto, 1989).

Thirty female Fischer 344 rats, weighing 130–200 g [age not specified], were subjected to partial hepatectomy and 24 h later were given 10 mg/kg bw NDEA by gastric instillation. After a two-week recovery period, nine rats were maintained on basal diet (controls), 11 rats were fed 250 mg/kg diet (ppm) tamoxifen [purity not specified] and 10 were fed 500 ppm tamoxifen in a semipurified diet for six months. At termination, livers were examined for altered hepatocellular foci with the help of a variety of histochemical markers. The numbers of foci per liver were 90 ± 30 in controls, and 5430 ± 310 in low-dose and 7280 ± 490 in high-dose tamoxifen-treated rats (Dragan et al., 1991a).

Groups of 6–12 female Fischer 344 rats weighing 125–150 g [age not specified] were subjected to partial hepatectomy and 24 h later were given 40 mg/kg bw tamoxifen [purity not specified] by gastric instillation. The animals were then maintained on a basal diet or a diet containing 500 mg/kg diet (ppm) phenobarbital. After six months, all rats were killed and slices of the three main lobes of the liver were used for enzymic histochemical demonstration of altered hepatocellular foci with the help of a variety of histochemical markers. The numbers of foci per liver were 100 ± 50 in controls, 130 ± 50 in those given tamoxifen alone and 370 ± 130 in those given tamoxifen followed by phenobarbital (Dragan et al., 1991b).

Three groups of 10 female Sprague-Dawley rats, seven weeks of age, were given 20 mg DMBA by gastric instillation in sesame oil; starting 92 days later, two of the groups were given 1.0 or 10.0 mg/kg bw tamoxifen by gastric instillation in 0.5% methylcellulose for seven days, while the third group received no further treatment. At 20 weeks, mammary tumours were found in 8/9 controls, 5/10 low-dose tamoxifen-treated rats and 7/9 high-dose tamoxifen-treated rats (Kawamura et al., 1991).

A group of 10 female Sprague-Dawley rats, weighing 200 g [age not specified], was given 0.5 mg/rat tamoxifen in peanut oil twice at a five-day interval by subcutaneous injection; one day after the last injection, the animals underwent partial hepatectomy and 24 h later received 10 mg/kg bw NDEA by gastric instillation. Another group of 10 rats was subjected to partial hepatectomy and NDEA treatment only (controls). At six weeks, the severity of altered hepatocellular foci [from graphic presentations] was graded as 1.8 in controls and 0 in tamoxifen-treated rats (Oredipe et al., 1992). [The Working Group noted that the evaluation of foci was semi-quantitative.]

Groups of female Sprague-Dawley rats [numbers not specified], 59 days of age, were given 5 mg/rat DMBA weekly by gastric instillation for four weeks. One group was also simultaneously given 10 mg/kg bw tamoxifen weekly by subcutaneous injection for four weeks. After 14 weeks, the incidence of mammary tumours was 100% and the multiplicity was 6.7 ± 0.8 tumours per animal in the DMBA-treated group. In the DMBA/-tamoxifen-treated group, the incidence was 49.5% and the multiplicity was 1.4 ± 0.2 tumours per animal. In a second experiment, two groups of rats were treated with DMBA by gastric instillation for four weeks. Beginning at week 9, one group was given 1 mg/kg bw tamoxifen twice daily by subcutaneous injection for three weeks. At 12 weeks, all animals were ovariectomized. A large percentage of tumours regressed. In the control group, 1.3 new tumours per rat appeared, whereas in the tamoxifen-treated rats 0.3 new tumours per rat developed. All new tumours that appeared in tamoxifen-treated rats were hormone-independent, whereas in controls, only 13% continued to grow (Fendl & Zimniski, 1992). It was subsequently reported that, following the cessation of tamoxifen treatment, some tumours resumed growth (Zimniski & Warren, 1993).

A group of 20 female Sprague-Dawley rats, 50 days of age, was given 50 mg/kg bw N-methyl-N-nitrosourea (MNU) as a single intravenous injection. When at least one mammary tumour had reached a diameter of 10 mm, the animals were given 6 mg/kg bw tamoxifen by gastric instillation on five days a week for four weeks. A positive control group of 50 female rats received the treatment with MNU alone. At the cessation of treatment (207 days), the multiplicity of mammary tumours was 1.1 in controls (median size, 10.2 cm^3) and 1.25 in the tamoxifen-treated group (median size, 2.5 cm^3) (Winterfeld et al., 1992).

Groups of female Sprague-Dawley rats, weighing 200–220 g [age not specified], received no treatment (control; 26 rats) or 1 mg/kg bw tamoxifen in propylene glycol by intraperitoneal injection 1 h (four rats) or 24 h (three rats) before a single intraperitoneal injection of 50 mg/kg bw NDEA. Other groups were subjected to partial hepatectomy (eight rats) or partial hepatectomy and 1 mg/kg bw tamoxifen (eight rats) 24 h before treatment with NDEA. Eight weeks after treatment, rats were killed and liver samples were examined for altered hepatocellular foci identified by glutathione S-transferase immunohistochemistry. Pretreatment for 1 h with tamoxifen increased the number of foci almost 2-fold and pretreatment for 24 h increased the number 3.4-fold (Servais & Galand, 1993).

Two groups of female OFA rats [number and age not specified], weighing 130–160 g, were given 20 mg/animal DMBA in sesame oil as a single gastric instillation. After seven weeks, one group was given 1 mg/kg bw tamoxifen in sesame oil or sesame oil alone by subcutaneous injection three times per week for six weeks. At 11 weeks, the mean number of mammary tumours in controls was 9.3 tumours per rat; in tamoxifen-treated rats, this was reduced by 17.2 ± 2.8% (Weckbecker *et al.*, 1994).

Groups of 34–35 male Sprague-Dawley rats, aged 25 days, were given 20 mg/kg bw 1,2-dimethylhydrazine weekly by subcutaneous injection for 20 weeks and were fed control diet or diets initially containing 4 mg/kg diet (ppm) tamoxifen [purity not specified], which was reduced to 2 ppm at 29 days, 1 ppm at 56 days and to 0.5 ppm at 65 days. Most animals were killed 65 days after the last injection of 1,2-dimethylhydrazine. Animals receiving tamoxifen displayed reduced body weights. Mortality was comparable in control and treated animals. The total number of colon adenocarcinomas and their distribution in the proximal and distal portions did not differ between the groups (Gershbein, 1994).

Groups of 16–20 female Fischer 344 rats, 130–150 g [age not specified], were subjected to partial hepatectomy and 24 h later were given 10 mg/kg bw NDEA in tricaprilyn or vehicle alone by gastric instillation. Two weeks later, groups of NDEA- or vehicle-exposed rats were fed 250 mg/kg diet (ppm) tamoxifen free base [purity not specified] in a semi-purified diet. Treatment with tamoxifen reduced body weights by 16–24%. Tamoxifen increased the incidence of liver tumours at 15 months in rats given NDEA (3/8 hepatocellular carcinomas versus 0/6 in rats given NDEA alone) (Dragan *et al.*, 1994).

In a study that also included toremifene, virgin Sprague-Dawley rats, aged 43 days, were randomized into groups of 20 and allocated to control diet or to diets containing 0.2 mg/kg diet (ppm) tamoxifen. Seven days later, groups were given either 50 mg/kg bw MNU or saline by intravenous injection. Animals were killed when moribund and the experiment was terminated at 180 days after MNU treatment. Tamoxifen did not affect the incidence, multiplicity or latency of mammary tumours compared with controls (Moon *et al.*, 1994). [The Working Group noted that the dose of MNU, producing 100% of tumours in the MNU- and MNU/tamoxifen-treated groups, may have been too high to allow the detection of a protective effect.]

In a tumour promotion study, in which toremifene was also studied, groups of 14–22 female Sprague-Dawley rats, weighing 130 ± 10 g [age not specified], were subjected to partial hepatectomy and 24 h later were given a single dose of 10 mg/kg bw NDEA in trioctanoin by gastric instillation. Two weeks later, the rats were given either basal diet or diet containing 250 or 500 mg/kg diet (ppm) tamoxifen for 18 months. All exposures to tamoxifen suppressed body-weight gain. Uterine weights were suppressed at six months. The number of altered hepatic foci identified by any of four histochemical markers as well as the volume of liver occupied by foci was increased by tamoxifen. At six months, the incidence of hepatic neoplastic nodules was: controls, 8/15; low-dose, 13/15; and high-dose, 11/15. At 18 months, the incidence of hepatocellular carcinomas in all groups approached 100% and the incidence of renal carcinomas was slightly increased by tamoxifen [$p = 0.008$, Cochran–Armitage trend test] (Table 8) (Dragan et al., 1995).

Table 8. Incidence of tumours in female Sprague-Dawley rats exposed to tamoxifen after NDEA

Exposure	Renal cell adenomas	Renal cell carcinomas	Hepatocellular carcinomas
None	5/19	0/19	2/17
Tamoxifen 250 ppm	5/18	0/18	11/18
Tamoxifen 500 ppm	5/8	2/8[a]	8/8

From Dragan et al. (1995)
[a] [$p = 0.008$, Cochran-Armitage trend test]

3.3.3 Hamster

Groups of 7–12 male Syrian hamsters, four to six weeks of age, received subcutaneous implants of one pellet containing either 25 mg 17β-oestradiol or 25 mg tamoxifen, or one pellet of each. All animals were killed after seven months. The number of kidney tumour-bearing animals was 3/3 oestradiol-treated hamsters examined, 2/8 oestradiol/tamoxifen-treated hamsters and 0/8 tamoxifen-treated hamsters. The multiplicity of kidney tumours was reduced from 6.5 with oestradiol to 1.0 in oestradiol/tamoxifen animals; tamoxifen alone produced no kidney tumour (Liehr et al., 1988).

Two groups of 5–20 male and female Armenian hamsters (*Cricetulus migratorius*), two to three months of age, received subcutaneous implants of 36-mg pellets of zeranol on study days 0 and 94. One group was given 5 mg/animal of tamoxifen by subcutaneous injection twice a week up to day 32 and then once a week until day 202, when the experiment was terminated. Among 9 males and 7 females receiving zeranol only, the incidence of hepatocellular carcinomas was about 60%, whereas in four males and four females also receiving tamoxifen, the incidence was reduced to 1–2% (Coe et al., 1992).

4. Other Data Relevant to an Evaluation of Carcinogenicity and its Mechanisms

In the studies reviewed here, tamoxifen citrate, if used, will be referred to as tamoxifen.

4.1 Absorption, distribution, metabolism and excretion

4.1.1 Humans

The absorption, distribution, metabolism and excretion of tamoxifen have been reviewed extensively (Furr & Jordan, 1984; Buckley & Goa, 1989; Wiseman, 1994). All studies have involved oral administration of tamoxifen citrate unless stated otherwise.

Tamoxifen is well absorbed after oral administration and appears to be more than 99% bound to plasma proteins (mostly to albumin) (Lien et al., 1989). Tamoxifen absorption shows wide interindividual variation, which is probably due to differences in liver metabolism and differences in absorption in the gastrointestinal tract. Administration of 40 mg/day for two months to patients with breast cancer produced steady-state mean plasma concentrations of tamoxifen of 186–214 ng/mL. The single maximum plasma concentrations in this study were about 70 ng/mL tamoxifen and about 20 or 40 ng/mL N-desmethyltamoxifen (the different values being with Tamoplex® and Nolvadex®, respectively) (McVie et al., 1986). Administration of a single 20-mg dose of tamoxifen to six male volunteers resulted in peak plasma concentrations of 42 ng/mL tamoxifen and 12 ng/mL N-desmethyltamoxifen. Maximal levels were achieved approximately 5 h after administration and area under the curve (AUC) was 2606 ng × h/mL (Adam et al., 1980). The distribution half-life (i.e. initial $t_{1/2}$) of tamoxifen is 7–14 h. The mean terminal half-life was 111 h, somewhat shorter than the previously reported seven days or more (Fromson et al., 1973a). Steady-state concentrations of tamoxifen and of N-desmethyltamoxifen were reached after three to four weeks of 20 mg b.i.d. (40 mg/day) administration (McVie et al., 1986) and after 4–8 weeks of 20 mg/day administration (Lien et al., 1995).

The apparent volume of distribution for tamoxifen in humans is 50–60 L/kg (Lien et al., 1989), indicating that most of the drug (99.9%) is present in peripheral compartments, which is suggestive of extensive tissue binding (Lien et al., 1991).

In healthy male volunteers given 40 mg tamoxifen, the plasma elimination half-life of tamoxifen during the first day was 10 h. However, after 34 h, appreciable levels of tamoxifen and N-desmethyltamoxifen were still present, suggesting a lengthening of half-life with increasing study duration or the existence of multiple half-lives (Guelen et al., 1987). The pharmacokinetics of tamoxifen appear to be biphasic, with a distribution phase of 7–14 h and an elimination phase of about seven days (Fromson et al., 1973a). The elimination half-life of N-desmethyltamoxifen is around seven days and 4-hydroxytamoxifen has a shorter half-life than tamoxifen (Buckley & Goa, 1989).

Tamoxifen and its metabolites are mostly excreted via bile into faeces as glucuronides and other conjugates. Urinary excretion is a very minor route of elimination (Furr & Jordan, 1984).

In seven premenopausal breast cancer patients and nine postmenopausal women with non-neoplastic diseases treated with tamoxifen for 56 days, the serum levels of N-didesmethyltamoxifen were higher in the postmenopausal women ($p < 0.02$). A similar trend was observed for N-desmethyltamoxifen ($p < 0.06$) (Lien et al., 1995).

Administration of 40 mg/day tamoxifen (20 mg twice a day) to primary breast cancer patients for 15–940 days (Daniel et al., 1981) resulted in plasma concentrations of 27–520 (mean, 300) ng/mL tamoxifen, 210–761 (mean, 462) ng/mL N-desmethyltamoxifen and 2.8–11.4 (mean, 6.7) ng/mL 4-hydroxytamoxifen. Concurrent tumour biopsy concentrations were 5.4–117 (mean, 25.1) ng tamoxifen/mg protein, 7.8–210 (mean, 52) ng N-desmethyltamoxifen/mg protein and 0.29–1.13 (mean, 0.53) ng 4-hydroxytamoxifen/mg protein.

After 14 daily doses of 40 mg tamoxifen, concentrations in plasma and in breast tumour cell nuclear and cytosolic fractions were measured in three patients (Murphy et al., 1987). The results are shown in Table 9.

Table 9. Concentrations of tamoxifen and its metabolites in plasma and breast tumour cells of three patients receiving 40 mg/day for 14 days

	Plasma (ng/mL)	Breast tumour cell fractions	
		Nucleus (ng/mg protein)	Cytosol (ng/mg protein)
Tamoxifen	363–745	8.0–11.1	8.1–18.5
N-Desmethyltamoxifen	185–422	3.6–7.9	6.6–26.8
4-Hydroxytamoxifen	1.4–3.1	0.16–0.26	0.02–0.36

From Murphy et al. (1987)

A number of metabolites (see Figure 1) have been identified in urine and plasma of human breast cancer patients by LC/MS/MS techniques. Plasma extracts contained tamoxifen, N-desmethyltamoxifen and tamoxifen-N-oxide (Poon et al., 1993). Glucuronides of four hydroxylated metabolites (4-hydroxytamoxifen, 4-hydroxy-N-desmethyltamoxifen, dihydroxytamoxifen and another monohydroxy- (possibly α-hydroxy-) N-desmethyltamoxifen) were detected in the patients' urine. In a more recent study, seven metabolites were identified in plasma (N-didesmethyltamoxifen, α-hydroxytamoxifen, 4-hydroxytamoxifen, tamoxifen-N-oxide, α-hydroxy-N-desmethyltamoxifen, 4-hydroxy-N-desmethyltamoxifen and 4-hydroxytamoxifen-N-oxide) (Poon et al., 1995).

In biopsy and autopsy samples taken from 14 patients, levels of tamoxifen and its metabolites (N-desmethyl, N-didesmethyl, 4-hydroxy and 4-hydroxy-N-desmethyl) were 10- to 60-fold higher in tissues (liver, lung, pancreas, brain, adipose) than in serum, being

Figure 1. Postulated metabolic pathways of tamoxifen

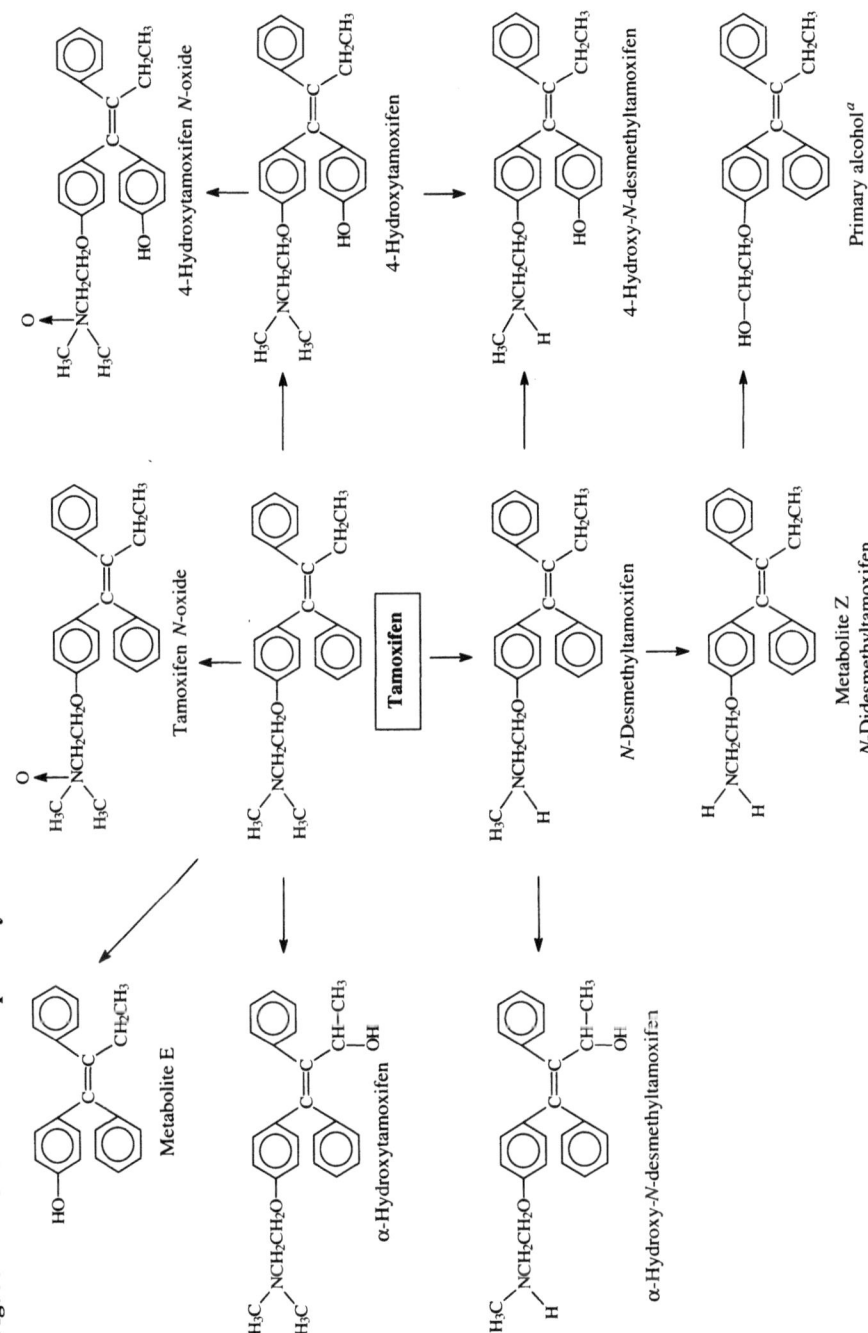

Adapted from Ruenitz & Nanavati (1990), Lien et al. (1991), Pongracz et al. (1995) and Poon et al. (1995)
[a] May be oxidized to the oxyacetic acid of tamoxifen and to 4-hydroxytamoxifen oxyacetic acid.

particularly high in liver and lung. Nine of the patients were in steady-state (treatment for more than 35 days), three had received tamoxifen for 7–13 days and two had received tamoxifen for 3–3.5 years (but had been tamoxifen-free for 28 days and 14 months, respectively, at the time of tissue sampling). Tissue samples from all other patients were obtained within 4–60 h. Tissues from the pancreas, pancreatic tumour, primary breast cancer and metastatic breast cancer in brain also retained large amounts of the drug. The amounts of N-demethylated and hydroxylated metabolites were high in most tissues except in fat, and tamoxifen and some of its metabolites were also present in specimens of skin and bone (Lien et al., 1991). Post-mortem and biopsy analysis of liver from tamoxifen-treated patients showed the presence of tamoxifen (0.14–15 nmol/g), 4-hydroxytamoxifen and N-desmethyltamoxifen (Martin et al., 1995).

4.1.2 Experimental systems

The kinetics, absorption, distribution, excretion and metabolism of tamoxifen in experimental animals have been reviewed (Furr & Jordan, 1984; Buckley & Goa, 1989; Wiseman, 1994).

In rats, mice, dogs and rhesus monkeys, tamoxifen is well absorbed following oral administration. Most of the dosed material appears in the faeces, but bile duct cannulation experiments with rats and dogs demonstrated that this was a result of biliary excretion (Fromson et al., 1973b).

In order to achieve similar plasma levels, much higher oral doses of tamoxifen are required by rats and mice than by human breast cancer patients: doses in rats over seven days of 3.0 mg/kg bw gave < 1 ng/mL and 200 mg/kg bw gave 1000 ng/mL; doses in mice over 7–10 days of 2.5 mg/kg bw gave < 10 ng/mL and 200 mg/kg bw gave 300 ng/mL; doses in human patients over 10 days of 4.9 mg/kg bw gave 1300 ng/mL (Robinson et al., 1991).

In rats given tamoxifen orally at 1 mg/kg bw per day for 3 or 14 days, essentially the same amounts of drug were found after three days and 14 days treatment (except for fat), suggesting that steady-state is obtained within three days. Concentrations of tamoxifen and its metabolites (N-desmethyl, N-didesmethyl, 4-hydroxy and 4-hydroxy-N-desmethyl) were 8–70-fold higher in tissues (brain, adipose, liver, heart, lung, kidney, uterus, testis) than in serum. The highest levels were found in lung and liver, but substantial amounts were also found in kidney and adipose tissue. Within one dosing interval (24 h), marked fluctuations in the tissue concentrations were observed in rats receiving the steady-state treatment, with maximum/minimum concentration (C_{max}/C_{min}) ratios for tamoxifen found in female rat lung and liver being 6.3 and 4.1, respectively (Lien et al., 1991).

Groups of female Fischer 344 rats were treated with a non-necrotic, subcarcinogenic dose of N-nitrosodiethylamine (10 mg/kg orally) and were given tamoxifen at 250 mg/kg of AIN-76A diet for 6 or 15 months (Dragan et al., 1994). Treatment with tamoxifen resulted in a decrease in body weight of 16–24% at serum levels comparable to the therapeutic level in humans. In serum, the ratio of tamoxifen/4-hydroxytamoxifen/N-desmethyltamoxifen was 1/0.1/0.5–1. Rat livers had 20–30 times more tamoxifen and

4-hydroxytamoxifen and at least 100 times more N-desmethyltamoxifen than the serum at both 6 and 15 months. The ratio in the liver after 6 or 15 months of continuous administration was 1/0.1/1.3–2.3.

Administration of [^{14}C]tamoxifen to dogs, rats, mice and rhesus monkeys has shown that tamoxifen has a long half-life in all of these species: in rats, the distribution half-life in blood was 53 h but the elimination half-life was 10 days. The route of excretion in rats, mice, rhesus monkeys and dogs is predominantly faecal, with virtually none of the recovered material being unchanged tamoxifen (Fromson et al., 1973b).

In rats, tamoxifen is eliminated in urine to a significant extent as the acidic metabolites. In one study, in the period 0–24 h after dosing with [^{14}C]tamoxifen, the radioactive components recovered (expressed as percentages of the administered dose) were: total radioactivity, 8.7%; tamoxifen acid, 1.02%; and 4-hydroxytamoxifen acid, 1.81%. In faeces, the corresponding values were 30.5%, 0.5% and 2.40%. In contrast to other tamoxifen metabolites, neither of these metabolites is excreted as glucuronic acid or glycine conjugates (Ruenitz & Nanavati, 1990).

Tamoxifen can be metabolized in vitro by both microsomal cytochrome P450 and flavin monooxygenase pathways to intermediates that bind irreversibly to microsomal proteins (Mani & Kupfer, 1991). Incubation of tamoxifen with rat liver microsomes yielded three major polar metabolites identified as the N-oxide, N-desmethyl and 4-hydroxy derivatives. Formation of the N-oxide was catalysed by flavin monooxygenase, while that of the N-desmethyl and 4-hydroxy metabolites was mediated by cytochrome P450. Tamoxifen N-demethylation appears to be catalysed in rats by CYP1A, CYP2C and CYP3A enzymes, while in man the evidence points to the CYP3A enzyme. However, these enzymes are not major contributors to the 4-hydroxylation of tamoxifen (Mani et al., 1993, 1994). Peroxidases may also metabolize tamoxifen to a reactive intermediate that binds covalently with protein (Davies et al., 1995) and DNA (Pathak & Bodell, 1994; Pathak et al., 1995).

Lim et al. (1994) compared the metabolism of tamoxifen in microsomes from female human, rat and mouse liver. The major metabolites formed by rat liver microsomes were 4-hydroxytamoxifen, 4′-hydroxytamoxifen, N-desmethyltamoxifen and tamoxifen N-oxide. In addition, it was suggested that two previously unreported epoxide metabolites, 3,4-epoxytamoxifen and 3′,4′-epoxytamoxifen, and their hydrolysed derivatives, 3,4-dihydroxytamoxifen and 3′,4′-dihydroxytamoxifen, had been identified, but these conclusions were based only upon mass spectral data; no synthetic standards were available. Jarman et al. (1995) were unable to confirm the existence of these dihydroxy compounds in microsomal incubates containing tamoxifen or deuterated analogues of tamoxifen. Using tamoxifen and [ethyl-D$_5$]tamoxifen, they showed a large isotope effect in the formation of α-hydroxytamoxifen (see Section 4.4). They confirmed the presence of α-hydroxytamoxifen-N-oxide and identified a new metabolite, α-hydroxy-N-desmethyltamoxifen.

Metabolites of tamoxifen were examined in human liver homogenate and a human hepatic G2 cell line treated with a mixture of tamoxifen and its deuterated analogues (Poon et al., 1995). In both the hepatic G2 cell line and the liver homogenate, α-hydroxytamoxifen, 4-hydroxytamoxifen, N-desmethyltamoxifen and tamoxifen N-oxide were detected. In the liver homogenate, N-didesmethyltamoxifen was also detected.

When primary cultures of human, rat and mouse hepatocytes were incubated with tamoxifen (10 µM) for 18–24 h, the concentration of α-hydroxytamoxifen in the medium was 50-fold lower in the human cultures (0.41 ± 0.55 ng/mL, two determinations) than in the rat (26.8 ± 10.1 ng/mL, three determinations) and mouse (18.9 ± 13.5 ng/mL, four determinations) cultures (Phillips et al., 1996a).

4.2 Toxic effects

4.2.1 Humans

The most reliable data regarding the association between tamoxifen and gynaecological symptoms come from randomized trials of tamoxifen versus placebo, in which some of these clinical data were collected prospectively.

The potential long-term toxicity of tamoxifen therapy has been reviewed. In large adjuvant trials, about 4% of recipients stop therapy because of side-effects (Love, 1989; Jaiyesimi et al., 1995). The most commonly reported side-effects of tamoxifen therapy are vasomotor symptoms, such as hot flushes and tachycardia, nausea and vomiting. A reduction over time in the vasomotor symptoms reported by patients receiving tamoxifen was observed in a randomized, double-blind, placebo-controlled clinical trial (Love & Feyzi, 1993). Atrophy is a common uterine response. Gynaecological adverse effects such as changes in vaginal discharge, bleeding, vaginal/external genitalia irritation, endometrial hyperplasia, polyps of the endometrium and, in premenopausal women, menstrual irregularities are summarized in Table 10.

Some evidence exists that tamoxifen may be associated with thromboembolic events in patients with advanced breast cancer. Table 11 summarizes studies regarding the effects of tamoxifen on blood coagulation. In general, the effects of tamoxifen on clotting factors are not clinically significant and probably do not persist during chronic (more than six months) administration or after cessation of therapy.

In a randomized trial of tamoxifen (20 mg/day for five years) versus placebo in pre- and postmenopausal women with breast cancer, thromboembolic disease was reported in 0.2% of women who received placebo versus 0.9% of those who received tamoxifen (Fisher et al., 1989a).

In a randomized controlled study, morbidity due to cardiac and thromboembolic disease was assessed in 2365 postmenopausal breast cancer patients with (40 mg/day, two or five years) or without tamoxifen therapy. The median follow-up period was six years. Tamoxifen therapy was associated with a statistically significantly reduced incidence of hospital admissions due to any cardiac disease, with a relative risk of 0.7 for tamoxifen for two and five years versus control (95% CI, 0.5–1.0; $p = 0.03$). In the randomized comparison of five versus two years of tamoxifen treatment, there was a statistically significant reduction in risk with longer treatment (relative risk, 0.4; 95% CI, 0.2–0.9; $p = 0.03$). Although the trend of reduced risk in the tamoxifen group was also evident in the analysis of specific subgroups of cardiac diseases such as myocardial infarct and ischaemic heart disease, the results failed to reach significance. There was no association between tamoxifen treatment and relative risk for admission to hospital due to thromboembolic disease (1.1; 95% CI, 0.7–1.6) (Rutqvist et al., 1993). In another study, a total of 1312 women who had undergone mastectomy for breast cancer were randomized to receive either adjuvant treatment with tamoxifen (20 mg/day) or a placebo, with tamoxifen given only on first recurrence of disease. The maximal duration of tamoxifen treatment was 14 years. Use of tamoxifen was associated with lower rates of myocardial infarction, the relative risk in the control group being 1.9 (95% CI, 1.0–3.7) compared with women allocated to tamoxifen treatment (McDonald et al., 1995).

Studies of beneficial effects of tamoxifen upon blood cholesterol levels, and increased levels of sex hormone-binding globulin and thyroid-binding globulin (Dewar et al., 1992; Love et al., 1994a) are summarized in Table 12. Tamoxifen and 4-hydroxytamoxifen have also been shown to protect human low-density lipoproteins in vitro against copper-ion dependent lipid peroxidation, a model system that is relevant to events occurring within atherosclerotic lesions (Wiseman et al., 1993; Wiseman, 1994). Tamoxifen also lowers the levels of atherogenic amino acid homocysteine in humans (see Table 12) (Anker et al., 1995).

Some studies of the effects of tamoxifen on bone mineral density suggest that tamoxifen acts as an oestrogen agonist to preserve bone density in postmenopausal breast cancer patients; however, the effects are weak and not consistent among the different studies (Table 13).

Over 20 years of use have made tamoxifen one of the most studied anti-cancer drugs (Jordan, 1993), and it is associated with less toxicity than other current endocrine treatments for breast cancer (Muss, 1992). While the potential additional benefits of treatment in breast cancer patients in terms of blood lipid and cholesterol levels and bone mineral density remain to be fully established, it is worthy of note that two well-designed randomized trials of tamoxifen versus no adjuvant endocrine therapy (described above) have shown significantly reduced numbers of hospital admissions for cardiac disease and no difference in deaths due to cardiac or thromboembolic disease (Rutqvist et al., 1993) and significantly reduced risks of myocardial infarction and cardiac deaths (McDonald et al., 1995) in women receiving tamoxifen.

Tamoxifen has been associated in case reports with changes in liver enzyme levels in the serum (Hayes et al., 1995) and on rare occasions a spectrum of more severe events including fatty liver (Noguchi et al., 1987), cholestasis and hepatitis (Cortez Pinto et al., 1995) and a fatal case of hepatocellular damage and agranulocytosis (Ching et al., 1992).

Several in-vitro studies have demonstrated the antioxidant action of tamoxifen on microsomal and liposomal lipid peroxidation. The effects of tamoxifen on serum malondialdehyde and several antioxidant components were evaluated in 64 postmenopausal breast cancer patients after three and six months of treatment with 20 mg/day tamoxifen (Thangaraju et al., 1994). Serum malondialdehyde levels decreased significantly from 7.64 ± 1.2 nmol/dL before treatment initiation to 6.04 ± 0.95 nmol/dL ($p < 0.001$) after three months to 5.83 ± 0.91 nmol/dL ($p < 0.001$) after six months of tamoxifen administration. The levels of blood glutathione slightly increased from 2.61 ± 0.50 μmol/mL red

Table 10. Tamoxifen-associated side-effects in the reproductive tract

Reference	Study groups and methods	Main results
Breast cancer patients		
Ferrazzi et al. (1977)	Karyopycnotic index in vaginal smear cells in 35 post-menopausal patients with advanced breast cancer before and after treatment with 30–40 mg/day tamoxifen for 30–45 days	Increase of the karyopycnotic index to 10–30%; in 4 cases, the index reached ≥ 50% and in 1 case 80%. Two months after cessation of therapy, karyopycnotic index had returned to atrophic pattern.
Boccardo et al. (1981)	Karyopycnotic index in vaginal smear cells in 28 post-menopausal patients with breast cancer before and after treatment with 20 mg/day tamoxifen at 4 and 8 weeks	Increase of karyopycnotic index in 68% of the study group. Mean values at 0, 4 and 8 weeks were 1, 5 and 10%. Large variation
Burke et al. (1987)	Comparative sonographic examination of the uterus in 30 postmenopausal women receiving 20–30 mg/day tamoxifen and 15 postmenopausal controls	Increased uterine volume in 26.6%; hyperechogenicity in 46.6% of the tamoxifen group compared to none in the controls
Ford et al. (1988)	Case report, 1 postmenopausal patient receiving tamoxifen for recurrent benign breast disease	After 5 months of treatment, stage IV endometriosis
Pons & Rigonnot (1988)	45 postmenopausal patients receiving tamoxifen for 12–90 months; cytology and clinical examination of vagina, cervix and uterus	Oestrogenization of cervix and vagina in 23 patients; endometrial hyperplasia in 11; polyploid hyperplasia in 5; glandular cystic hyperplasia in 4; polyps in 2; cervical early adenocarcinoma in 1 and endometrial early adenocarcinoma in 1; proliferative stimulation of pre-existing leiomyoma in 2
Cano et al. (1989)	Case report, one 33-year-old patient receiving 20 mg/day tamoxifen for two years after mastectomy	Endometrioma of the left ovary with multiple adherence to the uterus; grade IV endometriosis
Fisher et al. (1989a)	1326 post-operative breast cancer patients receiving tamoxifen (20 mg/day) for 5 years and 1318 post-operative breast cancer placebo controls	Hot flushes in 40% of controls versus 57% of tamoxifen; vaginal discharge in 12% of controls versus 23% of tamoxifen; irregular menses in 15% of controls versus 19% of tamoxifen
Nuovo et al. (1989)	Case report: 3 postmenopausal patients (one also with chronic lymphocytic leukaemia) with metastatic breast cancer receiving 20 mg/day tamoxifen; 2 cases for 6 years, 1 case for 2 years	Endometrial polyps (one patient with leiomyomata)

Table 10 (contd)

Reference	Study groups and methods	Main results
Neven et al. (1989)	14 breast cancer patients receiving tamoxifen (20 mg/day) examined for postmenopausal bleeding [duration of treatment not given]; 42 breast cancer patients with postmenopausal bleeding without tamoxifen treatment	Increased incidence of endometrial hyperplasia in the tamoxifen group (RR, 5.2; 95% CI, 2–13.9; $p < 0.05$) and increased frequency of endometrial polyps (RR, 3.5; 95% CI, 2–6.2; $p < 0.05$)
Neven et al. (1989)	30 breast cancer patients receiving 20 mg/day tamoxifen; 29 breast cancer patients without tamoxifen. Hysteroscopic findings	Higher relative risks for polyps for the tamoxifen group (RR, 6.7; 95% CI, 1.3–35.7; $p < 0.05$) and for proliferative uterine mucosa (RR, 2.9; 95% CI, 1.2–7.3; $p < 0.05$)
Neven et al. (1990)	16 breast cancer patients receiving 20 mg/day tamoxifen for 6–36 months; 10 postmenopausal, 4 with induced amenorrhoea, 2 premenopausal. Mean age, 55.8 ± 10.2; mean parity, 1.6 ± 1.1	Endometrial changes: mild proliferation of the mucosa (7 cases), polyps (4 cases), adenocarcinoma (1 case)
Le Bouëdec et al. (1990)	22 breast cancer patients with oestrogen receptor-positive tumour; 3 premenopausal, 19 postmenopausal; mean age, 62.5 years; treatment duration, 26 months; cumulative dose, 5.4–43.2 g	Examination for uterine bleeding revealed 12 cases of endometrial hyperplasia; 6 cases of endometrial polyps; 6 cases of uterine myomas; 1 case with adenocarcinoma of the uterus; 1 case with acanthoma; 3 cases with endometrial atrophy
Cross & Ismail (1990)	Case report: 54-year-old woman mastectomized for breast carcinoma 18 years earlier followed 9 years later by bilateral oophorectomy because of axillary metastatic node. Tamoxifen introduced at that time at 40 mg/day for 6 months and then reduced to 20 mg/day until this report	Uterine bleeding leading to hysterectomy; endometrial hyperplasia and no residual ovarian tissue identified; polyp; a few intramural tumours
Buckley (1990)	Case report: 44-year old breast cancer patient receiving 20 mg/day tamoxifen for 3 years	Severe simple endometrial hyperplasia
Le Bouëdec et al. (1991)	Case report: 69-year old breast cancer patient receiving 20 mg/day tamoxifen for 7 years	Severe endometriosis, large uterine adenomyoma
De Muylder et al. (1991)	46 breast cancer patients with hormone-receptor positive tumour receiving tamoxifen for 6–36 months; 34 postmenopausal; 12 premenopausal; tamoxifen dose-rate not indicated	13 cases with endometrial polyps, 8 with endometrial hyperplasia, 2 with uterine adenocarcinoma; the rate of endometrial hyperplasia correlated with the cumulative dose of tamoxifen

Table 10 (contd)

Reference	Study groups and methods	Main results
Lang-Avenous et al. (1991)	28 patients receiving tamoxifen [dose not stated] after diagnosis of breast cancer	11 cases with atrophic endometrium; 5 with atrophic endometrium associated with polyps; 3 with cystic glandular polyps; 2 with regressive glandular cystic hyperplasia
Corley et al. (1992)	Case reports: 3 postmenopausal breast cancer patients (aged 77, 72 and 58) and one premenopausal breast cancer patient (age 45) receiving 20 mg/day tamoxifen for 3, 6 and 10 years (postmenopausal patient) or for 2 years (premenopausal patient)	Endometrial polyps, in one case metastatic breast carcinoma was present in the polyp
Dilts et al. (1992)	49-year-old woman, gravida 3, para 1, bilaterally mastectomized for metachronous breast cancer at 1 year interval. Tamoxifen started after 2nd mastectomy for 3 months (20 mg/day)	Echographic diagnosis of leiomyoma and an ovarian cyst. Exploratory laparotomy revealed a marked oestrogen-stimulated pelvis similar to that seen with a term pregnancy.
Hulka & Hall (1993)	14 postmenopausal breast cancer patients receiving tamoxifen: duration and dose not stated; no control group; pelvic sonograms and endometrial biopsy	11 patients with abnormal (> 7 mm) endometrial thickening and abnormalities in the sonogram (hyperechoic and cystic zones); 9 cases of uterine polyps, 4 cases of endometrial hyperplasia, 2 cases of endometritis, 1 proliferative endometrium, 1 inactive endometrium, 1 endometrial carcinoma
Rayter et al. (1993)	49 breast cancer patients receiving tamoxifen (20 mg/day) for an average of 47.5 months (37% premenopausal; 63 post-menopausal; average age 54.5 years); 45 breast cancer patients without tamoxifen (42% premenopausal, 51% post-menopausal; average age, 54 years)	Clinical enlargement of the uterus in 8 tamoxifen patients versus 0 control ($r = 0.006$). Endometrial thickness seemed greater in the tamoxifen group but not so great as the effect of menopause (pre-menopausal, 9.2 mm; postmenopausal, 6.4 mm); more endometrial nuclear hyperplasia ($p = 0.047$).

Table 10 (contd)

Reference	Study groups and methods	Main results
Lahti et al. (1993)	51 postmenopausal breast cancer patients receiving 20–40 mg/day tamoxifen for an average of 30 months; 52 postmenopausal breast cancer patients without tamoxifen; groups matched for age, parity, age at menopause and body mass index	Thicker endometrium in the tamoxifen group (10.4 ± 5 versus 4.2 ± 2.7 mm, $p = 0.0001$) by transvaginal sonography; larger uterine volume in the tamoxifen group (45 ± 27 versus 25 ± 11 cm^3; $p = 0.001$) by transvaginal sonography; endometrial polyps more frequent in the tamoxifen group (36% versus 10%; $p = 0.004$). 1 atypical hyperplasia, 1 adenomatous hyperplasia and 1 endometrial adenocarcinoma in the tamoxifen group; two endometrial adenocarcinomas in the control group
Seoud et al. (1993)	Six postmenopausal breast cancer patients received tamoxifen (20 mg/day), 2 for < 2 years, 4 for > 2 years.	Three with endometrial adenocarcinoma; 1 with homologous mixed Müllerian sarcoma; 1 with primary fallopian tube carcinoma; 1 with endometrial polyps and glandular hyperplasia
Ugwumadu et al. (1993)	Case report: 58-year old breast cancer patient treated 13 years earlier by bilateral oophorectomy; 40 mg/day tamoxifen for 8 years	Postmenopausal bleeding, myometrial adenomyosis, cystic atrophy of the endometrium and endometrial polyp
Uzily et al. (1993)	95 breast cancer patients; mean age, 58 years, receiving 20 mg/day tamoxifen for median time of 24 (1–84) months: vaginal ultrasonography and endometrial biopsy. No control group	89% of tamoxifen users > 12 months had endometrial thickness of > 0.5 cm versus 71% of < 12 months therapy. Four cases with endometrial hyperplasia; 4 with benign endometrial polyp, 3 showed dysplasia and 3 with endometrial cancer; except for one patient with endometrial hyperplasia, all had received tamoxifen for more than 12 months.
Ismail (1994)	19 breast cancer patients receiving tamoxifen (either 20 or 40 mg/day) (2 patients died of other than gynaecological disease and necropsy was carried out; the remaining 17 tamoxifen-treated patients were examined because of gynaecological symptoms) and 15 patients with gynaecological symptoms without tamoxifen; matched for age and presentation	Tamoxifen versus control group; endometrial hyperplasia 11 versus 4; endometrial polyps: 11 versus 1; primary endometrial malignancies: 2 versus 4; endometrial polyp cancers: 4 versus 0; all carcinomas in the tamoxifen group were observed in cases with > 35 g cumulative doses.

Table 10 (contd)

Reference	Study groups and methods	Main results
Leo et al. (1994)	2 case reports: 36-year-old woman with mastectomy and axillary node dissection followed by chemotherapy (cyclophosphamide, methotrexate, 5-fluorouracil) cycles and tamoxifen 30 mg/day as adjuvant therapy	After 4 years, sudden increase of uterine volume and leiomyoma of the corpus uteri
	50-year-old woman, mastectomized for breast cancer followed by chemotherapy and tamoxifen 30 mg/day	After 4 years, admitted for severe abdominal pain; vaginal serography showed uterine fibroid of the corpus uteri and increased endometrial thickness.
Krause & Gerber (1994)	8 patients treated with tamoxifen following breast cancer	6 endometrial polyps, 1 adenosis uteri, 1 endometrial cancer
Ugwumadu & Harding (1994)	56-year-old woman underwent mastectomy and lymph node biopsy for invasive duct carcinoma, then received radiotherapy and tamoxifen 20 mg/day.	After 2 years of treatment, uterus was about the size of a 6–8-week gestation on physical examination and four years later the size of a 20-week gestation. Laparotomy revealed enlarged uterus with thickened endometrium, polypoid in places and multiple benign leiomyomata was confirmed.
	62-year-old patient treated by lumpectomy and radiotherapy for a poorly differentiated duct carcinoma. General and pelvic examinations were normal and tamoxifen was started at 20 mg/day.	2.5 years later, a uterus equivalent to a 14-week gestation was found, with a rather well oestrogenized vagina.
Healthy women		
Kedar et al. (1994)	111 postmenopausal healthy women (46–71 years) from the Pilot Breast Cancer Prevention Trial: 61 receiving 20 mg/day tamoxifen (average age, 56), 50 placebo controls (average age, 58 years)	The tamoxifen group had a larger uterus (34 versus 22.2 mL; $p < 0.001$), and increased endometrial thickness (9.1 versus 4.8 mm; $p < 0.001$); in addition 10 cases (16%) of atypical hyperplasia versus none in the placebo group and 5 cases (8%) of endometrial polyps in the tamoxifen group versus one in the placebo group.

Table 11. Tamoxifen-associated side-effects on blood coagulation

Reference	Study groups and methods	Main results
Breast cancer patients		
Nevasaari et al. (1978)	Case report: 4 patients (43, 57, 60 and 68 years old) with metastatic breast cancer receiving 20–40 mg tamoxifen for 2 weeks to 3½ months	Deep vein thrombosis
Lipton et al. (1984)	220 patients with metastatic breast cancer started on tamoxifen	7 venous thromboses within 6 months; 4 cases with phlebitis, 2 with phlebitis and pulmonary embolism, 1 with phlebitis
Enck & Rios (1984)	39 postmenopausal patients (average age: 64 years) with metastatic breast cancer: 24 receiving 20 mg/day tamoxifen for mean of 36 (2–87) weeks; 4 receiving 15 mg/day diethylstilboestrol; 11 controls	Lower concentrations of antithrombin-III in 42% (10/24) of the tamoxifen-treated (mean duration, 36 weeks) cases compared with 9% (1/11) in the control group
Hendrick & Subramanian (1980)	Case report: 72-year-old breast cancer patient with lung and bone metastasis receiving 20 mg/day tamoxifen	Death 4 weeks after start of tamoxifen treatment due to thrombosis of the superior mesenteric artery with no evidence of local metastasis in the artery and no sign of atheroma
Jordan et al. (1987)	25 premenopausal and 22 postmenopausal breast cancer patients receiving 20 mg/day tamoxifen for between 434 and 2592 days and between 91 and 1560 days respectively. 95 premenopausal and 8 postmenopausal breast cancer patients receiving only combination chemotherapy served as controls.	Antithrombin-III levels decreased compared to only chemotherapy controls ($p < 0.001$). However, in no case were the antithrombin-III values decreased by > 30%, which is considered the level of clinical significance.
Bertelli et al. (1988)	55 breast cancer patients receiving 20 mg/day tamoxifen for ≥ 3 months and 36 breast cancer patients without any treatment after mastectomy as controls	Decreased antithrombin-III levels in the tamoxifen group (26.6 ± 1 versus 30.2 ± 1.2 mg/dL; $p = 0.03$)
Love et al. (1992a)	140 women with axillary node-negative breast cancer, 70 receiving 20 mg/day tamoxifen, 70 placebo controls	Fibrinogen levels decreased by 15% in the tamoxifen group by 6 months ($p < 0.001$); antithrombin-III concentrations decreased significantly in the tamoxifen group but not to clinically significant levels. Decrease in platelet counts of 7–9%.

Table 11 (contd)

Reference	Study groups and methods	Main results
Cuzick et al. (1993)	153 breast cancer patients, 20 current tamoxifen users (mean duration of treatment 72 months), 73 ex-users (mean duration of treatment: 24 months, median time after cessation of tamoxifen administration: 58 months) and 60 breast cancer controls, who had never used tamoxifen.	No differences between controls and ex-users; in current users kaolin cephalin clotting times were marginally shorter, fibrinogen and fast alpha-2 antiplasmin levels were lower ($p = 0.03$, $p = 0.0001$ and $p = 0.009$ respectively) and plasminogen levels were higher ($p = 0.02$).
Love et al. (1994a)	30 breast cancer patients receiving 20 mg/day tamoxifen for 5 years and 32 breast cancer placebo control patients	After 5 years fibrinogen levels were 17% lower in the tamoxifen-treated group compared with base-line ($t = 0$) compared with the change in the placebo group ($p = 0.08$).
Healthy women		
Jones et al. (1992)	515 normal healthy premenopausal and postmenopausal women with a history of breast cancer, receiving tamoxifen (20 mg/day) as a chemopreventive agent; follow-up for 36 months every 6 months by determination of fibrinogen, antithrombin-III, protein C and protein S	Marginal reduction of antithrombin-III (postmenopause only) and protein S (a natural coagulation inhibitor) after 6 months, which was no longer observed after 12 months. No increase in the incidence of thromboembolic events

Table 12. Tamoxifen-associated side-effects on blood lipids, steroid hormone-binding globulin and thyroid function-associated parameters

Reference	Study groups and methods	Main results[a]
Gordon et al. (1986)	50 postmenopausal breast cancer patients receiving 20 mg/day tamoxifen (average treatment duration, 11 months; range, 1–42 months); 50 healthy (not breast cancer) postmenopausal women as control	Serum thyroxin levels were elevated in 10/50 tamoxifen cases versus 1/50 control cases ($p < 0.04$). No significant difference in triiodothyronine levels. Thyroid-binding globulin levels increased in 6/6 (> 30 mg/L) tamoxifen cases who had elevated serum thyroxin levels.
Bertelli et al. (1988)	55 breast cancer patients receiving 20 mg/d tamoxifen for ≥ 3 months and 36 breast cancer patients without any treatment after mastectomy as controls	Total cholesterol and LDL-cholesterol were significantly ($p < 0.05$) lower in the tamoxifen group. Total cholesterol: 212.6 ± 6 versus 254.3 ± 8 mg/dL and LDL-cholesterol 126.7 ± 62 versus 175.9 ± 9.6 mg/dL.
Bruning et al. (1988)	8 premenopausal (mean age, 43.3 years) and 46 postmenopausal (mean age, 63.2 years) receiving 20 mg/day tamoxifen for 6 months	No change in total cholesterol; significant ($p < 0.05$) increase in HDL and decrease ($p < 0.05$) in LDL. Significant increase in sex hormone binding globulin (SHBG) ($p < 0.001$)
Bagdade et al. (1990)	8 postmenopausal women receiving 20 mg/day tamoxifen for 3 months	No significant changes in total cholesterol or triglyceride levels; significant decrease in non-esterified free cholesterol levels ($p < 0.05$) and in LDL fraction; concentrations of cholesterol, free cholesterol and free cholesterol/lecithin ratio fell ($p < 0.025$; $p < 0.05$; $p < 0.025$). Significant increase in SHBG ($p < 0.005$)

Table 12 (contd)

Reference	Study groups and methods	Main results[a]
Cuzick et al. (1993)	153 breast cancer patients (116 postmenopausal); 20 (14) current tamoxifen users (mean duration of treatment, 72 months); 73 (55) ex-users (mean duration of treatment, 24 months; median time after cessation of tamoxifen administration, 58 months) and 60 (47) breast cancer controls who had never used tamoxifen	In the premenopausal groups, no difference between controls and ex-users. In the postmenopausal groups: Ex-users Controls Current users TC 7.00 6.63 5.81 $0.01 < p < 0.05$ LDL-C 5.20 4.82 3.75 $0.01 < p < 0.05$ TG 1.31 1.12 1.33 $0.01 < p < 0.05$ SHBG 62 55 105 $p < 0.001$ T3 1.81 1.81 2.15 $0.001 < p \leq 0.01$ T4 96.9 97.6 126.9 $0.001 < p \leq 0.01$
Dewar et al. (1992)	44 postmenopausal women (mean age, 59; range, 45–76) with breast cancer; 24 receiving 20 mg/day tamoxifen for 5 years and 20 placebo controls; after five years, 18 treated patients were randomly selected either to continue ($n = 10$) or stop ($n = 8$) treatment and followed for additional 3 years	Tamoxifen treatment consistently lowered total cholesterol levels but the effect ended after cessation of treatment: Year 1 2 3 4 5 Change (mmol/L) −0.52 −0.96 −0.96 −0.88 −1.02 p 0.013 0.003 0.022 0.005 0.001 Apparently no change in HDL

Table 12 (contd)

Reference	Study groups and methods	Main results[a]
Dnistrian et al. (1993)	24 breast cancer patients (11 premenopausal, 13 postmenopausal), mostly hormone receptor-positive, receiving 20 mg/day tamoxifen for 4–8 weeks (only 4 received tamoxifen alone, 20 also received chemotherapy.)	Tamoxifen induced 17% decrease in total cholesterol levels and 27% decrease in LDL-cholesterol. No clear change in HDL-cholesterol levels; significant decrease (33%) in LDL/HDL ratio.
Love et al. (1994a)	30 breast cancer patients receiving 20 mg/day tamoxifen for 5 years and 32 breast cancer placebo control patients	At baseline ($t = 0$) no differences between the two groups. Total cholesterol and LDL-cholesterol levels were significantly decreased in the tamoxifen-treated group at 5 years ($p = 0.001$) and the changes were significantly greater than in the placebo control ($p = 0.01$ versus $p = 0.001$).
Anker et al. (1995)	31 postmenopausal breast cancer patients (mean age, 65 years) receiving 20–30 mg tamoxifen for 1–> 19 months. Levels of plasma homocysteine (a risk factor for atherosclerotic disease) and serum cholesterol were determined at various time points.	Plasma homocysteine was suppressed by a mean value of 29.8% after 9–12 months and by 24.5% after 13–18 months of treatment. Cholesterol levels decreased by mean values varying between 7.2% and 17.6% after 5–9 months of treatment.
Grey et al. (1995a)	23 healthy postmenopausal women randomly assigned to receive tamoxifen (20 mg/day) for 2 years (mean age, 58 ± 6 years) compared with 23 similar women receiving placebo (mean age, 60 ± 5 years)	Tamoxifen lowered serum cholesterol by 12 ± 2% and LDL-cholesterol by 19 ± 3%; HDL-cholesterol not altered.
Mamby et al. (1995)	14 postmenopausal breast cancer patients participating in a longitudinal, double-blind, randomized placebo-controlled study of tamoxifen (20 mg/day) and 14 placebo controls.	Significant increases in the tamoxifen group after 3 months in thyroid-binding globulin levels (from 21.26 ± 1.06 to 26.94 ± 1.81), thyroxine (T4) levels (from 7.02 ± 0.3 to 8.39 ± 0.46) and thyroxine uptake (from 127.71 ± 5.61 to 142.43 ± 6.82). No change in thyroid-stimulating hormone levels or free thyroxine index

LDL, low-density lipoprotein; HDL, high-density lipoprotein; SHBG, sex hormone binding globulin (nmol/L); TC, total cholesterol (mmol/L); LDL-C, low-density lipoprotein-cholesterol (mmol/L); TG, triglycerides (mmol/L); T3, triiodothyronine (nmol/L); T4, thyroxine (nmol/L)

Table 13. Effects of tamoxifen on bone mineralization

Reference	Study groups and methods	Main results
Love et al. (1988)	48 women with breast cancer treated with tamoxifen for at least 2 years and 37 women not treated with tamoxifen	No difference in bone mineral density (BMD) between the two groups
Fentiman et al. (1989)	Premenopausal women taking tamoxifen (20 mg/day for 36 months) for mastalgia, compared with placebo group (50 mg/day vitamin C)	No change from baseline levels in either treated or placebo group after 3 months treatment, and no change in tamoxifen group after 6 months
Fornander et al. (1990)	75 recurrence-free postmenopausal breast cancer patients taking tamoxifen (40 mg/day for 2 or 5 years) compared with control patients taking no adjuvant endocrine therapy	BMD similar in treated and control groups, measured about 7 years after initial randomization. Cortical bone: 1.03 g/cm^2 in tamoxifen versus 1.03 g/cm^2 in controls; trabecular bone: 0.74 g/cm^2 versus 0.73 g/cm^2
Love et al. (1994b)	Two-year, randomized, double-blind trial of tamoxifen (20 mg/day) in 70 treated women with breast cancer compared with 70 placebo controls	Mean BMD of lumbar spine increased by 0.6% per year in treated group and decreased by 1.00% per year in placebo group ($p < 0.001$). Radial BMD decreased to same extent in both groups.
Ward et al. (1993)	15 early postmenopausal women with stage I or II breast cancer taking tamoxifen (20 mg/day) and 21 healthy postmenopausal controls. Serum sex hormone-binding globulin and antithrombin III levels measured, and BMD at various sites measured	Tamoxifen prevented bone loss at femoral neck (+ 1.4% gain in BMD/year versus −1.8% in control group; $p = 0.03$) and lumbar spine (+0.09%/year versus −2.3%; $p = 0.04$), and reduced bone turnover. Sex hormone binding globulin was increased and antithrombin III reduced in treated group.
Kristensen et al. (1994)	20 women receiving tamoxifen (30 mg/day) for 2 years and 23 untreated controls. All patients postmenopausal with primary breast cancer, classified as low risk after surgery	Lumbar BMD increased by about 3% in first year in tamoxifen group and then stabilized. Lumbar BMD decreased by about 2.5% in control group in the first year ($p = 0.00074$), continued to decrease to about 4.5% after two years. BMD at forearms stable in tamoxifen but declined in control group ($p = 0.024$).
Wright et al. (1994)	41 women with breast cancer, 22 treated with tamoxifen for ≥ 15 months (mean, 33 months) and 19 untreated. Transiliac crest bone biopsies analysed by histomorphometry	No statistically significant difference between treated and control groups in bone area, osteoid perimeter and area, or osteoid width. Tissue-based bone formation significantly lower ($p = 0.05$) and remodelling period significantly longer ($p < 0.05$) in treated group
Grey et al. (1995b)	23 healthy postmenopausal women randomly assigned to receive tamoxifen (20 mg/day) for 2 years (mean age, 58 ± 6 years) compared with 23 similar women receiving placebo (mean age, 60 ± 5 years)	1.4% increase in lumbar spine BMD in the tamoxifen group versus 0.7% decline in the placebo group ($p < 0.01$). This small protective effect was comparable in magnitude to calcium supplementation and less than that of either oestrogen or bisphosphonates.

cells to 2.86 ± 0.43 μmol/mL ($p < 0.01$) to 2.91 ± 0.47 μmol/mL ($p < 0.01$) and slight increases were also observed in serum levels of ceruloplasmin, uric acid, vitamins A, C and E and selenium. [Except for concentrations of malondialdehyde, the changes in all parameters were ≤ 10% of the initial value.]

Ocular toxicity has been reported following tamoxifen treatment, the first published reports of retinopathy and corneal changes being associated with particularly high doses of tamoxifen of at least 240 mg/day (Kaiser-Kupfer & Lippman, 1978). It is characterized by white refractile intraretinal deposits distributed mainly at the posterior pole. Ocular toxicity also appears to be an infrequent but serious complication of tamoxifen therapy at doses of 20–40 mg/day (Griffiths, 1987; De Jong-Busnac, 1989). In the study by Pavlidis *et al.* (1992), four of 63 patients administered 20 mg tamoxifen per day displayed retinopathy and/or keratopathy 10, 27, 31 and 35 months, respectively, after the start of therapy. However, in another controlled study, no ocular toxicity was found in 79 breast cancer patients taking tamoxifen in conventional doses (10–20 mg two or three times a day) for an average of two years and three months (Longstaff *et al.*, 1989). Ocular toxicity has not been reported in any of the major adjuvant breast cancer studies involving tamoxifen (Fisher *et al.*, 1989a; Ribeiro & Swindell, 1992; Fornander *et al.*, 1991). Where retinopathy was reported in patients, it was reversible on cessation of tamoxifen treatment if the condition was detected at an early stage (Ashford *et al.*, 1988; Chang *et al.*, 1992).

Leukopenia and neutropenia (Glick *et al.*, 1981; Boccardo *et al.*, 1994b; Miké *et al.*, 1994) have been reported on rare occasions following the administration of tamoxifen.

4.2.2 *Experimental systems*

In single-dose toxicity studies, the oral LD_{50} of tamoxifen was approximately 3 g/kg for mice and 2.5 g/kg for rats (Furr & Jordan, 1984). Tamoxifen is well tolerated upon chronic administration to mice, rats and dogs at large multiples of the pharmacologically active dose (approximately 0.1 mg/kg), the pharmacological properties of tamoxifen (behaving as an oestrogen in some species and tissues and as an antioestrogen in others) accounting for many of the effects described in toxicology studies (Tucker *et al.*, 1984). Tamoxifen is an antioestrogen with complex pharmacology encompassing variable species-, tissue-, cell-, gene- and duration of administration-specific effects from oestrogen-like agonist actions to complete blockage of oestrogenic action (Jordan & Robinson, 1987). In short-term laboratory assays, tamoxifen is usually classified as oestrogenic in mice but as a partial agonist/antagonist in rats. The concept that tamoxifen is oestrogenic in mice may not provide a complete description of the effects in this species, as prolonged administration to ovariectomized mice results in the uterus becoming refractory to oestrogen administration (Jordan *et al.*, 1990). Whilst the initial response of the uterus to tamoxifen is oestrogen-like, as administration continues, uterine weight returns to initial values. In immature rats, administration of tamoxifen increases uterine weight in a dose-dependent manner without attaining the same maximal effect as obtained with 17β-oestradiol; administration of tamoxifen together with oestradiol provides a partial but incomplete antagonism of the uterotrophic action of 17β-oestradiol (Harper &

Walpole, 1967a,b). The increase in uterine weight is largely due to hypertrophy of the luminal epithelium, with little change in the myometrium and stroma. This hypertrophic effect was not associated with any change in thymidine incorporation or cell division typical of uterine response to 17β-oestradiol treatment (Jordan *et al.*, 1980). More recent studies have confirmed the hypertrophic effect of tamoxifen and other antioestrogens on the luminal and glandular epithelium of the rat uterus and contrasted this effect with that of oestrogens (Branham *et al.*, 1993).

In mice, repeated administration of doses up to 50 mg/kg for 13–15 months caused atrophy of gonads and accessory sex organs, with cystic endometrial hyperplasia in the uterus, elongation of the vertebrae and a marked increase in bone density with resorption and new bone formation in irregular patterns. These changes are consistent with the pharmacological action in this species. In the liver, there were fatty changes and a swelling of the parenchymal cells (Tucker *et al.*, 1984).

In rats, administration of tamoxifen for 6–24 months at doses between 35 and 100 mg/kg per day caused atrophy of the gonads and accessory sex organs, whilst, at lower doses (2 mg/kg per day), the uterine endometrium showed an absence of glands, flattening of the epithelium and occasional squamous metaplasia (Tucker *et al.*, 1984; Greaves *et al.*, 1993). After six months' treatment with 35 mg/kg per day, there was nodular hyperplasia in the liver (Greaves *et al.*, 1993). The lysosomal lipidosis seen in a number of tissues, including retina and cornea, after chronic administration of 100–130 mg/kg per day is consistent with the cationic amphiphilic structure of tamoxifen (Lüllmann & Lüllmann-Rauch, 1981); the higher incidence of cataracts may be related to changes in sex hormone status (Greaves *et al.*, 1993).

In dogs, repeated administration of up to 75 mg/kg tamoxifen per day for three months resulted in cessation of ovulation and hyperplasia of the germinal epithelium of the ovary and severe endometritis with squamous metaplasia, as well as biliary stasis with no other morphological change in the liver at the highest-dose level only (Tucker *et al.*, 1984).

Six months' administration of tamoxifen at doses up to 8 mg/kg per day to marmosets produced a slight increase in ovarian follicular cyst weight and number, probably as a result of its antioestrogenic effect in this species (Furr *et al.*, 1979; Tucker *et al.*, 1984).

Rat, chicken and human microsomes exhibited low tamoxifen-binding activity compared with hamster and mouse microsomes (Mani *et al.*, 1994). In another study (White *et al.*, 1995), covalent binding of tamoxifen to microsomal proteins was observed with human, rat and mouse microsomes; the activity of mouse microsomes was highest (17-fold higher than human microsomes), while rat microsomes had intermediate activity (3.8-fold higher than human microsomes).

White *et al.* (1993) showed that, while the total hepatic microsomal cytochrome P450 content of rats given tamoxifen intraperitoneally (0.12 mmol/kg or 45 mg/kg per day for four days) was not increased (and, indeed, was transiently decreased), there were 30–60-fold increases in the metabolism of benzyloxy- and pentoxyresorufin; the metabolism of ethoxyresorufin was only slightly increased. Immunoblotting experiments revealed two- to three-fold increases in CYP2B1, CYP2B2 and CYP3A1 proteins. Induction of these proteins was centrilobular. None of these monooxygenase activities was induced in C57Bl/6 mice and only small increases in benzyloxy- and pentoxyresorufin metabolism were seen in DBA/2 mice. There has been independent confirmation of the induction of CYP2B1, CYP2B2 and CYP3A in the liver of Fischer 344 rats (particularly females) administered tamoxifen orally for seven days. In addition, microsomal epoxide hydrolase was induced. These were selective inductions, there being no increased expression of CYP1A1, CYP1A2 or γ-glutamyl transpeptidase (Nuwaysir et al., 1995).

4.3 Reproductive and developmental effects

4.3.1 Humans

Tamoxifen is contraindicated during pregnancy (Vidal, 1995; Medical Economics, 1996).

Cullins et al. (1994) reported the birth of an infant with Goldenhar's syndrome (oculoauriculovertebral dysplasia) delivered by Caesarian section at 26 weeks to a 35-year-old woman with breast cancer who had received 20 mg/day tamoxifen throughout pregnancy. They noted that 50 pregnancies reported to the manufacturer had been associated with tamoxifen administration. There were 19 normal births, 8 terminations, 13 unknown outcomes and 10 associated with a fetal or neonatal disorder. Two infants had congenital craniofacial defects. [The Working Group noted that details of these 50 cases were not available in this secondary reference.]

Zemlickis et al. (1992) reported on three women with breast cancer who received treatment during the first trimester of pregnancy. One woman received tamoxifen with cyclophosphamide, methotrexate, fluorouracil and vincristine sulfate; the pregnancy ended in live birth, and the baby was alive and well at the time of follow-up. The other two women did not receive tamoxifen and the pregnancy ended in miscarriage. Two further women with breast cancer received chemotherapy during the third trimester. One received tamoxifen with fluorouracil, doxorubicin and cyclophosphamide, and a live-born infant was delivered who was alive and well at the time of follow-up. The other woman did not receive tamoxifen but also delivered a live birth with some intrauterine growth retardation; this child was well at the time of the follow-up.

Lai et al. (1994) reported the birth of a normal male infant with a birthweight of 3340 g at term following six months' daily therapy with 30 mg tamoxifen and 160 mg megestrol acetate for adenocarcinoma of the endometrium and three months' treatment with a combined oestrogen/gestagen oral contraceptive pill.

Two studies have been made of the effect of tamoxifen on reproductive parameters in healthy female volunteers. In the first, 16 women with regular menstrual cycles were followed during one control cycle, one treatment cycle during which women received 20 mg tamoxifen twice daily from cycle day 18 until day 30 or onset of menstruation, whichever came first, and one follow-up cycle (Swahn et al., 1989). The length of the treatment cycle (28.5 days ± 2.0 days) was significantly longer than that of the control (27.2 ± 2.0 days) or follow-up (27.5 ± 1.9 days) cycles, owing to a prolonged luteal phase. Levels of follicle-stimulating hormone (FSH), progesterone, 17-hydroxyprogesterone, 20-dihydroprogesterone, oestrone, oestrone sulfate and 17β-oestradiol were significantly elevated during the treatment cycle compared with the control cycle. Levels of pregnanediol glucuronide remained unchanged during the treatment cycle, whereas the concentrations during the follow-up cycle were approximately double those of the control cycle. Prolactin levels decreased slightly during tamoxifen treatment, but the effect was not statistically significant. There was a positive correlation between plasma levels of tamoxifen and 17-hydroxyprogesterone ($r = 0.72$; $p < 0.05$), but not with plasma levels of the other hormones during treatment or follow-up cycles. The treatment did not cause any major disturbance of the bleeding pattern.

In the second study, Mäentausta et al. (1993) studied the effects of tamoxifen on endometrial 17β-hydroxysteroid dehydrogenase and progesterone and oestrogen receptors during the luteal phase of the menstrual cycle in 11 healthy female volunteers. The study included one control and two treatment cycles. During the first treatment cycle, the subjects received 200 mg mifepristone two days after the peak serum luteinizing hormone (LH) concentration. During the second treatment cycle, the subjects received 40 mg tamoxifen on the second and third days after the peak serum LH concentration. The time interval between these treatments was about a month, and the authors state that this ensured that the effects of each treatment modality had disappeared before the next treatment. 17β-Hydroxysteroid dehydrogenase and progesterone and oestrogen receptors were examined immunohistochemically in endometrial tissue specimens taken on the sixth to eighth day after the peak serum LH concentration. Tamoxifen did not have any significant effect on staining of 17β-hydroxysteroid dehydrogenase or the abundance of receptors. The authors state that serum concentrations of 17β-oestradiol, progesterone and LH were not significantly affected by the administration of tamoxifen.

Six women were treated for uterine fibroids for at least three months with 10 mg tamoxifen twice daily starting between days 1 and 3 of the menstrual period. Increased variability in the length of the menstrual and ovarian cycle was associated with significant lengthening of the luteal phase from 12.5 ± 1.5 days to 16.9 ± 3.5 days ($p < 0.02$; Lumsden et al., 1989). A significant increase in the excretion of oestrone and pregnanediol glucuronide in the urine was associated with increased concentrations of 17β-oestradiol and progesterone in plasma, reflecting multiple follicular development and ovulation. A significant rise in the concentration of FSH occurred during the luteal phase of the cycle.

A number of studies of endocrine parameters have been carried out in pre- and postmenopausal women receiving tamoxifen therapy (for review, see Sunderland & Osborne, 1991). Most studies report that in postmenopausal women levels of gonadotrophins, FSH and LH decrease with tamoxifen therapy, although remaining within the normal postmenopausal range. 17β-Oestradiol and progesterone levels do not change in postmenopausal women receiving tamoxifen. In contrast, in premenopausal women receiving tamoxifen, 17β-oestradiol and progesterone levels show a striking elevation, often to two or three times the normal level. The elevated hormone levels follow a pattern consistent with the normal menstrual cycle. Despite these supraphysiological levels of 17β-oestradiol, FSH and LH levels remain unchanged or only slightly increased. Many premenopausal women receiving long-term tamoxifen therapy continue to have regular ovulation and menstrual cycles, although as many as one third may develop temporary amenorrhoea or oligomenorrhoea.

In a study of the pregnancy outcome in the partners of men who had been treated with tamoxifen ($n = 22$) or clomiphene ($n = 12$) for oligozoospermia, no important difference in the course of pregnancy was found between the groups (Salata *et al.*, 1993).

Gooren (1989) reported a patient with incomplete androgen insensitivity syndrome (hypospadias, unilateral cryptorchidism and pubertal gynaecomastia, all surgically corrected) and plasma FSH levels below the reference range for adult men. After treatment with 10 mg tamoxifen twice daily, his plasma FSH level rose, spermatogenesis improved and his wife conceived three times within a period of five years.

In a number of uncontrolled studies, treatment with tamoxifen has been reported to be associated with an increase in sperm count of men with idiopathic oligozoospermia. However, in addition to the fact that these studies were not randomized controlled trials, a limitation of the studies was that patients who would be considered fertile were included (Kotoulas *et al.*, 1994). Krause *et al.* (1992) reported a randomized trial of tamoxifen in the treatment of idiopathic oligozoospermia. The sperm output and pregnancy rate was somewhat higher in the group of 39 patients who received 30 mg tamoxifen daily than in the 37 patients who received the placebo. [The numbers of subjects assigned to each group of the trial in the reporting of the pregnancy rates conflict with the numbers assigned to therapy recorded earlier in the paper.] Kotoulas *et al.* (1994) reported that 122 men randomly assigned to treatment with 10 mg tamoxifen twice daily for a period of three months had improved sperm density and number of live spermatozoa compared with 117 men who received the placebo therapy for the same period of time. The improvement in sperm density was more marked in the subgroups who were oligozoospermic than in normozoospermic men. In addition, there was a statistically significant decrease in the number of abnormal sperm after tamoxifen treatment, but the authors comment that this decrease was observed in only 12 patients in the tamoxifen group compared with eight patients in the placebo group.

4.3.2 *Experimental systems*

(a) *Effects on the fetus*

Cunha *et al.* (1987) assessed the potential oestrogenicity and teratogenicity of tamoxifen in 54 genital tracts isolated from 4–19-week-old human female fetuses and grown from one to two months in untreated athymic nude mice. After grafting of the human fetal genital tracts, the hosts were given subcutaneous implants of 20-mg pellets of tamoxifen, clomiphene or diethylstilboestrol, or were sham operated. In all mice that received tamoxifen, the vaginal epithelia of the hosts were thickened and cornified, and the uteri exhibited cystic hyperplasia. In specimens of human genital tract grown to a gestational age equivalent of 15 weeks or less, the vagina and urogenital sinus were lined with an immature squamous epithelium, which was similar in drug-treated and untreated specimens. The authors noted that the absence of oestrogenic response in these specimens correlated with the apparent absence of oestrogen receptors. Two of the four tamoxifen-treated specimens grown to a gestational age equivalent of 16 weeks or more exhibited epithelial hyperplasia and maturation. Untreated specimens were unstimulated. Formation of endometrial and cervical glands proceeded in 13/15 (87%) control specimens grown to a gestational age equivalent to 13 weeks or more in untreated hosts. The results from tamoxifen-treated specimens were similar to those obtained with clomiphene-treated specimens, and therefore were pooled. Glands were present in only 6/13 (46%) age-matched specimens treated with tamoxifen or clomiphene. In the developing uterine corpus of untreated controls, the uterine mesenchyme segregated into inner (endometrial stroma) and outer (myometrial) layers, whereas, in specimens treated with tamoxifen, condensation and segregation of the mesenchyme were greatly impaired. The epithelium of the fallopian tubes of specimens treated with tamoxifen was hyperplastic and disorganized, and the complex mucosal plications characteristic of the fallopian tube were also distorted.

As tamoxifen is an antifertility agent in rats, it has proved difficult to conduct studies of possible teratogenic effects in this species (Furr & Jordan, 1984). Tucker *et al.* (1984) reported that 0.025 mg/kg bw tamoxifen was the highest dose that could be given throughout pregnancy in Alpk/AP rats without completely preventing implantation. At this dose, about 50% of matings gave rise to successful pregnancies. These authors also stated that in several teratogenic studies in rats, all doses above 2 mg/kg bw produced an incidence of irregular ossification of ribs in the fetus. They considered that this was secondary to a tamoxifen-induced reduction in the size of the uterus of the dam and noted that the effect disappeared in the early neonatal period. In rabbits, administration of 0.1 and 0.2 mg/kg bw tamoxifen throughout pregnancy did not produce any effect on implantation or on the fetus. In marmosets, doses of up to 10 mg/kg bw tamoxifen from days 25 to 35 of pregnancy did not produce any effect in the fetus. [The Working Group noted that few details of these studies were reported.]

Twenty adult female cynomolgus monkeys (*Macaca fascicularis*) with two spontaneous menstrual cycles of normal duration during an initial two- to three-month period of observation were randomly assigned to receive a low dose of tamoxifen (0.5 mg/kg bw per day; $n = 6$), a high dose of tamoxifen (3.0 mg/kg bw per day; $n = 7$) or lactose ($n = 7$) by gastric instillation daily for 12 days, starting four days after the mid-cycle 17β-oestradiol peak (Olive *et al.*, 1990). The luteal phase of the menstrual cycle was prolonged in the groups receiving tamoxifen compared with the control group, but no difference between the groups receiving low-dose and high-dose tamoxifen was observed. No noteworthy difference in hormonal characteristics between the groups was observed. The authors concluded that administration of tamoxifen during the luteal phase did not alter pituitary gonadotropin secretion or corpus luteum function. They suggested that the prolongation by tamoxifen of the length of the luteal phase in a subset of monkeys was perhaps due to a direct effect on the endometrium. In a study of 26 female *Macaca fascicularis* with proven fertility and normal menstrual cycles, 13 were treated with a single oral dose of 5 mg/kg bw tamoxifen and 13 with vehicle only on postovulation day 4 (Tarantal *et al.*, 1993). Serum progesterone and tamoxifen concentrations were evaluated on postovulation days 4, 8, 12, 16 and 18. There was no effect of tamoxifen on serum progesterone levels or on the fertility rate — 6/13 (46%) treated females and 4/13 controls (31%) became pregnant. In the centre in which the study was carried out, the conception rate for the *Macaca fascicularis* colony was approximately 50% per mated cycle. Among the six pregnant animals treated with tamoxifen, one aborted spontaneously on gestational day 40 (after detection of severe growth retardation and embryonic death on gestational day 38) and five delivered live births naturally during gestational days 160–163. Among the control females who became pregnant, one had an early embryonic loss (at or before gestational day 18), one had a still birth at gestional day 162 and two delivered live births. None of the live births exhibited any abnormality. Neither tamoxifen nor any of its metabolites was detected in maternal serum and urine. The authors postulated that either absorption of tamoxifen was negligible or its metabolism and excretion occurred at an extremely rapid rate.

Beyer *et al.* (1989) assessed the embryotoxic potential of tamoxifen by studying its effect on cultured whole rat embryos in the presence and absence of a NADPH-supplemented post-mitochondrial supernatant fraction from Aroclor 1254-induced male rat liver (S9). Embryos were obtained from pregnant animals on gestational day 10. Only viable embryos, as determined by the presence of visible heart beat and active vitelline circulation, were evaluated. At the time of explantation, conceptuses were up to 10 ± 2 somite stage and were exposed to tamoxifen added directly to the culture medium at the beginning of the 24-h culture period. The results are presented in Table 14. In order to explore further the possible role of oestrogenicity, the interactive effects of tamoxifen with diethylstilboestrol and 17β-oestradiol were investigated. At 0.19 mM diethylstilboestrol or 0.1 mM 17β-oestradiol, in the presence of S9, a series of four tamoxifen concentrations ranging from 0.05 to 0.19 mM were added to the culture medium at the onset of the culture period. In all cases, the effect of tamoxifen appeared to be additive rather than antagonistic. Thus, the effect of tamoxifen was to exacerbate the embryotoxic/dysmorphogenic effects of both diethylstilboestrol and 17β-oestradiol.

Table 14. Embryotoxicity of tamoxifen to rat embryos

Tamoxifen concentration	Exogenous metabolic activation system (S9)	No. of embryos tested	Embryo-lethality (%)	Rotation defects (%)	Neural tube defects (%)	All other defects combined[a] (%)
0.19 mM	+	20	20	27.5	6.3	93.8
0.19 mM	−	17	64.7	43.4	0	100
0	+	261	1.9	8.4	0.7	6.1
0	−	111	2.6	5.4	0.9	2.7

From Beyer *et al.* (1989)
[a]Relatively inconsistent and so combined for analysis

In a preliminary experiment, groups of two or three rabbits were given 0.25, 0.5, 1.0, 2.0 or 4.0 mg/kg bw tamoxifen daily by gastric instillation from day 6 to day 18 of gestation (Esaki & Sakai, 1980). Abortions were observed in both rabbits treated with 4 mg/kg bw and one of the three rabbits treated with 2 mg/kg died. In a following experiment, groups of 10–14 rabbits were given 0.125, 0.5 or 2.0 mg/kg bw tamoxifen daily by gastric instillation from day 6 to day 18 of gestation. In the groups receiving 0.5 and 2.0 mg/kg doses, body-weight gain in the dams was suppressed. Abortions occurred in one animal in each of the lower-dose groups and in five animals in the group receiving 2.0 mg/kg bw. Fetal death rates, defined as the total number of resorption sites for dead embryos divided by the total number of implantations, were 11.6% in the control group, 16.7% in the low-dose group, 39.4% in the mid-dose group and 32.7% in the high-dose group. No effect of tamoxifen on the body weight of live fetuses was observed. On external observation of the live-born fetuses, one exencephaly was observed in the control group and one brain hernia [*sic*] in the group receiving 0.125 mg/kg and one abdominal hernia with brain hernia [*sic*] in the group receiving 2.0 mg/kg. On internal examination, four anomalies were observed in the control group, one in the group receiving the lowest dose of tamoxifen and two in each of the other groups. There were 11 instances of minor malformations of the skull, sternum, caudal vertebrae or ribs in the control group, 12 in the group receiving 0.125 mg/kg tamoxifen and 9 in each of the other two groups.

Groups of four pregnant rabbits were given 2 mg/kg bw tamoxifen per day orally, beginning on gestational day 10 or 20, or vehicle only (Furr *et al.*, 1976). Administration of the drug from gestational day 10 resulted in considerable embryonic loss; only two rabbits gave birth and the average number of young born was 1.75 ± 1.2 compared with 5.8 ± 1.6 for vehicle-treated controls. Since the number of implantation sites was similar, a major effect of the drug was to induce fetal resorption. Administration of the drug from day 20 caused premature parturition and abortion: the length of gestation in the group receiving tamoxifen was 26.8 ± 1.3 days compared with 32.5 ± 0.3 days in controls, and the percentage of young born alive was 65% as compared to 96%. Both of these effects were associated with a significant reduction in plasma progesterone concentration. The differences in plasma progesterone concentrations were not due to differences in the numbers of corpora lutea in the different groups.

Pregnant guinea-pigs (n = 6) of the Hartley albino strain were given 2 mg/kg bw tamoxifen by subcutaneous injection for three or six days (Gulino *et al.*, 1984). Uteri of the fetuses (n = 10) were weighed 24 h after the last administration. Compared with control fetuses, a dose-related increase in uterine wet weight was observed, such that the uterine weight of fetuses of the dam that had received injections for a six-day period was 2.5 times that of controls. This uterotropic effect was associated with a significant increase in uterine DNA content. Tamoxifen also induced an increase in the size of the uterine stroma and myometrium in the fetus. Luminal epithelial cell height was increased by 67 ± 2% after six days of treatment of the dam and luminal epithelial cell number was increased by 160 ± 20%. Uterine epithelial downgrowths invading the stroma were observed in 26 ± 4% of tamoxifen-treated fetuses. In a subsequent study from the same laboratory, groups of 6–10 pregnant guinea-pigs of the Hartley albino strain were given 5 mg/kg bw tamoxifen per day by subcutaneous injection for 12 days or the vehicle alone (Pasqualini & Lecerf, 1986). The uterine epithelial cells of the fetal guinea-pigs were examined by transmission electron microscopy for ultrastructural changes. The fetuses were at 60–64 days of gestation at the time of necropsy. A moderate increase in the height of the fetal uterine epithelial cells and moderate effects on the Golgi system, the rough endoplasmic reticulum and mitochondria were observed. No change in the number of microvilli or cell degeneration was apparent. When the same dose of tamoxifen was administered in combination with 1 mg/kg bw 17β-oestradiol per day for 12 days, the effects on mitochondria were greater than when either compound was given on its own, while the increase in number of microvilli apparent when 17β-oestradiol was given on its own was reduced to the basal level. Therefore, although tamoxifen has antioestrogenic properties, in this species it acted as an agonist in the uterus during fetal development.

Pregnant pigs (sows) were fed diets containing 0 or 10 mg/kg diet (ppm) tamoxifen from gestational day 30 until weaning (Yang et al., 1995). No significant differences in sow body weight, litter size, live births per litter, piglet mortality, piglet sex ratio or piglet birth or weaning weight were observed between the groups. At the age of 21 days, female piglets exposed to tamoxifen in utero and during lactation had smaller ovaries and enlarged uteri compared with controls, but no histological abnormality. Corresponding male piglets had testes 15% lighter than those produced by sows fed the control diet; no consistent histological difference was observed between the groups. Subsequent breeding performance was not affected.

In two trials, approximately 500 eggs from single comb White Leghorn hens were injected on the day of set with either 100 μL tamoxifen (2 mg/μL) or vehicle (corn oil) into the albumen (Coco et al., 1992). Based on phenotypic sexing, the sex ratio of male to female chicks was 76 : 24 for those exposed to tamoxifen compared with 47 : 53 in those treated with vehicle only. When a subset of these chicks was sexed at three weeks of age by identification of gonadal type at necropsy, these ratios were corrected to 46 : 54 and 52 : 48, respectively. In the second trial, the sex ratio based on phenotypic sexing was 62 : 38 for tamoxifen-exposed chicks and 45 : 55 for vehicle-exposed chicks. Gonadal sexing corrected these ratios to 44 : 56 and 45 : 55, respectively. Thus, the genital sexing errors were 27% in the first trial and 18% in the second for tamoxifen-exposed chicks, significantly higher than those treated with vehicle (2 and 0.6%, respectively). Therefore, phenotypic genital sexual differentiation was altered by administration of tamoxifen.

(b) Effects on the dam of gestational exposure to tamoxifen

O'Grady et al. (1974) investigated the effect of doses of tamoxifen known to delay implantation (0.1 mg/kg bw) or to inhibit implantation (0.2 mg/kg bw) on mitosis in the uterus. Tamoxifen was administered to rats on the morning of gestational day 2 and mitosis of the luminal and glandular epithelial and subepithelial stroma was assessed on days 2–5 of the pre-implantation period. The authors considered the delay in implantation induced by the lower dose of tamoxifen to be mediated by an observed delay in oestrogen-supported stromal mitosis. In a study from the same laboratory, Watson et al. (1975) showed that the lower dose of 0.1 mg/kg bw tamoxifen in rats delayed the increase in plasma 17β-oestradiol level by 20 h, a time interval identical to the delay in implantation. While the absolute concentration of 17β-oestradiol reached was lower than that in control animals, the rate of decline was slower and therefore the exposure of the uterus to an increased peak of 17β-oestradiol was more prolonged. A dose of 0.2 mg/kg bw, which prevented implantation, completely eliminated the increase in plasma 17β-oestradiol level and caused a decrease in pituitary LH and a marked rise in plasma LH levels. Neither dose of tamoxifen affected levels of progesterone.

Pugh and Sumano (1979) investigated the effect of tamoxifen on the occurrence of the trophoblastic surface coat change which is associated with implantation in mouse embryos. Groups of 19–26 embryos were cultured in a collagen-containing culture system. Tamoxifen (2.8×10^{-10} M) totally prevented the surface coat change and implantation. When this level of tamoxifen was added to a culture containing 10^{-8} M 17β-oestradiol, the percentage of blastocysts which became attached to collagen decreased from 90.5% to 39.1%.

Gupta and Roy (1987) assessed the effects of tamoxifen on concentrations of cytosolic oestrogen receptor in different parts of the fallopian tube and uterus during ovum transplant in New Zealand albino rabbits. Half of the animals were given 0.03 mg/kg bw tamoxifen orally and the other half were not treated. Groups of animals were killed at normal oestrus stage and at 14, 24, 34, 48, 72, 144 or 168 h *post coitum*. In the tamoxifen-treated animals, the concentration of cytosol receptor was reduced in the ampulla and ampullary isthmic junction but not in the isthmus or uterine isthmic junction, compared with untreated animals. In the treated animals, the ampullary concentration of cytosol receptor increased during 14–34 h post coitum, and suddenly decreased at 48 h post coitum, whereas, from 72 h to 144 h post coitum, it increased gradually. The authors concluded that tamoxifen modulates tubal cytosolic oestrogen receptors during egg transport. [Details of the timing of tamoxifen administration are unclear.]

Treatment of pregnant pigs with 0.7 ($n = 4$) or 7.0 ($n = 2$) mg/kg bw tamoxifen per day did not affect the development of mammary structures or the ability to lactate at parturition (Lin & Buttle, 1991a). Sows were fed diets containing 0 or 10 mg/kg (ppm) tamoxifen from gestational day 30 until weaning (Yang *et al.*, 1995). No significant difference was observed between sows exposed to tamoxifen and unexposed sows in ovarian or uterine weights 21 days after lactation, although there was a trend towards ovarian atrophy and uterine enlargement in exposed sows. The ovaries of exposed sows contained predominantly small and degenerated follicles, whereas numerous large follicles were observed in the ovaries of control sows. The histological appearance of the uteri and ovaries of the treated sows was similar to controls.

(c) *Effects of exposure of neonates and immature animals to tamoxifen on development of the reproductive system*

Uterotropic effects of tamoxifen have been observed in mice, rats and guinea-pigs (Table 15). In rats, these effects are seen in neonatal rats only after short periods of treatment, prolonged treatment appearing to inhibit uterine development. In guinea-pigs, these effects are much stronger when the dose is administered to neonates rather than to immature animals (Gulino *et al.*, 1984).

Irisawa and Iguchi (1990) reported that neonatal treatment of mice with tamoxifen initially caused an increase in uterine weight and height of the uterine epithelium as well as an increase in the thickness of the vaginal epithelium. Tamoxifen treatment also

Table 15. Effect of administration of tamoxifen to neonatal or immature animals on subsequent development of the uterus

Species	Controls	Tamoxifen dose	Age (or weight) at administration	Age when outcome assessed	Effects on uterus — Uterine weight relative to body weight	Other effects	Reference
Rat	Vehicle	100 µg s.c.	Day 5	Day 9	Increased 1.5-fold	Epithelial hypertrophy	Clark et al. (1981)
	Vehicle	5 µg s.c.	Days 1, 3 and 5	ca. Day 120	All uteri were atrophic.	90% replacement of luminal lining and glands by squamous metaplasia	Chamness et al. (1979)
	Saline	0.01, 0.1, 1.0, 10.0 mg/kg bw, orally or s.c. for 3 days	35–45 g	Days 4 or 7	Increased with increasing dose; more marked change with oral dose; continuing treatment for a further 3 days reduced uterine weight		Wakeling et al. (1983)
	Untreated	10 µg/day for 5 days s.c.	Days 1–5	Day 26	Significantly decreased compared with controls	Cross-sectional areas of uterine glands, luminal epithelium and endometrial stroma were substantially reduced. Little change in cell density in any cell population, except for a marked reduction in the cell density of the luminal epithelium.	Branham et al. (1988)
	Vehicle	100 or 200 µg for 5 days s.c.	Days 1–5	Day 60	Significantly decreased	Uterine lumen of the greater part of the horns was narrow and lined with cuboidal epithelial cells. In about half the rats given the larger doses, some parts of the luminal epithelium disappeared.	Ohta et al. (1989)
Mouse	Saline vehicle	2, 20 or 100 µg for 5 days s.c.	Days 1–5	Days 35 or 150	Decreased at day 35 in mice receiving the 2 or 20 µg dose; increased in mice receiving the 100 µg dose. At day 150, all treated groups had lower uterine weights than controls.	In 40%, 90% and 100% of the groups receiving 2, 20 or 100 µg, respectively, the circular musculature of the myometrium exhibited involution. The number of uterine glands per section was significantly reduced.	Iguchi et al. (1986)

Table 15 (contd)

Species	Controls	Tamoxifen dose	Age (or weight) at administration	Age when outcome assessed	Effects on uterus — Uterine weight relative to body weight	Other effects	Reference
	Saline	100 µg for 5 days s.c.	Days 1–5	Days 5, 10, 15, 20, 30 and 60	Increased at days 5, 15 and 20 — lighter at day 60; increased weight resulted from oedematous change in stromal tissue	Cell heights of luminal epithelium greater at days 5–30 than controls; shorter at day 60	Irisawa & Iguchi (1990)
Guinea-pig	Vehicle	0.6 µg/g bw for 3 or 6 days s.c.	Days 6 or 27	24 h after last injection	Increased with administration at day 6 but only weakly with administration at day 27[a]	Increased uterine DNA content, luminal epithelial cell height. Luminal epithelial cell number increased with administration at day 6 but only slightly with administration at day 27.	Gulino et al. (1984)
	Vehicle	100 µg for 2 or 12 days s.c.	Newborn (2–15 days old)	24 h after last injection	—	Electron microscopy showed moderate effects on epithelial cell height, microvilli number, Golgi system, rough endoplasmic reticulum and mitochondria. The longer period of dosage produced a 'very intensive effect' on mitochondria.	Pasqualini & Lecerf (1986)
		100 µg for 2 or 12 days s.c.	Day 2		Increased[a]	Cell heights increased 2–3 fold.	Pasqualini et al. (1986)
Pig	Vehicle	0.1 or 1 mg/kg bw per day for 7 days i.m.	6 weeks old	24 h after last injection	Dose-related increase in wet weight: 6, 12, 28 g	DNA expressed as mg/g tissue decreased ca. 50%; RNA and protein stable	Lin & Buttle (1991)

s.c., subcutaneous injection; i.m., intramuscular injection
[a]Absolute weight

caused poor formation of the uterine gland and development of the mesenchymal stroma. However, by 60 days of age, the weights of the uteri of the tamoxifen-treated mice were lower and the cell heights of the uterine luminal epithelium were smaller than those of controls. The number of uterine glands and the number of mice having a well developed tunica muscularis remained smaller than those in controls of the same age. Thus, neonatal treatment with tamoxifen resulted in a permanent alteration in both the uterine epithelial and stromal compartments. The critical period for induction of these uterine abnormalities was determined to be within three to seven days after birth.

The genital organs of female C57Bl/Tw mice given five daily injections of 100 μg tamoxifen from the day of birth were examined at 5, 10, 15, 20, 30 and 60 days of age (Irisawa & Iguchi, 1990). Adenosis-like lesions were found in the vaginae of 5–30-day-old mice exposed to tamoxifen. These lesions were not detected at 60 days of age. The number of polyovular follicles containing two to four oocytes per follicle markedly increased from 10 to 15 days of age in mice exposed to tamoxifen, and the incidence was twice as high as that in age-matched controls. Corpora lutea were found in the ovaries of 60-day-old controls, whereas no corpora lutea were found in age-matched mice exposed to tamoxifen. In order to determine the critical period of induction by tamoxifen of abnormalities of the female genital organs, other groups of mice were also given five daily injections of 100 μg tamoxifen or of vehicle alone starting on the day of birth, or 3, 5, 7 and 10 days after birth. Tamoxifen injections starting within five days of birth caused a high incidence of polyovular follicles in the ovary and of aplasia of tunica muscularis in the uterus. Atrophy of the uterine luminal epithelium was also induced when the treatment was started within seven days of birth. However, in mice given tamoxifen from day 10, uterine weights were greater than in those given tamoxifen from zero to seven days, and the authors concluded that the postnatal limit of the critical period for the female genital organs lies within seven days of birth.

In female C57Bl/Tw mice given five daily injections of 2, 20 or 100 μg tamoxifen starting on the day of birth, uterine hypoplasia, myometrial involution and suppression of uterine-gland genesis were found at 35 and 150 days of age (Iguchi *et al.*, 1986). About half of the mice killed when 150 days old were ovariectomized at 90 days. Vaginal hypoplasia and hypospadia were observed in most treated animals at 150 days of age. Vaginal adenosis was found in 40% of the 35-day-old mice treated with 2 μg tamoxifen, 70% of those treated with 20 μg and 100% of those treated with 100 μg, whereas none of the controls showed these lesions. Adenosis was not observed in any of the 150-day-old mice. In both age groups, the weight of ovaries was significantly lower following injections of 20 or 100 μg tamoxifen than in controls. At 150 days of age, hernia of the urinary bladder, located under or below the symphysis pubis, was found in 56% and 100% of non-ovariectomized mice in the mid- and high-dose groups. The urinary bladders of the group receiving the lowest dose and the control group were situated normally in the abdominal cavity. The authors suggested that the tamoxifen treatment caused a long-lasting suppression of the development of the pubic bone and ligament, resulting in looseness of the symphysis pubis which allowed the bladder to descend through the extended subpubic space.

In NMRI mice treated neonatally with tamoxifen, adenosis-like lesions observed in the vagina and cervix were similar to those induced by neonatal treatment with diethylstilboestrol, but differed in that the tamoxifen-induced lesions regressed with time (Forsberg, 1985).

Fifteen male NMRI/Tg mouse pups were given 20 μg tamoxifen by subcutaneous injection daily for three days, starting approximately 24 h after birth. Ten control pups were given injections of saline. At three months of age, all mice were housed with normal females for two weeks to investigate reproductive capacities. All tamoxifen-exposed males were sterile and did not impregnate any female during the mating period, whereas all control males were able to impregnate one or both females with which they were housed. When killed at eight months of age, the exposed male pups had multiple reproductive tract lesions including testicular hypoplasia, undescended testes, epididymal cysts and squamous metaplasia of the seminal vesicle; two of the exposed mice had squamous metaplasia of the median prostate (Taguchi, 1987).

In addition to inhibiting uterine development, administration of 5 μg tamoxifen by subcutaneous injection to newborn female Sprague-Dawley rats on days 1, 3 and 5 of age produced early vaginal opening and absent cycles (Chamness et al., 1979). At four months of age, all ovaries were atrophic and the oviducts showed severe squamous metaplasia with abscess formation. Corporea lutea were uniformly absent except for a few that were found in one animal. The vaginal observations were stated to be unremarkable, except that one animal had a vaginal adenosis suggestive of that observed in women whose mothers received diethylstilboestrol during pregnancy.

Branham et al. (1993) gave 20–24-day-old rats five daily subcutaneous injections of tamoxifen (0.01–100 μg/rat/day) and then examined the uteri 2 h after the last dose. Uterine weights increased only slightly, whereas luminal epithelium hypertrophy increased 3-fold at 10 μg/rat and glandular epithelium hypertrophy increased 2-fold at the same dose. In contrast, oestrogens (17β-oestradiol, ethinyloestradiol, diethylstilboestrol) tested over the same dose range produced substantial increases in uterine weight and no glandular epithelium hypertrophy; the luminal epithelium response to 17β-oestradiol was similar to that of tamoxifen, while the other oestrogens required a 100-fold lower dose to elicit the same response. The greater hypertrophic response in luminal epithelium to both oestrogens and antioestrogens does not correlate with the oestrogen receptor content, which is greatest in the endometrial stroma and glandular epithelium in mouse, rat and macaque (Martin, 1980; Korach et al., 1988; Tse & Goldfarb, 1988; McClellan et al., 1984). It was suggested by Branham et al. (1993) that the high concentrations of tamoxifen (and other antioestrogens) required to elicit glandular epithelial hypertrophy is consistent with either a nonoestrogen-receptor-mediated response or a stromal mediation of epithelial responses.

Female rats of the T strain given single daily injections of 100 or 200 μg tamoxifen for five days beginning on the day of birth exhibited continued vaginal dioestrus when sacrificed on day 60, whereas vehicle-treated controls showed regular oestrus cycles (Ohta et al., 1989). Ovaries from the tamoxifen-treated rats were polyfollicular without corpora lutea, whereas ovaries from controls contained both follicles and corpora lutea.

The vaginae of tamoxifen-treated rats ovariectomized on days 10 or 60 failed to respond to a three-day priming with 0.1 µg 17β-oestradiol, showing no oestrus smears. The authors concluded, therefore, that continued vaginal dioestrus in tamoxifen-treated rats may be accounted for by changed sensitivity of the ovary to gonadotropin and/or of the vagina to sex hormones. Lack of cyclicity and corpora lutea in the ovaries in rats was also reported by Irisawa and Iguchi (1990) and in NMRI mice by Forsberg (1985). Thus, tamoxifen appears to impair the female genital organs directly and/or indirectly through the hypothalamus.

In a study of the regulation of reproductive behaviour in rats (Ulibarri & Micevych, 1993), male rat pups were castrated, given sham surgeries or implanted with tamoxifen [dose not specified] within 3 h of birth. Female animals were implanted with a similar dose of tamoxifen or with empty capsules. All capsules were removed on postnatal day 10. Tamoxifen treatment was toxic to pups and only nine males and two females survived to surgery on day 90. Tamoxifen-treated females had large green ovarian growths and smaller growths throughout their peritonea. Tamoxifen-treated males had significantly smaller testes at adult surgery than sham-treated males. Tamoxifen-treated males and sham-operated males did not show appreciable lordosis behaviour. The authors noted that this finding differs from results with other oestrogen antagonists. The authors speculated that the antioestrogenic *trans*-isomer of tamoxifen may have been converted to the oestrogenic *cis*-isomer or that the *trans*-isomer of tamoxifen may have acted oestrogenically.

Pasqualini *et al.* (1986) reported that 100 µg tamoxifen administered subcutaneously to two-day-old guinea-pigs for two or 12 days substantially increased the weight and the protein and DNA content of the uterus and vagina; the weight increase was 3–4-fold in the group receiving prolonged treatment. Progesterone did not block this action. Tamoxifen caused a strong increase in the content of progesterone receptor in cytosol and nuclei of the cells of the vagina after prolonged treatment.

In immature, six-week-old pigs given 0.1 or 1.0 mg/kg bw tamoxifen per day for seven days, significant dose-related increases were seen in uterine weight, in the total content of uterine DNA, RNA and protein and in levels of progesterone receptor per milligram DNA (Lin & Buttle, 1991). The total duct area in the mammary glands increased about three-fold in the groups treated with either dose of tamoxifen, compared with vehicle-treated controls. The concentration of progesterone receptors in cytosol extracts of mammary tissue was very heterogeneous and independent of treatment with tamoxifen. Concurrent administration of tamoxifen with oestradiol benzoate induced significant increases in total uterine protein and in the concentration of progesterone receptors compared with treatment with oestradiol benzoate alone. However, concurrent administration partially inhibited the effect of oestradiol benzoate in stimulating an increase in mammary duct area. Thus, tamoxifen acts as an oestrogen agonist in the uterus of immature pigs, but as an antagonist in the mammary gland.

In rabbits, tamoxifen appears to act as an oestrogen antagonist when administered to sexually immature animals (Foster *et al.*, 1993). Female New Zealand white rabbits were given 10 mg/kg bw tamoxifen per day by subcutaneous injection from day 22 of age for a total of 108 days, while control rabbits were given the vehicle only. Tamoxifen treatment impaired sexual development profoundly, as assessed by ovarian weight, diameter of growing follicles, diameter of anthral follicles and number of such follicles. There was profound suppression of pituitary gonadotropin levels in the group receiving tamoxifen, but no difference in the circulating levels of plasma 17β-oestradiol between control and tamoxifen-treated rabbits. These differences were associated with suppression of the developmental shift from smooth to rough gonadotropin-releasing hormone cell types in the hypothalamus.

(d) *Effects of exposure of neonates and immature animals to tamoxifen on bone development*

Neonatal treatment of female mice with tamoxifen induces permanent chondrification of the pubic bones and, in consequence, expansion of the pubic ligament, leading to urinary bladder hernia [exstrophy] with or without caecum hernia [dilatated] (see above) (Iguchi et al., 1986). Subsequently, Iguchi et al. (1988) examined sequential changes in the pelvic bone of male and female C57Bl/TW mice following neonatal treatment with tamoxifen and sought to determine a critical period for the induction by tamoxifen of bladder hernia with or without caecum hernia. Mice were given five daily subcutaneous injections of 100 μg tamoxifen or of the vehicle alone, starting on the day of birth or at 3, 5, 7 or 10 days of age. Untreated mice showed completely calcified pelvic bone after 30 days of age, whereas, in age-matched tamoxifen-treated mice, the greater part of the junctional regions in the pelvis remained cartilaginous. Treatment with tamoxifen starting within five days of age caused bladder hernia with or without caecum hernia. The pubic ligament in tamoxifen-treated mice aged 30–540 days was markedly expanded as compared with age-matched controls. Permanent chondrification in the pelvis was found in all mice given tamoxifen starting before 10 days of age. Neonatal treatment of mice with similar doses of clomiphene and nafoxidine did not induce permanent chondrification of the pelvis, expansion of the pubic ligaments or hernia. Therefore, the authors conclude that tamoxifen has a specific effect on the pubic symphysis and on some junctional regions of the developing pelvis in mice when given neonatally. In a study from the same laboratory, Uesugi et al. (1993) carried out a morphometric analysis of the pelvis of C57Bl/TW mice given five daily injections of 100 μg tamoxifen or saline alone starting at birth, and killed at 120 days of age. The total areas of the pelvis, ilium, ischium, and pubis were significantly smaller in tamoxifen-treated mice than in the controls. Differences were also observed in the shape of the pelvis, reflected by the lengths of the ilium and pubis, and the widths of the ilium, pubis and ischium were smaller in tamoxifen-treated mice than in controls. The numbers of osteoblasts and osteoclasts per 200 μm trabecular surface length and per 10 000 μm^2 subperiosteal area of pubic bone section were smaller in tamoxifen-treated females than in control females. The authors concluded that neonatal administration of tamoxifen retards the growth of the ilium and pubis in mice by changing the activities of osteoclasts and osteoblasts and that the drug acts directly on the pubis of the neonatal mouse to inhibit its ossification.

Tamoxifen has been reported to have oestrogen agonist effects, namely effects on rat bone in immature or ovariectomized animals, and antagonistic effects in intact mature animals. As the different effects may be due to differences in ovarian status, oestrogen levels and tamoxifen dose, Moon et al. (1991) investigated the effects of different doses of tamoxifen on the long bones of intact and ovariectomized female rats, with or without oestrogen treatment. Pellets containing 0, 1.5, 3, 5, 15 or 30 mg tamoxifen were implanted subcutaneously into intact, young adult female Sprague-Dawley rats. An untreated baseline control group was available. Tamoxifen treatment resulted in a dose-dependent decrease in overall growth rate and a dose-dependent increase in the periosteal bone formation rate in both ovariectomized and intact rats. It also prevented a decrease in cancellous bone balance after ovariectomy, although the highest dose of tamoxifen caused a small decrease in the cancellous bone balance in intact female rats. In order to determine whether tamoxifen alters the skeletal response of ovariectomized rats to oestrogen, rats were implanted with pellets containing 5 mg tamoxifen or 0.1 mg 17β-oestradiol, or both drugs or none. Tamoxifen treatment did not alter the effects of 17β-oestradiol on the periosteal bone formation rate in ovariectomized rats, but reduced the increase in cancellous bone balance to values similar to those in intact rats. The authors concluded that tamoxifen behaves as a partial oestrogen agonist on rat bone.

(e) *Effects of exposure of adult non-pregnant animals to tamoxifen on reproductive parameters*

In mature, virgin female Spague-Dawley rats which had been bilaterally ovariectomized, a single subcutaneous injection of 1 mg/kg bw tamoxifen increased uterine wet weight and blood flow (Marshall & Senior, 1987). The uterotrophic response lasted for between 35 and 42 days. Twenty-four hours after tamoxifen treatment, cytosolic oestrogen receptor levels were markedly reduced compared with control values and remained depressed until 21 days after injection, when they began to increase towards control values. The concentration of nuclear receptors reached a maximum at 27 h after injection, then declined to a plateau by 21 days after injection, but this was still above control values. Weights of uteri and vaginae in ovariectomized adult female C57Bl/Tw mice given three daily subcutaneous injections of 100 µg tamoxifen were significantly greater than those in ovariectomized untreated mice (Chou et al., 1992). The uterine weight increase was associated with increased DNA and protein contents of the uterus, and in the cell heights of uterine luminal epithelial cells.

Gill-Sharma et al. (1993) investigated the effects of oral administration of doses of 40, 200 or 400 µg/kg bw per day tamoxifen for 60, 70, 80 or 90 days on the circulating concentrations of plasma hormones, tissue weights and reproductive performance of adult male Holtzman rats. Tamoxifen produced a dose-related reduction in testosterone concentration. Concentrations of FSH, prolactin and 17β-oestradiol were unaffected. The plasma level of LH was significantly lower after treatment with 200 and 400 µg/kg bw tamoxifen per day than in controls, but the 40 µg/kg dose had no effect. Tamoxifen given at 40 µg/kg bw per day for 90 days did not affect the weights of testes, seminal vesicles, epididymes, ventral prostate glands or the pituitary glands. At higher doses, the weights of the ventral prostate glands, seminal vesicles and epididymes were significantly lower than those of controls. Histological examination of testes from tamoxifen-exposed animals showed marked disorganization of the cytoarchitecture of the tubule and obliteration of the lumen. The potency, fecundity, number of implantation sites, fertility index and litter size of male rats treated with tamoxifen were significantly lower than those of controls, and these effects were more marked for the highest dose than for the lowest dose. Reversibility studies were performed with 200 µg/kg bw tamoxifen per day. All the effects of tamoxifen on weights of seminal vesicles, ventral prostate glands, epididymes, concentrations of LH and testosterone in plasma, potency, fecundity, fertility index and litter size were reversed 90 days after drug withdrawal.

In female guinea-pigs given 10 mg tamoxifen by subcutaneous injection daily from days 11 to 14 of the cycle, uterine output of prostaglandin F_2 was not inhibited and luteal regression was not delayed (Poyser, 1993). The uteri were removed on day 15. In homogenates of endometrium and myometrium, prostaglandin synthesis was redirected in the uteri from tamoxifen-treated animals from prostaglandin I_2 to F_2, showing tamoxifen to be an oestrogen agonist in guinea-pigs.

Groups of 12 female mink were fed diets containing 0 or 10 mg/kg (ppm) tamoxifen for two months before breeding (Yang *et al.*, 1995). Treated females were placed with untreated males. All the exposed females rejected the advances of the males and often attacked them. The females were provided with an opportunity to mate at four-day intervals during a 20-day period, but none mated. Upon necropsy four days later, the uteri showed various degrees of pyometra in one or both horns. Histological examination of two females from each group showed ovarian follicular atrophy and degeneration, mild to severe uterine atrophy, pyometra and endometritis in tamoxifen-exposed animals, whereas the reproductive tracts from the control females appeared normal.

4.4 Genetic and related effects

4.4.1 *Humans*

No data were available to the Working Group.

4.4.2 *Experimental systems* (see also Table 16 for references and Appendices 1 and 2)

Mutation and allied effects

Reports available to the Working Group for a lack of tamoxifen activity in a *Salmonella typhimurium* mutation test and a rat dominant lethal assay were not suitable for evaluation.

Unscheduled DNA synthesis was induced in primary cultures of rat hepatocytes treated with tamoxifen, but only in cells isolated from animals that had been pretreated with three daily doses of tamoxifen itself (45 mg/kg orally).

Tamoxifen induced significant morphological transformation of Syrian hamster embryo cells.

Tamoxifen induced micronucleus formation in a number of in-vitro studies with MCL-5 cells, a genetically-engineered human lymphoblastoid cell line that expresses five human cytochrome P450s (CYP1A1, CYP1A2, CYP2A6, CYP2E1 and CYP3A4) and epoxide hydrolase. Kinetochore staining (Crofton-Sleigh *et al.*, 1993) showed that, at

Table 16. Genetic and related effects of tamoxifen

Test system	Result[a]		Dose[b] (LED/HID)	Reference
	Without exogenous metabolic system	With exogenous metabolic system		
URP, Unscheduled DNA synthesis, rat primary hepatocytes	−[c]	NT	1.86	White et al. (1992)
TCS, Cell transformation, Syrian hamster embryo cells, clonal assay	+	NT	0.037	Metzler & Schiffmann (1991)
MIH, Micronucleus test, human lymphoblastoid MCL-5 cells in vitro	+[d]	NT	0.74	White et al. (1992)
MIH, Micronucleus test, human lymphoblastoid MCL-5 cells in vitro	+[d]	NT	2	Crofton-Sleigh et al. (1993)
MIH, Micronucleus test, AHH-1 cells in vitro	−	NT	8	Crofton-Sleigh et al. (1993)
MIH, Micronucleus test, human lymphoblastoid MCL-5 cells in vitro	+[d]	NT	1	Phillips et al. (1994b)
MIH, Micronucleus test, human lymphoblastoid MCL-5 cells in vitro	+[d]	NT	0.5	Styles et al. (1994)
MIH, Micronucleus test, human lymphoblastoid h1A1 cells expressing CYP1A1 in vitro	−	NT	1.5	Styles et al. (1994)
MIH, Micronucleus test, human lymphoblastoid n1A2 cells expressing CYP1A2 in vitro	−	NT	1.5	Styles et al. (1994)
MIH, Micronucleus test, human lymphoblastoid h2E1 cells expressing CYP2E1 in vitro	+	NT	0.125	Styles et al. (1994)
MIH, Micronucleus test, human lymphoblastoid h3A4 cells expressing CYP3A4 in vitro	+	NT	0.25	Styles et al. (1994)
MIH, Micronucleus test, human lymphoblastoid h2D6 cells expressing CYP2D6 in vitro	(+)	NT	3	Styles et al. (1994)
CVA, Chromosomal aberrations, rat hepatocytes in vivo	+		0.3 po × 1	Sargent et al. (1994)
AVA, Aneuploidy, rat hepatocytes in vivo	+		0.3 po × 1	Sargent et al. (1994)
BID, Binding (covalent) to DNA, primary rat hepatocytes in vitro (^{32}P-postlabelling)	+	NT	0.37	Phillips et al. (1994a)
BID, Binding (covalent) to DNA, human lymphocytes in vitro	+	NT	10	Hemminki et al. (1995)
BID, Binding (covalent) to DNA, phenobarbital-treated rat liver microsomes in vitro (^{32}P-postlabelling)	NT	+	37	Pathak et al. (1995)

Table 16 (contd)

Test system	Result[a]		Dose[b] (LED/HID)	Reference
	Without exogenous metabolic system	With exogenous metabolic system		
BID, Binding (covalent) to DNA, calf thymus in vitro	NT	+	37	Moorthy et al. (1996)
BID, Binding (covalent) to DNA, primary rat hepatocytes in vitro (^{32}P-postlabelling)	+		0.37	Phillips et al. (1996a)
BID, Binding (covalent) to DNA, primary mouse hepatocytes in vitro (^{32}P-postlabelling)	+		3.7	Phillips et al. (1996a)
BID, Binding (covalent) to DNA, primary human hepatocytes in vitro (^{32}P-postlabelling)	–		3.7	Phillips et al. (1996a)
BID, Binding (covalent) to DNA, human endometrium in vitro	–		186	Carmichael et al. (1996)
BVD, Binding (covalent) to DNA, male and female SD rat liver in vivo (^{32}P-postlabelling)	+		20 ip × 1	Han & Liehr (1992)
BVD, Binding (covalent) to DNA, female SD rat kidney in vivo (^{32}P-postlabelling)	(+)[c]		20 ip × 6	Han & Liehr (1992)
BVD, Binding (covalent) to DNA, Syrian hamster liver in vivo (^{32}P-postlabelling)	+		5 ip × 1	Han & Liehr (1992)
BVD, Binding (covalent) to DNA, Fischer 344/N rat liver in vivo (^{32}P-postlabelling)	+[f]		5 po × 7	White et al. (1992)
BVD, Binding (covalent) to DNA, female Sprague-Dawley rat liver in vivo (^{32}P-postlabelling)	+		3.7 × 10	Montandon & Williams (1994)
BVD, Binding (covalent) to DNA, female Syrian hamster liver in vivo	+		6.9 × 7	Montandon & Williams (1994)
BVD, Binding (covalent) to DNA, Fischer 344 rat liver in vivo	+		22 po × 1	Phillips et al. (1994b)
BVD, Binding (covalent) to DNA, female ICR mice liver in vivo (^{32}P-postlabelling)	+		45 po × 1	Randerath et al. (1994a)
BVD, Binding (covalent) to DNA, female ICR mice liver, lung and kidney in vivo (^{32}P-postlabelling)	+		45 ip × 4	Randerath et al. (1994b)
BVD, Binding (covalent) to DNA, female Sprague-Dawley rat liver in vivo (^{32}P-postlabelling)	+		45 ip × 4	Randerath et al. (1994b)
BVD, Binding (covalent) to DNA, female Wistar rat liver in vivo (^{32}P-postlabelling)	+		20 diet × 3 mo	Carthew et al. (1995a)

Table 16 (contd)

Test system	Result[a]		Dose[b] (LED/HID)	Reference
	Without exogenous metabolic system	With exogenous metabolic system		
BVD, Binding (covalent) to DNA, female Wistar, Fischer 344 and Lewis LEW rat liver in vivo	+		20 diet × 1 mo	Carthew et al. (1995b)
BVD, Binding (covalent) to DNA, female Sprague-Dawley rat liver in vivo (^{32}P-postlabelling)	+		20 ip × 7	Pathak et al. (1995)
BVD, Binding (covalent) to DNA, female ICR mice liver in vivo (^{32}P-postlabelling)	+		45 ip × 4	Moorthy et al. (1996)
BVD, Binding (covalent) to DNA, DBA/2 and C57Bl/6 mouse liver in vivo	+		45 po × 4	White et al. (1992)
BVD, Binding (covalent) to DNA, female SD rat liver in vivo (^{32}P-postlabelling)	+		45 po × 7	Hard et al. (1993)
BHD, Binding (covalent) to DNA, female human breast cancer patient liver (^{32}P-postlabelling)	–		0.5 daily 2–39 mo	Martin et al. (1995)
BHD, Binding (covalent) to DNA, female human breast cancer patients, white blood cells (^{32}P-postlabelling)	–		0.36 daily 3–72 mo	Phillips et al. (1996b)
BHD, Binding (covalent) to DNA, female human breast cancer patients endometrium (^{32}P-postlabelling)	–		0.73 daily 3–108 mo	Carmichael et al. (1996)

[a] +, positive; (+), weak positive; –, negative; NT, not tested; ?, inconclusive
[b] LED, lowest effective dose; HID, highest ineffective dose; in-vitro tests, μg/mL; in-vivo tests, mg/kg bw/day
[c] Positive when rats were pretreated orally with tamoxifen (45 mg/kg bw/day × 3); hepatocyte cultures established 24 h after the last dose and then exposed to tamoxifen
[d] Expressing native CYP1A1 and transfected CYPs 1A2, 2A6, 3A4 and 2E1 and microsomal epoxide hydrolase; cytochalasin B-arrested
[e] No adducts detected in uterine tissue
[f] No adduct formation in duodenum, kidney, lung, spleen, uterus or peripheral lymphocyte DNA at 45 mg/kg bw/day po × 7

every dose tested, an excess of micronuclei without kinetochores was induced, a result indicating that the micronuclei were probably induced by clastogenic events. Tamoxifen has also been tested in cell lines expressing each of the isozymes singly. The frequencies of micronucleus occurrence fell in the order MCL-5 > CYP2E1 > CYP3A4 > CYP2D6; micronuclei were not significantly induced in cells expressing only CYP1A1 or CYP1A2 (Styles et al., 1994).

In hepatocytes isolated from female Sprague-Dawley rats given a single dose of tamoxifen by gavage, aneuploidy was observed in 70% of the cells, even at the lowest dose level of 0.3 mg/kg bw (Sargent et al., 1994). Premature condensation (2–10%) and endoreduplication (5–10%) were also observed in the hepatocytes from tamoxifen-treated rats. Chromosome exchanges as well as breakages were observed and examination of the cells by electron microscopy revealed both unipolar and incompletely elongated spindles.

p53 Mutations

DNA from hepatocarcinomas of female Sprague-Dawley rats treated with tamoxifen was examined for the presence of mutations in exons 5–9 of the *p53* gene (Vancutsem et al., 1994). Mutations were found in 12 out of 24 tumours; a total of 13 mutations were clustered at two specific sites, codons 231 (exon 6–7) and 294 (exon 8). Nine were A → G transitions at the second base of codon 231 (CAC), which resulted in a histidine to arginine substitution. Four tumours contained a silent C → T transition in the third base of codon 294 (TGC); one tumour contained both mutations.

DNA adducts

Several studies have demonstrated that tamoxifen forms DNA adducts when incubated with DNA in the presence of microsomal systems, in cells in culture and in rodents, but not in humans. In all of the studies, ^{32}P-postlabelling analysis was the detection method used.

Incubation of tamoxifen with DNA in the presence of rat or human liver microsomes resulted in the formation of DNA adducts, with the pattern of adducts depending on whether cumene hydroperoxide or nicotinamide-adenine dinucleotide phosphate (NADPH) was included in the incubation as the cofactor for peroxidase or cytochrome P450 enzyme-mediated reactions, respectively (Pathak & Bodell, 1994). With tamoxifen at a concentration of 100 μM, total adduct levels of 2.97 adducts per 10^8 nucleotides were obtained with human microsomes when NADPH was the cofactor and 11.1 adducts per 10^8 nucleotides when cumene hydroperoxide was used. With uninduced rat liver microsomes, the corresponding adduct levels were 0.86 and 6.5 adducts per 10^8 nucleotides, respectively.

In another study, somewhat lower levels of microsome-mediated DNA modification by tamoxifen at a concentration of 1 mM were achieved (Hemminki et al., 1995). In the presence of NADP and glucose-6-phosphate, the adduct levels were 0.24 adducts per 10^8 nucleotides with rat microsomes and 0.043 adducts per 10^8 nucleotides with human microsomes.

Covalent binding of tamoxifen to DNA can also be mediated by horseradish peroxidase/hydrogen peroxide (Davies et al., 1995).

In primary cultures of hepatocytes from uninduced female Fischer 344 rats treated with 1 µM or 10 µM [0.37 or 3.7 µg/mL] tamoxifen for 18 h, the levels of DNA adducts were 18.7 ± 7.5 and 115.1 ± 16.4 per 10^8 nucleotides, respectively (Phillips et al., 1994a).

The metabolic activation of tamoxifen in primary cultures of rat, mouse and human hepatocytes has been compared (Phillips et al., 1996a). DNA adducts were readily detected in rat hepatocytes treated with 1 µM or 10 µM tamoxifen (mean levels, 18.2 and 89.8 adducts per 10^8 nucleotides, respectively) and mouse hepatocytes (15.0 ± 1.8 adducts per 10^8 nucleotides) treated with 10 µM tamoxifen. However, DNA adducts were not detected in tamoxifen-treated human hepatocytes with a detection limit for the assay of 0.04 adducts per 10^8 nucleotides.

Low levels of DNA adducts (up to 0.16 adducts per 10^8 nucleotides) were detected in cultured human lymphocytes treated with 10–100 µg/mL tamoxifen but not at lower (2.5 and 5 µg/mL) doses (Hemminki et al., 1995).

Han and Liehr (1992) demonstrated the formation of DNA adducts in the livers of Sprague-Dawley rats given 20 mg/kg bw tamoxifen by intraperitoneal injection daily for one, three or six days. Lower levels of adducts were detected in the kidneys of both sexes. No adducts were detected in uterine tissue. Adducts were also detected in the liver DNA of female hamsters treated with single intraperitoneal injections of 5 or 10 mg/kg bw tamoxifen.

Liver DNA adducts were also detected in Fischer 344 rats treated orally with tamoxifen (White et al., 1992). The DNA adducts in rats reached levels of $\geq 100/10^8$ nucleotides and were dose-related in the range 5–45 mg/kg bw tamoxifen per day for seven days. DNA adducts were not detected in the duodenum, kidney, lung, spleen, uterus or peripheral lymphocytes of treated rats.

C57Bl/6 and DBA/2 mice were given 45 mg/kg bw tamoxifen per day orally for four days. Tamoxifen–DNA adduct levels in the liver were 17 ± 5.7 and 28 ± 6.8 adducts per 10^8, respectively, compared with 116 ± 29 adducts per 10^8 in rats treated at the same dose. Dietary exposure of C57Bl/6 mice to tamoxifen (450 mg/kg of diet (ppm)) for 30 days resulted in about one third of the level of total adducts (69 ± 21 adducts per 10^8 nucleotides) seen in correspondingly treated Fischer rats (approximately 200 adducts per 10^8 nucleotides) (White et al., 1992).

DNA adduct formation in rat liver was also demonstrated, but not quantified, in female Crl:CD(BR) rats given 45 mg/kg bw tamoxifen orally for seven days (Hard et al., 1993). In a subsequent study (Montandon & Williams, 1994), Sprague-Dawley rats were given ten daily doses of 10, 30 and 90 µmol/kg (6, 17 and 51 mg/kg bw per day) tamoxifen and 2, 30 and 40.9 adducts per 10^8 nucleotides were measured [these values are the means of two different methods used by the authors to quantitate adducts]. Parallel studies in Syrian hamsters given 17, 53 and 160 µmol/kg bw/day (10, 30 and 90 mg/kg per day, respectively) for seven days produced adduct levels of 1.8, 3.5 and 13.6 adducts per 10^8 nucleotides [mean values of two quantitation methods used].

In three female Wistar (Alderley Park) rats given tamoxifen in the diet at 420 mg/kg (ppm) for three months, the level of liver adducts was 721 ± 420 per 10^8 nucleotides, which fell to 443 ± 38 per 10^8 nucleotides after a further three months on basal diet. In control rats, the background adduct levels ranged from 75 to 80 per 10^8 nucleotides (Carthew et al., 1995a). In three other strains of rats (Fischer 344, Wistar LAC-P and Lewis LEW) fed diets containing 420 mg/kg diet (ppm) tamoxifen for up to 180 days, the adducts levels were about 500 per 10^8 nucleotides after 30 days, rising to about 3000 per 10^8 nucleotides after 180 days (Carthew et al., 1995b).

In a pilot study, DNA adducts levels were compared in liver samples from seven women (37–91 years of age) who had been treated with tamoxifen (at either 20 mg or 2 × 20 mg/day) up to the time of sampling for 2–39 months, with those of seven women (42–74 years of age) not receiving tamoxifen (Martin et al., 1995). Mean DNA adduct levels were 18–60 per 10^8 nucleotides in the tamoxifen-treated women and 38–80 per 10^8 nucleotides in the samples from women who had not received the drug. The adduct patterns observed did not show the characteristics of those seen with DNA from the livers of tamoxifen-treated rats.

In another small study, DNA from white blood cells of seven women receiving tamoxifen (serum concentrations, 34–178 ng/mL) as adjuvant therapy for breast cancer and of three women who served as healthy controls was analysed by ^{32}P-postlabelling (Phillips et al., 1996b). With a limit of detection of 0.08 adducts per 10^8 nucleotides, adducts having the chromatographic properties of tamoxifen–DNA adducts formed in rodent liver cells were not detected in any of the individuals and no difference between the chromatograms of samples from the exposed and control women was observed.

Carmichael et al. (1996) analysed endometrial DNA from 18 patients receiving daily treatment with 10–40 mg tamoxifen for three months to nine years. Although all chromatograms of ^{32}P-labelled DNA digests displayed a background of low-level DNA damage, no evidence for the formation of tamoxifen–DNA adducts was found, and the adduct patterns were indistinguishable from those of endometrial DNA from unexposed controls.

The potential of tamoxifen to form DNA adducts in human endometrium *in vitro* has also been investigated using explant cultures incubated with 20–200 μM tamoxifen (Carmichael et al., 1996). The viability of the metabolizing enzyme systems of the endometrial samples was demonstrated by the detection of expected DNA adducts after incubation with benzo[a]pyrene; however, no adducts were seen after incubation with tamoxifen, in spite of the generation of a metabolite with LC–MS analysis characteristics of α-hydroxytamoxifen.

4.4.3 *Metabolites of tamoxifen*

4-Hydroxytamoxifen caused morphological transformation of Syrian hamster embryo (SHE) cells. Treatment of SHE cells with 10 μM 4-hydroxytamoxifen for 48 h resulted in the emergence of immortalized cells in 3 out of 5 flasks; these cells were able to form fibrosarcomas when injected into thymus-aplastic mice (Metzler & Schiffmann, 1991).

Treatment of rat primary hepatocyte cultures with α-hydroxytamoxifen resulted in 15- to 63-fold higher levels of adducts (and the same pattern of adducts detected by ^{32}P-postlabelling) than with comparable concentrations of tamoxifen (Phillips et al., 1994a; 1996a). A similar level of adducts (173.9 ± 4.1 adducts per 10^8 nucleotides) was seen in mouse hepatocytes treated with α-hydroxytamoxifen at a concentration of 1 μM. Treatment of human cells with α-hydroxytamoxifen resulted in DNA adduct formation at levels (1.94 ± 0.89 and 18.9 ± 17.9 adducts per 10^8 nucleotides at 1 μM and 10 μM, respectively) about 300-fold lower than those in rat hepatocytes. Concentrations of α-hydroxytamoxifen in the culture medium of cells incubated with tamoxifen were approximately 50-fold lower in experiments with human hepatocytes than in those with rat or mouse hepatocytes (Phillips et al., 1996a).

The hypothesis has been advanced that tamoxifen is activated to a DNA-binding species through oxidation at the α-position of the ethyl group (Potter et al., 1994). This proposal is supported by studies with the deuterated compound [ethyl-D$_5$]tamoxifen, which showed lower DNA-binding activity in rat liver in vivo than the non-deuterated compound (Phillips et al., 1994b). It also had a lower ability to induce micronucleus formation in MCL-5 cells. The magnitude of the reduction in genotoxicity (two- to three-fold) correlated well with the comparative rates of metabolism of the deuterated and non-deuterated compounds in rat liver microsomal incubations (Jarman et al., 1995). Thus, the reduced genotoxicity of [ethyl-D$_5$]tamoxifen is the result of its lower rate of oxidation due to the greater bond energy of the C–D bond compared with the C–H bond, implying that metabolic activation involves metabolism at the ethyl group of the molecule. This is supported by the observation of higher DNA-binding activity of α-hydroxytamoxifen in primary cultures of hepatocytes, in which DNA adducts were formed at between 25 and 49 times the level seen with equimolar concentrations of tamoxifen and which gave the same pattern of major adducts by ^{32}P-postlabelling (Phillips et al., 1994a).

Studies on the nature of the DNA adducts formed from tamoxifen in vivo and in vitro provide evidence for this and other pathways of activation of tamoxifen to form DNA-binding products. The demonstration that tamoxifen–DNA adduct formation in mice was altered by pretreatment with pentachlorophenol, a sulfotransferase inhibitor, suggested the existence of two pathways of activation (Randerath et al., 1994a,b). The levels of some of the major adducts were unaffected by pentachlorophenol, but levels of one major and several minor ones were increased 13–17-fold (Randerath et al., 1994a). However, another sulfotransferase inhibitor, 2,6-dichloro-4-nitrophenol, did not enhance the levels of these adducts (Randerath et al., 1994b). The metabolite 4-hydroxytamoxifen was found to give rise to adducts of the pentachlorophenol-inducible type (Randerath et al., 1994b; Moorthy et al., 1996).

α-Hydroxytamoxifen has low chemical reactivity towards DNA, but the synthetic compound α-acetoxytamoxifen is much more reactive. The DNA adducts formed with α-acetoxytamoxifen showed the same pattern on ^{32}P-postlabelling analysis as those from DNA treated with α-hydroxytamoxifen and those found in the DNA of rat hepatocytes treated with tamoxifen or of the livers of rats treated with tamoxifen in vivo. The major α-acetoxytamoxifen–DNA adduct was also isolated as a nucleoside and characterized by ultraviolet, mass and proton magnetic resonance spectroscopy and assigned the structure

(E)-α-(N^2-deoxyguanosinyl)tamoxifen, in which the α-ethyl position of tamoxifen is linked covalently to the exocyclic amino group of deoxyguanosine (Osborne et al., 1996).

When incubated with rat liver microsomal fractions or with peroxidase enzymes in the presence of DNA, the metabolite 4-hydroxytamoxifen forms DNA adducts. The principal adduct formed in each case co-migrated on thin-layer chromatography with a minor adduct formed in the liver of tamoxifen-treated rats (Pathak et al., 1995). In another study, two minor DNA adducts formed by rat microsomal activation of tamoxifen in the presence of DNA co-migrated in several thin-layer chromatography systems with the products of the reaction of (Z)-1,2-diphenyl-1-(4-hydroxyphenyl)but-1-ene ('metabolite E', see Figure 1) with DNA in the presence of silver(I) oxide (Pongracz et al., 1995).

4.5 Mechanistic considerations

4.5.1 *Genotoxicity*

The ability of tamoxifen to form DNA adducts in rodent liver cells *in vivo* and *in vitro* suggests a genotoxic mechanism for carcinogenicity in rat liver. This hypothesis is supported by the dose–response relationship for both tumour formation (in both male and female rats) and adduct formation. Although adducts are also formed in mouse and hamster liver, the levels are lower and these species have not been tested adequately for carcinogenesis by tamoxifen. Tamoxifen also possesses tumour-promoting activity in rat liver. An unusual aspect of tamoxifen–DNA adduct formation is that, in the rat, little or no adduct formation occurs in other tissues following oral administration. Although some information is available on the nature of the reactive intermediates of tamoxifen, the enzymes involved in their formation have not been clearly identified. The possibility that tamoxifen is inactive in most assays for mutagenic activity (gene mutations) because of failures of in-vitro metabolizing systems and/or transport of the reactive intermediate to the target site has not been excluded.

Studies on human hepatocytes indicate that they have a much lower ability to activate tamoxifen to DNA-binding products than those of rodents. In addition, limited information indicates that tamoxifen–DNA adducts are not formed in either the liver or endometrium of women taking tamoxifen as adjuvant therapy for breast cancer. These findings suggest that humans are less susceptible to the genotoxicity of tamoxifen than rodents.

4.5.2 *Tamoxifen–oestrogen receptor interactions*

Tamoxifen acts as an oestrogen agonist and/or antagonist by binding directly to the oestrogen receptor. In some tissues, including breast, tamoxifen exerts antioestrogenic effects by binding to the oestrogen receptor with high affinity. The tamoxifen–oestrogen receptor complex is incapable of binding to DNA-responsive elements, and therefore fails to induce normal transcriptional activity (Pasqualini et al., 1987). In other tissues, such as bone (Love et al., 1992b), uterus (Jordan & Prestwich, 1977) and liver, tamoxifen acts as a partial agonist, possibly because cells from those tissues contain a different array of DNA-binding sites, thereby leading to typical oestrogen-mediated changes in gene expression and subsequent biological effects on growth and differentiation.

Uterus

Several studies have demonstrated that tamoxifen exhibits agonistic properties in the uterus. Sustained occupancy of receptor–oestrogen complexes in the nucleus appears to be required for oestrogen-induced stimulation of DNA replication, an early event in cell division. For example, nuclear occupancy of the oestrogen receptor for 10–15 h is required to stimulate uterine cell division (Korach et al., 1985). Assuming that tamoxifen–oestrogen receptor complexes are capable of interactions with oestrogen-response elements on DNA, then tamoxifen could enhance mitotic activity leading to biological changes which increase cancer risk. However, little is known about the sequence of events proceeding from interactions of DNA with the oestrogen receptor to biological changes.

Alternatively, tamoxifen could produce a partially antagonistic response by blocking oestrogen access to the receptor in tissues where there are appropriate DNA-responsive elements for the tamoxifen–oestrogen receptor complex. Because tamoxifen is not as potent as 17β-oestradiol, there is a diminished response in oestrogen-deficient tissue. This is likely to occur in tissues that are oestrogen receptor-positive and have oestrogen levels high enough to elicit a response, but low enough for tamoxifen to block oestrogen access to a sufficient number of receptors, thereby decreasing normal oestrogen responsiveness (Jordan & Prestwich, 1977). In any oestrogen receptor-positive tissues with very low levels of oestrogen, tamoxifen would act as an agonist, because there would be no tissue-specific oestrogen response to diminish.

Breast

Neoplasia of the breast appears to progress from a relatively differentiated state which is dependent on steroid hormones for growth to an undifferentiated state which is hormone independent. This progression is reflected by the presence of receptors for oestrogen and progesterone in the dependent state, whereas few or no receptors are present in the independent state. Several effects of tamoxifen in mammary cells have been documented. Consistent with antioestrogenic activity, it decreased c-*myc* expression in the VHB$_1$ cell line derived from an infiltrating duct-cell carcinoma (Collyn-d'Hooghe et al., 1991). A decrease in c-*myc* and c-*erb*B-2 mRNA levels has also been observed in breast tumour cells of patients treated with tamoxifen (Le Roy et al., 1991). Another effect of tamoxifen is the induction of the autocrine secretion of transforming growth factor β (TGF-β) detected in human mammary ductal carcinoma biopsies. TGF-β is localized between and around stromal fibroblasts (Butta et al., 1992). This was observed with both oestrogen receptor-positive and -negative tumours, suggesting an oestrogen-receptor independent mechanism of action for tamoxifen. TGF-β acts as a growth inhibitor in human breast cancer cells (Knabbe et al., 1987), hence, its induction may be a mechanism of growth inhibition by tamoxifen that takes account of its efficacy against both oestrogen receptor-positive and -negative tumours.

Liver

Increased incidence of liver adenomas, total nodular hyperplasia and hepatocellular carcinomas is observed in women following prolonged use of oral contraceptives, as used in the 1960s (IARC, 1987b). It is generally considered that ethinyloestradiol, the oestrogenic component of oral contraceptives, is responsible for their hepatocarcinogenic activity and that the hepatic oestrogen receptor is involved (Goldfarb, 1976; Mastri *et al.*, 1985).

Several studies have shown that the liver contains significant quantities of oestrogen receptors in hepatocytes, Kupffer cells and endothelial cells. Since tamoxifen possesses at least partial agonist activity in liver, tamoxifen-mediated increases in liver tumour incidences in rodents may reflect, in part, oestrogen-receptor-dependent responses. Occupancy of hepatic oestrogen receptors is associated with stimulation of growth factors involved in hepatocyte mitogenesis (Vickers & Lucier, 1991). The human hepatic oestrogen receptor appears to be quantitatively and qualitatively similar to that of rodents.

Thus, tamoxifen-mediated increases in liver tumour incidence in rodents may involve both DNA damage leading to increased numbers of initiated cells and oestrogen-receptor-mediated clonal expansion of those initiated cells.

5. Summary of Data Reported and Evaluation

5.1 Exposure data

Tamoxifen has been available since the early 1970s for the first-line treatment of metastatic breast cancer in postmenopausal women. Since the 1980s, it has become the therapy of choice for this condition. Tamoxifen has also become the adjuvant therapy of choice for treatment of postmenopausal, node-positive women with positive oestrogen-receptor or progesterone-receptor levels and, since the early 1990s, for the treatment of postmenopausal, node-negative women with positive oestrogen-receptor or progesterone-receptor levels. It is also widely used in treating postmenopausal receptor-negative women and premenopausal women with node-negative, receptor-positive disease. When used as adjuvant therapy, tamoxifen reduces the annual rates of both death from and recurrence of breast cancer by about 25%. Tamoxifen is commonly given at doses of 20 mg daily for periods of two to five years in the adjuvant setting, although doses of up to 40 mg daily have been used in the past. Several clinical trials are in progress to study the efficacy of tamoxifen in preventing breast cancer in healthy women believed to be at high risk of developing the disease.

Tamoxifen has been widely adopted as the first-line therapy of choice for hormone-responsive male breast cancer and is frequently used as adjuvant therapy for oestrogen receptor- or progesterone receptor-positive male breast cancer.

Tamoxifen is registered for use in nearly 100 countries and cumulative use since 1973 is estimated at 7 million patient-years.

5.2 Human carcinogenicity data

The potential effect of tamoxifen in increasing the risk of endometrial cancer has been reported in one adequate cohort study, four adequate case–control studies and 14 randomized controlled trials.

In the cohort study, based on follow-up of registered cases of breast cancer in the population-based Surveillance, Epidemiology and End Results (SEER) database in the United States, the only available data on therapy were those reported at the time of initial registration. Both groups of women with reported tamoxifen use and those with no such reported use had elevated rates of endometrial cancer compared with the rates expected from the SEER database as a whole. The risk was significantly greater for women with reported tamoxifen use. The similar stage distribution in the two groups suggests a lack of serious detection bias in this study. The absence of hysterectomies could not be confirmed in this study.

The case–control studies were based on the identification of a series of women with breast cancer who had subsequently been diagnosed with endometrial cancer, with tamoxifen exposure assessed in comparison with breast cancer patients who had not developed endometrial cancer. In two of these, case and control selection was based on the records of population-based cancer registries, and two used the same source as well as hospital-based cancer registries. For the Swedish study, although an increased risk of endometrial cancer for tamoxifen use was found, the only information on treatment was that recorded in the cancer registry. Further, the absence of hysterectomy in the control series could not be confirmed. For the remaining three case–control studies, more detailed data on treatment and on hysterectomies were obtained from medical records. In the studies in France and the Netherlands, a nonsignificant elevation of risk for endometrial cancer with use of tamoxifen was found, with a significant increase in risk with increasing duration of therapy in one. In the United States study, which reported on shorter duration of use, the point estimate of risk was less than unity.

Although several potential confounders were not systematically addressed in most studies, the Working Group considered that these were unlikely to have had a major effect on the reported relative risks.

In most of the randomized trials, small numbers of endometrial cancers were reported, and for many the data were not reported in a way that corrected for the greater survival time in most trials of the tamoxifen-treated patients compared to the control series. In two of the largest trials, however, there was a strong and statistically significant association between risk for endometrial cancer and use of tamoxifen. Although there may have been a tendency for publication bias and there is some possibility of a detection bias as a result of investigations in women with side-effects from tamoxifen, the magnitude of the risk found in the two large trials is unlikely to be explained by such biases. Further, for the trials that reported deaths in women with endometrial cancer, to date there have been eight deaths in women allocated to tamoxifen treatment groups and one in those not allocated to tamoxifen.

One case series reported significantly more high-grade endometrial tumours in tamoxifen-treated cancer patients than in patients without prior tamoxifen use. However, in at least six other studies, this difference was not found.

The SEER-based cohort study found a significantly reduced risk for contralateral breast cancers in the tamoxifen-treated women, compared with women with no reported tamoxifen use. The case–control study from the United States also reported a significant reduction of risk for contralateral cancers of the breast following tamoxifen use.

Although for some small trials there seemed to be little difference in the numbers of contralateral breast cancers in tamoxifen-treated women compared with controls, for the large trials, there was a substantially and significantly reduced risk for contralateral breast cancer in tamoxifen-treated women compared with controls. Further, in an overview analysis of nearly all trials published in 1992 with data available to 1990, there was a significant reduction of 39% in contralateral breast cancers in the tamoxifen-treated groups.

For all other cancer sites, no significant excess of any cancer has been found in either the cohort study or the trials. Although an excess of gastrointestinal cancer was reported following a combined analysis of three Scandinavian trials, this has not yet been confirmed by other studies.

5.3 Animal carcinogenicity data

Tamoxifen was tested for carcinogenicity by oral administration in one study in mice and in eight studies in rats, only one of which was a formal two-year study. In mice, the incidences of benign ovarian and testicular tumours were increased. In rats, tamoxifen induced preneoplastic liver lesions and benign or malignant liver tumours. In one study, the incidence of some tumours in hormone-dependent tissues was decreased, including in the mammary gland, although reduced weight gain may have been a contributing factor. In two studies in which tamoxifen was tested by subcutaneous implantation in intact or ovariectomized female mice, it inhibited mammary tumour development in both.

In mice, tamoxifen was reported to inhibit 3-methylcholanthrene-induced cervical cancer and virus-induced leukaemia. In several studies in both male and female rats, tamoxifen enhanced the hepatocarcinogenicity of previously administered N-nitrosodiethylamine. In one study in rats, tamoxifen enhanced the development of N-nitrosodiethylamine-induced kidney tumours. In a number of studies in rats, tamoxifen inhibited 7,12-dimethylbenz[a]anthracene-induced mammary tumour development. In two studies in hamsters, tamoxifen inhibited hormonal carcinogenesis induced by 17β-oestradiol in the kidney and zeranol in the liver.

5.4 Other relevant data

Orally administered tamoxifen is well absorbed and maximum plasma levels are reached in about 5 h. Steady-state concentrations of tamoxifen in humans are reached in 3–4 weeks and those of the primary metabolite, *N*-desmethyltamoxifen, in about eight weeks. Tissue concentrations tend to be higher than plasma concentrations. Metabolism involves phenyl hydroxylation, alkyl hydroxylation, demethylation and *N*-oxide formation. Metabolism results in more products in man and rats than in mice. Much higher oral doses of tamoxifen are required for rats or mice to achieve plasma concentrations similar to human levels.

Tamoxifen is an antioestrogen with complex pharmacology encompassing variable species-, tissue-, cell-, gene-, age- and duration of administration-specific effects from oestrogen-like agonist actions to complete blockade of oestrogen action. This complexity is consistent with the various, and sometimes paradoxical, effects that have been associated with tamoxifen administration in animals and humans

The most frequent side-effects of tamoxifen administration are hot flushes and vaginal discharge. Tamoxifen has effects on the human uterus, inducing atrophy, hyperplasia and, less frequently, polyps. Randomized placebo-controlled trials revealed a slight increase of thromboembolic events, but also a protective effect regarding myocardial diseases, according to hospital admission rates and deaths. Tamoxifen administration has been shown to decrease blood total cholesterol and low-density lipoprotein-cholesterol concentrations in a number of studies. Several preliminary trials have suggested mildly positive effects of tamoxifen in preserving bone mineral density in postmenopausal women, but much longer follow-up is required to confirm this potentially beneficial effect.

The acute toxicity of tamoxifen in experimental animals is low. In repeated-dose studies in rats, tamoxifen induced hypertrophy, but not cell proliferation, in the endometrial epithelium; endometrial hyperplasia was, however, reported in mice. Furthermore squamous metaplasia and atrophy of the uterine epithelium was observed in chronic studies in rats. Induction of cytochrome P450s and preneoplastic lesions have been detected in the livers of rats.

Ocular toxicity, including lipidosis of the retina and cornea and increased incidence of cataracts, was reported in studies in rats of chronic exposure to tamoxifen.

In the presence of human, mouse, rat and hamster microsomes, tamoxifen binds covalently to protein.

Tamoxifen has oestrogenic effects on human fetal genital tracts grown in athymic mice. In rats, doses above 2 mg/kg body weight produce irregular ossification of ribs in the fetus, which is thought to be secondary to reduction of the size of the uterus of the dam. No effects on the fetus have been reported in rabbits, marmosets or cynomolgus monkeys.

There is no direct evidence that tamoxifen is active in tests for gene mutation. Evidence for the genotoxic potential of tamoxifen is supported by data obtained on DNA adduct formation in rodent liver cells *in vitro* and *in vivo*, and in rodent and human liver microsomal systems; on unscheduled DNA synthesis in rat hepatocytes *in vitro*; and on the induction of clastogenic events both *in vitro*, in genetically-engineered human cells, and *in vivo* in rat liver.

There is evidence from ^{32}P-postlabelling studies that three metabolites, α-hydroxytamoxifen, 4-hydroxytamoxifen and (Z)-1,2-diphenyl-1-(4-hydroxyphenyl)but-1-ene (metabolite E) can be further metabolized to products that react with DNA. The major DNA adduct formed in rodent liver cells has been identified as (E)-α-$(N^2$-deoxyguanosinyl)tamoxifen. Human hepatocytes do not form detectable DNA adducts when treated *in vitro* with tamoxifen; they form 300-fold lower levels of adducts than rat and mouse hepatocytes when treated with α-hydroxytamoxifen.

Preliminary studies indicate that tamoxifen does not give rise to detectable levels of DNA adducts in human liver *in vivo* or in human endometrium *in vitro* and *in vivo*.

Mechanistic considerations

Tamoxifen increases liver tumour incidence in rats, which may involve both DNA damage leading to increased numbers of initiated cells and oestrogen receptor-mediated clonal expansion of those initiated cells.

The available evidence suggests that tamoxifen is carcinogenic in rat liver by a genotoxic mechanism. Preliminary information from studies of human tissues suggests that humans are less susceptible to the genotoxicity of tamoxifen. Tamoxifen also possesses tumour-promoting activity in the rat liver.

Several studies have shown that the liver contains significant quantities of oestrogen receptor in hepatocytes, Kupffer cells and endothelial cells.

Tamoxifen acts as an oestrogen agonist and/or antagonist by binding directly to the oestrogen receptor. In some tissues, such as breast, tamoxifen exhibits antioestrogenic properties by binding to the oestrogen receptor with high affinity. The tamoxifen–oestrogen receptor complex is incapable of binding to DNA-responsive elements. Thus, oestrogen receptor binding does not result in normal transcriptional activity. In other tissues, such as bone and liver, tamoxifen acts as a partial agonist, possibly because cells from those tissues contain a different array of DNA binding sites, thereby leading to typical oestrogen-mediated changes in gene expression and subsequent biological effects on growth and differentiation. Therefore, tissue-specific effects of tamoxifen–oestrogen receptor on gene expression may be involved in the ability of tamoxifen to increase or decrease tumour risk.

5.5 Evaluation[1,2]

There is *sufficient evidence* in humans for the carcinogenicity of tamoxifen in increasing the risk for endometrial cancer and there is conclusive evidence that tamo-

---

[1] Dr Cuzick dissociated himself from the evaluation process because he considered that the range of evaluation statements available within the framework of the *Monographs* was not suitable for this agent.
[2] For definition of the italicized terms, see Preamble, pp. 22–25.

xifen reduces the risk for contralateral breast cancer in women with a previous diagnosis of breast cancer.

There is *inadequate evidence* in humans for the carcinogenicity of tamoxifen in other organs.

There is *sufficient evidence* in experimental animals for the carcinogenicity of tamoxifen.

Overall evaluation

Tamoxifen is *carcinogenic to humans (Group 1)* and there is conclusive evidence that tamoxifen reduces the risk of contralateral breast cancer.

6. References

Adam, H.K., Patterson, J.S. & Kemp, J.V. (1980) Studies on the metabolism and pharmacokinetics of tamoxifen in normal volunteers. *Cancer Treatment Rep.*, **64**, 761–764

Ahotupa, M., Hirsimäki, P., Pärssinen, R. & Mäntylä, E. (1994) Alterations of drug metabolizing and antioxidant enzyme activities during tamoxifen-induced hepatocarcinogenesis in the rat. *Carcinogenesis*, **15**, 863–868

Akhtar, S.S., Allan, S.G., Rodger, A., Chetty, U.D.I., Smyth, J.F. & Leonard, R.C.F. (1991) A 10-year experience of tamoxifen as primary treatment of breast cancer in 100 elderly and frail patients. *Eur. J. surg. Oncol.*, **17**, 30–35

Altaras, M.M., Aviram, R.,, Cohen, I., Cordoba, M., Yarkoni, S. & Beyth, Y. (1993) Role of prolonged stimulation of tamoxifen therapy in the etiology of endometrial sarcomas. *Gynecol. Oncol.*, **49**, 255–258

Andersson, M., Storm, H.H. & Mouridsen, H.T. (1991) Incidence of new primary cancers after adjuvant tamoxifen therapy and radiotherapy for early breast cancer. *J. natl Cancer Inst.*, **83**, 1013–1017

Andersson, M., Storm, H.H. & Mouridsen, H.T. (1992) Carcinogenic effects of adjuvant tamoxifen treatment and radiotherapy for early breast cancer. *Acta oncol.*, **31**, 259–263

Anker, G., Lønning, P.E., Ueland, P.M., Refsum, H. & Lien, E.A. (1995) Plasma levels of the antherogenic amino acid homocysteine in post-menopausal women treated with tamoxifen. *Int. J. Cancer*, **60**, 365–368

Ashford, A.R., Donev, I., Tiwari, R.P. & Garrett, T.J. (1988) Reversible ocular toxicity related to tamoxifen therapy. *Cancer*, **61**, 33–35

Atlante, G., Pozzi, M., Vincenzoni, C. & Vocaturo, G. (1990) Four case reports presenting new acquisitions on the association between breast and endometrial carcinoma. *Gynecol.Oncol.*, **37**, 378–380

Bagdade, J.D., Wolter, J., Subbaiah, P.V. & Ryan, W. (1990) Effects of tamoxifen treatment on plasma lipids and lipoprotein lipid composition. *J. clin. Endocrinol. Metab.*, **70**, 1132–1135

Baltuch, G., Shenouda, G., Langleben, A. & Villemure, J.-G. (1993) High dose tamoxifen in the treatment of recurrent high grade glioma: a report of clinical stabilization and tumour regression. *Can. J. neurol. Sci.*, **20**, 168–170

Barakat, R.R. & Hoskins, W.J. (1994) Current management of endometrial cancer. *Contemporary Ob./Gyn.*, **39**, 13–34

Barakat, R.R., Wong, G., Curtin, J.P., Vlamis, V. & Hoskins, W.J. (1994) Tamoxifen use in breast cancer patients who subsequently develop corpus cancer is not associated with a higher incidence of adverse histologic features. *Gynecol. Oncol.*, **55**, 164–168

Bardi, M., Arnoldi, E., Pizzocchero, G., Pezzica, E., Mattioni, D. & Perotti, M. (1994) Endometrioid carcinoma in pelvic endometriosis in a postmenopausal woman with tamoxifen adjuvant therapy for breast cancer. A case report. *Eur. J. Gynaec. Oncol.*, **15**, 393–395

Bates, T., Riley, D.L., Houghton, J., Fallowfield, L. & Baum, M. (on behalf of the Elderly Breast Cancer Working Party) (1991) Breast Cancer in elderly women: a Cancer Research Campaign trial comparing treatment with tamoxifen and optimal surgery with tamoxifen alone. *Br. J. Surg.*, **78**, 591–594

Baum, M., Houghton, J. & Riley, D. (1992) Results of the Cancer Research Campaign Adjuvant Trial for Perioperative Cyclophosphamide and Long-Term Tamoxifen in Early Breast Cancer reported at the tenth year of follow-up. *Acta oncol.*, **31**, 251–257

Bedford, G.R. & Richardson, D.N. (1966) Preparation and identification of *cis* and *trans* isomers of a substituted triarylethylene. *Nature*, **212**, 733–734

Beer, T.W., Buchanan, R. & Buckley, C.H. (1995) Uterine stromal sarcoma following tamoxifen treatment (Letter to the Editor). *J. clin. Pathol.*, **48**, 596

Beggs, W.H. (1993) Anti-candida activity of the anti-cancer drug tamoxifen. *Res. Comm. chem. Pathol. Pharmacol.*, **80**, 125–128

Bertelli, G., Pronzato, P., Amoroso, D., Cusimano, M.P., Conte, P.F., Montagna, G., Bertolini, S. & Rosso, F. (1988) Adjuvant tamoxifen in primary breast cancer: influence on plasma lipids and antithrombin III levels. *Breast Cancer Res. Treat.*, **12**, 307–310

Berthou, F. & Dréano, Y. (1993) High-performance liquid chromatographic analysis of tamoxifen, toremifene and their major human metabolites. *J. Chromatogr.*, **616**, 117–127

Beyer, B.K., Stark, K.L., Fantel, A.G. & Juchau, M.R. (1989) Biotransformation, estrogenicity and steroid structure as determinants of dysmorphogenic and generalized embryotoxic effects of steroidal and nonsteroidal estrogens. *Toxicol. appl. Pharmacol.*, **98**, 113–127

Boccardo, F., Bruzzi, P., Rubagotti, A., Nicolò, G. & Rosso, R. (1981) Estrogen-like action of tamoxifen on vaginal epithelium in breast cancer patients. *Oncology*, **38**, 281–285

Boccardo, F., Amoroso, D., Rubagotti, A., Capellini, M., Pacini, P., Castagnetta, L., Traina, A., Farris, A., Iacobelli, S., Mustacchi, G., Nenci, I., Piffanelli, A., Sismondi, P., De Sanctis, C., Mesiti, M., Gallo, L., Villa, E. & Schieppati, G. (1994a) Prolonged tamoxifen treatment of early breast cancer: the experience of the Italian Cooperative Group for chemohormonal therapy of early breast cancer. In: Jordan, V.C., ed., *Long-Term Tamoxifen Treatment for Breast Cancer*, Madison, WI, The University of Wisconsin Press

Boccardo, F., Rubagotti, A., Perrotta, A., Amoroso, D., Balestrero, M., De Matteis, A., Zola, P., Sismondi, P., Francini, G., Petrioli, R., Sassi, M., Pacini, P. & Galligioni, E. (1994b) Ovarian ablation versus goserelin with or without tamoxifen in pre-perimenopausal patients with advanced breast cancer: results of a multicentric Italian study. *Ann. Oncol.*, **5**, 337–342

Bocklage, T., Lee, K.R. & Belinson, J.L. (1992) Uterine Müllerian adenosarcoma following adenomyoma in a woman on tamoxifen therapy. *Gynecol. Oncol.*, **44**, 104–109

Branham, W.S., Zehr, D.R., Chen, J.J. & Sheehan, D.M. (1988) Alterations in developing rat uterine cell populations after neonatal exposure to estrogens and antiestrogens. *Teratology*, **38**, 271–279

Branham, W.S., Zehr, D.R. & Sheehan, D.M. (1993) Differential sensitivity of rat uterine growth and epithelium hypertrophy to estrogens and antiestrogens. *Proc. Soc. exp. Biol. Med.*, **203**, 297–303

Breast Cancer Chemotherapy Consensus Conference (1985) Adjuvant chemotherapy for breast cancer. *J. Am. med. Assoc.*, **254**, 3461–3463

Breast Cancer Trials Committee (1987) Adjuvant tamoxifen in the management of operable breast cancer: the Scottish Trial. *Lancet*, **ii**, 171–175

British Medical Association/Royal Pharmaceutical Society of Great Britain (1994) *British National Formulary Number 27 (March 1994)*, London, p. 329

British Pharmacopoeial Commission (1993) *British Pharmacopoeia 1993*, Vols. I & II, London, Her Majesty's Stationery Office, pp. 650–651, 1119–1120

Brooks, M.D., Ebbs, S.R., Colletta, A.A. & Baum, M. (1992) Desmoid tumours treated with triphenylethylenes. *Eur. J. Cancer*, **28A**, 1014–1018

Bruning, P.F., Bonfrer, J.M.G., Hart, A.A.M., de Jong-Bakker, M., Linders, D., van Loon, J. & Nooyen, W.J. (1988) Tamoxifen, serum lipoproteins and cardiovascular risk. *Br. J. Cancer*, **58**, 497–499

Buchanan, R.B., Blamey, R.W., Durrant, K.R., Howell, A., Paterson, A.G., Preece, P.E., Smith, D.C., Williams, C.J. & Wilson, R.G. (1986) A randomized comparison of tamoxifen with surgical oophorectomy in premenopausal patients with advanced breast cancer. *J. clin. Oncol.*, **4**, 1326–1330

Buckley, C.H. (1990) Tamoxifen and endometriosis. Case report. *Br. J. Obstet. Gynaecol.*, **97**, 645–646

Buckley, M.M.-T. & Goa, K.L. (1989) Tamoxifen: a reappraisal of its pharmacodynamic and pharmacokinetic properties and therapeutic use. *Drugs*, **37**, 451–490

Budavari, S., ed. (1995) *The Merck Index*, 12th Ed., Rahway, NJ, Merck & Co.

Burke, P., Fasciano, F., Frigerio, A., Temporelli, A. & Fortunati, N. (1987) Ultrasonography study of postmenopausal uterus in patients treated with tamoxifen. *Min. gin.*, **39**, 453–457 (in Italian)

Butta, A., MacLennan, K., Flanders, K.C., Sacks, N.P.M., Smith, I., McKinna, A., Dowsett, M., Wakefield, L. M., Sporn, M.B., Baum, M. & Colletta, A.A. (1992) Induction of transforming growth factor β1 in human breast cancer *in vivo* following tamoxifen treatment. *Cancer Res.*, **52**, 4261–4264

Cano, A., Matallin, P., Legua, V., Tortajada, M. & Bonilla-Musoles, F. (1989) Tamoxifen and endometriosis (Letter to the Editor). *Lancet*, **i**, 376

Carmichael, P.L., Ugwumadu, A.H.N., Neven, P., Hewer, A.J., Poon, G.K. & Phillips, D.H. (1996) Lack of genotoxicity of tamoxifen in human endometrium. *Cancer Res.*, **56**, 1475–1479

Carthew, P., Martin, E.A., White, I.N.H., De Matteis, F., Edwards, R.E., Dorman, B.M., Heydon, R.T. & Smith, L.L. (1995a) Tamoxifen induces short-term cumulative DNA damage and liver tumors in rats: promotion by phenobarbital. *Cancer Res.*, **55**, 544–547

Carthew, P., Rich, K.J., Martin, E.A., De Matteis, F., Lim, C.-K., Manson, M.M., Festing, M.F.W., White, I.N.H. & Smith, L.L. (1995b) DNA damage as assessed by ^{32}P-postlabelling in three rat strains exposed to dietary tamoxifen: the relationship between cell proliferation and liver tumour formation. *Carcinogenesis*, **16**, 1299–1304

Castiglione, M., Gelber, R.D. & Goldhirsch, A. (1990) Adjuvant systemic therapy for breast cancer in the elderly: competing causes of mortality. *J. clin. Oncol.*, **8**, 519–526

Chamart, S., Hanocq, M., Helson, M., Devleeschouwer, N. & Leclercq, G. (1989) Determination of 2-methyl derivatives of tamoxifen in cell culture medium using high-performance liquid chromatography and electrochemical detection. *J. Chromatogr.*, **496**, 365–375

Chamness, G.C., Bannayan, G.A., Landry, L.A., Jr, Sheridan, P.J. & McGuire, W.L. (1979) Abnormal reproductive development in rats after neonatally administered antioestrogen (tamoxifen). *Biol. Reprod.*, **21**, 1087–1090

Champion, P.E., Nabholtz, M., Jenkins, H., MacLean, G., Allen, S. & Lees, A. (1991) Is tamoxifen increasing the risk of uterine malignancy in women treated for breast cancer ? (Abstract). *Breast Cancer Res. Treat.*, **19**, 195

Chang, T., Gonder, J.R. & Ventresca, M.R. (1992) A case-report. Low-dose tamoxifen retinopathy. *Can. J. Ophthalmol.*, 27, 148–149

Ching, C.K., Smith, P.G. & Long, R.G. (1992) Tamoxifen-associated hepatocellular damage and agranulocytosis (Letter to the Editor). *The Lancet*, **339**, 940

Chou, Y.-C., Iguchi, T. & Bern, H.A. (1992) Effects of antiestrogens on adult and neonatal mouse reproductive organs. *Reprod. Toxicol.*, **6**, 439–446

Clark, J.H., Guthrie, S.C. & McCormack, S.A. (1981) Neonatal stimulation of the uterus by clomiphene, tamoxifen and nafoxidine: relationship to the development of reproductive tract abnormalities. *Adv. exp. Med. Biol.*, **138**, 87–98

Clarke, M.R. (1993) Uterine malignant mixed Müllerian tumor in a patient on long-term tamoxifen therapy for breast cancer. *Gynecol. Oncol.*, **51**, 411–415

Coco, C.M., Hargis, B.M. & Hargis, P.S. (1992) Effect of in ovo 17β-estradiol or tamoxifen administration on sexual differentiation of the external genitalia. *Poultry Sci.*, **71**, 1947–1951

Coe, J.E., Ishak, K.G., Ward, J.M. & Ross, M.J. (1992) Tamoxifen prevents induction of hepatic neoplasia by zeranol, an estrogenic food contaminant. *Proc. natl Acad. Sci. USA*, **89**, 1085–1089

Cohen, I., Altaras, M.M., Lew, S., Tepper, R., Beyth, Y. & Ben-Baruch, G. (1994) Case Report. Ovarian endometrioid carcinoma and endometriosis developing in a postmenopausal breast cancer patient during tamoxifen therapy: a case report and review of the literature. *Gynecol. Oncol.*, **55**, 443–447

Cole, M.P., Jones, C.T.A. & Todd, I.D.H. (1971) A new anti-oestrogenic agent in late breast cancer. An early clinical appraisal of ICI 46 474. *Br. J. Cancer*, **25**, 270–275

Collyn-d'Hooghe, M., Vandewalle, B., Hornez, L., Lantoine, D., Revillion, F., Lefebvre, J. & Kerckaert, J. P. (1991) c-*myc* Overexpression, c-*mil*, c-*myb* expression in a breast tumor cell line. Effects of estrogen and antiestrogen. *Anticancer Res.*, **11**, 2175–2180

Cook, L.S., Weiss, N.S., Schwartz, S.M., White, E., McKnight, B., Moore, D.E. & Daling, J.R. (1995) Population-based study of tamoxifen therapy and subsequent ovarian, endometrial, and breast cancers. *J. natl Cancer Inst.*, **87**, 1359–1364

Corley, D., Rowe, J., Curtis, M.T., Hogan, W.M., Noumoff, J.S. & LiVolsi, V.A. (1992) Postmenopausal bleeding from unusual endometrial polyps in women on chronic tamoxifen therapy. *Obstet. Gynecol.*, **79**, 111–116

Cortez Pinto, H., Baptista, A., Ermelinda Camilo, M., Bruno de Costa, E., Valente, A. & Carneiro de Moura, M. (1995) Tamoxifen-associated steatohepatitis — report of three cases. *J. Hepatol.*, **23**, 95–97

Costa, A., Sacchini, V., Boranni, B., Luini, A., Boyle, P., Rofmensz, N., Veronesi, U. & the Italian Tamoxifen Trial Units (1996) Breast cancer chemoprevention with tamoxifen. The Italian trial (Abstract). *Breast Cancer Res. Treat.*, **37**, 348

Council of Europe (1995) *European Pharmacopoeia*, 2nd Ed., Part II, 19th fasc., Sainte-Ruffine, France, Maisonneuve S.A., pp. 1046-1–1046-4

Crofton-Sleigh, C., Doherty, A., Ellard, S., Parry, E.M. & Venitt, S. (1993) Micronucleus assays using cytochalasin-blocked MCL-5 cells, a proprietary human cell line expressing five human cytochromes P-450 and microsomal epoxide hydrolase. *Mutagenesis*, **8**, 363–372

Cross, S.S. & Ismail, S.M. (1990) Endometrial hyperplasia in an oophorectomized women receiving tamoxifen therapy. Case report. *Br. J. Obstet. Gynaecol.*, **97**, 190–192

Cullins, S.L., Pridjian, G. & Sutherland, C.M. (1994) Goldenhar's syndrome associated with tamoxifen given to the mother during gestation. *J. Am. med. Assoc.*, **271**, 1905–1906

Cummings, F.J., Gray, R., Tormey, D.C., Davis, T.E., Volk, H., Harris, J., Falkson, G. & Bennett, J.M. (1993) Adjuvant tamoxifen versus placebo in elderly women with node-positive breast cancer: long-term follow-up and causes of death. *J. clin. Oncol.*, **11**, 29–35

Cunha, G.R., Taguchi, O., Namikawa, R., Nishizuka, Y. & Robboy, S.J. (1987) Teratogenic effects of clomiphene, tamoxifen, and diethylstilbestrol on the developing human female genital tract. *Hum. Pathol.*, **18**, 1132–1143

Curtis, R.E., Boice, J.D., Jr, Shriner, D.A., Hankey, B.F. & Fraumeni, J.F., Jr (1996) Second cancers after adjuvant tamoxifen therapy for breast cancer. Brief communication. *J. natl Cancer Inst.* (in press)

Cuzick, J., Allen, D., Baum, M., Barrett, J., Clark, G., Kakkar, V., Melissari, E., Moniz, C., Moore, J., Parsons, V., Pemberton, K., Pitt, P., Richmond, W., Houghton, J. & Riley, D. (1993) Long term effects of tamoxifen. Biological Effects of Tamoxifen Working Party. *Eur. J. Cancer*, **29A**, 15–21

Dallenbach-Hellweg, G. & Hahn, U. (1995) Mucinous and clear cell adenocarcinomas of the endometrium in patients receiving antiestrogens (tamoxifen) and gestagens. *Int. J. gynecol. Pathol.*, **14**, 7–15

Daniel, P., Gaskell, S.J., Bishop, H., Campbell, C. & Nicholson, R.I. (1981) Determination of tamoxifen and biologically active metabolites in human breast tumour and plasma. *Eur. J. Cancer clin. Oncol.*, **17**, 1183–1189

Dauplat, J., Le Bouëdec, G. & Achard, J.L. (1990) Adenocarcinoma of the endometrium in two patients treated with tamoxifen. *Presse méd.*, **19**, 380–381 (in French)

Davies, A.M., Martin, E.A., Jones, R.M., Lim, C.K., Smith, L.L. & White, I.N.H. (1995) Peroxidase activation of tamoxifen and toremifene resulting in DNA damage and covalently bound protein adducts. *Carcinogenesis*, **16**, 539–545

De Jong-Busnac, M. (1989) Ophthamological complications of low-dose tamoxifen in the treatment of breast cancer. *Ned. Tijdschr. Geneesk.*, **133**, 514–516 (in Dutch)

De Muylder, X., Neven, P., De Somer, M., Van Belle, Y., Vanderick, G. & De Muylder, E. (1991) Endometrial lesions in patients undergoing tamoxifen therapy. *Int. J. gynecol. Obstet.*, **36**, 127–130

Deprest, J., Neven, P. & Ide, P. (1992) An unusual type of endometrial cancer, related to tamoxifen? *Eur. J. Obstet. Gynecol. reprod. Biol.*, **46**, 147–150

Dewar, J.A., Horobin, J.M., Preece, P.E., Tavendale, R., Tunstall-Pedoe, H. & Wood, R.A.B. (1992) Long term effects of tamoxifen on blood lipid values in breast cancer. *Br. med. J.*, **305**, 225–226

Dilts, P.V., Jr, Hopkins, M.P., Chang, A.E. & Cody, R.L. (1992) Rapid growth of leiomyoma in patient receiving tamoxifen. *Am. J. Obstet. Gynecol.*, **166**, 167–168

Dnistrian, A.M., Schwartz, M.K., Greenberg, E.J,. Smith, C.A. & Schwartz, D.C. (1993) Effect of tamoxifen on serum cholesterol and lipoproteins during chemohormonal therapy. *Clin. chim. Acta*, **223**, 43–52

Dragan, Y.P., Rizvi, T., Xu, Y.-H., Hully, J.R., Bawa, N., Campbell, H.A., Maronpot, R.R. & Pitot, H.C. (1991a) An initiation-promotion assay in rat liver as a potential complement to the 2-year carcinogenesis bioassay. *Fundam. appl. Toxicol.*, **16**, 525–547

Dragan, Y.P., Xu, Y.-D. & Pitot, H.C. (1991b) Tumor promotion as a target for estrogen/antiestrogen effects in rat hepatocarcinogenesis. *Prev. Med.*, **20**, 15–26

Dragan, Y.P., Fahey, S., Street, K., Vaughan, J., Jordan, V.C. & Pitot, H.C. (1994) Studies of tamoxifen as a promoter of hepatocarcinogenesis in female Fischer F344 rats. *Breast Cancer Res. Treat.*, **31**, 11–25

Dragan, Y.P., Vaughan, J., Jordan, V.C. & Pitot, H.C. (1995) Comparison of the effects of tamoxifen and toremifene on liver and kidney tumor promotion in female rats. *Carcinogenesis*, **16**, 2733–2741

Early Breast Cancer Trialists' Collaborative Group (1988) Effects of adjuvant tamoxifen and of cytotoxic therapy on mortality in early breast cancer. An overview of 61 randomized trials among 28,896 women. *New Engl. J. Med.*, **319**, 1681–1692

Early Breast Cancer Trialists' Collaborative Group (1992) Systemic treatment of early breast cancer by hormonal, cytotoxic, or immune therapy: 133 randomized trials involving 31 000 recurrences and 24 000 deaths among 75 000 women. *Lancet*, **339**, 1–15, 71–85

Enck, R.E. & Rios, C.N. (1984) Tamoxifen treatment of metastatic breast cancer and antithrombin III levels. *Cancer*, **53**, 2607–2609

Enevoldson, T.P. & Harding, A.E. (1992) Improvement in the POEMS syndrome after administration of tamoxifen (Letter to the Editor). *J. Neurol. Neurosurg. Psychiat.*, **55**, 71–72

Esaki, K. & Sakai, Y. (1980) Tamoxifen; influence of oral administration of tamoxifen on the rabbit fetus. *Jitchukan Zenrinsho Kenkyuho*, **6**, 217–231 (in Japanese)

Evans, M.J., Langlois, N.E.I., Kitchener, H.C. & Miller, I.D. (1995) Is there an association between long-term tamoxifen treatment and the development of carcinosarcoma (malignant mixed Müllerian tumor) of the uterus? *Int. J. Gynecol. Cancer*, **5**, 310–313

Farmindustria (1993) *Repertorio Farmaceutico Italiano* (Italian Pharmaceutical Directory), 7th Ed., Milan, Associazione Nazionale dell'Industria Farmaceutica, CEDOF, S.P.A., pp. A-794–A795; A-1101–A-1102

Fendl, K.C. & Zimniski, S.J. (1992) Role of tamoxifen in the induction of hormone-independent rat mammary tumours. *Cancer Res.*, **52**, 235–237

Fentiman, I.S., Caleffi, M., Rodin, A., Murby, B. & Fogelman, I. (1989) Bone mineral content of women receiving tamoxifen for mastalgia. *Br. J. Cancer*, **60**, 262–264

Ferrazzi, E., Cartei, G., Mattarazzo, R. & Fiorentino, M. (1977) Oestrogen-like effect of tamoxifen on vaginal epithelium (Letter to the Editor). *Br. med. J.*, **i**, 1351–1352

Fisher, B., Redmond, C., Brown, A., Fisher, E.R., Wolmark, N., Bowman, D., Plotkin, D., Wolter, J., Bornstein, R., Legault-Poisson, S., Saffer, E.A. & Other NSABP Investigators (1986) Adjuvant chemotherapy with and without tamoxifen in the treatment of primary breast cancer: 5-year results from the National Surgical Adjuvant Breast and Bowel Project Trial. *J. clin. Oncol.*, **4**, 459–471

Fisher, B., Costantino, J., Redmond, C., Poisson, R., Bowman, D., Couture, J., Dimitrov, N.V., Wolmark, N., Wickerham, D.L., Fisher, E.R., Margolese, R., Robidoux, A., Shibata, H., Terz, J., Paterson, A.H.G., Feldman, M.I., Fararr, W., Evans, J., Lickley, H.L. & Ketner, R.N. (1989a) A randomized clinical trial evaluating tamoxifen in the treatment of patients with node-negative breast cancer who have estrogen-receptor-positive tumors. *New Engl. J. Med.*, **320**, 479–484

Fisher, B., Redmond, C., Wickerham, L., Wolmark, N., Bowman, D., Couture, J., Dimitrov, N.V., Margolese, R., Legault-Poisson, S. & Robidoux, A. (1989b) Systemic therapy in patients with node-negative breast cancer. A commentary based on two National Surgical Adjuvant Breast and Bowel Project (NSABP) clinical trials. *Ann. intern. Med.*, **111**, 703–712

Fisher, B., Costantino, J.P., Redmond, C.K., Fisher, E.R., Wickerham, D.L. & Cronin, W.M. (1994) Endometrial cancer in tamoxifen-treated breast cancer patients: findings from the National Surgical Adjuvant Breast and Bowel Project (NSABP) B-14. *J. natl Cancer Inst.*, **86**, 527–537

Folk, J.J., Mazur, M.T., Eddy, G.L. & Musa, A.G. (1995) Secretory endometrial adenocarcinoma in a patient on tamoxifen for breast cancer: a report of a case. *Gynecol. Oncol.*, **58**, 133–135

Ford, M.R., Turner, M.J., Wood, C. & Soutter, W.P. (1988) Endometriosis developing during tamoxifen therapy. *Am. J. Obstet. Gynecol.*, **158**, 119

Fornander, T., Rutqvist, L.E., Cedermark, B., Glas, U., Mattsson, A., Silfverswärd, C., Skoog, L., Somell, A., Theve, T., Wilking, N., Askergren, J. & Hjalmar, M.-L. (1989) Adjuvant tamoxifen in early breast cancer: occurrence of new primary cancers. *Lancet*, **i**, 117–120

Fornander, T., Rutqvist, L.E., Sjöberg, H.E., Blomqvist, L., Mattsson, A. & Glas, U. (1990) Long term adjuvant tamoxifen in early breast cancer: effect on bone mineral density in postmenopausal women. *J. clin. Oncol.*, **8**, 1019–1024

Fornander, T., Rutqvist, L.E., Cedermark, B., Glas, U., Mattsson, A., Skoog, L., Somell, A., Theve, T., Wilking, N., Askergren, J., Rotstein, S., Hjalmar, M.-L. & Perbeck, L. (1991) Adjuvant tamoxifen in early-stage breast cancer: effects on intercurrent morbidity and mortality. *J. clin. Oncol.*, **9**, 1740–1748

Fornander, T., Hellström, A.-C. & Moberger, B. (1993) Descriptive clinicopathologic study of 17 patients with endometrial cancer during or after adjuvant tamoxifen in early breast cancer. *J. natl Cancer Inst.*, **85**, 1850–1855

Forsberg, J.G. (1985) Treatment with different antioestrogens in the neonatal period and effects in the cervicovaginal epithelium and ovaries of adult mice: a comparison to estrogen-induced changes. *Biol. Reprod.*, **32**, 427–441

Foster, W.G., Jarrell, J.F. & YoungLai, E.V. (1993) Developmental changes in the gonadotropin releasing hormone neuron of the female rabbit: effects of tamoxifen citrate and pregnant mare serum gonadotropin. *Can. J. Physiol. Pharmacol.*, **71**, 761–767

Fried, K.M. & Wainer, I.W. (1994) Direct determination of tamoxifen and its four major metabolites in plasma using coupled column high-performance liquid chromatography. *J. Chromatogr. B*, **655**, 261–268

Fromson, J.M., Pearson, S. & Bramah, S. (1973a) The metabolism of tamoxifen (ICI 46,474). Part II: In female patients. *Xenobiotica*, **3**, 711–714

Fromson, J.M., Pearson, S. & Bramah, S. (1973b) The metabolism of tamoxifen (ICI 46,474). Part I: In laboratory animals. *Xenobiotica*, **3**, 693–709

Furr B.J.A. & Jordan, V.C. (1984) The pharmacology and clinical uses of tamoxifen. *Pharmacol. Ther.*, **25**, 127–205

Furr, B.J.A., Valcaccia, B. & Challis, J.R.G. (1976) The effects of nolvadex (tamoxifen citrate; ICI 46,474) on pregnancy in rabbits. *J. Reprod. Fert.*, **48**, 367–369

Furr, B.J.A., Patterson, J.S., Richardson, D.N., Slater, S.R. & Wakeling, A.E. (1979) Tamoxifen. In: Goldberg, M.E., ed., *Pharmacological and Biochemical Properties of Drug Substances*, Washington, American Pharmacological Association, Vol. II, pp. 355–399

Gennaro, A.R., ed. (1995) *Remington: The Science and Practice of Pharmacy*, 19th Ed., Vol. II, Easton, PA, Mack Publishing Co., p. 1094

Gershbein, L.L. (1994) Induction of colon adenocarcinomas in rats fed trypsin and tamoxifen diets by parenteral and intragastric 1,2-dimethylhydrazine. *Res. Comm. mol. Pathol. Pharmacol.*, **85**, 347–350

Gherman, R.B., Parker, M.F. & Macri, C.I. (1994) Granulosa cell tumor of the ovary associated with antecedent tamoxifen use. *Obstetr. Gynecol.*, **84**, 717–719

Ghia, M. & Mereto, E. (1989) Induction and promotion of γ-glutamyltranspeptidase-positive foci in the liver of female rats treated with ethinyl estradiol, clomiphene, tamoxifen and their associations. *Cancer Lett.*, **46**, 195–202

Gibson, L.E., Barakat, R.R., Curtin, J.P., Jones, W.B., Lewis, J.L., Jr & Hoskins, W.J. (1994) Tamoxifen effects on the endometrium: a retrospective comparative study (Abstract no. 837). *Proc. ASCO*, **13**, 263

Gill-Sharma, M.K., Gopalkrishnan, K., Balasinor, N., Parte, P., Jayaraman, S. & Juneja, H.S. (1993) Effects of tamoxifen on the fertility of male rats. *J. Reprod. Fert.*, **99**, 395–402

Gillett, D. (1995) Leiomyosarcoma of the uterus in a woman taking adjuvant tamoxifen therapy (Letter to the Editor). *Med. J. Aust.*, **163**, 160–161

Glick, J.H., Creech, R.H., Torri, S., Holdroyde, C., Brodovsky, H., Catalano, R.B. & Varano, M. (1981) Randomized clinical trial of tamoxifen plus sequential CMF chemotherapy versus tamoxifen alone in postmenopausal women with advanced breast cancer. *Breast Cancer Res. Treat.*, **1**, 59–68

Glick, J.H., Gelber, R.D., Goldhirsch, A. & Senn, H.-J. (1992) Meeting highlights: adjuvant therapy for primary breast cancer. *J. natl Cancer Inst.*, **84**, 1479–1485

Goldfarb, S. (1976) Sex hormones and hepatic neoplasia. *Cancer Res.*, **36**, 2584–2588

Goldhirsch, A., Wood, W.C., Senn, H.-J., Glick, J.H. & Gelber, R.D. (1995) Meeting highlights: international consensus panel on the treatment of primary breast cancer. *J. natl Cancer Inst.*, **87**, 1441–1445

Goodwin, J.W., Crowley, J., Eyre, H.J., Stafford, B., Jaeckle, K.A. & Townsend, J.J. (1993) A phase II evaluation of tamoxifen in unresectable or refractory meningiomas: a southwest oncology group study. *J. Neuro-Oncol.*, **15**, 75–77

Gooren, L. (1989) Improvement of spermatogenesis after treatment with the antiestrogen tamoxifen in a man with the incomplete androgen insensitivity syndrome. *J. clin. Endocrinol. Metab.*, **68**, 1207–1210

Gordon, D., Beastall, G.H., McArdle, C.S. & Thomson, J.A. (1986) The effect of tamoxifen therapy on thyroid function tests. *Cancer*, **58**, 1422–1425

Gray, R. (1993) Tamoxifen: how boldly to go where no women have gone before. *J. natl Cancer Inst.*, **85**, 1358–1360

Greaves, P., Goonetilleke, R., Nunn, G., Topham, J. & Orton, T. (1993) Two-year carcinogenicity study of tamoxifen in Alderley Park Wistar-derived rats. *Cancer Res.*, **53**, 3919–3924

Grey, A.B., Stapleton, J.P., Evans, M.C. & Reid, I.R. (1995a) The effects of the antiestrogen tamoxifen on cardiovascular risk factors in normal postmenopausal women. *J. clin. Endocrinol. Metabol.*, **80**, 3191–3195

Grey, A.B., Stapleton, J.P., Evans, M.C., Tatnell, M.A., Ames, R.W. & Reid, I.R. (1995b) The effects of the antiestrogen tamoxifen on bone mineral density in normal late postmenopausal women. *Am. J. Med.*, **99**, 636–641

Griffiths, M.F.P. (1987) Tamoxifen retinopathy at low dosage (Letter to the Editor). *Am. J. Ophthalmol.*, **104**, 185–186

Guelen, P.J.M., Stevenson, D., Briggs, R.J. & de Vos, D. (1987) The bioavailability of Tamoplex (tamoxifen). Part 2. A single dose cross-over study in healthy male volunteers. *Meth. Find. exp. clin. Pharmacol.*, **9**, 685–690

Guetta, V., Lush, R.M., Figg, W.D., Waclawiw, M.A. & Cannon, R.O., III (1995) Effects of the antiestrogen tamoxifen on low-density lipoprotein concentrations and oxidation in postmenopausal women. *Amer. J. Cardiol.*, **76**, 1072–1073

Gulino, A., Screpanti, I. & Pasqualini, J.R. (1984) Differential estrogen and antiestrogen responsiveness of the uterus during development in the fetal, neonatal and immature guinea pig. *Biol. Reprod.*, **31**, 371–381

Gupta, J.S. & Roy, S.K. (1987) Effect of tamoxifen on cytosolic estrogen receptor in the different parts of fallopian tube and uterus during ovum transport. *Exp. clin. Endocrinol.*, **90**, 293–300

Gylling, H., Pyrhonen, S., Mäntylä, E., Mäenpää, H., Kangas, L. & Miettinen, T.A. (1995) Tamoxifen and toremifene lower serum cholesterol by inhibition of Δ^8-cholesterol conversion to lathosterol in women with breast cancer. *J. clin. Oncol.*, **13**, 2900–2905

Han, X. & Liehr, J.G. (1992) Induction of covalent DNA adducts in rodents by tamoxifen. *Cancer Res.*, **52**, 1360–1363

Hard, G.C., Iatropoulos, M.J., Jordan, K., Radi, L., Kaltenberg, O.P., Imondi, A.R. & Williams, G.M. (1993) Major difference in the hepatocarcinogenicity and DNA adduct forming ability between toremifene and tamoxifen in female Crl:CD(BR) rats. *Cancer Res.*, **53**, 4534–4541

Hardell, L. (1988a) Tamoxifen as risk factor for carcinoma of corpus uteri (Letter to the Editor). *Lancet*, **ii**, 563

Hardell, L. (1988b) Pelvic irradiation and tamoxifen as risk factors for carcinoma of corpus uteri (Letter to the Editor). *Lancet*, **ii**, 1432

Harper, M.J.K. & Walpole, A.L. (1966) Contrasting endocrine activities of *cis* and *trans* isomers in a series of substituted triphenylethylenes. *Nature*, **212**, 87

Harper, M.J.K. & Walpole, A.L. (1967a) A new derivative of triphenylethylene: effect on implantation and mode of action in rats. *J. Reprod. Fertil.*, **13**, 101–119

Harper, M.J.K. & Walpole, A.L. (1967b) Mode of action of ICI 46,474 in preventing implantation in rats. *J. Endocrinol.*, **39**, 83–92

Harrison, J.D., Morris, D.L., Ellis, I.O., Jones, J.A. & Jackson, I. (1989) The effect of tamoxifen and estrogen receptor status on survival in gastric carcinoma. *Cancer*, **64**, 1007–1010

Hasmann, M., Rattel, B. & Löser, R. (1994) Preclinical data for droloxifene. *Cancer Lett.*, **84**, 101–116

Hatch, K.D., Beecham, J.B., Blessing, J.A. & Creasman, W.T. (1991) Responsiveness of patients with advanced ovarian carcinoma to tamoxifen. A gynecologic oncology group study of second-line therapy in 105 patients. *Cancer*, **68**, 269–271

Hayes, D.F., Van Zyl, J.A., Hacking, A., Goedhals, L., Bezwoda, W.R., Mailliard, J.A., Jones, S.E., Vogel, C.L., Berris, R.F., Shemano, I. & Schoenfelder, J. (1995) Randomized comparison of tamoxifen and two separate doses of toremifene in postmenopausal patients with metastatic breast cancer. *J. clin. Oncol.*, **13**, 2556–2566

Hemminki, K., Widlak, P. & Hou, S.-M. (1995) DNA adducts caused by tamoxifen and toremifene in human microsomal system and lymphocytes *in vitro*. *Carcinogenesis*, **16**, 1661–1664

Hendrick, A. & Subramanian, V.P. (1980) Tamoxifen and thromboembolism (Letter to the Editor). *J. Am. med. Assoc.*, **243**, 514–515

Hirsimäki, P., Hirsimäki, Y., Nieminen, L. & Payne, B.J. (1993) Tamoxifen induces hepatocellular carcinoma in rat liver: a 1-year study with two antiestrogens. *Arch. Toxicol.*, **67**, 49–54

Hulka, C.A. & Hall, D.A. (1993) Endometrial abnormalities associated with tamoxifen therapy for breast cancer: sonographic and pathologic correlation. *Am. J. Roentgentol.*, **160**, 809–812

IARC (1987a) *IARC Monographs on the Evaluation of Carcinogenic Risks to Humans*, Suppl. 7, *Overall Evaluations of Carcinogenicity: An Update of* IARC Monographs *Volumes 1 to 42*, Lyon, pp. 82–83, 182–184, 210–211, 239–240, 241–242

IARC (1987b) *IARC Monographs on the Evaluation of Carcinogenic Risks to Humans*, Suppl. 7, *Overall Evaluations of Carcinogenicity: An Update of* IARC Monographs *Volumes 1 to 42*, Lyon, pp. 272–310

Iguchi, T., Hirokawa, M. & Takasugi, N. (1986) Occurrence of genital tract abnormalities and bladder hernia in female mice exposed neonatally to tamoxifen. *Toxicology*, **42**, 1–11

Iguchi, T., Irisawa, S., Uchima, F.-D.A. & Takasugi, N. (1988) Permanent chondrification in the pelvis and occurrence of hernias in mice treated neonatally with tamoxifen. *Reprod. Toxicol.*, **2**, 127–134

Ingle, J.N. (1984) Additive hormonal therapy in women with advanced breast cancer. *Cancer*, **53**, 766–777

Ingle, J.N., Ahmann, D.L., Green, S.J., Edmonson, J.H., Bisel, H.F., Kvols, L.K., Nichols, W.C., Creagan, E.T., Hahn, R.G., Rubin, J. & Frytak, S. (1981) Randomized clinical trial of diethylstilbestrol versus tamoxifen in postmenopausal women with advanced breast cancer. *New Engl. J. Med.*, **304**, 16–21

Ingle, J.N., Krook, J.E., Green, S.J., Kubista, T.P., Everson, L.K., Ahman, D.L., Chang, M.N., Bisel, H.F., Windschitl, H.E., Twito, D.I. & Pfeifle, D.M. (1986) Randomized trial of bilaterial oophorectomy versus tamoxifen in premenopausal women with metastatic breast cancer. *J. clin. Oncol.*, **4**, 178–185

Irisawa, S. & Iguchi, T. (1990) Critical period of induction by tamoxifen of genital organ abnormalities in female mice. *In Vivo*, **4**, 175–180

Ismail, S.M. (1994) Pathology of endometrium treated with tamoxifen. *J. clin. Pathol.*, **47**, 827–833

Jaiyesimi, I.A., Buzdar, A.U., Sahin, A.A. & Ross, M.A. (1992) Carcinoma of the male breast. *Ann. intern. Med.*, **117**, 771–777

Jaiyesimi, I.A., Buzdar, A.U., Decker, D.A. & Hortobagyi, G.N. (1995) Use of tamoxifen for breast cancer : 28 years later. *J. clin. Oncol.*, **13**, 513–529

Jarman, M., Poon, G.K., Rowlands, M.G., Grimshaw, R.M., Horton, M.N., Potter, G.A. & McCague, R. (1995) The deuterium isotope effect for the α-hydroxylation of tamoxifen by rat liver microsomes accounts for the reduced genotoxicity of [D_5-ethyl]tamoxifen. *Carcinogenesis*, **16**, 683–688

Johnstone, A.J., Sarkar, T.K. & Hussey, J.K. (1991) Primary hepatocellular carcinoma in a patient with breast carcinoma. *Clin. Oncol.*, **3**, 180–181

Jones, A.L., Powles, T.J., Treleaven, J.G., Burman, J.F., Nicolson, M.C., Chung, H.-I. & Ashley, S.E. (1992) Haemostatic changes and thromboembolic risk during tamoxifen therapy in normal women. *Br. J. Cancer*, **66**, 744–747

Jordan, V.C. (1978) Use of the DMBA-induced rat mammary carcinoma system for the evaluation of tamoxifen as a potential adjuvant therapy. *Rev. Endocrinol. rel. Cancer (October Supplement)*, 49–55

Jordan, V.C. (1988) The development of tamoxifen for breast cancer therapy: a tribute to the late Arthur L. Walpole. *Breast Cancer Res. Treat.*, **11**, 197–209

Jordan, V.C. (1993) A current view of tamoxifen for the treatment and prevention of breast cancer. *Br. J. Pharmacol.*, **110**, 507–517

Jordan, V.C. & Prestwich, G. (1977) Binding of [^{3}H]tamoxifen in rat uterine cytosols: a comparison of swinging bucket and vertical tube rotor sucrose density gradient analysis. *Mol. Cell Endocrinol.*, **8**, 179–188

Jordan, V.C. & Robinson, S.P. (1987) Species-specific pharmacology of antiestrogens: role of metabolism. *Fed. Proc.*, **46**, 1870–1874

Jordan, V.C., Dix, C.J. & Allen, K.E. (1979) The effectiveness of long-term treatment in a laboratory model for adjuvant hormone therapy of breast cancer. In: Salmon, S.E. & Jones, S.E., eds, *Adjuvant Therapy of Cancer*, Vol. 2, New York, Grune and Stratton, pp. 19–26

Jordan, V.C., Allen, K.E. & Dix, C.J. (1980) Pharmacology of tamoxifen in laboratory animals. *Cancer Treat. Rep.*, **64**, 745–759

Jordan, V.C., Fritz, N.F. & Tormey, D.C. (1987) Long-term adjuvant therapy with tamoxifen: effects on sex hormone binding globulin and antithrombin III. *Cancer Res.*, **57**, 4517–4519

Jordan, V.C., Lababidi, M.K. & Mirecki, D.M. (1990) Anti-oestrogenic and anti-tumour properties of prolonged tamoxifen therapy in C3H/OUJ mice. *Eur. J. Cancer*, **26**, 718–721

Jordan, V.C., Lababidi, M.K. & Langan-Fahey, S. (1991) Suppression of mouse mammary tumorigenesis by long-term tamoxifen therapy. *J. natl Cancer Inst.*, **83**, 492–496

Jose, R., Kekre, A.N., George, S.S. & Seshadri, L. (1995) Endometrial carcinoma in a tamoxifen-treated breast cancer patient. *Aust. N.Z. J. Obstet. Gynaecol.*, **35**, 201

Kaiser-Kupfer, M.I. & Lippman, M.E. (1978) Tamoxifen retinopathy. *Cancer Treat. Rep.*, **62**, 315–320

Kangas, L., Nieminen, A.-L., Blanco, G., Grönroos, M., Kallio, S., Karjalainen, A., Perilä, M., Södervall, M. & Toivola, R. (1986) A new triphenylethylene compound, Fc-1157a. II. Antitumor effects. *Cancer Chemother. Pharmacol.*, **17**, 109–113

Kawamura, I., Mizota, T., Kondo, N., Shimomura, K. & Kohsaka, M. (1991) Antitumor effects of droloxifene, a new antiestrogen drug, against 7,12-dimethylbenz(a)anthracene-induced mammary tumors in rats. *Jpn. J. Pharmacol.*, **57**, 215–224

Kedar, R.P., Bourne, T.H., Powles, T.J., Collins, W.P., Ashley, S.E., Cosgrove, D.O. & Campbell, S. (1994) Effects of tamoxifen on uterus and ovaries of postmenopausal women in a randomised breast cancer prevention trial. *Lancet*, **343**, 1318–1321

Kenny, A.M., Prestwood, K.M., Pilbeam, C.C. & Raisz, L.G. (1995) The short term effects of tamoxifen on bone turnover in older women. *J. clin. Endocrinol. Metabol.*, **80**, 3287–3291

Killackey, M.A., Hakes, T.B. & Pierce, V.K. (1985) Endometrial adenocarcinoma in breast cancer patients receiving antiestrogens. *Cancer Treat. Rep.*, **69**, 237–238

Kitaichi, M., Nishimura, K., Itoh, H. & Izumi, T. (1995) Pulmonary lymphangioleiomyomatosis: a report of 46 patients including a clinicopathologic study of prognostic factors. *Am. J. respir. crit. Care Med.*, **151**, 527–533

Knabbe, C., Lippman, M.E., Wakefield, L.M., Flanders, K.C., Kasid, A., Derynck, R. & Dickson, R.B. (1987) Evidence that TGF-β is a hormonally regulated negative growth factor in human breast cancer cells. *Cell*, **48**, 417–428

Kohigashi, K., Fukuda, Y. & Imura, H. (1988) Inhibitory effect of tamoxifen on diethylstilbestrol-promoted hepatic tumorigenesis in male rats and its possible mechanism of action. *Jpn. J. Cancer Res. (Gann)*, **79**, 1335–1339

Korach, K.S., Fox-Davies, C., Quarmby, V.E. & Swaisgood, M.H. (1985) Diethylstilbestrol metabolites and analogs. Biochemical probes for differential stimulation of uterine estrogen responses. *J. biol. Chem.*, **260**, 15420–15426

Korach, K.S., Horigome, T., Tomooka, Y., Yamashita, S., Newbold, R.R. & McLachlan, J.A. (1988) Immunodetection of estrogen receptor in epithelial and stromal tissues of neonatal mouse uterus. *Proc. natl Acad. Sci.*, **85**, 3334–3337

Kotoulas, I.-G., Mitropoulos, D., Cardamakis, E., Dounis, A. & Michopoulos, J. (1994) Tamoxifen treatment in male infertility. I. Effect on spermatozoa. *Fert. Ster.*, **61**, 911–914

Krause, A. & Gerber, B. (1994) Postmenopausal hemorrhage and endometrial carcinoma during tamoxifen therapy. *Zbl. Gynakol.*, **116**, 44–47 (in German)

Krause, W., Holland-Moritz, H. & Schramm, P. (1992) Treatment of idiopathic oligozoospermia with tamoxifen — a randomized controlled study. *Int. J. Androl.*, **15**, 14–18

Kristensen, B., Ejlersten, B., Dalgaard, P., Larsen, L., Nistrup Holmegaard, S., Transbøl, I. & Mouridsen, H.T. (1994) Tamoxifen and bone metabolism in postmenopausal low-risk breast cancer patients: a randomized study. *J. clin. Oncol.*, **12**, 992–997

Lahti, E., Blanco, G., Kauppila, A., Apaja-Sarkkinen, M., Taskinen, P.J. & Laatikainen, T. (1993) Endometrial changes in postmenopausal breast cancer patients receiving tamoxifen. *Obstet. Gynecol.*, **81**, 660–664

Lai, C.-H., Hsueh, S., Chao, A.-S. & Soong, Y.-K. (1994) Successful pregnancy after tamoxifen and megestrol acetate therapy for endometrial carcinoma. *Br. J. Obstet. Gynaecol.*, **101**, 547–549

Lang-Avérous, G., Rupp, K., Wehner, H. & Dallenbach-Hellweg, G. (1991) The role of steroid hormones and related biological substances in the etiology of endometrial carcinoma. *Verh. Dtsch. ges. Pathol.*, **75**, 366–369 (in German)

Lanza, A., Alba, E., Re, A., Tessarolo, M., Leo, Bellino, R., Lauricella, A. & Wierdis, T. (1994) Endometrial carcinoma in breast cancer patients treated with tamoxifen. Two case reports and review of the literature. *Eur. J. Gynaec. Oncol.*, **15**, 455–459

Le Bouëdec, G. & Dauplat, J. (1992) Cancer of the endometrium caused by antiestrogens. *Rev. Fr. Gynécol. Obstét.*, **87**, 345–348 (in French)

Le Bouëdec, G., De Latour, M., Feillel, V. & Dauplat, J. (1990) Metrorrhagia and tamoxifen. 22 patients treated for breast cancer. *J. Gynécol. Obstét. Biol. Reprod.*, **19**, 889–894 (in French)

Le Bouëdec, G., Kauffmann, P., De Latour, M., Fondrinier, E., Curé, H. & Dauplat, J. (1991) Metastases of cancer of the breast in the uterus. 8 case histories. *J. Gynécol. Obstét. Biol. Reprod.*, **20**, 349–354 (in French)

van Leeuwen, F.E., Benraadt, J., Coebergh, J.W.W., Kiemeney, L.A.L.M., Gimbrère, C.H.F., Otter, R., Schouten, L.J., Damhuis, R.A.M., Bontenbal, M., Diepenhorst, F.W., van den Belt-Dusebout, A.W. & van Tinteren, H. (1994) Risk of endometrial cancer after tamoxifen treatment of breast cancer. *Lancet*, **343**, 448–452

Le Roy, X., Escot, C., Brouillet, J.-P., Theillet, C., Maudelonde, T., Simony-Lafontaine, J., Pujol, H. & Rochefort, H. (1991) Decrease of c-*erb*B-2 and c-*myc* RNA levels in tamoxifen-treated breast cancer. *Oncogene*, **6**, 431–437

Lentz, S.S. (1994) Advanced and recurrent endometrial carcinoma: hormonal therapy. *Sem. Oncol.*, **21**, 100–106

Leo, L., Lanza, A., Re, A., Tessarolo, M., Bellino, R., Lauricella, A. & Wierdis, T. (1994) Leiomyomas in patients receiving Tamoxifen. *Clin. exp. Obstet. Gynecol.*, **21**, 94–98

Leslie, W.D., Cowden, E.A. & MacLean, J.P. (1995) Oestrogen and bone density: a comparison of tamoxifen and hypo-oestrogenaemia. *Nuclear Med. Commun.*, **16**, 698–702

Liehr, J.G., Sirbasku, D.A., Jurka, E., Randerath, K. & Randerath, E. (1988) Inhibition of estrogen-induced renal carcinogenesis in male Syrian hamsters by tamoxifen without decrease in DNA adduct levels. *Cancer Res.*, **48**, 779–783

Lien, E.A., Solheim, E., Lea, O.A., Lundgren, S., Kvinnsland, S. & Ueland P.M. (1989) Distribution of 4-hydroxy-*N*-desmethyltamoxifen and other tamoxifen metabolites in human biological fluids during tamoxifen treatment. *Cancer Res.*, **49**, 2175–2183

Lien, E.A., Solheim, E. & Ueland, P.M. (1991) Distribution of tamoxifen and its metabolites in rat and human tissues during steady-state treatment. *Cancer Res.*, **51**, 4837–4844

Lien, E.A., Anker, G. & Ueland, P.M. (1995) Pharmacokinetics of tamoxifen in premenopausal and postmenopausal women with breast cancer. *J. Steroid Biochem. mol. Biol.*, **55**, 229–231

Lim, C.K., Chow, L.C.L., Yuan, Z.-X. & Smith, L.L. (1993) High performance liquid chromatography of tamoxifen and metabolites in plasma and tissues. *Biomed. Chromatogr.*, **7**, 311–314

Lim, C.K., Yuan, Z.-X., Lamb, J.H., White, I.N.H., De Matteis, F. & Smith, L.L. (1994) A comparative study of tamoxifen metabolism in female rat, mouse and human liver microsomes. *Carcinogenesis*, **15**, 589–593

Lin, C.L. & Buttle, H.L. (1990) Progesterone receptor in the mammary tissue of pregnant and lactating gilts and the effect of tamoxifen treatment during late gestation. *J. Endocrinol.*, **130**, 251–257

Lin, C.L. & Buttle, H.L. (1991) Effect of oestradiol benzoate and tamoxifen on the growth of and induction of progesterone receptors in the uterus and mammary gland of immature pigs. *J. Endocrinol.*, **130**, 259–265

Lipton, A., Harvey, H.A. & Hamilton, R.W. (1984) Venous thrombosis as a side effect of tamoxifen treatment. *Cancer Treat. Rep.*, **68**, 887–889

LiVolsi, V.A., Salhany, K.E. & Dowdy, Y.G. (1995) Endocervical adenocarcinoma in tamoxifen-treated patient (Letter to the Editor). *Am. J. Obstet. Gynecol.*, **172**, 1065

Longstaff, S., Sigurdsson, H., O'Keefe, M., Ogston, S. & Preece, P. (1989) A controlled study of the ocular effects of tamoxifen in conventional dosage in the treatment of breast carcinoma. *Eur. J. Cancer clin. Oncol.*, **25**, 1805–1808

Love, R. (1989) Tamoxifen therapy in primary breast cancer: biology, efficacy and side effects. *J. clin. Oncol.*, **7**, 803–815

Love, R.R. & Feyzi, J.M. (1993) Reduction in vasomotor symptoms from tamoxifen over time. *J. natl Cancer Inst.*, **85**, 673–674

Love, R.R., Mazess, R.B., Tormey, D.C., Barden, H.S., Newcomb, P.A. & Jordan, V.C. (1988) Bone mineral density in women with breast cancer treated with adjuvant tamoxifen for at least two years. *Breast Cancer Res. Treat.*, **12**, 297–302

Love, R.R., Newcomb, P.A., Wiebe, D.A., Surawicz, T.S., Jordan, V.C., Carbone, P.P. & DeMets, D.L. (1990) Effects of tamoxifen therapy on lipid and lipoprotein levels in postmenopausal patients with node-negative breast cancer. *J. natl Cancer Inst.*, **82**, 1327–1332

Love, R.R., Wiebe, D.A., Newcomb, P.A., Cameron, L., Leventhal, H., Jordan, V.C., Feyzi, J. & DeMets, D.L. (1991) Effects of tamoxifen on cardiovascular risk factors in postmenopausal women. *Ann. intern. Med.*, **115**, 860–864

Love, R.R., Surawicz, T.S. & Williams, E.C. (1992a) Antithrombin III level, fibrinogen level, and platelet count changes with adjuvant tamoxifen therapy. *Arch. intern. Med.*, **152**, 317–320

Love, R.R., Mazess, R.B., Barden, H.S., Epstein, S., Newcombe, P.A., Jordan, V.C., Carbone, P.P. & DeMets, D.L. (1992b) Effect of tamoxifen on bone mineral density in post-menopausal women with breast cancer. *New Engl. J. Med.*, **326**, 852–856

Love, R.R., Wiebe, D.A., Feyzi, J.M., Newcombe, P.A. & Chappell, R.J. (1994a) Effects of tamoxifen on cardiovascular risk factors in postmenopausal women after 5 years of treatment. *J. natl Cancer Inst.*, **86**, 1534–1539

Love, R.R., Barden, H.S., Mazess, R.B., Epstein, S. & Chappell, R.J. (1994b) Effect of tamoxifen on lumbar spine bone mineral density in postmenopausal women after 5 years. *Arch. intern. Med.*, **154**, 2585–2588

Lüllmann, H. & Lüllmann-Rauch, R. (1981) Tamoxifen-induced generalised lipidosis in rats subchronically treated with high doses. *Toxicol. appl. Pharmacol.*, **61**, 138–146

Lumsden, M.A., West, C.P. & Baird, D.T. (1989) Tamoxifen prolongs luteal phase in premenopausal women but has no effect on the size of uterine fibroids. *Clin. Endocrinol.*, **31**, 335–343

Mäentausta, O., Svalander, P., Danielsson, K.G., Bygdeman, M. & Vihko, R. (1993) The effects of an antiprogestin, mifepristone, and an antiestrogen, tamoxifen, on endometrial 17β-hydroxysteroid dehydrogenase and progestin and estrogen receptors during the luteal phase of the menstrual cycle: an immunohistochemical study. *J. clin. Endocrinol. Metab.*, **77**, 913–918

Magriples, U., Naftolin, F., Schwartz, P.E. & Carcangiu, M.L. (1993) High-grade endometrial carcinoma in tamoxifen-treated breast cancer patients. *J. clin. Oncol.*, **11**, 485–490

Malfetano, J.H. (1990) Tamoxifen-associated endometrial carcinoma in postmenopausal breast cancer patients. *Gynecol. Oncol.*, **39**, 82–84

Mamby, C.C., Love, R.R. & Lee, K.E. (1995) Thyroid function test changes with adjuvant tamoxifen therapy in postmenopausal women with breast cancer. *J. clin. Oncol.*, **13**, 854–857

Mani, C. & Kupfer, D. (1991) Cytochrome P-450-mediated activation and irreversible binding of the antioestrogen tamoxifen to proteins in rat and human liver: possible involvement of flavin-containing mono-oxygenases in tamoxifen activation. *Cancer Res.*, **51**, 6052–6058

Mani, C., Gelboin, H.V., Park, S.S., Pearce, R., Parkinson, A. & Kupfer D. (1993) Metabolism of the antimammary cancer antioestrogenic agent tamoxifen 1. Cytochrome P-450-catalyzed N-demethylation and 4-hydroxylation. *Drug Metab. Dispos.*, **21**, 645–656

Mani, C., Pearce, R., Parkinson, A. & Kupfer D. (1994) Involvement of cytochrome P4503A in catalysis of tamoxifen activation and covalent binding to rat and human liver microsomes. *Carcinogenesis*, **15**, 2715–2720

Manni, A., Trujillo, J.E., Marshall, J.S., Brodkey, J. & Pearson, O.H. (1979) Antihormone treatment of stage IV breast cancer. *Cancer*, **43**, 444–450

Mäntylä, E.T.E., Nieminen, L.S. & Karlsson, S.H. (1995) Endometrial cancer induction by tamoxifen in the rat (Abstract no. 61). *Eur. J. Cancer*, **31A** (Suppl. 5), S14

Mäntylä, E.T.E., Karlsson, S.H. & Nieminen, L.S. (1996) Induction of endometrial cancer by tamoxifen in the rat. In: Li, J.J., Li, S.A., Gustafsson, J.-Å., Nandi, S. & Sekely, L.I., eds., *Hormonal Carcinogenesis. II. Proceedings of the Second International Symposium*, New York, Springer Verlag, pp. 442–445

Marshall, K. & Senior, J. (1987) A study on the effect of a single dose of tamoxifen on uterine hyperaemia and growth in the rat. *Br. J. Pharmacol.*, **92**, 429–435

Martin, L. (1980) Estrogens, anti-estrogens and the regulation of cell proliferation in the female reproductive tract *in vivo*. In: McLachlan, J.A., Korach, K. & Lamb, J.C., eds, *Estrogens in the Environment*, New York, Elsevier/North Holland, pp. 103–129

Martin, E.A., Rich, K.J., White, I.N.H., Woods, K.L., Powles, T.J. & Smith, L.L. (1995) ^{32}P-Postlabelled DNA adducts in liver obtained from women treated with tamoxifen. *Carcinogenesis*, **16**, 1651–1654

Martínez Cerezo, F.J., Tomás, A., Donoso, L., Enríquez, J., Guarner, C., Balanzó, J., Martínez Nogueras, A. & Vilardell, F. (1994) Controlled trial of tamoxifen in patients with advanced hepatocellular carcinoma. *J. Hepatol.*, **20**, 702–706

Mastri, C., Mistry, P. & Lucier, G.W. (1985) In vivo oestrogenicity and binding characteristics of alpha-zearalanol (P-1496) to different classes of oestrogen binding proteins in rat liver. *J. Steroid Biochem.*, **23**, 279–289

Mathew, A., Chabon, A.B., Kabakow, B., Drucker, M. & Hirschman, R.J. (1990) Endometrial carcinoma in five patients with breast cancer on tamoxifen therapy. *N.Y. State J. Med.*, **90**, 207–208

McAuliffe, F.M. & Foley, M.E. (1993) Tamoxifen and endometrial lesions (Letter to the Editor). *Lancet*, **342**, 1124

McClay, E.F. & McClay, M.E.T. (1994) Tamoxifen: is it useful in the treatment of patients with metastatic melanoma ? *J. clin. Oncol.*, **12**, 617–626

McClay, E.F., Albright, K.D., Jones, J.A., Christen, R.D. & Howell, S.B. (1993) Tamoxifen modulation of cisplatin cytotoxicity in human malignancies. *Int. J. Cancer*, **55**, 1018–1022

McClellan, M.C., West, N.B., Tacha, D.E., Greene, G.L. & Brenner, R.M. (1984) Immunocytochemical localization of estrogen receptors in the macaque reproductive tract with monoclonal antiestrophilins. *Endocrinol.*, **114**, 2002–2014

McDermott, M.T., Hofeldt, F.D. & Kidd, G.S. (1990) Tamoxifen therapy for painful idiopathic gynecomastia. *South. med. J.*, **83**, 1283–1285

McDonald, C.C. & Stewart, H.J. (1991) Fatal myocardial infarction in the Scottish adjuvant tamoxifen trial. *Br. med. J.*, **303**, 435–437

McDonald, C.C., Alexander, F.E., Whyte, B.W., Forrest, A.P. & Stewart, H.J. (1995) Cardiac and vascular morbidity in women receiving adjuvant tamoxifen for breast cancer in a randomised trial. *Br. med. J.*, **311**, 977–980

McVie, J.G., Simonetti, G.P.C., Stevenson, D., Briggs, R.J., Guelen, P.J.M. & de Vos, D. (1986) The bioavailability of Tamoplex (tamoxifen). Part 1. A pilot study. *Meth. Find. exp. clin. Pharmacol.*, **8**, 505–512

Medical Economics (1996) *PDR®: Physicians' Desk Reference*, 50th Ed., Montvale, NJ, Medical Economics Data Production Co., pp. 2842–2844

Metzler, M. & Schiffmann, D. (1991) Structural requirements for the in vitro transformation of Syrian hamster embryo cells by stilbene estrogens and triphenylethylene-type antiestrogens. *Am. J. clin. Oncol.*, **14** (Suppl. 2), S30–S35

Mignotte, H., Sasco, A.J., Lasset, C., Saez, S. & Rivoire, M. (1992) Adjuvant therapy of breast cancer with tamoxifen and endometrial carcinoma. *Bull. Cancer*, **79**, 969–977 (in French)

Miké, V., Currie, V.E. & Gee, T.S. (1994) Fatal neutropenia associated with long-term tamoxifen therapy. *Lancet*, **344**, 541–542

Mishkin, S.Y., Farber, E., Ho, R., Mulay, S. & Mishkin, S. (1985) Tamoxifen alone or in combination with estradiol-17β inhibits the growth and malignant transformation of hepatic hyperplastic nodules. *Eur. J. Cancer clin. Oncol.*, **21**, 615–623

Montandon, F. & Williams, G.M. (1994) Comparison of DNA reactivity of the polyphenylethylene hormonal agents diethylstilbestrol, tamoxifen and toremifene in rat and hamster liver. *Arch. Toxicol.*, **68**, 272–275

Moon, L.Y., Wakley, G.K. & Turner, R.T. (1991) Dose-dependent effects of tamoxifen on long bones in growing rats: influence of ovarian status. *Endocrinology*, **129**, 1568–1574

Moon, R.C., Steele, V.E., Kelloff, G.J., Thomas, C.F., Detrisac, C.J., Mehta, R.G. & Lubet, R.A. (1994) Chemoprevention of MNU-induced mammary tumorigenesis by hormone response modifiers: toremifene, RU 16117, tamoxifen, aminoglutethimide and progesterone. *Anticancer Res.*, **14**, 889–894

Moorthy, B., Sriram, P., Pathak, D.N., Bodell, W.J. & Randerath, K. (1996) Tamoxifen metabolic activation: comparison of DNA adducts formed by microsomal and chemical activation of tamoxifen and 4-hydroxytamoxifen with DNA adducts formed *in vivo*. *Cancer Res.*, **56**, 53–57

Mouridsen, H.T., Rose, C., Overgaard, M., Dombernowsky, P., Panduro, J., Thorpe, S., Rasmussen, B.B., Blichert-Toft, M. & Andersen, K.W. (1988) Adjuvant treatment of postmenopausal patients with high risk primary breast cancer. *Acta oncol.*, **27**, 699–705

Mühlemann, K., Cook, L.S. & Weiss, N.S. (1994) The incidence of hepatocellular carcinoma in US white women with breast cancer after the introduction of tamoxifen in 1977. *Breast Cancer Res. Treat.*, **30**, 201–204

Murphy, C., Fotsis, T., Pantzer, P., Aldercreutz, H. & Martin, F. (1987) Analysis of tamoxifen, N-desmethyltamoxifen and 4-hydroxytamoxifen levels in cytosol and KCl-nuclear extracts of breast tumours from tamoxifen treated patients by gas chromatography-mass spectometry (GC-MS) using selected ion monitoring (SIM). *J. Steroid Biochem.*, **28**, 609–618

Muss, H.B. (1992) Endocrine therapy for advanced breast cancer: a review. *Breast Cancer Res. Treat.*, **21**, 15–26

Mustacchi, G., Milani, S., Pluchinotta, A., De Matteis, A., Rubagotti, A. & Perrota, A. (1994) Tamoxifen or surgery plus tamoxifen as primary treatment for elderly patients with operable breast cancer. The G.R.E.T.A. (Group for Research on Endocrine Therapy in the Elderly) Trial. *Anticancer Res.*, **14**, 2197–2200

National Institutes of Health Consensus Development Panel (1992) Consensus statement: treatment of early-stage breast cancer. *J. natl Cancer Inst.*, **11**, 1–5

National Surgical Adjuvant Breast and Bowel Project (1992) *NSABP Protocol P-1: A Clinical Trial to Determine the Worth of Tamoxifen for Preventing Breast Cancer*, Pittsburgh, PA, University of Pittsburgh, January 24

Nayfield, S.G., Karp, J.E., Ford, L.G., Dorr, F.A. & Kramer, B.S. (1991) Potential role of tamoxifen in prevention of breast cancer. *J. natl Cancer Inst.*, **83**, 1450–1459

Nevasaari, K., Heikkinen, M. & Taskinen, P.J. (1978) Tamoxifen and thrombosis. *Lancet.*, **ii**, 946–947

Neven, P., De Muylder, X., Van Belle, Y., Vanderick, G. & De Muylder, E. (1989) Tamoxifen and the uterus and endometrium (Letter to the Editor). *Lancet*, **i**, 375

Neven, P., De Muylder, X., Van Belle, Y., Vanderick, G. & De Muylder, E. (1990) Hysteroscopic follow-up during tamoxifen treatment. *Eur. J. Obstet. Gynecol. reprod. Biol.*, **35**, 235–238

Noguchi, M., Taniya, T., Tarjiri, K., Miwa, K., Miyazaki, I., Koshino, H., Mabuchi, H. & Nomomura, A. (1987) Fatal hyperlipaemia in a case of metastatic breast cancer treated by tamoxifen. *Br. J. Surg.*, **74**, 586–587

Nolvadex Adjuvant Trial Organisation (NATO) (1983) Controlled trial of tamoxifen as adjuvant agent in the management of early breast cancer. Interim analysis at four years. *Lancet*, **i**, 257–261

Nolvadex Adjuvant Trial Organisation (NATO) (1988) Controlled trial of tamoxifen as a single adjuvant agent in the management of early breast cancer. *Br. J. Cancer*, **57**, 608–611

Nuovo, M.A., Nuovo, G.J., McCaffrey, R.M., Levine, R.U., Barron, B. & Winkler, B. (1989) Endometrial polyps in postmenopausal patients receiving tamoxifen. *Int. J. gynecol. Pathol.*, **8**, 125–131

Nuwaysir, E.F., Dragan, Y.P., Jefcoate, C.R., Jordan, V.C. & Pitot, H.C. (1995) Effects of tamoxifen administration on the expression of xenobiotic metabolising enzymes in rat liver. *Cancer Res.*, **55**, 1780–1786

O'Dea, J.P.K. & Davis, E.H. (1990) Tamoxifen in the treatment of menstrual migraine. *Neurology*, **40**, 1470–1471

O'Grady, J.E., Armstrong, E.M., Moore, I.A.R. & Vass, M.A. (1974) Effect of tamoxifen (ICI-46,474) on mitosis in the uterus of the rat during the early stages of pregnancy. *J. Endocrinol.*, **63**, 19P

O'Halloran, M.J. & Maddock, P.G. (1974) ICI 46,474 in breast cancer. *J. Irish med. Assoc.*, **67**, 38–39

Ohta, Y., Iguchi, T. & Takasugi, N. (1989) Deciduoma formation in rats treated neonatally with the anti-estrogens, tamoxifen and MER-25. *Reprod. Toxicol.*, **3**, 207–212

Olive, D.L., Groff, T.R., Schultz, N., Schenken, R.S. & Riehl, R.M. (1990) Effects of tamoxifen on corpus luteum function and luteal phase length in cynomolgus monkeys. *Fert. Ster.*, **54**, 333–338

O'Neill, E. & Rodríguez Mojica, W. (1992) Asymptomatic carcinoma of the endometrium in a patient on adjunctive tamoxifen therapy for carcinoma of the breast. *Bol. Asoc. Med P.R.*, **84**, 74–77

Oredipe, O.A., Barth, R.F., Dwivedi, C. & Webb, T.E. (1992) Dietary glucarate-mediated inhibition of initiation of diethylnitrosamine-induced hepatocarcinogenesis. *Toxicology*, **74**, 209–222

Osborne, M.R., Hewer, A., Hardcastle, I.R., Carmichael, P.L. & Phillips, D.H. (1996) Identification of the major tamoxifen-deoxyguanosine adduct formed in the liver DNA of rats treated with tamoxifen. *Cancer Res.*, **56**, 66–71

Palacios, A., Pertusa, S., Montoya, A. & Martínez San Pedro, R. (1993) Breast cancer, tamoxifen, and uterus (Letter to the Editor). *Med. clin. Barc.*, **100**, 479 (in Spanish)

Palshof, T. (1988) *Adjuvant Endocrine Therapy in Premenopausal and Postmenopausal Women with Breast Cancer. Report of the Copenhagen Breast Cancer Trials 1975–1987*, Thesis, Copenhagen, Medi-book

Parry, B.R., Hung, N.A., McCall, J.L. & Phipps, R.F. (1993) Apparent regression of rectal polyps in a patient with Gardner's syndrome receiving concomitant tamoxifen therapy. *Aust. N.Z. J. Surg.*, **63**, 578–579

Pasqualini, J.R. & Lecerf, F. (1986) Ultrastructural modifications provoked by tamoxifen either alone or combined with oestradiol in the uteri of fetal or newborn guinea-pigs. *J. Endocrinol.*, **110**, 197–202

Pasqualini, J.R., Nguyen, B.-L., Sumida, C., Giambiagi, N. & Mayrand, C. (1986) Tamoxifen and progesterone effects in target tissues during the perinatal period. *J. Steroid Biochem.*, **25**, 853–857

Pasqualini, J.R., Sumida, C., Giambiagi, N.A. & Nguyen, B.L. (1987) The complexity of antioestrogen responses. *J. Steroid. Biochem.*, **27**, 883–889

Pathak, D.N. & Bodell, W.J. (1994) DNA adduct formation by tamoxifen with rat and human liver microsomal activation systems. *Carcinogenesis*, **15**, 529–532

Pathak, D.N., Pongracz, K. & Bodell, W.J. (1995) Microsomal and peroxidase activation of 4-hydroxytamoxifen to form DNA adducts: comparison with DNA adducts formed in Sprague-Dawley rats treated with tamoxifen. *Carcinogenesis*, **16**, 11–15

Pavlidis, N., Petris, C., Briassoulis, E., Klouvas, G., Psilas, C., Rempapis, J. & Petroutsos, G. (1992) Clear evidence that long-term, low dose tamoxifen treatment can induce ocular toxicity. *Cancer*, **69**, 2961–2964

Perry, R.R., Kang, Y. & Greaves, B. (1985) Effects of tamoxifen on growth and apoptosis of estrogen-dependent and -independent human breast cancer cells. *Ann. surg. Oncol.*, **2**, 238–245

Phillips, D.H., Carmichael, P.L., Hewer, A., Cole, K.J. & Poon, G.K. (1994a) α-Hydroxytamoxifen, a metabolite of tamoxifen with exceptionally high DNA-binding activity in rat hepatocytes. *Cancer Res.*, **54**, 5518–5522

Phillips, D.H., Potter, G.A., Horton, M.N., Hewer, A., Crofton-Sleigh, C., Jarman, M. & Venitt, S. (1994b) Reduced genotoxicity of [D_5-ethyl]tamoxifen implicates α-hydroxylation of the ethyl group as a major pathway of tamoxifen activation to a liver carcinogen. *Carcinogenesis*, **15**, 1487–1492

Phillips, D.H., Carmichael, P.L., Hewer, A., Cole, K.J., Hardcastle, I.R., Poon, G.K., Keogh, A. & Strain, A.J. (1996a) Activation of tamoxifen and its metabolite α-hydroxytamoxifen to DNA-binding products: comparisons between human, rat and mouse hepatocytes. *Carcinogenesis*, **17**, 89–94

Phillips, D.H., Hewer, A., Grover, P.L., Poon, G.K. & Carmichael, P.L. (1996b) Tamoxifen does not form detectable DNA adducts in white blood cells of breast cancer patients. *Carcinogenesis*, **17**, 1149–1152

Planting, A.S.T., Alexieva-Figusch, J., Blonk-v.d.Wijst, J. & van Putten, W.L.J. (1985) Tamoxifen therapy in premenopausal women with metastatic breast cancer. *Cancer Treat. Rep.*, **69**, 363–368

Pongracz, K., Pathak, D.N., Nakamura, T., Burlingame, A.L. & Bodell, W.J. (1995) Activation of the tamoxifen derivative metabolite E to form DNA adducts: comparison with the adducts formed by microsomal activation of tamoxifen. *Cancer Res.*, **55**, 3012–3015

Pons, J.Y. & Rigonnot, L. (1988) Hyperplasia of the endometrium in menopausal patients treated with tamoxifen for a breast cancer. *J. Gynecol. Obstet. Biol. reprod.*, **17**, 11–20 (in French)

Poon, G.K., Chui, Y.C., McCague, R., Lønning, P.E., Feng, R., Rowlands, M.G. & Jarman, M. (1993) Analysis of Phase I and Phase II metabolites of tamoxifen in breast cancer patients. *Drug Metab. Disp.*, **21**, 1119–1124

Poon, G.K., Walter, B., Lønning, P.E., Horton, M.N. & McCague, R. (1995) Identification of tamoxifen metabolites in human HEP G2 cell line, human liver homogenate, and patients on long-term therapy for breast cancer. *Drug Metab. Disp.*, **23**, 377–382

Potter, G.A., McCague, R. & Jarman, M. (1994) A mechanistic hypothesis for DNA adduct formation by tamoxifen following hepatic oxidative metabolism. *Carcinogenesis*, **15**, 439–442

Powles, T.J., Tillyer, C.R., Jones, A.L., Ashley, S.E., Treleaven, J., Davey, J.B. & McKinna, J.A. (1990) Prevention of breast cancer with tamoxifen — an update on the Royal Marsden Hospital pilot programme. *Eur. J. Cancer*, **26**, 680–684

Poyser, N.L. (1993) Effects of onapristone, tamoxifen and ICI 182780 on uterine prostaglandin production and luteal function in nonpregnant guinea-pigs. *J. Reprod. Fert.*, **98**, 307–312

Pritchard, K.I., Thomson, D.B., Myers, R.E., Sutherland, D.J.A., Mobbs, B.G. & Meakin, J.W. (1980) Tamoxifen therapy in premenopausal patients with metastatic breast cancer. *Cancer Treat. Rep.*, **64**, 787–796

Pritchard, K.I., Meakin, J.W., Boyd, N.F., DeBoer, G., Paterson, A.H.G., Ambus, U., Dembo, A.J., Sutherland, D.J.A., Wilkinson, R.H., Bassett, A.A., Evans, W.K., Beale, F.A., Clark, R.M. & Keane, T.J. (1987) Adjuvant tamoxifen in postmenopausal women with axillary node positive breast cancer: an update. In: Salmon, S.E. & Jones, S.E., eds, *Adjuvant Therapy of Cancer*, New York, Grune & Stratton, pp. 391–400

Pugh, D.M. & Sumano, H.S. (1979) The effects of oestradiol-17β and tamoxifen on the development of mouse embryos cultured over collagen. *Br. J. Pharmocol.*, **67**, 458

Qinn, M.A. & Campbell, J.J. (1989) Tamoxifen therapy in advanced/recurrent endometrial carcinoma. *Gynecol. Oncol.*, **32**, 1–3

Ralph, D.J., Brooks, M.D., Bottazzo, G.F. & Pryor, J.P. (1992) The treatment of Peyronie's disease with tamoxifen. *Br. J. Urol.*, **70**, 648–651

Randerath, K., Bi, J., Mabon, N., Sriram, P. & Moorthy, B. (1994a) Strong intensification of mouse hepatic tamoxifen DNA adduct formation by pretreatment with the sulfotransferase inhibitor and ubiquitous environmental pollutant pentachlorophenol. *Carcinogenesis*, **15**, 797–800

Randerath, K., Moorthy, B., Mabon, N. & Sriram, P. (1994b) Tamoxifen: evidence by ^{32}P-postlabeling and use of metabolic inhibitors for two distinct pathways leading to mouse hepatic DNA adduct formation and identification of 4-hydroxytamoxifen as a proximate metabolite. *Carcinogenesis*, **15**, 2087–2094

Rasmussen, K.L. & Nielsen, K.M. (1991) Development of endometrial cancer during tamoxifen therapy. *Ugeskr. Laeger.*, **153**, 2638 (in Danish)

Rayter, Z., Shepherd, J., Gazet, J.-C., Trott, P., Svensson, W. & A'Hern, R. (1993) Tamoxifen and endometrial lesions. *Lancet.*, **342**, 1124

Redmond, C.K., Wickerham, D.L., Cronin, W., Fisher, B., Costantino, J. & NSABP Participants (1993) The NSABP Breast Cancer Prevention Trial (BCPT): a progress report (Abstract no. 78). *Proc. Am. Soc. clin. Oncol.*, **12**, 69

Reynolds, J.E.F., ed. (1993) *Martindale: The Extra Pharmacopoeia*, 30th Ed., London, The Pharmaceutical Press, pp. 500–502

Ribeiro, G. & Swindell, R. (1985) The Christie Hospital tamoxifen (Nolvadex) adjuvant trial for operable breast carcinoma: 7-yr results. *Eur. J. Cancer clin. Oncol.*, **21**, 897–900

Ribeiro, G. & Swindell, R. (1992) The Christie Hospital adjuvant tamoxifen trial. *J. natl Cancer Inst. Monogr.*, **11**, 121–125

Rivkin, S.E., Green, S., Metch, B., Cruz, A.B., Abeloff, M.D., Jewell, W.R., Costanzi, J.J., Farrar, W.B., Minton, J.P. & Osborn, C. K. (1994) Adjuvant CMFVP versus tamoxifen versus concurrent CMFVP and tamoxifen for postmenopausal, node-positive, and estrogen receptor-positive breast cancer patients: a Southwest Oncology Group study. *J. clin. Oncol.*, **12**, 2078–2085

Robinson, S.P., Mauel, D.A. & Jordan, V.C. (1988) Antitumor actions of toremifene in the 7,12-dimethylbenzanthracene (DMBA)-induced rat mammary tumor model. *Eur. J. Cancer clin. Oncol.*, **24**, 1817–1821

Robinson, S.P., Langan-Fahey, S.M., Johnson, D.A. & Jordan, V.C. (1991) Metabolites, pharmacodynamics, and pharmacokinetics of tamoxifen in rats and mice compared to the breast cancer patient. *Drug Metab. Dispos.*, **19**, 36–43

Robinson, D.C., Bloss, J.D. & Schiano, M.A. (1995) A retrospective study of tamoxifen and endometrial cancer in breast cancer patients. *Gynecol. Oncol.*, **59**, 186–190

Rodier, J.F., Camus, E., Janser, J.C., Renaud, R. & Rodier, D. (1990) Tamoxifen and endometrial adenocarcinoma. *Bull. Cancer*, **77**, 1207–1210 (in French)

Ruenitz, P.C. & Nanavati, N.T. (1990) Identification and distribution in the rat of acidic metabolites of tamoxifen. *Drug Metab. Dispos.*, **18**, 645–648

Rutqvist, L.E. (1993) Long-term toxicity of tamoxifen. *Recent Results Cancer Res.*, **127**, 257–266

Rutqvist, L.E. & Mattsson (1993) Cardiac and thromboembolic morbidity among postmenopausal women with early-stage breast cancer in a randomized trial of adjuvant tamoxifen. *J. natl Cancer Inst.*, **85**, 1398–1406

Rutqvist, L.E., Cedermark, B., Glas, U., Johansson, H., Rotstein, S., Skoog, L., Somell, A., Theve, T., Wilking, N., Askergren, J., Hjalmar, M.-L., Ringborg, U. & Participating Members of the Stockholm Breast Cancer Study Group (1992) Randomized trial of adjuvant tamoxifen in node negative postmenopausal breast cancer. *Acta oncol.*, **31**, 265–270

Rutqvist, L.E., Johansson, H., Signomklao, T., Johansson, U., Fornander, T. & Wilking, N., for the Stockholm Breast Cancer Study Group (1995) Adjuvant tamoxifen therapy for early stage breast cancer and second primary malignancies. *J. natl Cancer Inst.*, **87**, 645–651

Rydén, S., Fernö, M., Möller, T., Aspegren, K., Bergljung, L., Killander, D. & Landberg, T. (1992) Long-term effects of adjuvant tamoxifen and/or radiotherapy. The South Sweden Breast Cancer Trial. *Acta oncol.*, **31**, 271–274

Salata, I., Kowalski, J., Czechowski, B., Ochedalski, T., Karowicz, A. & Kowalska-Koprek, U. (1993) Does treatment with antioestrogens in men with oligozoospermia influence the pregnancy course in women after artificial insemination by husband. *Gin. Pol.*, **64**, 493–497 (in Polish)

Samelis, S.F., Stathopoulos, G.P., Malamos, N.A., Kondili, E., Moschopoulos, N.P. & Papacostas, P. (1992) Toxicity of long-term treatment with tamoxifen in breast cancer patients (Abstract no. 300). *Ann. Oncol.*, **3** (Suppl. 5), 78

Sargent, L.M., Dragan, Y.P., Bahnub, N., Wiley, J.E., Sattler, C.A., Schroeder, P., Sattler, G. L., Jordan, V.C. & Pitot, H.C. (1994) Tamoxifen induces hepatic aneuploidy and mitotic spindle disruption after a single in vivo administration to female Sprague-Dawley rats. *Cancer Res.*, **54**, 3357–3360

Sasco, A.J., Raffi, F., Satgé, D., Goburdhun, J., Fallouh, B. & Leduc, B. (1995) Endometrial Müllerian carcinosarcoma after cessation of tamoxifen therapy for breast cancer. *Int. J. gynecol. Obstet.*, **48**, 307–310

Sasco, A.J., Chaplain, G., Amoros, E. & Saez, S. (1996) Endometrial cancer following breast cancer: effect of tamoxifen and castration by radiotherapy. *Epidemiology*, **7**, 9–13

Sawka, C.A., Pritchard, K.I., Paterson, A.H.G., Sutherland, D.J.A., Thomson, D.B., Shelley, W.E., Myers, R.E., Mobbs, B.G., Malkin, A. & Meakin, J.W. (1986) Role and mechanism of action of tamoxifen in premenopausal women with metastatic breast carcinoma. *Cancer Res.*, **46**, 3152–3156

Segna, R.A., Dottino, P.R., Deligdisch, L. & Cohen, C.J. (1992) Tamoxifen and endometrial cancer. *Mt Sinai. J. Med.*, **59**, 416–418

Sengupta, A., Dutta, S. & Mallick, R. (1991) Modulation of cervical carcinogenesis by tamoxifen in a mouse model system. *Oncology*, **48**, 258–261

Seoud, M.A.-F., Johnson, J. & Weed, J.C., Jr (1993) Gynecologic tumors in tamoxifen-treated women with breast cancer. *Obstet. Gynecol.*, **82**, 165–169

Servais, P. & Galand, P. (1993) Increased yield in GST-P-positive liver pre-neoplastic foci induced by DENA or ENU in rats pre-treated with estradiol or tamoxifen. *Int. J. Cancer*, **54**, 996–1001

Shewmon, D.A., Stock, J.L., Abusamra, L.C., Kristan, M.A., Baker, S. & Heiniluoma, K.M. (1994) Tamoxifen decreases lipoprotein (a) in patients with breast cancer. *Metabolism*, **43**, 531–532

Silva, E.G., Tornos, C.S. & Follen-Mitchell, M. (1994) Malignant neoplasms of the uterine corpus in patients treated for breast carcinoma: the effects of tamoxifen. *Int. J. gynecol. Pathol.*, **13**, 248–258

Sonnendecker, H.E.M., Cooper, K. & Kalian, K.N. (1994) Case report. Primary Fallopian tube adenocarcinoma *in situ* associated with adjuvant tamoxifen therapy for breast carcinoma. *Gynecol. Oncol.*, **52**, 402–407

Spinelli, G., Bardazzi, N., Citernesi, A., Fontanarosa, M. & Curiel, P. (1991) Endometrial carcinoma in tamoxifen-treated breast cancer patients. *J. Chemother.*, **3**, 267–270

Stephens, C.J.M., Wojnarowska, F.T. & Wilkinson, J.D. (1989) Autoimmune progesterone dermatitis responding to tamoxifen. *Br. J. Dermatol.*, **121**, 135–137

Sterzik, K., Rosenbusch, B., Mogck, J., Heyden, M. & Lichtenberger, K. (1993) Tamoxifen treatment of oligozoospermia: a reevaluation of its effects including additional sperm function tests. *Arch. Gynecol. Obstet.*, **252**, 143–147

Stewart, H.J. (for the Scottish Cancer Trials Breast Group) (1992) The Scottish trial of adjuvant tamoxifen in node-negative breast cancer. *Monogr. natl Cancer Inst.*, **11**, 117–120

Stewart, H.J. & Knight, G.M. (1989) Tamoxifen and the uterus and endometrium (Letter to the Editor). *Lancet*, **i**, 375–376

Styles, J.A., Davies, A., Lim, C.K., De Matteis, F., Stanley, L.A., White, I.N.H., Yuan, Z.-X. & Smith, L.L. (1994) Genotoxicity of tamoxifen, tamoxifen epoxide and toremifene in human lymphoblastoid cells containing human cytochrome P450s. *Carcinogenesis*, **15**, 5–9

Sunderland, M.C. & Osborne, C.K. (1991) Tamoxifen in premenopausal patients with metastatic breast cancer: a review. *J. clin. Oncol.*, **9**, 1283–1297

Swahn, M.I., Bygdeman, M., Matlin, S.A. & Wu, Z.Y. (1989) The effect of tamoxifen on the function and lifespan of the corpus luteum and on subsequent ovarian function. *Acta endocrinol.*, **121**, 417–425

Swenerton, K.D., Chrumka, K., Paterson, A.H.G. & Jackson, G.C. (1984) Efficacy of tamoxifen in endometrial cancer. In: Bresciani, ed., *Progress in Cancer Research and Therapy*, Vol. 31, New York, Raven, pp. 417–424

Sydow, G. & Wunderlich, V. (1994) Effects of tamoxifen, droloxifene and 17β-estradiol on Rauscher mouse leukemogenesis. *Cancer Lett.*, **82**, 89–94

Taguchi, O. (1987) Reproductive tract lesions in male mice treated neonatally with tamoxifen. *Biol. Reprod.*, **37**, 113–116

Tarantal, A.F., Hendrickx, A.G., Matlin, S.A., Lasley, B.L., Gu, Q.-Q., Thomas, C.A.A., Vince, P.M. & van Look, P.F.A. (1993) Tamoxifen as an antifertility agent in the long-tailed macaque. *Contraception*, **47**, 307–316

Taylor, O.M., Benson, E.A., McMahon, M.J. & the Yorkshire Gastrointestinal Tumour Group (1993) Clinical trial of tamoxifen in patients with irresectable pancreatic adenocarcinoma. *Br. J. Surg.*, **80**, 384–386

Thangaraju, M., Kumar, K., Gandhirajan, R. & Sachdanandam, P. (1994) Effect of tamoxifen on plasma lipids and lipoproteins in postmenopausal women with breast cancer. *Cancer*, **73**, 659–663

Thomas, J., ed. (1991) *Prescription Products Guide 1991*, 20th Ed., Victoria, Australian Pharmaceutical Publishing Co. Ltd., pp. 1218–1220

Tormey, D.C., Gray, R., Falkson, H.C., Gilchrist, K., Abeloff, M.D., Falkson, G. & Participating Investigators (1993) Maintenance tamoxifen after induction postoperative chemotherapy in node-positive breast cancer patients: the Eastern Cooperative Oncology Group Trials. *Recent Results Cancer Res.*, **127**, 185–196

Tse, J. & Goldfarb, S. (1988) Immunohistochemical demonstration of estrophilin in mouse tissues using a biotinylated monoclonal antibody. *J. Histochem. Cytochem.*, **36**, 1527–1531

Tucker, M.J., Adam, H.K. & Patterson, J.S. (1984) Tamoxifen. In: Laurence, D.R., McLean, A.E.M. & Weatherall, M., eds, *Safety Testing of New Drugs*, New York, Academic Press, pp. 125–162

Uesugi, Y., Sato, T. & Iguchi, T. (1993) Morphometric analysis of the pelvis in mice treated neonatally with tamoxifen. *Anat. Rec.*, **235**, 126–130

Ugwumadu, A.H.N. & Harding, K. (1994) Uterine leimyomata and endometrial proliferation in postmenopausal women teated with the anti-oestrogen tamoxifen. *Eur. J. Obstet. Gynecol.*, **54**, 153–156

Ugwumadu, A.H.N., Bower, D. & Ho, P.K.-H. (1993) Tamoxifen induced adenomyosis and adenomyomatous endometrial polyp. *Br. J. Obstet. Gynaecol.*, **100**, 386–392

Ulibarri, C. & Micevych, P.E. (1993) Role of perinatal estrogens in sexual differentiation of the inhibition of lordosis by exogenous cholecystokinin. *Physiol. Behav.*, **54**, 95–100

United States Library of Medicine (1996) *RTECS Database*, Bethesda, MD

United States Pharmacopeial Convention (1994) *The 1995 US Pharmacopeia*, 23rd Rev./*The National Formulary*, 18th Rev., Rockville, MD, pp. 1477–1479

Uziely, B., Lewin, A., Brufman, G., Dorembus, D. & Mor-Yosef, S. (1993) The effect of tamoxifen on the endometrium. *Breast Cancer Res. Treat.*, **26**, 101–105

Vanchieri, C. (1993) European tamoxifen studies moving ahead. *J. natl Cancer Inst.*, **85**, 1450–1451

Vancutsem, P.M., Lazarus, P. & Williams, G.M. (1994) Frequent and specific mutations of the rat *p53* gene in hepatocarcinomas induced by tamoxifen. *Cancer Res.*, **54**, 3864–3867

Vargas Roig, L.M., Lotfi, H., Olcese, J.E., Lo Castro, G. & Ciocca, D.R. (1993) Effects of short-term tamoxifen administration in patients with invasive cervical carcinoma. *Anticancer Res.*, **13**, 2457–2464

Vickers, A.E. & Lucier, G.W. (1991) Estrogen receptor, epidermal growth factor and cellular ploidy in elutriated subpopulations of hepatocytes during liver tumor promotion by 17 alpha-ethinylestradiol in rats. *Carcinogenesis*, **12**, 391–399

Vidal (1995) *Dictionnaire Vidal*, 71st Ed., Paris, Editions du Vidal, p. 144

de Vos, D., Guelen, P.J.M. & Stevenson, D. (1989) The bioavailability of Tamoplex (tamoxifen). Part 4. A parallel study comparing Tamoplex and four batches of Nolvadex in healthy male volunteers. *Meth. Find. exp. clin. Pharmacol.*, **11**, 647–655

Wakeling, A.E., O'Connor, K.M. & Newboult, E. (1983) Comparison of the biological effects of tamoxifen and a new antioestrogen (LY 117018) on the immature rat uterus. *J. Endocrinol.*, **99**, 447–453

Ward, H.W.C. (1973) Anti-oestrogen therapy for breast cancer: a trial of tamoxifen at two dose levels. *Br. med. J.*, **i**, 13–14

Ward, R.L., Morgan, G., Dalley, D. & Kelly, P.J. (1993) Tamoxifen reduces bone turnover and prevents lumbar spine and proximal femoral bone loss in early postmenopausal women. *Bone Min.*, **22**, 87–94

Watson, J., Anderson, F.B., Alam, M., O'Grady, J.E. & Heald, P.J. (1975) Plasma hormones and pituitary luteinizing hormone in the rat during the early stages of pregnancy and after postcoital treatment with tamoxifen (ICI 46,474). *J. Endocrinol.*, **65**, 7–17

Weckbecker, G., Tolcsvai, L., Stolz, B., Pollak, M. & Bruns, C. (1994) Somatostatin analogue octreotide enhances the antineoplastic effects of tamoxifen and ovariectomy on 7,12-dimethylbenz(*a*)anthracene-induced rat mammary carcinomas. *Cancer Res.*, **54**, 6334–6337

West, C.M.L., Reeves, S.J. & Brough, W. (1990) Additive interaction between tamoxifen and rifampicin in human biliary tract carcinoma cells. *Cancer Lett.*, **55**, 159–163

White, I.N.H., De Matteis, F., Davies, A., Smith, L.L., Crofton-Sleigh, C., Venitt, S., Hewer, A. & Phillips, D.H. (1992) Genotoxic potential of tamoxifen and analogues in female Fischer F344/n rats, DBA/2 and C57Bl/6 mice and in human MCL-5 cells. *Carcinogenesis*, **13**, 2197–2203

White, I.N.H., Davies, A., Smith, L.L., Dawson, S. & De Matteis, F. (1993) Induction of CYP2B1 and 3A1, and associated monooxygenase activities by tamoxifen and certain analogues in the livers of female rats and mice. *Biochem. Pharmacol.*, **45**, 21–30

White, I.N.H., de Matteis, F., Gibbs, A.H., Lim, C.K., Wolf, C.R., Henderson, C. & Smith, L.L. (1995) Species differences in the covalent binding of [^{14}C]tamoxifen to liver microsomes and the forms of cytochrome P450 involved. *Biochem. Pharmacol.*, **49**, 1035–1042

Williams, G.M., Iatropoulos, M.J., Djordjevic, M.V. & Kaltenberg, O.P. (1993) The triphenylethylene drug tamoxifen is a strong liver carcinogen in the rat. *Carcinogenesis*, **14**, 315–317

Winterfeld, G., Hauff, P., Görlich, M., Arnold, W., Fichtner, I. & Staab, H.J. (1992) Investigations of droloxifene and other hormone manipulations on *N*-nitrosomethylurea-induced rat mammary tumours. I. Influence on tumour growth. *J. Cancer Res. clin. Oncol.*, **119**, 91–96

Wiseman, H. (1994) *Tamoxifen: Molecular Basis of Use in Cancer Treatment and Prevention*, Chichester, John Wiley

Wiseman, H., Paganga, G., Rice-Evans, C. & Halliwell, B. (1993) Protective actions of tamoxifen and 4-hydroxytamoxifen against oxidative damage to human low-density lipoproteins: a mechanism accounting for the cardioprotective action of tamoxifen. *Biochem. J.*, **292**, 635–638

Wolter, J., Ryan, W.G., Subbaiah, P.V. & Bagdade, J.D. (1988) Apparent beneficial effects of tamoxifen on serum lipoprotein subfractions and bone mineral content in patients with breast cancer (Abstract no. 34). *Proc. Am. Soc. clin. Oncol.*, **7**, 10

Wong, A. & Chan, A. (1993) Survival benefit of tamoxifen therapy in adenocarcinoma of pancreas. A case–control study. *Cancer*, **71**, 2200–2203

Wright, C.D.P., Garrahan, N.J., Stanton, M., Gazet, J.-C., Mansell, R.E. & Compston, J.E. (1994) Effect of long-term tamoxifen therapy on cancellous bone remodeling and structure in women with breast cancer. *J. Bone min. Res.*, **9**, 153–159

Yager, J.D. & Shi, Y.E. (1991) Synthetic estrogens and tamoxifen as promoters of hepatocarcinogenesis. *Prev. Med.*, **20**, 27–37

Yager, J.D., Roebuck, B.D., Paluszcyk, T.L. & Memoli, V.A. (1986) Effects of ethinyl estradiol and tamoxifen on liver DNA turnover and new synthesis and appearance of gamma glutamyl transpeptidase-positive foci in female rats. *Carcinogenesis*, **7**, 2007–2014

Yagoda, A., Abi-Rached, B. & Petrylak, D. (1995) Chemotherapy for advanced renal-cell carcinoma: 1983-1993. *Sem. Oncol.*, **22**, 42–60

Yang, H.-H., Aulerich, R.J., Helferich, W., Yamini, B., Chou, K.C., Miller, E.R. & Bursian, S.J. (1995) Effects of zearalenone and/or tamoxifen on swine and mink reproduction. *J. appl. Toxicol.*, **15**, 223–232

Zemlickis, D., Lishner, M., Degendorfer, P., Panzarella, T., Sutcliffe, S.B. & Koren, G. (1992) Fetal outcome after in utero exposure to cancer chemotherapy. *Arch. intern. Med.*, **152**, 573–576

Zimniski, S.J. & Warren, R.C. (1993) Induction of tamoxifen-dependent rat mammary tumors. *Cancer Res.*, **53**, 2937–2939

TOREMIFENE

1. Exposure Data

1.1 Chemical and physical data

1.1.1 Nomenclature

Toremifene

Chem. Abstr. Serv. Reg. No.: 89778-26-7
Deleted CAS Reg. No.: 98644-21-4
Chem. Abstr. Name: (Z)-2-[4-(4-Chloro-1,2-diphenyl-1-butenyl)phenoxy]-*N,N*-dimethylethanamine
IUPAC Systematic Name: 2-[*para*-[(Z)-4-Chloro-1,2-diphenyl-1-butenyl]phenoxy]-*N,N*-dimethylethylamine
Synonyms: (Z)-4-Chloro-1,2-diphenyl-1-(4-(2-(*N,N*-dimethylamino)ethoxy)phenyl)-1-butene; Z-toremifene; toremifene base

Toremifene citrate

Chem. Abstr. Serv. Reg. No.: 89778-27-8
Chem. Abstr. Name: (Z)-2-[4-(4-Chloro-1,2-diphenyl-1-butenyl)phenoxy]-*N,N*-dimethylethanamine, 2-hydroxy-1,2,3-propanetricarboxylate (1:1)
IUPAC Systematic Name: 2-[*para*-[(Z)-4-Chloro-1,2-diphenyl-1-butenyl]phenoxy]-*N,N*-dimethylethylamine citrate (1:1)
Synonyms: (Z)-4-Chloro-1,2-diphenyl-1-[4-[2-(*N,N*-dimethylamino)ethoxy]phenyl]-1-butene citrate (1:1)

1.1.2 Structural and molecular formulae and relative molecular mass

Toremifene

$C_{26}H_{28}ClNO$ Relative molecular mass: 405.87

Toremifene citrate

$C_{26}H_{28}ClNO \cdot C_6H_8O_7$ Relative molecular mass: 598.10

1.1.3 *Chemical and physical properties of the pure substances*

Toremifene

Melting-point: 108–110 °C (Budavari, 1995)

Toremifene citrate

(a) *Description*: White crystals (Orion, 1996)

(b) *Melting-point*: 160–162 °C (Budavari, 1995)

(c) *Spectroscopy*: Ultraviolet, infrared, nuclear magnetic resonance and mass spectrometric data have been reported (Orion, 1996)

(d) *Solubility*: Sparingly soluble in methanol; slightly soluble in ethanol; very slightly soluble in water (0.44 mg/mL at 37 °C), acetone and chloroform; practically insoluble in octanol and diethyl ether (Budavari, 1995; Orion, 1996)

(e) *Stability*: Sensitive to ultraviolet light (Orion, 1996)

(f) *Dissociation constant*: pK_a, ~ 8.0 (Orion, 1996)

(g) *Octanol/water partition coefficient (P)*: log P, 3.3 (Orion, 1996)

1.1.4 *Technical products and impurities*

Toremifene in pharmaceutical preparations is invariably present as its citrate salt.

Toremifene citrate is available as an 88.5-mg tablet (equivalent to 60 mg toremifene base), which may also contain maize starch, lactose, polyvinylpyrrolidone (povidone), sodium starch glycolate, magnesium stearate, microcrystalline cellulose and colloidal anhydrous silica (Orion, 1996).

The *E*-isomer may be present as a minor impurity (≤ 0.3%) (Orion, 1996).

Trade names and designations for toremifene citrate and its pharmaceutical preparations include: FC 1157a; Fareston; NK 622.

1.1.5 *Analysis*

Toremifene and its metabolites can be analysed in biological fluids by liquid chromatography–atmospheric pressure ionization mass spectrometry (Watanabe *et al.*, 1989) and high-performance liquid chromatography (Holleran *et al.*, 1987; Hasan *et al.*, 1990; Webster *et al.*, 1991; Berthou & Dréano, 1993; Lim *et al.*, 1994).

1.2 Production and use

1.2.1 *Production*

Toremifene was first synthesized in 1981. Toremifene was first marketed commercially in 1990; production in 1995 was about 100 kg (Orion, 1996).

The synthesis of toremifene citrate consists of four process phases. In the first phase, 4-hydroxybenzophenone is O-alkylated with 2-chloroethyl dimethylamine yielding the first intermediate [4-(2-dimethylaminoethoxy)phenyl]phenylmethanone. This intermediate is condensed with a complex formed of cinnamaldehyde and lithium aluminium hydride and the second intermediate 1-[4-(2-dimethylaminoethoxy)phenyl]-1,2-diphenyl-butane-1,4-diol is obtained. This intermediate is treated with thionyl chloride yielding toremifene base which is converted to toremifene citrate by the addition of citric acid in water/ethanol (Orion, 1996).

1.2.2 *Use*

Toremifene, an antioestrogenic compound and a chlorinated analogue of tamoxifen, has been investigated for the treatment of metastatic breast cancer in postmenopausal women. It has been studied in animal experiments (Kangas *et al.*, 1986) and in clinical phase I (Kivinen & Mäenpää, 1990; Hamm *et al.*, 1991) and phase II (Valavaara *et al.*, 1988; Valavaara & Pyrhönen, 1989; Hietanen *et al.*, 1990; Valavaara, 1990; Jönsson *et al.*, 1991; Pyrhönen *et al.*, 1994) trials (see Glossary, p. 449).

Toremifene is being studied, in comparison with tamoxifen, in at least five different phase III trials (see Glossary, p. 449) in women with metastatic breast cancer. In order to clarify the dose-dependence of its action, daily doses of 60–240 mg are being used, in comparison with 20–40-mg daily doses of tamoxifen (Pyrhönen, 1990). One worldwide three-armed randomized phase III trial of tamoxifen (20 mg daily) versus toremifene (60 mg daily) or toremifene (200 mg daily) in postmenopausal women with metastatic breast cancer showed similar response rates and survival in all three arms (Hayes *et al.*, 1995). Results from other comparative phase III trials will soon be available. Three trials of toremifene as adjuvant therapy are also in progress: two performed by the International Breast Cancer Study Group, and one by the Finnish Breast Cancer Group (Orion, 1996).

Like tamoxifen, toremifene has also been tested for use in several other malignant diseases including endometrial carcinoma (Horvath *et al.*, 1990; Mäenpää *et al.*, 1992a), ovarian carcinoma (Mäenpää *et al.*, 1992b) and melanoma (Kleeberg *et al.*, 1993). Studies in patients with advanced breast cancer show some response to treatment and minimal side-effects. This seems to be similar to tamoxifen and there appears to be major cross-resistance between the two drugs (Jönsson *et al.*, 1991; Nomura *et al.*, 1993; Stenbygaard *et al.*, 1993; Vogel *et al.*, 1993; Pyrhönen *et al.*, 1994). Toremifene has beneficial effects on cardiovascular lipid profiles in postmenopausal women with breast cancer (Gylling *et al.*, 1995).

Thus, although toremifene is not yet registered for use in most countries, it is under extensive investigation for therapy of metastatic breast cancer as well as in the adjuvant setting.

Toremifene was developed in Finland and has been available there since 1990. It has been available in Sweden, Russia and the Ukraine since 1994, and became available in Japan in 1995 (Anon., 1995a; Orion, 1996).

1.3 Occurrence

Toremifene is not known to occur as a natural product.

1.4 Regulations and guidelines

A Health Registration Application for toremifene was filed with the European Union's Committee for Proprietary Medicinal Products in December 1994. A New Drug Application for toremifene was filed with the United States Food and Drug Administration in January 1995 (Anon., 1995b). Toremifene was subsequently recommended for approval by the United States Food and Drug Administration (Anon., 1995a) and the European Union's Committee for Proprietary Medicinal Products in October 1995 (Anon., 1995a). It was approved in February 1996 in the European Union for treatment of hormone-dependent metastatic breast cancer in postmenopausal patients (European Commission, 1996).

2. Studies of Cancer in Humans

No report of carcinogenicity or chemopreventive activity of toremifene in humans has been published.

3. Studies of Cancer in Experimental Animals

3.1 Oral administration

Rat: In a study that also included tamoxifen, groups of 57, 84 and 75 female Sprague-Dawley [Crl:CD(BR)] rats, six weeks of age, were given 0 (control), 12 and 24 mg/kg bw toremifene citrate (purity, 99%) per day by gastric instillation in 0.5% carboxymethylcellulose on seven days per week for up to 12 months. Nine rats in each group were killed at three and six months. At 12 months, 18 control, 36 low-dose and 10 high-dose rats were killed and, at 15 months, 13, 20 and 13 animals in the respective groups were killed; 8, 10 and 34 respectively died during the experiment. All rats, including those found dead or moribund, were subjected to necropsy; organs examined histopathologically included liver, ovaries, uterus, mammary gland, adrenal glands, tail bone, sternum, brain and pituitary. Weight gain in both groups receiving toremifene citrate was less than that in controls. At three months, the incidence of placental-type glutathione S-transferase-positive altered hepatocellular foci was 5/9 (56%) control, 3/9 (33%) low-dose and 1/9 (11%) high-dose rats. No liver tumour was found at 12 or 15 months. At 12 months, the incidence of granulosa-cell tumours of the ovary was 1/34 low-dose and 1/10 high-dose rats compared with 0/17 controls. In rats killed at 15 months, three months after cessation of exposure, no ovarian tumour was found. The incidence of hyperplasia, adenoma or carcinoma in the mammary gland and that of pituitary adenoma or carcinoma were zero in toremifene citrate-treated rats (Hard *et al.*, 1993). [The Working Group noted that exposure was limited to 12 months and that the study was terminated at 15 months.]

In a study that also included tamoxifen, groups of 20 female Sprague-Dawley rats, six weeks of age, were given 0 (control), 12 or 48 (MTD, maximum tolerated dose) mg/kg bw toremifene citrate (purity > 99%) per day by gastric instillation in 0.5% carboxymethylcellulose for up to one year. All surviving animals were observed without further exposure for an additional 13 weeks. Five animals from each group were killed after 26 weeks and 52 weeks of treatment; all surviving rats (8 controls, 9 low-dose and 3 high-dose animals) were killed 65 weeks after the beginning of treatment. Weight gain was reduced in both toremifene citrate-treated groups. No liver tumour was found in animals at interim or terminal kills. Findings in tissues other than the liver were not reported (Hirsimäki *et al.*, 1993). [The Working Group noted the small number of animals, that exposure was of 12 months' duration and that the study was terminated at 65 weeks.]

In a study that also included tamoxifen, groups of 10 female Sprague-Dawley rats, six weeks of age, were given 0, 12 or 48 (MTD) mg/kg bw toremifene citrate (purity > 99%) per day by gastric instillation in 0.5% carboxymethylcellulose for 12 months. Groups of five animals were killed at 12 months or after a further 13 weeks of recovery. No liver tumour occurred in any group (Ahotupa *et al.*, 1994). [The Working Group noted the small number of animals and that the study was terminated at 65 weeks.]

As part of a tumour promotion study that also included tamoxifen, groups of 36–37 female Fischer rats, weighing 130 ± 10 g [age not specified], were subjected to partial hepatectomy and three weeks later exposed to toremifene [purity not specified] in the diet at concentrations of 0 (control), 250, 500 or 750 mg/kg diet (ppm) for 6 or 18 months. All exposures to toremifene suppressed body-weight gain in animals killed at six months, and uterine weights were reduced. At this time, no increase was found in either the number or volume of hepatocellular altered foci identified by staining for the placental form of glutathione *S*-transferase or adenosine triphosphatase, whereas γ-glutamyltranspeptidase-positive foci were increased at all doses (dose-related). One hepatic neoplastic nodule was found in controls compared with none in the treated animals. At the terminal kill at 18 months, there was no increase in liver tumours (see Table 1). No kidney tumour was found (Dragan *et al.*, 1995). [The Working Group noted the small numbers of animals and the short duration.]

Groups of 50 male and 50 female Sprague-Dawley rats, six weeks of age, were given toremifene citrate (purity > 98%) in the diet for two years. The rats received mean daily intakes of 0 (control), 0.12, 1.2, 5.0 or 12 mg/kg bw per day. The concentrations of toremifene in the diet were adjusted to maintain constant dose levels in terms of mg/kg bw per day. Toremifene citrate caused decreases in food consumption and body-weight gain in a dose-dependent manner, with high-dose females having 79% food consumption and 58% body weight compared with controls and high-dose males having 73% and 40%, respectively. Toremifene citrate reduced mortality, principally in the two highest dose groups. Mortality was 2% in the females receiving 12 mg/kg and 16% in those receiving 5 mg/kg, compared with 66% in controls, and 10% and 8% in the corresponding groups of males compared with 40% in controls. No increase in tumours was found. In females, the incidences of mammary and pituitary tumours were reduced, while, in males, the incidences of pituitary and testicular tumours were reduced (see Table 2) (Karlsson et al., 1996). [The Working Group noted that some of the reduced tumour incidences may have been related to body-weight reduction.]

Table 1. Incidences of liver neoplasms in female Sprague-Dawley rats exposed to toremifene

Exposure (mg/kg diet (ppm))	Neoplastic nodules	Hepatocellular carcinomas
None	16/22	0/22
Toremifene, 250	6/22	0/22
Toremifene, 500	4/21	1/21
Toremifene, 750	15/22	0/22

From Dragan et al. (1995)

Table 2. Incidence (%) of certain tumours in Sprague-Dawley rats exposed to toremifene citrate

	Dose (mg/kg bw per day)				
	0	0.12	1.2	5.0	12.0
Females					
Mammary tumours	60	14[a]	4[b]	2[b]	4[b]
Pituitary tumours	86	52[b]	2[b]	2[b]	0[b]
Males					
Pituitary tumours	54	38[b]	4[b]	2[b]	4[b]
Testicular tumours	10	12	0	0	0

From Karlsson et al. (1996)
[a] $p < 0.01$
[b] $p < 0.001$

In a study that also included tamoxifen, in a compilation of three experiments reported in the proceedings of a meeting, groups of 38, 62 or 64 female Sprague-Dawley rats [age unspecified] were given daily doses of 3, 12 or 48 mg/kg bw by gastric instillation for up to 52 weeks. No tumours of the uterus were seen (Mäntylä et al., 1996).

3.2 Administration with known carcinogens

Rat: Groups of 5–10 (32 in controls) female Sprague-Dawley rats, 50 ± 2 days of age, were given 12 mg/animal 7,12-dimethylbenz[a]anthracene (DMBA) as a single gastric instillation in sesame oil. After six weeks, when mammary tumours had reached about 1 cm in diameter, groups were treated with 0, 0.3, 1.0, 3.0, 7.5, 15.0 or 30.0 mg/kg bw toremifene citrate (purity > 98%) [vehicle not specified] per day by gastric instillation for at least five weeks. The numbers of new tumours per animal were 3.0 ± 2.6 in controls and 1.4 ± 1.2 in the 0.3-mg/kg bw, 0.6 ± 0.7 in the 1.0-mg/kg bw, 0.7 ± 1.1 in the 3.0-mg/kg bw, 1.6 ± 2.0 in the 7.5-mg/kg bw, 1.8 ± 2.4 in the 15.0-mg/kg bw and 0.6 ± 1.4 in the 30.0-mg/kg bw toremifene citrate-treated groups, a significant decrease ($p < 0.005$) at all doses, except 0.3 and 15 mg/kg bw (Kangas *et al.*, 1986).

Groups of 20 Sprague-Dawley rats [females], 50 days of age, were given 20 mg per animal DMBA in peanut oil as a single gastric instillation. Twenty-eight days later, groups were given 50, 200 or 800 μg/animal toremifene citrate in peanut oil daily by gastric instillation for four months. By 100 days after DMBA administration, 75% of rats given DMBA alone had developed mammary tumours, many having multiple tumours, whereas, in the group also receiving toremifene (200 or 800 μg), less than 20% had tumours [percentages derived from graphs] and only single tumours. Cessation of toremifene treatment (200 or 800 μg) after four months led to the development of mammary tumours, so that by 4.5 months about 70% of animals had tumours (Robinson *et al.*, 1988).

Two groups of female Sprague-Dawley rats, 50 days old, received 12 mg/animal DMBA [vehicle not specified] as a single gastric instillation. After seven weeks, the animals were given 0 (five rats with 16 mammary tumours) or 3 (six rats with 25 mammary tumours) mg/kg bw toremifene [purity not specified] per day by gastric instillation for five weeks. During treatment, 32 new mammary tumours appeared in the control group and 16 in the treated group (Huovinen & Collan, 1994).

In a tumour promotion study, in which tamoxifen was also studied, groups of 14–22 female Fischer rats, weighing 130 ± 10 g [age not specified], were subjected to partial hepatectomy and 24 h later were given 10 mg/kg bw *N*-nitrosodiethylamine (NDEA) in trioctanoin as a single gastric instillation. Two weeks later, rats were given either basal diet or diet containing 250, 500 or 750 mg/kg diet (ppm) toremifene for 6 or 18 months. All exposures to toremifene depressed body-weight gain in animals killed at six months and uterine weights were depressed. The number and volume fraction of liver occupied by altered hepatic foci identified by any of the histochemical markers used was increased by toremifene. At six months, the incidences of hepatic neoplastic nodules in all groups were 53, 20, 20 and 43% in controls, low-, mid- and high-dose, respectively. At 18 months, the incidence of liver tumours in all groups approached 100%. Toremifene increased the incidence of hepatocellular carcinomas in the high-dose group (2/17, 2/18, 7/16 and 11/18 in the controls, low-, mid- and high-dose respectively). The incidence of kidney tumours was increased by toremifene at the highest dose (Table 3) (Dragan *et al.*, 1995).

Table 3. Incidences of kidney neoplasms in female Fischer rats exposed to toremifene after NDEA

Exposure (mg/kg diet (ppm))	Renal cell adenomas	Renal cell carcinomas
None	5/19[a]	0/19
Toremifene, 250	0/18	0/18
Toremifene, 500	7/16	2/16[b]
Toremifene, 750	12/20[c]	5/20[c]

From Dragan et al. (1995)
[a] [$p = 0.002$; Cochran Armitage test for trend]
[b] [not significant; Fisher's exact test]
[c] [$p = 0.03$; Fisher's exact test]

In a study that also included tamoxifen, groups of virgin female Sprague-Dawley rats aged 43 days were randomized into groups of 20 and allocated to control diet or a diet containing 100 mg/kg diet (ppm) toremifene citrate (reduced to 50 mg/kg at 71 days of age because of reduced body-weight gain). Seven days later, groups were given either 50 mg/kg bw N-methyl-N-nitrosourea or saline by intravenous injection. Animals were killed when moribund and the experiment was terminated at 180 days. Toremifene citrate reduced the incidence of mammary tumours to 46% compared with 100% in controls ($p < 0.05$); the multiplicity was reduced to 0.7 ± 0.2 from 10.6 ± 1.2 ($p < 0.05$) and latency was increased to 166 ± 8 days from 53 ± 4 days ($p < 0.05$) in the controls (Moon et al., 1994).

4. Other Data Relevant to an Evaluation of Carcinogenicity and its Mechanisms

4.1 Absorption, distribution, metabolism and excretion

4.1.1 Humans

In a study with 70 postmenopausal female volunteers, Anttila et al. (1990) found that toremifene was well absorbed and over 99% bound to plasma proteins. Peak serum concentration was usually reached within 4 h and the mean half-life of distribution was generally around 4 h. A further study (Anttila et al., 1995) was conducted on 10 healthy subjects (7 men and 3 women; body weight, 80.9 ± 20.3 kg) given a single oral dose of 120 mg toremifene, following an overnight fast. Measured pharmacokinetic parameters for toremifene, N-desmethyltoremifene and deaminohydroxytoremifene in serum, respectively, were: maximum concentrations (C_{max}), 414 ± 173 ng/mL, 130 ± 53 ng/mL and 38 ± 24 ng/mL at median times of 2 h, 72 h and 2 h, the areas under the integrated time × concentration curves (AUC) being 28.4 ± 12.3, 94.1 ± 77.5 and 0.48 ± 0.66 (μg × h/mL).

Elimination half-life ($t_{1/2}$) values were 6.2 ± 2.2 days for toremifene and 21.0 ± 24.1 days for N-desmethyltoremifene. Apparent clearance of toremifene after oral dosing was 5.1 L/h and its apparent volume of distribution was 958 ± 309 L. Multiple dosing with 60 mg toremifene per day resulted in an average steady-state serum level of 800 ng/mL within six weeks after the start of therapy (Anttila et al., 1990). Postmenopausal patients (19 women) receiving high doses of toremifene (240–780 mg/day) for advanced breast cancer showed plasma concentrations ranging from 1.5 to 4.0 µg/mL (Bishop et al., 1992). In 70 postmenopausal patients with advanced breast cancer receiving single oral daily doses of either 10, 20, 40, 60, 200 or 400 mg toremifene for eight weeks, the time to reach steady-state plasma concentrations was between one and five weeks (one to two weeks for the 200 and 400 mg doses). The time to peak concentration was 1.5–4.5 h. The peak toremifene concentrations were 1117–1270 ng/mL (at a dose of 60 mg/day) and 198–669 ng/mL (at a dose of 20 mg/day). Plasma concentrations of 4-hydroxytoremifene were detectable only at high doses (200–400 mg per day) of toremifene, typical peak concentrations being 383–515 ng/mL after a 400 mg-dose. The peak concentrations of N-desmethyltoremifene were 538–2622 ng/mL (at a dose of 20 mg/day), 2709–5769 ng/mL (at a dose of 60 mg/day) and 7937–9135 ng/mL (at a dose of 400 mg/day) (Wiebe et al., 1990).

Toremifene undergoes extensive demethylation and hydroxylation to active and inactive metabolites via hepatic mixed function oxidases (see Figure 1). In human urine, four unconjugated and three glucuronide-conjugated metabolites were detected in one study, but only 4-hydroxytoremifene glucuronide was identified (Watanabe et al., 1989). In the study of Anttila et al. (1990), N-desmethyltoremifene was the major metabolite in serum and was present at a concentration twice that of toremifene; other metabolites included 4-hydroxytoremifene, deaminohydroxytoremifene (one tenth of toremifene concentration (Anttila et al., 1990)) and didesmethyltoremifene (Kangas, 1990).

Elimination of toremifene is slow, with a mean half-life of five days (Anttila et al., 1990). The terminal half-lives for elimination of toremifene, N-desmethyltoremifene and 4-hydroxytoremifene are five, six and five days, respectively (Wiebe et al., 1990).

Enterohepatic recirculation of toremifene has been reported in humans (Wiebe et al., 1990). The majority of a dose of toremifene is excreted as metabolites in faeces (Anttila et al., 1990) and the long half-life of toremifene may be due to both plasma protein binding and enterohepatic recirculation (Wiebe et al., 1990).

4.1.2 Experimental systems

Following administration of [^{3}H]toremifene to female Sprague-Dawley rats by intravenous injection, 70% of the total radioactivity was eliminated within 13 days, with more than 90% of this appearing in the faeces. Toremifene metabolites have been identified in rats and others have been postulated (see Figure 1). 4-Hydroxytoremifene is a major metabolite in rats and is present in urine at twice the level of N-desmethyltoremifene (Sipilä et al., 1990). Toremifene is metabolized and excreted by isolated perfused rat liver, but a significant amount binds to the reperfusion circuit. Furthermore, clinically relevant doses of toremifene do not appear to inhibit hepatic mixed function

Figure 1. Postulated metabolic pathways of toremifene

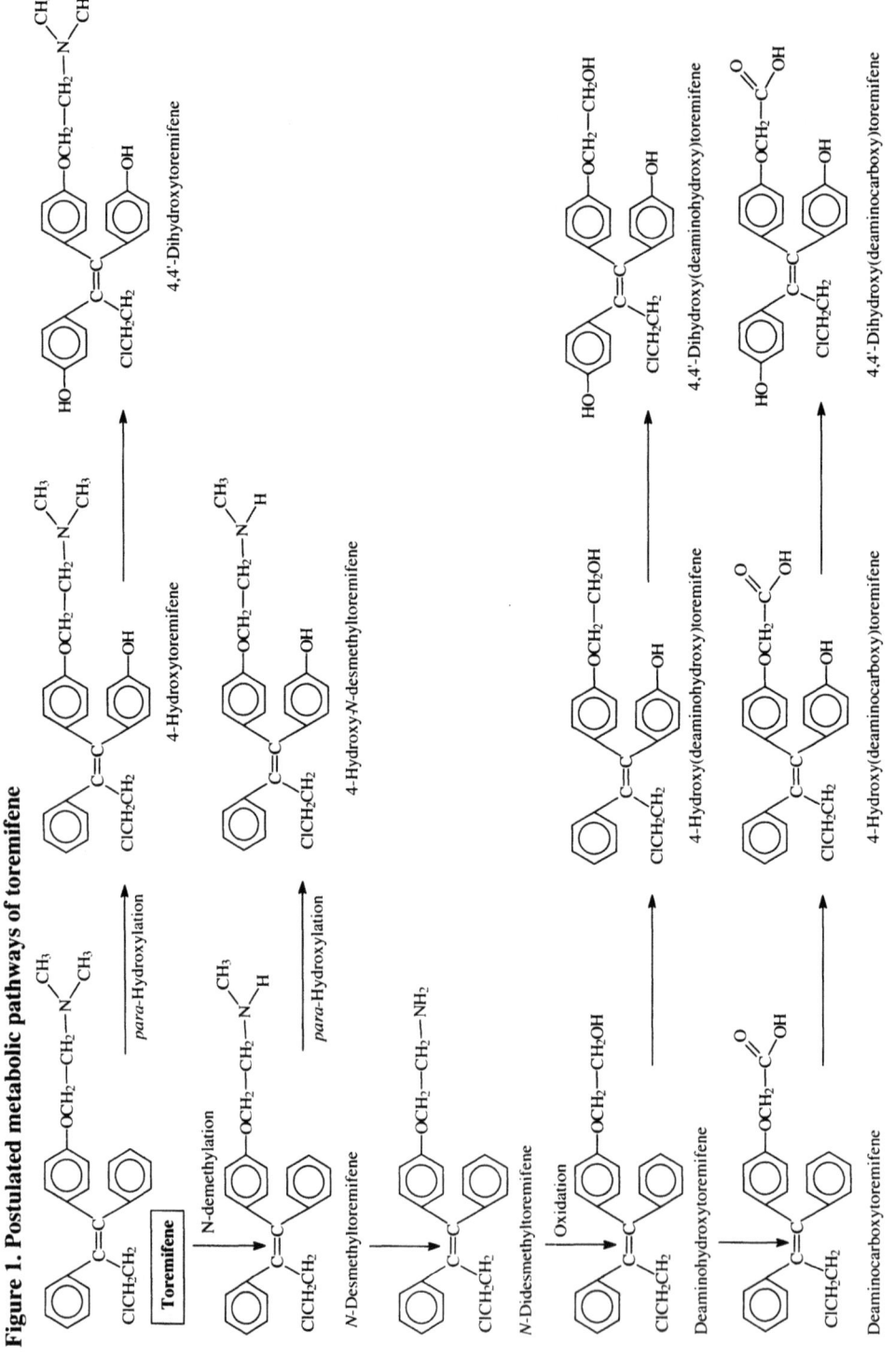

Adapted from Kangas (1990)

oxidase activity, as indicated by elimination of antipyrine (Webster *et al.*, 1993). Enterohepatic recirculation of toremifene has been reported in rats and small amounts of unchanged toremifene have been found in the faeces, suggesting biliary secretion (Sipilä *et al.*, 1990).

The major pathways of toremifene metabolism are mediated mainly by a CYP3A4 enzyme in human liver microsomes (Berthou *et al.*, 1994).

Administration to rats of 0.12 mmol/kg bw toremifene per day for four days by gastric instillation increased the metabolism of benzyloxy- and pentoxyresorufin 10–80-fold, while ethoxyresorufin metabolism hardly changed (White *et al.*, 1993).

4.2 Toxic effects

4.2.1 *Humans*

In a phase I clinical trial of 107 cancer patients (74 with breast cancer), toremifene was administered at doses from 10 to 400 mg per day for eight weeks to groups of 11–26 patients (age range, 25–80 years; mean, 58 years) (Kohler *et al.*, 1990). In general, toremifene was well tolerated at all doses tested. Gastrointestinal complaints were the most common side-effects (at all dose levels). Nausea and vomiting, usually mild, were reported by 43% of patients. Antioestrogenic side-effects included hot flushes (29%), vaginal discharge (8.4%) and vaginal bleeding (2.8%). Other effects observed were related to the central nervous system and included dizziness/vertigo (12%), lethargy/-fatigue (10%), headaches (7%), insomnia (4%), anxiety (3%) and irritability (2%). The only ophthalmological finding was dry eye (reduced tearing), which was reported by three patients at higher doses. There was no change in electrolytes, liver function, renal function or serum lipids. No dose-related change in total leukocytes, granulocytes or platelets was found. A moderate decrease in antithrombin III activity was found. A decline in luteinizing hormone (LH) and follicle-stimulating hormone (FSH) levels (but only at concentrations equal to or greater than 40 mg/day) and an increase in sex hormone-binding globulin (SHBG) were noted. No change was observed in cortisol, prolactin, oestrone or 17β-oestradiol levels or in thyroid function tests. Similar results were reported from a phase I study in 72 healthy postmenopausal volunteers in which toremifene was given within the dose range of 3–680 mg as a single dose or on five consecutive days (Kivinen & Mäenpää, 1990). Other effects of 60 mg/day toremifene given to breast cancer patients for 3, 6 or 12 months included a stimulatory effect on cell-mediated immunity, according to a positive effect on mitogen-stimulation tests (Valavaara *et al.*, 1990) [The Working Group noted that the control group consisted of healthy women.]

Thirty-one gynaecologically asymptomatic postmenopausal breast cancer patients with intact uteri were randomized to receive 20 mg tamoxifen or 60 mg toremifene as adjuvant treatment (Tomás *et al.*, 1995). Pap smear, endometrial biopsy, hysteroscopy and curettage were performed before treatment and at the end of 6 and 12 months of treatment. In the toremifene group, endometrial thickness increased from 3.9 mm before treatment to 6.0 mm at six months and 7.0 mm at 12 months. Proliferation in endometrial cytology in the toremifene group at the three observation times, respectively, occurred in 0/13, 3/11 and 2/10 patients. There was no significant difference between toremifene and tamoxifen in any of the parameters investigated.

A three-armed randomized comparison was performed with toremifene at 60 mg/day ($n = 221$) and 200 mg/day ($n = 212$) and tamoxifen at 20 mg/day ($n = 215$) in postmenopausal patients with hormone receptor-positive or unknown metastatic breast cancer (Hayes et al., 1995). The group receiving 200 mg/day toremifene experienced significantly more nausea ($p = 0.027$), but no other significant difference in toxicity or quality of life was reported among the three arms of the trial. Clinical tumour flare (a transient increase in bone and/or musculoskeletal pain within two weeks of starting the drug) occurred in 16% of the 60-mg toremifene and 19% of the 200-mg toremifene groups (and 19% of the tamoxifen group). Seventeen patients died during the study or within 30 days of the last dose due to causes believed not to be secondary to metastatic breast disease. These were similarly distributed, with no significant differences among the three arms (nine and six in the 60-mg and 200-mg toremifene groups, respectively, and two in the tamoxifen group). Serious but non-lethal adverse events in the 60-mg and 200-mg toremifene and tamoxifen groups, respectively, included pulmonary embolism (5, 2, 2), cerebrovascular accidents (0, 3, 0), thrombosis (1, 0, 1), impaired liver function texts (alanine transaminase $\geq$ 100 IU/L, 11, 22, 4; total bilirubin $\geq$ 2 mg/dL, 3, 7, 4) and corneal keratopathies (4, 8, 2). Twenty-one patients withdrew from the study because of toxicity; 6 and 12 in the 60-mg and 200-mg toremifene groups, respectively, and 3 in the tamoxifen group.

4.2.2 *Experimental systems*

In a preliminary toxicity study in which toremifene was administered to rats at doses of up to 48 mg/kg bw for 26 weeks, no ocular or hepatic changes were observed (Kangas et al., 1986). [No further details were given.]

Toremifene at a steady-state concentration of 10 μg/mL (a high, but clinically relevant concentration) caused a significant decrease in bile flow in isolated perfused rat liver and therefore appears to impair liver function, but it did not have any effect on antipyrine elimination (Webster et al., 1993).

In Sprague-Dawley rats given 250–750 mg/kg of diet (ppm) toremifene for 18 months, uterine weights were depressed (Dragan et al., 1995).

4.3 Reproductive and developmental effects

4.3.1 *Humans*

No data were available to the Working Group.

4.3.2 *Experimental systems*

In a study reported only as an abstract, Hirsimäki et al. (1990) stated that pregnancy was not compromised in rats given oral doses of up to 50 mg/kg bw toremifene per day, although toxic effects occurred in the dam at doses of 10 mg/kg bw per day or higher. In rabbits, abortion occurred with doses of 10 mg/kg bw per day and total litter loss with 50 mg/kg bw per day. Fertility of male rats was reduced after 10 weeks of oral treatment with 25 mg/kg bw per day, but not at lower levels. This reduction in fertility was accompanied by a reduction in the weight of the reproductive organs. Females became acyclic when treated with doses of 0.2 mg/kg bw per day or higher and, although they mated, they did not become pregnant. At a dose of 0.04 mg/kg bw per day, the oestrus cycle was normal, and mating and pregnancy were successful. Oestrus cycles recovered within two weeks and mating occurred, but treatment could not be recommenced until day 6 of gestation, otherwise implantation was prevented. At doses of 1 mg/kg bw per day or more, parturition difficulties occurred.

4.4 Genetic and related effects

4.4.1 *Humans*

No studies were available to the Working Group.

4.4.2 *Experimental systems*

Mutagenicity (see also Table 4 for references and Appendices 1 and 2)

Toremifene induced micronucleus formation in MCL-5 cells, a genetically engineered human lymphoblastoid cell line that expresses native CYP1A1 and transfected CYP1A2, CYP2A6, CYP2E1 and CYP3A4 and epoxide hydrolase, and also weakly in similar cell lines that expressed CYP2E1 or 3A4 but not in a line expressing CYP2D6.

DNA adducts in vivo

A very low level of DNA adducts (0.85 ± 0.1 adducts per 10^8 nucleotides) was detected by ^{32}P-postlabelling in the livers of female Fischer 344 rats given 0.12 mmol/kg toremifene per day by gastric instillation for four days and killed 24 h after the final treatment (White *et al.*, 1992).

Treatment of female Sprague-Dawley rats with up to 90 μmol/kg toremifene per day by gastric instillation for 10 days did not lead to formation of detectable DNA adducts in the liver (Montandon & Williams, 1994). Similarly, DNA adducts were not detected in the livers of Crl:CD(BR) rats (Sprague-Dawley) given 48 mg/kg toremifene (0.12 mmol/kg) per day by gastric instillation for seven days and killed 24 h later (Hard *et al.*, 1993).

A very low level of DNA adducts (0.02 adducts per 10^8 nucleotides) was detected by ^{32}P-postlabelling in cultured human lymphocytes treated with 100 μg/mL toremifene (Hemminki *et al.*, 1995). Adducts were not detected at lower concentrations.

A low level of microsome-mediated DNA adduct formation by toremifene was detected by ^{32}P-postlabelling (Hemminki *et al.*, 1995). In the presence of NADP and glucose-6-phosphate, toremifene concentrations of 1 mM gave adduct levels of 0.04 adducts per 10^8 nucleotides with rat microsomes and 0.012 adducts per 10^8 nucleotides with human microsomes.

Table 4. Genetic and related effects of toremifene

Test system	Result[a]		Dose[b] (LED/HID)	Reference
	Without exogenous metabolic system	With exogenous metabolic system		
MIH, Micronucleus test, human lymphoblastoid MCL-5 cells *in vitro*	+[c]	NT	0.5	Styles *et al.* (1994)
MIH, Micronucleus test, human lymphoblastoid h1A1 cells expressing CYP1A1 *in vitro*	–	NT	1.5	Styles *et al.* (1994)
MIH, Micronucleus test, human lymphoblastoid h1A2 cells expressing CYP1A2 *in vitro*	–	NT	1.5	Styles *et al.* (1994)
MIH, Micronucleus test, human lymphoblastoid h2E1 cells expressing CYP2E1 *in vitro*	(+)	NT	0.75	Styles *et al.* (1994)
MIH, Micronucleus test, human lymphoblastoid h3A4 cells expressing CYP3A4 *in vitro*	(+)	NT	0.75	Styles *et al.* (1994)
MIH, Micronucleus test, human lymphoblastoid h2D6 cells expressing CYP2D6 *in vitro*	–	NT	1.5	Styles *et al.* (1994)
BID, Binding (covalent) to DNA, human lymphocytes *in vitro*	(+)	NT	100	Hemminki *et al.* (1995)
BVD, Binding (covalent) to DNA, female Fischer 344/N rat liver *in vivo* (^{32}P-postlabelling)	(+)		50 po × 4	White *et al.* (1992)
BVD, Binding (covalent) to DNA, female SD rat liver *in vivo* (^{32}P-postlabelling)	–		48 po × 7	Hard *et al.* (1993)
BVD, Binding (covalent) to DNA, female SD rat liver *in vivo* (^{32}P-postlabelling)	–		33 po × 10	Montandon & Williams (1994)

[a] +, positive; (+), weak positive; –, negative; NT, not tested; ?, inconclusive
[b] LED, lowest effective dose; HID, highest ineffective dose; in-vitro tests, μg/mL; in-vivo tests, mg/kg bw/day
[c] Expressing native CYP1A1 and transfected CYPs 1A2, 2A6, 3A4 and 2E1 and epoxide hydrolase; cytochalasin B-arrested

Horseradish peroxidase activated toremifene to a reactive intermediate which bound covalently to both DNA and protein (Davies *et al.*, 1995).

4.5 Hormonal effects

4.5.1 *Humans*

The effects of toremifene on endocrine parameters in healthy postmenopausal women and in women with advanced breast cancer have been studied. Oestrogenic effects were evaluated by measuring concentrations of LH, FSH, SHBG and prolactin, and antioestrogenicity in 17β-oestradiol-primed postmenopausal women by vaginal cornification index. During eight weeks of treatment with 60 or 200 mg/day toremifene, FSH levels decreased by a mean of 29 and 53%, respectively, and LH levels by approximately 20 and 50%. SHBG concentrations increased about two-fold at both dose levels (Hamm *et al.*, 1991). Prolactin concentrations in serum did not change, although, in patients with basal prolactin, a decrease to the normal level was seen (Számel *et al.*, 1994). The no-effect dose level of toremifene in the vaginal cornification antioestrogenic assay was 10 mg daily. There was no clear dose–response relationship of the vaginal cornification index at doses of 20–200 mg/day (Hamm *et al.*, 1991).

4.5.2 *Experimental systems*

Toremifene bound to oestrogen receptors in rat uterus competitively with [^{3}H]17β-oestradiol, the IC_{50} concentration being 0.5 μmol/L and the dissociation constant 1 nM (Kallio *et al.*, 1986; Simberg *et al.*, 1990). It induced binding of oestrogen receptors to the nuclear compartment and increased progesterone receptor concentrations in the rat uterus *in vivo* during five days of administration (Kallio *et al.*, 1986).

The oestrogenic and antioestrogenic actions of toremifene were studied by a uterotrophic assay in immature and ovariectomized adult mice and rats given toremifene daily for three days (oestrogenicity) and together with 17β-oestradiol (antioestrogenicity). Significant oestrogenic and antioestrogenic responses were observed in mice at the lowest test dose reported, 0.05 mg/kg. In rats, the lowest dose inducing a significant oestrogenic response was 0.1 mg/kg, while an antioestrogenic response was observed at 0.01 mg/kg (Kallio *et al.*, 1986; Kangas, 1990; di Salle *et al.*, 1990).

The hormonal effects of toremifene were studied in rat liver by measurement of cytosolic (reduction) and nuclear (increase) oestrogen receptors. Toremifene produced an oestrogen agonistic effect (Kendall & Rose, 1992).

Triphenylethylene antioestrogens have tissue- and species-specific hormonal effects. Toremifene is predominantly oestrogenic in mice, antioestrogenic in rats and humans (Kangas, 1992) and both oestrogenic and antioestrogenic in monkeys (Wood *et al.*, 1992).

5. Summary of Data Reported and Evaluation

5.1 Exposure data

Toremifene, a chlorinated analogue of tamoxifen, was first marketed in 1990 and by 1995 was registered in five countries. It is currently undergoing further clinical trials for the treatment of metastatic breast cancer as well as trials for use as adjuvant therapy.

5.2 Human carcinogenicity data

No data were available to the Working Group.

5.3 Animal carcinogenicity data

Toremifene was tested for carcinogenicity in one study by oral administration to male and female rats and in four studies of limited duration in female rats. No increase in tumour incidence was observed in these studies. In the one study of long duration, toremifene decreased the incidence of tumours in some hormone-dependent tissues, notably mammary gland.

In one study in female rats, toremifene increased the incidence of kidney tumours and the proportion of malignant liver tumours induced by N-nitrosodiethylamine.

In four other experiments in rats, toremifene inhibited the development of 7,12-dimethylbenz[a]anthracene- or N-methyl-N-nitrosourea-induced mammary tumours.

5.4 Other relevant data

Toremifene is well absorbed in humans. The major metabolites result from N-demethylation, hydroxylation and deamination, and are excreted predominantly in faeces. The elimination half-life is about six days. The metabolism is qualitatively similar, but quantitatively different, in rats.

In a single study, no teratogenic effect of toremifene was found in rats.

Toremifene induced micronucleus formation in one study that used genetically engineered cell lines. Low levels of DNA adducts were detected in rat liver in one of three studies. Low levels of DNA adduct formation have also been reported in human lymphocytes *in vitro*.

5.5 Evaluation[1]

There is *inadequate evidence* in humans for the carcinogenicity of toremifene.

There is *inadequate evidence* in experimental animals for the carcinogenicity of toremifene.

Overall evaluation

Toremifene is *not classifiable as to its carcinogenicity to humans (Group 3)*.

---

[1] For definition of the italicized terms, see Preamble, pp. 22–25.

6. References

Ahotupa, M., Hirsimäki, P., Pärssinen, R. & Mäntylä, E. (1994) Alterations of drug metabolizing and antioxidant enzyme activities during tamoxifen-induced hepatocarcinogenesis in the rat. *Carcinogenesis*, **15**, 863–868

Anon. (1995a) European OK for Fareston. *Scrip*, **2073**, 22

Anon. (1995b) Scherling-Plough granted U.S. marketing rights for Fareston. *Drug News Perspectives*, **April 18**

Anttila, M., Valavaara, R., Kivinen, S. & Mäenpää, J. (1990) Pharmacokinetics of toremifene. *J. Steroid Biochem.*, **36**, 249–252

Anttila, M., Laakso, S., Nyländen, P. & Sotaniemi, E.A. (1995) Pharmacokinetics of the novel antiestrogenic agent toremifene in subjects with altered liver and kidney function. *Clin.Pharmacol.Ther.*, **57**, 628–635

Berthou, F. & Dréano, Y. (1993) High-performance liquid chromatographic analysis of tamoxifen, toremifene and their major human metabolites. *J. Chromatogr.*, **616**, 117–127

Berthou, F., Dréano, Y., Belloc, C., Kangas, L., Gautier, J.-C. & Beaune, P. (1994) Involvement of cytochrome P450 3A enzyme family in the major metabolic pathways of toremifene in human liver microsomes. *Biochem. Pharmacol.*, **47**, 1883–1895

Bishop, J., Murray, R., Webster, L., Pitt, P., Stokes, K., Fennessy, A., Olver, I. & Leber, G. (1992) Phase I clinical and pharmacokinetics study of high-dose toremifene in post-menopausal patients with advanced breast cancer. *Cancer Chemother. Pharmacol.*, **30**, 174–178

Budavari, S., ed. (1995) *The Merck Index*, 12th Ed., Rahway, NJ, Merck & Co.

Davies, A.M., Martin, E.A., Jones, R.M., Lim, C.K., Smith, L.L. & White, I.N.H. (1995) Peroxidase activation of tamoxifen and toremifene resulting in DNA damage and covalently bound protein adducts. *Carcinogenesis*, **16**, 539–545

Dragan, Y.P., Vaughan, J., Jordan, V.C. & Pitot, H.C. (1995) Comparison of the effects of tamoxifen and toremifene on liver and kidney tumor promotion in female rats. *Carcinogenesis*, **16**, 2733–2741

European Commission (1996) *Fareston Containing Toremifene*, Directorate General III, Brussels

Gylling, H., Pyrhönen, S., Mäntylä, E., Mäenpää, H., Kangas, L. & Miettinen, T.A. (1995) Tamoxifen and toremifene lower serum cholesterol by inhibition of Δ^8-cholesterol conversion to lathosterol in women with breast cancer. *J. clin. Oncol.*, **13**, 2900–2905

Hamm, J.T., Tormey, D.C., Kohler, P.C., Haller, D., Green, M. & Shemano, I. (1991) Phase I study of toremifene in patients with advanced cancer. *J. clin. Oncol.*, **9**, 2036–2041

Hard, G.C., Iatropoulos, M.J., Jordan, K., Radi, L., Kaltenberg, O.P., Imondi, A.R. & Williams, G.M. (1993) Major difference in the hepatocarcinogenicity and DNA adduct forming ability between toremifene and tamoxifen in female Crl:CD(BR) rats. *Cancer Res.*, **53**, 4534–4541

Hasan, S.A., Wiebe, V.J., Cadman, K.S. & DeGregorio, M.W. (1990) Quantitative analysis of toremifene metabolites in biological specimens using high-performance liquid chromatography. *Analyt. Lett.*, **23**, 327–334

Hayes, D.F., Van Zyl, J.A., Hacking, A., Goedhals, L., Bezwoda, W.R., Mailliard, J.A., Jones, S.E., Vogel, C.L., Berris, R.F., Shemano, I. & Schoenfelder, J. (1995) Randomized comparison of tamoxifen and two separate doses of toremifene in postmenopausal patients with metastatic breast cancer. *J. clin. Oncol.*, **13**, 2556–2566

Hemminki, K., Widlak, P. & Hou, S.-M. (1995) DNA adducts caused by tamoxifen and toremifene in human microsomal system and lymphocytes *in vitro*. *Carcinogenesis*, **16**, 1661–1664

Hietanen, T., Baltina, D., Johansson, R., Numminen, S., Hakala, T., Helle, L. & Valavaara, R. (1990) High dose toremifene (240 mg daily) is effective as first line hormonal treatment in advanced breast cancer. An ongoing phase II multicenter Finnish-Latvian cooperative study. *Breast Cancer Res. Treat.*, **16** (Suppl.), S37–S40

Hirsimäki, Y., Beltrame, D., McAnulty, P., Tesh, J. & Wong, L. (1990) Preliminary investigations of the reproductive consequences of toremifene citrate treatment (Abstract no. 890). *Toxicologist*, **10**, 223

Hirsimäki, P., Hirsimäki, Y., Nieminen, L. & Payne, B.J. (1993) Tamoxifen induces hepatocellular carcinoma in rat liver: a 1-year study with two antiestrogens. *Arch. Toxicol.*, **67**, 49–54

Holleran, W.M., Gharbo, S.A. & DeGregorio, M.W. (1987) Quantitation of toremifene and its major metabolites in human plasma by high-performance liquid chromatography following fluorescent activation. *Analyt. Lett.*, **20**, 871–879

Horvath, G., Stendahl, U., Kalling, M., Fernö, M., Himmelmann, A. & Hajba, A. (1990) Antiestrogenic treatment of advanced and recurrent carcinoma corporis uteri — A phase II study of toremifene. *Anticancer Res.*, **10**, 323–326

Huovinen, R. & Collan, Y. (1994) Cell loss in dimethylbenz(a)anthracene-induced rat mammary carcinoma treated with toremifene and ovariectomy. *Tumor Biol.*, **15**, 345–353

Jönsson, P.-E., Malmberg, M., Bergljung, L., Ingvar, C., Ericsson, M., Ryden, S., Nilsson, I., & Johansson Terje, I. (1991) Phase II study of high dose toremifene in advanced breast cancer progressing during tamoxifen treatment. *Anticancer Res.*, **11**, 873–875

Kallio, S., Kangas, L., Blanco, G., Johansson, R., Karjalainen, A., Perilä, M., Pippo, I., Sundquist, H., Södervall, M. & Toivola, R. (1986) A new triphenylethylene compound, Fc-1157a. I. Hormonal effects. *Cancer Chemother. Pharmacol.*, **17**, 103–108

Kangas, L. (1990) Biochemical and pharmacological effects of toremifene metabolites. *Cancer Chemother. Pharmacol.*, **27**, 8–12

Kangas, L. (1992) Agonistic and antagonistic effects of antioestrogens in different target organs. *Acta oncol.*, **31**, 143–146

Kangas, L., Nieminen, A.-L., Blanco, G., Grönroos, M., Kallio, S., Karjalainen, A., Perilä, M., Södervall, M. & Toivola, R. (1986) A new triphenylethylene compound, Fc-1157a. II. Antitumor effects. *Cancer Chemother. Pharmacol.*, **17**, 109–113

Karlsson, S., Hirsimäki, Y., Mäntylä, E., Nieminen, L., Kangas, L., Hirsimäki, P., Perry, C.J., Mulhern, M., Millar, P., Handa, J. & Williams, G.M. (1996) A two-year dietary carcinogenicity study of the antiestrogen toremifene in Sprague-Dawley rats. *Drug chem. Toxicol.* (in press)

Kendall, M.E. & Rose, D.P. (1992) The effects of diethylstilbestrol, tamoxifen, and toremifene on estrogen-inducible hepatic proteins and estrogen receptor proteins in female rats. *Toxicol. appl. Pharmacol.*, **144**, 127–131

Kivinen, S. & Mäenpää, J. (1990) Effect of toremifene on clinical chemistry, hematology and hormone levels at different doses in healthy postmenopausal volunteers: phase I study. *J. Steroid Biochem.*, **36**, 217–220

Kleeberg, U.R., Engel, E., Bröcker, E.B., Avril, F., Israels, P., Weiss, J., Kangas, L., van Glabbeke, M. & Lentz, M.A. (1993) Effect of toremifene in patients with metastatic melanoma: a phase II study of the EORTC melanoma cooperative group. *Melanoma Res.*, **3**, 123–126

Kohler, P.C., Hamm, J.T., Wiebe, V.J., DeGregorio, M.W., Shemano, I. & Tormey, D.C. (1990) Phase I study of the tolerance and pharmacokinetics of toremifene in patients with cancer. *Breast Cancer Res. Treatment*, **16** (Suppl.), S19–S26

Lim, C.K., Yuan, Z.-X., Ying, K.-C. & Smith, L.L. (1994) High-performance liquid chromatography of toremifene and metabolites. *J. liq. Chromatogr.*, **17**, 1773–1783

Mäenpää, J.U., Sipilä, P.E.-H. & Hajba, A. (1992a) Toremifene for recurrent and advanced endometrial carcinoma (Letter to the Editor). *Eur. J. Cancer*, **28A**, 1768

Mäenpää, J.U., Sipilä, P.E.-H., Kangas, L., Karnani, P. & Grönroos, M. (1992b) Chemosensitizing effect of an antiestrogen, toremifene, on ovarian cancer. *Gynecol. Oncol.*, **46**, 292–297

Mäntylä, E.T.E., Karlsson, S.H. & Nieminen, L.S. (1996) Induction of endometrial cancer by tamoxifen in the rat. In: Li, J.J., Li, S.A., Gustafsson, J.-Å., Nandi, S. & Sekely, L.I., eds, *Hormonal Carcinogenesis II*, Proceedings of the Second International Symposium, New York, Springer-Verlag

Montandon, F. & Williams, G.M. (1994) Comparison of DNA reactivity of the polyphenylethylene hormonal agents diethylstilbestrol, tamoxifen and toremifene in rat and hamster liver. *Arch. Toxicol.*, **68**, 272–275

Moon, R.C., Steele, V.E., Kelloff, G.J., Thomas, C.F., Detrisac, C.J., Mehta, R.G. & Lubet, R.A. (1994) Chemoprevention of MNU-induced mammary tumorigenesis by hormone response modifiers: toremifene, RU 16117, tamoxifen, aminoglutethimide and progesterone. *Anticancer Res.*, **14**, 889–893

Nomura, Y., Tominaga, T., Abe, O., Izuo, M. & Ogana, N. (1993) Clinical evaluation of NK 622 (toremifene citrate) in advanced or recurrent breast cancer — A comparative study by a double blind method with tamoxifen. *Jpn. J. Cancer Chemother.*, **20**, 247–258 (in Japanese)

Orion (1996) *Toremifene*, Orion-Farmos, Turku, Finland

Potter, G.A., McCague, R. & Jarman, M. (1994) A mechanistic hypothesis for DNA adduct formation by tamoxifen following hepatic oxidative metabolism. *Carcinogenesis*, **15**, 439–442

Pyrhönen, S.O. (1990) Phase III studies of toremifene in metastatic breast cancer. *Breast Cancer Res. Treat.*, **16** (Suppl.), S41–S46

Pyrhönen, S.O., Valavaara, R., Heikkinen, M., Rissanen, P., Blanco, G., Nordman, E., Holsti, L.R. & Hajba, A. (1990) Treatment of advanced breast cancer with 20 mg toremifene, a phase II study. Preliminary communication. *J. Steroid Biochem.*, **36**, 227–228

Pyrhönen, S.O., Valavaara, R., Vuorinen, J. & Hajba, A. (1994) High dose toremifene in advanced breast cancer resistant to or relapsed during tamoxifen treatment. *Breast Cancer Res. Treat.*, **29**, 223–228

Robinson, S.P., Mauel, D.A. & Jordan, V.C. (1988) Antitumor actions of toremifene in the 7,12-dimethylbenzanthracene (DMBA)-induced rat mammary tumor model. *Eur. J. Cancer clin. Oncol.*, **24**, 1817–1821 di Salle, E., Zaccheo, T. & Ornati, G. (1990) Antiestrogenic and antitumor properties of the new triphenylethylene derivative toremifene in the rat. *J. Steroid Biochem.*, **36**, 203–206

Simberg, N.H., Murai, J.T. & Siiteri, P.K. (1990) In vitro and in vivo binding of toremifene and its metabolites in rat uterus. *J. Steroid Biochem.*, **36**, 197–202

Sipilä, H., Kangas, L., Vuorilehto, L., Kalapudas, A., Eloranta, M., Södervall, M., Toivola, R. & Anttila, M. (1990) Metabolism of toremifene in the rat *J. Steroid Biochem.*, **36**, 211–215

Stenbygaard, L.E., Herrstedt, J., Thomsen, J.F., Svendsen, K.R., Engelholm, S.A. & Dombernowsky, P. (1993) Toremifene and tamoxifen in advanced breast cancer — a double-blind cross-over trial. *Breast Cancer Res. Treat.*, **25**, 57–63

Styles, J.A., Davies, A., Lim, C.K., De Matteis, F., Stanley, L.A., White, I.N.H., Yuan, Z.-X. & Smith, L.L. (1994) Genotoxicity of tamoxifen, tamoxifen epoxide and toremifene in human lymphoblastoid cells containing human cytochrome P450s. *Carcinogenesis*, **15**, 5–9

Számel, I., Hindy, I., Vincze, B., Eckhardt, S., Kangas, L. & Hajba, A. (1994) Influence of toremifene on the endocrine regulation in breast cancer patients. *Eur. J.Cancer*, **30A**, 154–158

Tomás, E., Kauppila, A., Blanco, G., Apaja-Sarkkinen, M. & Laatikainen, T. (1995) Comparison between the effects of tamoxifen and toremifene on the uterus in postmenopausal breast cancer patients. *Gynecol. Oncol.*, **59**, 261–266

Valavaara, R. (1990) Phase II trials with toremifene in advanced breast cancer: a review. *Breast Cancer Res. Treat.*, **16** (Suppl.), S31–S35

Valavaara, R. & Pyrhönen, S.O. (1989) Low-dose toremifene in the treatment of estrogen-receptor-positive advanced breast cancer in postmenopausal women. *Current ther. Res.*, **46**, 966–973

Valavaara, R., Pyrhönen, S.O., Heikkinen, M., Rissanen, P., Blanco, G., Thölix, E., Nordman, E., Taskinen, P., Holsti, L. & Hajba, A. (1988) Toremifene, a new anti-estrogenic compound for treatment of advanced breast cancer. Phase II study. *Eur. J. Cancer clin. Oncol.*, **24**, 785–790

Valavaara, R., Tuominen, J. & Toivanen, A. (1990) The immunological status of breast cancer patients during treatment with a new antiestrogen, toremifene. *Cancer Immunol. Immunother.*, **31**, 381–386

Vogel, C.L., Shemano, I., Schoenfelder, J., Gams, R.A. & Green, M.R. (1993) Multicenter phase II efficacy trial of toremifene in tamoxifen-refractory patients with advanced breast cancer. *J. clin. Oncol.*, **11**, 345–350

Watanabe, N., Irie, T., Koyama, M. & Tominaga, T. (1989) Liquid chromatographic-atmospheric pressure ionization mass spectrometric analysis of toremifene metabolites in human urine. *J. Chromatogr.*, **497**, 169–180

Webster, L.K., Crinis, N.A., Stokes, K.H. & Bishop, J.F. (1991) High-performance liquid chromatographic method for the determination of toremifene and its major human metabolites. *J. Chromatogr.*, **565**, 482–487

Webster, L.K., Ellis, A.G. & Bishop, J.F. (1993) Effect of toremifene on antipyrine elimination in the isolated perfused rat liver. *Cancer Chemother. Pharmacol.*, **31**, 319–323

White, I.N.H., De Matteis, F., Davies, A., Smith, L.L., Crofton-Sleigh, C., Venitt, S., Hewer, A. & Phillips, D.H. (1992) Genotoxic potential of tamoxifen and analogues in female Fischer F344/n rats, DBA/2 and C57Bl/6 mice and in human MCL-5 cells. *Carcinogenesis*, **13**, 2197–2203

White, I.N.H., Davies, A., Smith, L.L., Dawson, S. & De Matteis, F. (1993) Induction of CYP2B1 and 3A1, and associated monooxygenase activities by tamoxifen and certain analogues in the livers of female rats and mice. *Biochem. Pharmacol.*, **45**, 21–30

Wiebe, V.J., Benz, C.C., Shemano, I., Cadman, T.B. & DeGregorio, M.W. (1990) Pharmacokinetics of toremifene and its metabolites in patients with advanced breast cancer. *Cancer Chemother. Pharmacol.*, **25**, 247–251

Wood, J.D., Glaister, J.R., Goodyer, M.J., Yamashita, T. & Nakamori, K. (1992) Week oral toxicity study of toremifene citrate (NK622) in female monkeys. *Pharmacometrics* (Japan), **44**(4), 375–387

HYPOLIPIDAEMIC DRUGS

CLOFIBRATE

This substance was considered by previous working groups, in February 1980 (IARC, 1980) and March 1987 (IARC, 1987). Since that time, new data have become available, and these have been incorporated in the monograph and taken into consideration in the evaluation.

1. Exposure Data

1.1 Chemical and physical data

1.1.1 *Nomenclature*

Chem. Abstr. Serv. Reg. No.: 637-07-0

Chem. Abstr. Name: 2-(4-Chlorophenoxy)-2-methylpropanoic acid, ethyl ester

IUPAC Systematic Name: Ethyl 2-(*para*-chlorophenoxy)-2-methylpropionate

Synonyms: *para*-Chlorophenoxyisobutyric acid ethyl ester; 2-(*para*-chlorophenoxy)-2-methylpropionic acid ethyl ester; ethyl *para*-chlorophenoxyisobutyrate; ethyl 2-(*para*-chlorophenoxy)isobutyrate; ethyl 2-(4-chlorophenoxy)isobutyrate; ethyl α-(*para*-chlorophenoxy)isobutyrate; ethyl α-(4-chlorophenoxy)isobutyrate; ethyl α-(*para*-chlorophenoxy)-α-methylpropionate; ethyl α-(4-chlorophenoxy)-α-methylpropionate; ethyl 2-(4-chlorophenoxy)-2-methylpropionate; ethyl clofibrate

1.1.2 *Structural and molecular formulae and relative molecular mass*

$C_{12}H_{15}ClO_3$ 	Relative molecular mass: 242.70

1.1.3 *Chemical and physical properties of the pure substance*

(a) *Description*: Colourless to pale-yellow liquid (Gennaro, 1995)

(b) *Boiling-point*: 158–160 °C (at 25 mm Hg) (Gennaro, 1995)

(c) *Density*: 1.138–1.144 at 25 °C (Hassan & Elazzouny, 1982)

(d) *Spectroscopy data*: Infrared, ultraviolet, nuclear magnetic resonance and mass spectral data have been reported (Hassan & Elazzouny, 1982).

(e) *Solubility*: Practically insoluble in water; miscible with acetone, chloroform, diethyl ether and ethanol (Budavari, 1995; Gennaro, 1995)

1.1.4 *Technical products and impurities*

Clofibrate is available as 500-mg capsules which may also contain gelatin, D&C Red 28, D&C Red 30, D&C Yellow 10 (Quinoline Yellow), FD&C Blue 1 (Brilliant Blue FCF), FD&C Red 3 (Erythrosine) or FD&C Yellow 6 (Sunset Yellow FCF) (Thomas, 1991; Medical Economics, 1996).

Trade names and designations of the chemical and its pharmaceutical preparations include: Amotril; Anparton; Apolan; Arterioflexin; Artes; Artevil; Ateculon; Ateriosan; Aterosol; Atheromide; Atheropront; Atrofort; Atrolen; Atromid; Atromid-S; Atromidin; Atrovis; AY 61123; Azionyl; Bioscleran; Cartagyl; Citiflus; Clarípex; Claripex CPIB; Cloberat; Clobrat; Clobren SF; Clof; Clofibral; Clofibrat; Clofinit; Clofipront; Clofirem; CPIB; Deliva; ECPIB; EPIB; Estaprol; Geromid; Healthstyle; Hyclorate; ICI 28257; Ipolipid; Klofiran; Levatrom; Lipavil; Lipavlon; Lipilim; Lipomid; Liponorm; Liporan; Liprinal; Lobetrin; Lostat; MG 46; Miscleron; Misclerone; Neo-Atromid; NSC 79389; Normet; Normolipol; Novofibrate; Recolip; Regelan; Sclerovasal; Serotinex; Sklerolip; Skleromexe; Sklero-Tablinen; Ticlobran; Xyduril; Yoclo.

1.1.5 *Analysis*

Methods for the analysis of clofibrate have been reviewed (Hassan & Elazzouny, 1982).

Several international pharmacopoeias specify high-performance liquid chromatography (HPLC) or titration with hydrochloric acid as the assays for purity of clofibrate, and HPLC or gas chromatography with flame ionization detection (GC/FID) for determining impurities and decomposition products. Methods are also specified for determining acid, heavy metal, arsenic and *para*-chlorophenol content. The assays for clofibrate in capsules apply titration with hydrochloric acid, or HPLC or GC/FID methods using standards (Council of Europe, 1984; Society of Japanese Pharmacopoeia, 1992; British Pharmacopoeial Commission, 1993; United States Pharmacopeial Convention, 1994).

1.2 Production and use

1.2.1 *Production*

Clofibric acid was first synthesized in 1947 (Windholz, 1976), but the ethyl ester, clofibrate, was not reported until 1961 (Budavari, 1995). Clofibrate is prepared by condensing phenol with ethyl 2-chloro-2-methylpropionate in the presence of a suitable dehydrochlorinating agent and then chlorinating the aromatic ring (Gennaro, 1995).

1.2.2 *Use*

The efficacy of clofibrate in reducing serum cholesterol levels was first reported in 1962 (Thorp & Waring, 1962). Clofibrate was first marketed in the United States of America in 1967 (Wysowski *et al.*, 1990).

Clofibrate is used as a hypolipidaemic drug. It reduces elevated plasma concentrations of triglycerides by reduction of elevated concentrations of very low-density lipoproteins (VLDLs) within two to five days after initiation of therapy. It is less effective in reducing low-density lipoprotein (LDL) cholesterol and the plasma concentration of total cholesterol. It is mostly effective in the treatment of type III hyperlipoproteinaemia. It may also be helpful in some patients with type IIb, type IV or type V hyperlipoproteinaemia (see Glossary, p. 448) (Goodman Gilman et al., 1990; Reynolds, 1993; Larsen et al., 1994).

The usual daily dose is 2 g (20–30 mg/kg bw per day) taken orally in two or three divided doses (Reynolds, 1993; Vidal, 1995).

The cellular mechanisms responsible for the hypolipidaemic effects of fibrate drugs have not been clarified fully but include: activation of lipoprotein lipase, suppression of free fatty acid release from adipose tissue, inhibition of hepatic triglyceride synthesis and increased secretion of cholesterol (see IARC, 1983) into bile. Therapy with clofibrate does not significantly reduce the rate of synthesis of VLDL triglycerides, but such treatment is associated with an increase in the rate of catabolism of VLDL particles (Larsen et al., 1994). The mobilization of deposits of cholesterol in tissues is accompanied by regression and disappearance of xanthomas (Goodman Gilman et al., 1990).

Clofibrate has been used in the prophylaxis of ischaemic heart diseases but it is no longer recommended for this purpose, because of adverse effects seen during long-term treatment: increased incidences of cholecystitis, gallstones and in some cases of certain cardiovascular disorders and excess deaths found in the WHO Cooperative Trial on the use of clofibrate in the primary prevention of ischaemic heart disease (Reynolds, 1993). Some patients have also shown a paradoxical rise in LDL (Goodman Gilman et al., 1990).

Clofibrate has been used in the treatment of neonatal jaundice (Gabilan et al., 1990; Erkul et al., 1991; Gabilan et al., 1991).

Following the report of a WHO-sponsored cooperative study of the use of clofibrate in the primary prevention of ischaemic heart disease (Committee of Principal Investigators, 1978), it was withdrawn in the Federal Republic of Germany and Norway in early 1979. In a number of other countries, including France, Italy, Sweden, Switzerland, the United Kingdom and the United States, practitioners were advised to reserve its use for patients with high plasma lipid concentrations that are refractory to dietary measures and to consider carefully the risks and benefits of the treatment (United States Food and Drug Administration, 1979; WHO, 1979a; Expert Panel, 1988). It was reintroduced in the Federal Republic of Germany in August 1979 (WHO, 1979b). In the United Kingdom, clofibrate is now rarely prescribed (Dunnigan, 1992).

In the United States, clofibrate represented 80.9% of the cholesterol-lowering medications used in 1978, 41.2% in 1983 and 3.5% in 1988. Gemfibrozil (see monograph, pp. 428–429), lovastatin and cholestyramine are now used more commonly (Wysowski et al., 1990).

1.3 Occurrence

Clofibrate is not known to occur as a natural product.

No quantitative data on occupational exposure levels were available to the Working Group.

The National Occupational Exposure Survey conducted between 1981 and 1983 in the United States by the National Institute for Occupational Safety and Health indicated that about 325 employees were potentially occupationally exposed to clofibrate. The estimate was based on a survey of companies and did not involve measurements of actual exposure (United States National Library of Medicine, 1996).

1.4 Regulations and guidelines

Clofibrate is listed in the following pharmacopoeias: British, Brazilian, Chinese, Czech, Egyptian, European, French, Greek, Hungarian, Indian, Italian, Japanese, Netherlands, Nordic, Portuguese, Romanian, Swiss and United States (Reynolds, 1993).

2. Studies of Cancer in Humans

2.1 Case–control study

A population-based case–control study in Kansas, United States, investigated a large number of possible risk factors for soft-tissue sarcoma (Hoar Zahm *et al.*, 1989). One of the factors examined was medical treatment with cholesterol-lowering drugs (among which was clofibrate). Among white males, aged 21 years or older, a total of 139 newly diagnosed (1976–82) and histologically confirmed cases of soft-tissue sarcomas were identified through the University of Kansas Cancer Data Service (50% deceased). Deceased cases were not excluded from the study. Three controls were matched to each case by age and vital status. For living cases, controls were selected either from the Health Care Financing Administration files or by telephone random digit dialling. For deceased cases, controls were selected from Kansas state mortality files. Exposure information was obtained from interviews with study subjects or with their next-of-kin. The response rate was 93%. The distribution of proxy type was similar among the cases and controls. Among users of cholesterol-lowering drugs (5 cases and 20 controls), a nonsignificant excess of soft-tissue sarcoma was seen (odds ratio, 1.7; 95% confidence interval (CI), 0.5–5.0). The increased risk was found only among deceased subjects (odds ratio, 1.9; 95% CI, 0.5–6.4; 4 cases, 15 controls). [The Working Group noted that no adjustment was made for confounders, that all medical data, such as on use of cholesterol-lowering drugs, were self- or proxy-reported and that the inclusion of deceased controls may have overrepresented the prevalence of their use.]

2.2 Clinical trials

A randomized trial of the World Health Organization, started in 1965 to determine whether clofibrate would lower the incidence of ischaemic heart disease in men, raised concern over a nonsignificant excess of cancer deaths in treated subjects (58 versus 42 in placebo-treated controls) (Committee of Principal Investigators, 1978, 1980; IARC, 1980). The greatest excesses were for cancers of the gastrointestinal and respiratory tracts. Results of a further four years of follow-up of this trial to the end of 1982 subsequently became available (Committee of Principal Investigators, 1984). On average, the total follow-up period was 13.2 years, 5.3 of which were during the actual treatment phase (range, four to eight years) and 7.9 thereafter. Three groups of men, divided according to their cholesterol level, were studied, comprising 208 000 man–years of observation. The first two groups included subjects in the upper third of the serum cholesterol distribution, randomly allocated either to treatment with clofibrate (1.6 g daily) or to receive an olive oil-containing placebo. The third group was composed of half of the men in the lowest third of the distribution, who received an olive oil-containing placebo. At the conclusion of follow-up, the age-standardized rates of death from malignant neoplasms per 1000 per annum were 2.4, 2.4 and 2.3, respectively (based on 206, 197 and 173 deaths from malignant neoplasms). However, the age-standardized death rates for malignant neoplasms during the treatment phase had been 2.0 (42 deaths), 1.2 (25 deaths) and 1.7 (30 deaths), respectively.

The Coronary Drug Project, a randomized and double blind trial in the United States and Puerto Rico, started in 1966, investigated the effects of lipid-lowering drugs on 8341 men, aged 30–64 years with a history of myocardial infarction. The first results, with a mean follow-up of 6.2 years study (5–8.5 years), showed no increase in the cancer death rate in the clofibrate (1.8 g/day)-treated group (10 deaths in 1103 patients) compared with that of a placebo-treated group (24 deaths in 2789 patients) (Coronary Drug Project Research Group, 1975). After a mean follow-up of 15 years (including 8.8 years after termination of the trial), with definite information about vital status for 98.9% of subjects, the clofibrate group had somewhat lower cancer mortality (3.4%) than did the placebo group (4.4%). This was also the case for lung cancer (13 deaths in 1103 clofibrate-treated men (12/1000) and 53 deaths in 2789 placebo-treated men (19/1000)) and for cancer of the gastrointestinal tract (4/1000 versus 6/1000) (Canner et al., 1986).

In the Stockholm Ischaemic Heart Disease study (Carlson & Rosenhamer, 1988), 555 patients with ischaemic heart disease, under 70 years of age, were treated with clofibrate and nicotinic acid ($n = 279$) or with a placebo ($n = 276$) (not blind). Because of cancer, 10 subjects among the treated group and 6 among the controls withdrew from the trial. The numbers of cancer deaths during the five years of treatment were four in the treatment group and six in the control group.

Recently, Law et al. (1994) conducted a meta-analysis to assess whether low serum cholesterol concentration increases mortality from causes other than ischaemic heart disease. The data were derived from the 10 largest cohort studies, two international studies and 28 randomized trials, supplemented by unpublished data. Only the trials provided information about cholesterol-lowering drugs. Extended observation after the trial period had ended was available for six of the trials and provided information on the risk for cancer 5–10 years after treatment with cholesterol-lowering drugs (about 15 years after the start of treatment). The overall relative odds estimate of the risk for cancer was 0.9 (95% CI, 0.7–1.1; based on 232 treated patients. The meta-analysis did not provide estimates of relative risk for cancer mortality for the clofibrate trial separately. [The Working Group noted that the numbers of cancer deaths provided cannot be compared directly because of differences in survival between clofibrate-treated subjects and those who did not receive the drug.]

3. Studies of Cancer in Experimental Animals

3.1 Oral administration

3.1.1 Mouse

In a study reported as a summary in a monograph, groups of 25 male and 25 female Alderley Park mice [age not specified] were given 0 (control), 1000 (therapeutic level in humans), 2500 or 5000 (maximum tolerated dose, MTD) mg/kg diet (ppm) clofibrate [purity not specified] in the diet for 18 months. Major organs and abnormalities were examined histologically. Mortality was similar in all groups. No difference in the incidence of any tumour type between control and treated groups was reported (Tucker & Orton, 1995).

In another study reported as a summary in a monograph, groups of 51 male and 51 female C57Bl/10J mice, six weeks of age, were given clofibrate [purity not specified] at daily dose levels of 150, 250 and 350 mg/kg bw in the diet for 18 months. The untreated control groups comprised 151 males and 151 females. There was body-weight reduction of about 10% the higher-dose group. Mortality was similar in all groups (70–80% survival at 18 months). There was a significant increase in liver weights in treated males and females in the two higher-dose groups. Full necropsy and histological examinations were carried out on all animals. No difference in tumour incidence between treated and control groups was reported (Tucker & Orton, 1995).

3.1.2 Rat

A group of 15 male Fischer 344 rats, weighing 84–100 g [age not specified], was given 0.5% (v/w) clofibrate [purity not specified; equivalent to about 250 mg/kg bw per day] in the diet for up to 28 months. A group of 15 untreated males served as controls. Of the treated animals, one rat was killed at 13 months and three more between 17 and 21 months. The remaining 11 rats were killed between 24 and 28 months. One or more hepatocellular carcinoma developed in 10/11 rats compared with 0/14 controls which survived to 28 months ($p < 0.001$); five of the animals with hepatocellular carcinomas showed pulmonary metastases. In addition, among the treated animals, pancreatic exocrine acinar carcinomas were found in 2/11 rats, whereas none was found in controls (Reddy & Qureshi, 1979). [The Working Group noted the small number of animals.]

A group of 25 male weanling Fischer 344 rats, weighing approximately 100 g, was fed 5000 mg/kg diet (ppm) clofibrate [purity not specified] in the diet for 72 (when the first tumour appeared)–97 weeks (total intake, 25–33 g/rat). A group of 25 untreated males served as controls. The study was terminated at 129 weeks, when all surviving animals were killed. Among the treated rats, malignant tumours developed at various sites. Hepatocellular carcinomas were found in 4/25 treated rats; among the other tumours observed in treated rats were a pancreatic exocrine acinar carcinoma in one rat and pancreatic exocrine acinar adenomas in three rats. Treated and control rats developed similar numbers of leukaemias and tumours of the testis (Svoboda & Azarnoff, 1979).

Groups of 70 (control) and 74 (continuous treatment) male Sprague-Dawley rats, seven weeks of age, were given 0 or 400 mg/kg bw clofibrate [purity not specified] daily in the diet for up to 113 weeks. A third group of 28 (recovery group) male Sprague-Dawley rats was given 400 mg/kg bw clofibrate in the diet for 42–95 weeks and then held for a further 16–18 weeks before killing. Three to five rats in each group were sacrificed at 4–10-week intervals beginning at week 4 and ending at week 113, when zero to five animals remained per group. Only the liver and abnormal organs were examined histologically. Hyperplastic (neoplastic) nodules did not occur before week 68 of treatment. In rats treated for 68 weeks or longer, the incidence of hyperplastic (neoplastic) nodules was: controls, 0/36; continuous treatment, 19/36; and recovery group, 1/16. The only hepatocellular carcinomas found were in two rats in the continuous treatment group at week 95 (Greaves et al., 1986).

3.1.3 Marmoset

In a study reported as a summary in a monograph, groups of 11–16 male and 11–16 female marmosets were given clofibrate [purity not specified] in water containing 0.5% w/w polysorbate 80 by gastric instillation at intended dose levels of 100, 150, 250 and 300 mg/kg bw per day. Effective doses were 94, 157, 213 and 263 mg/kg bw per day. Groups of 20 males and 20 females were untreated or treated with the vehicle only. The study was terminated after 6.5 years due to premature deaths. Necropsy was performed and all major organs were examined histologically. Causes of death varied and were not related to clofibrate treatment. There was no effect on liver weight in any of the clofibrate-treated groups. A statistically significant ($p < 0.01$) increase in kidney weight was seen in the higher-dose groups. There were no histological changes in the liver that could be attributed to clofibrate. No liver tumour or other treatment-related tumour was found in clofibrate-treated marmosets (Tucker & Orton, 1995).

3.2 Administration with known carcinogens

3.2.1 Mouse

Groups of 7–20 male C3H/Hen, C57Bl/6N and BALB/cA mice, six weeks of age, were subjected to partial hepatectomy. After 24 h, mice were given 20 mg/kg bw *N*-nitrosodiethylamine (NDEA) by intraperitoneal injection. Six hours later, they were given basal diet or a diet containing 1000 mg/kg diet (ppm) clofibrate [purity not specified] until week 20, at which time the experiment was terminated and all surviving animals were killed. Livers were analysed for the number and size distribution of glucose-6-phosphatase-deficient enzyme-altered islands by a stereological method (for statistical comparisons, Welch's test was used). NDEA alone induced many more and larger enzyme-altered islands in C3H mice than in the other two strains. In C3H mice, administration of clofibrate in addition to NDEA increased the number and volume of enzyme-altered islands. In the other two strains, clofibrate had no enhancing effect (Lee et al., 1989). [The Working Group noted the absence of a group given clofibrate alone.]

3.2.2 Rat

Groups of 30 male Fischer rats weighing 135–150 g [age not specified] were given 100 mg/L (ppm) NDEA in the drinking-water for two weeks. One week later the rats were fed 0 or 5000 mg/kg diet (ppm) clofibrate [purity not specified] in the diet for 48 weeks, at which time the experiment was terminated. Clofibrate significantly ($p < 0.001$) enhanced the development of liver tumours in rats previously exposed to NDEA: 25/28 rats given NDEA plus clofibrate had liver-cell tumours [type not specified] versus 5/18 (three hepatocellular carcinomas) in the group given NDEA alone (Reddy & Rao, 1978). [The Working Group noted the absence of a group given clofibrate alone.]

A group of 54 female rats [strain and age not specified] was treated twice with 50 mg/kg bw N-methyl-N-nitrosourea (MNU) in citrate buffer (pH 6.0) intravenously at one-week intervals. Twenty-six treated rats were given 20.8 mg/day clofibrate in milk [route and volume not specified] on five days per week for one year. The remaining 28 animals received milk only. One year after the first injection of MNU, all animals were killed. Complete necropsy and histological examination were performed. The authors reported that clofibrate had no effect on the incidence of tumours induced by MNU (Anisimov et al., 1981).

A group of 68 female rats [strain and age not specified] was treated intravenously with 1.5 mg 7,12-dimethylbenz[a]anthracene (DMBA) in water/lipid emulsion three times at one-week intervals. Thirty-six rats were then given 20.8 mg/day per rat clofibrate in milk [route and volume not specified] five days per week for one year at which time the experiment was terminated. The remaining 32 DMBA-treated animals were given milk only. One year after the first DMBA injection, animals were killed and complete necropsy and histological examination were performed. There was a decreased incidence (1.8 times lower) and a decreased multiplicity of mammary adenocarcinoma in clofibrate-treated animals compared with the animals treated with DMBA alone (1.21 versus 1.77, respectively). There was no difference in the incidence of other tumour types between the two groups (Anisimov et al., 1981).

Three groups of 13–17 male rats [strain and age not specified], weighing 200–220 g, were given 14 mg/kg bw dimethylhydrazine dihydrochloride (DMH) weekly by subcutaneous injection for 20 weeks. Two of these groups were given 25 mg/animal clofibrate [purity not specified] by gastric instillation on five days per week either beginning 10 days before or concomitantly with DMH treatment, and the third group was given water. All rats were killed 25 weeks after the start of DMH treatment. The incidence of intestinal tumours was 100% in all three groups. There was no difference in the number of intestinal tumours per animal. The mean volume of intestinal tumours was significantly smaller in groups treated with DMH and clofibrate compared with the group treated with DMH alone ($p < 0.05$, Student's t test). The percentage of tumours without invasion was considerably higher in animals that began clofibrate treatment before DMH treatment than in those only treated concomitantly or given no clofibrate (Berstein et al., 1982). [The Working Group noted that the strong carcinogenic effect of DMH in all groups may have precluded the detection of modulating effects.]

Groups of 15–25 male Fischer 344 rats, weighing 80–90 g [age not specified], were given 40 mg/L (ppm) NDEA in the drinking-water for five weeks (total dose, 32 mg/rat). One week later, the rats were given 0, 1000, 2500, 5000 or 10 000 mg/kg diet (ppm) clofibrate [purity not specified] in the diet for 19 weeks. At the end of clofibrate treatment, all surviving animals were killed. Body-weight gain was depressed, especially in the two highest-dose groups. Livers were fixed and sliced at 2 mm intervals and tumours larger than 1 mm in diameter were counted visually. At the lower-dose levels, clofibrate significantly increased the multiplicity of liver tumours initiated by NDEA: 12.5 ± 5.7 (0% clofibrate, 20/20 survivors), 22.2 ± 15.1 ($p < 0.025$, Student's t test) (1000 ppm clofibrate, 13/15 survivors) and 19.1 ± 8.3 ($p < 0.005$) (2500 ppm clofibrate, 23/25 survivors); 5000 ppm clofibrate had no effect (12.0 ± 4.6, 11/15 survivors) and 10 000 ppm clofibrate significantly decreased ($p < 0.05$) the multiplicity of liver tumours (7.8 ± 5.3, 17/20 survivors) (Mochizuki et al., 1982). [The Working Group noted the absence of a group given clofibrate alone and that the counting technique used is susceptible to multiple counting of large lesions.]

Three groups of 10 male Fischer 344 rats, weighing 90–100 g [age not specified], were concomitantly given 40 mg/L (ppm) NDEA in the drinking-water and fed 0, 1000 or 2500 mg/kg diet (ppm) clofibrate [purity not specified] for five weeks. The total intake of NDEA was 31, 26.5 and 25.9 mg/rat, respectively, in the three groups. All rats survived and were killed 25 weeks after the start of the experiment. Livers were fixed and sliced at 2 mm intervals and tumours larger than 1 mm in diameter were counted visually. Clofibrate significantly increased the multiplicity of liver tumours initiated by NDEA: 12.4 ± 5.4 (0% clofibrate), 25.3 ± 14.1 ($p < 0.025$, Student's t test) (1000 ppm clofibrate) and 22.6 ± 8.7 ($p < 0.01$) (2500 ppm clofibrate) (Mochizuki et al., 1983). [The Working Group noted the absence of a group given clofibrate alone and that the counting technique used is susceptible to multiple counting of large lesions.]

Two groups of 15 male Fischer 344 rats, eight weeks of age, were given basal diet containing 200 mg/kg diet (ppm) 2-acetylaminofluorene (2-AAF) for eight weeks, then maintained on basal diet for a further two weeks, after which the animals received 730 mg/kg diet (ppm) clofibrate [purity not specified] for 24 weeks or the basal diet. Another two groups of 9 or 12 rats were given basal diet without 2-AAF for 10 weeks and then given 730 ppm clofibrate in the diet for 24 weeks or the basal diet. Some animals from each group were killed at six weeks after the start of clofibrate treatment and the remainder were killed after 24 weeks of clofibrate treatment. The livers were analysed for altered foci and neoplasms. Clofibrate slightly enhanced the incidence of 2-AAF-induced foci at week 34. The incidence of foci/cm^2 was 5.4 ± 1.5 in animals given 2-AAF and clofibrate and 4.3 ± 2.2 in those given 2-AAF only. No significant increase in the incidence of liver neoplasms (nodules) was observed in the clofibrate-treated group (2/9 versus 0/9 in controls) (Numoto et al., 1984)

Groups of 20 male Fischer 344 rats, five weeks of age, were given 0 or 500 mg/kg diet (ppm) N-nitrosoethylhydroxyethylamine in the diet for two weeks, followed by 3500 mg/kg diet (ppm) clofibrate [purity not specified] in the diet for 24 weeks. All animals survived to the end of the experiment at week 27 when they were killed. Clofibrate did not increase the incidence or multiplicity of renal tubular-cell adenomas and adenocarcinomas (Kurokawa et al., 1988).

Groups of 60–70 male Fischer 344 rats, four weeks of age, were given 0 or 200 mg/kg bw NDEA as a single intraperitoneal injection in physiological saline. Two weeks later, the animals were fed diets containing 0 or 3000 mg/kg diet (ppm) clofibrate [purity not specified] for up to 64 weeks. All animals were subjected to partial hepatectomy at week 3. At weeks 8, 20, 32, 49 and 64, 7–22 rats were killed from the various groups. Clofibrate alone did not induce hepatocellular carcinomas and only a few, small preneoplastic foci were observed at the end of the study. However, in animals treated with NDEA, clofibrate increased the total number of glutathione S-transferase placental form (GST-P)-positive and -negative preneoplastic lesions from week 32 onward ($p < 0.05$, Student's t test) and the incidence of hepatocellular carcinomas: 12/26 (NDEA plus 3000 ppm clofibrate) versus 4/17 (NDEA alone) (Hosokawa et al., 1989).

Groups of 15 male Fischer 344 rats, six weeks of age, were given 0 or 500 mg/L (ppm) N-nitrosobutyl(4-hydroxybutyl)amine (NBHBA) in the drinking-water for four weeks. Subsequently, rats were given 2500, 5000 or 10 000 mg/kg diet (ppm) clofibrate [purity not specified] in the diet for four weeks, followed by a three-week interval during which they were fed 30 000 mg/kg (ppm) uracil in the diet. The clofibrate treatment was then resumed for a further nine weeks. A further group of animals treated with NBHBA and uracil only served as controls. The experiment was terminated at 20 weeks. The incidence of urinary bladder hyperplasias and papillomas in control animals (NBHBA only) and in animals treated with NBHBA and clofibrate was similar. The density of hyperplasias (number of lesions/10 cm basement membrane) was significantly increased ($p < 0.01$, Student's t test) in all clofibrate-treated groups (Hagiwara et al., 1990).

Groups of male Fischer 344 rats [exact numbers not specified], seven weeks of age, were given 0 or 3000 mg/kg diet (ppm) clofibrate [purity not specified] in the diet for 30 weeks, followed by a basal diet or a diet containing 100 ppm 2-AAF for up to 78 weeks. Three weeks after the start of the experiment, partial hepatectomy was performed on all animals. Five rats fed clofibrate were killed at week 30 and three to seven rats from each group were killed at week 48; all surviving animals were killed at 78 weeks. The authors reported that clofibrate inhibited the development of GST-P-positive focal lesions and hepatocellular carcinomas induced by subsequent feeding of 2-AAF (Mutai et al., 1990). [The Working Group noted the unusual design.]

Groups of 13–14 male Nagase analbuminaemic and 13–14 Sprague-Dawley rats, seven weeks of age, were given 200 mg/kg bw NDEA as a single intraperitoneal injection. Two weeks later, the rats were given 0 or 10 000 mg/kg diet (ppm) clofibrate [purity not specified] in the diet for six weeks. Four Nagase analbuminaemic and five

Sprague-Dawley rats were given the diet containing clofibrate without prior treatment with NDEA. Three weeks after the start of the experiment, partial hepatectomy was performed on all animals. The rats were killed at week 8. No GST-P-positive foci were found in the animals fed clofibrate without prior treatment with NDEA. NDEA alone induced significantly more and larger GST-P-positive foci in Nagase analbuminaemic rats than in Sprague-Dawley rats ($p < 0.001$, Student's t test). Clofibrate significantly decreased the number of GST-P-positive foci induced by NDEA in both strains ($p < 0.002$) (de Camargo *et al.*, 1993). [The Working Group noted that some studies suggest that peroxisome proliferators inhibit the histochemical detection of foci.]

Groups of 7–10 male Fischer 344 rats, 12 weeks of age, were given 150 mg/kg bw NDEA as a single intraperitoneal injection or were given 200 mg/kg diet (ppm) 2-AAF in the diet for eight weeks or were untreated. Two weeks later, rats were fed 1000 mg/kg diet (ppm) clofibrate [purity not specified] in the diet for up to 37 weeks or received no further treatment. Clofibrate increased the incidence of hepatocellular adenomas following treatment with NDEA (4/8 versus 0/8; $p < 0.05$, Fisher's exact test), but not after treatment with 2-AAF (Cattley *et al.*, 1994).

Groups of four male Sprague-Dawley rats, seven weeks of age, were given 200 mg/kg bw NDEA as a single intraperitoneal injection. After two weeks on basal diet, they were given 200 mg/kg diet (ppm) 2-AAF in the diet for two weeks and were subjected to partial hepatectomy at week 3. Subsequently, two groups of animals were given 3000 mg/kg diet (ppm) clofibrate [purity not specified] for two or four weeks. Another two groups were given basal diet for either two or four weeks. The numbers and areas of GST-P-positive foci of diameter greater than 0.2 mm were measured. Administration of clofibrate for two or four weeks significantly reduced the number and areas of GST-P-positive foci (Yokoyama *et al.*, 1993). [The Working Group noted that some studies have suggested that peroxisome proliferators inhibit the histochemical detection of foci.]

3.2.3 *Hamster*

Groups of 16–22 male Syrian golden hamsters, six weeks of age, were given 500 mg/kg bw *N*-nitrosobis(2-hydroxypropyl)amine (NBHPA) or 0.9% NaCl by subcutaneous injection weekly for five weeks, after which they were given 0, 2500 or 5000 mg/kg diet (ppm) clofibrate [purity not specified] in the diet for 30 weeks, at which time the experiment was terminated. Clofibrate significantly ($p < 0.001$) increased the multiplicity of hepatocellular lesions (including hyperplastic nodules and hepatocellular carcinomas) as measured by the number of lesions/cm^2 in histological sections: 0.5 ± 0.3 (NBHPA alone, 17 hamsters), 1.4 ± 0.5 (NBHPA plus 2500 ppm clofibrate, 16 hamsters) and 1.0 ± 0.3 (NBHPA plus 5000 ppm clofibrate, 17 hamsters). In contrast, 5000 ppm clofibrate significantly ($p < 0.05$) inhibited the development of pancreatic adenocarcinomas and lung neoplasms induced by NBHPA (Mizumoto *et al.*, 1988).

4. Other Data Relevant to an Evaluation of Carcinogenicity and its Mechanisms

4.1 Absorption, distribution, metabolism, and excretion

4.1.1 Humans

Absorption of clofibrate is typically monitored as circulating clofibric acid (2-(4-chlorophenoxy)isobutyric acid), since the ethyl ester is rapidly hydrolysed by tissue and serum esterases, both *in vivo* and *in vitro*, to the acid (Thorp, 1962). Gugler and Hartlapp (1978) evaluated plasma levels of clofibric acid following single and repeated doses of clofibrate in human volunteers (four men and one woman). Single oral doses of 500–2000 mg [7–28 mg/kg bw est.] resulted in mean peak plasma concentrations of 53–151 µg/mL, that were observed 4–6 h after dosing. At doses of 1000 mg [14 mg/kg bw est.] given twice daily for eight days, peak plasma concentrations of clofibric acid ranged between 200 and 240 µg/mL on the last day. Elimination appeared to be similar for a single dose and for multiple dosing regimens, with mean half-lives of 15–18 h following single doses of 500–2000 mg and 1000 mg twice daily for eight days. Similar plasma levels of clofibric acid were observed in seven male volunteers receiving a single oral administration of 1.3 g [19 mg/kg bw est.] clofibrate (Harvengt & Desager, 1976) and in four men and six women after single oral dosing of 500 mg [7 mg/kg bw est.] clofibrate (Männistö *et al.*, 1975). Cayen *et al.* (1977) reported protein binding levels of 98.5% and 96.8% at serum concentrations of 10 and 100 µg/mL clofibric acid, respectively.

Clofibric acid can undergo conjugation with glucuronic acid in man (Thorp, 1962). The metabolism and elimination of clofibrate and clofibric acid in three and five male subjects, respectively, were described by Emudianughe *et al.* (1983). Elimination was mainly via the urine, with 48-h recoveries of 56% (clofibrate, 565 mg oral dose) [8 mg/kg bw est.] and 80% (clofibric acid, 500 mg oral dose) [7 mg/kg bw est.]. The principal urinary metabolite was clofibryl glucuronide, with only approximately 2% of the dose excreted as clofibric acid. In four male and one female subjects, the total plasma clearance of clofibric acid was greater (6.8 mL/min) following a single oral dose of 2000 mg [29 mg/kg bw est.] than following a single oral dose of 500 mg [7 mg/kg bw est.] (5.6 mL/min) (Gugler & Hartlapp, 1978). The more rapid elimination following the higher dose of clofibrate was attributed to reduced plasma protein binding at higher plasma concentrations (see Figure 1).

4.1.2 Experimental systems

The absorption and distribution of orally administered clofibrate in rats appear to be similar to those in humans. Cayen *et al.* (1977) studied the serum levels of radioactivity in male albino Charles River rats given a single oral dose of 0.3 mmol/kg [73 mg/kg] bw [^{14}C]clofibrate or 0.3 mmol/kg [64 mg/kg] bw [^{14}C]clofibric acid. Peak serum concentrations of clofibric acid equivalents between 500 and 1000 nmol/mL (approximately 100–200 µg/mL) were similar to those in humans following single oral doses of

Figure 1. Postulated metabolic pathways of clofibrate

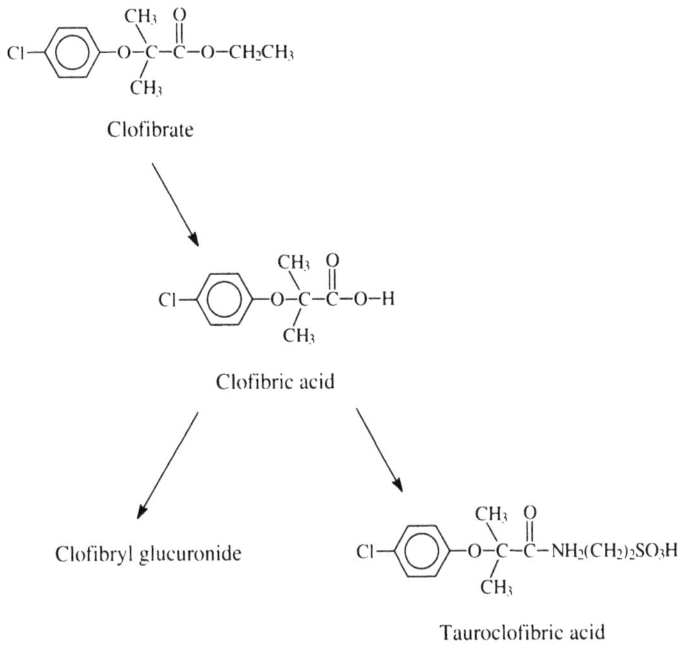

Clofibrate

Clofibric acid

Clofibryl glucuronide

Tauroclofibric acid

From Emudianughe et al. (1983)
Clofibryl glucuronide is the only conjugated form observed in rat, guinea pig, rabbit and man. In the dog and ferret, tauroclofibric acid is also formed, which in cat, was the only conjugate excreted.

clofibrate. Analysis of serum in rats given oral doses of [^{14}C]clofibrate indicated that over 90% of the drug was in the form of unconjugated clofibric acid, consistent with results after oral administration to humans. Groups of five male and five female rats aged three weeks and similar groups aged eight weeks were given 100 or 250 mg/kg bw clofibrate per day by gastric instillation for 16 days (Tucker & Orton, 1995). Blood concentrations of clofibric acid 4 h after the final dose (Table 1) were higher in the older rats than in the weanlings, possibly because of differences in esterase activity. The lack of an intravenous formulation of clofibrate precludes total plasma clearance determinations.

Table 1. Blood clofibric acid (μg/mL) concentrations in rats after clofibrate administration

Dose (mg/kg)	Three-week-old rats		Eight-week-old rats	
	Male	Female	Male	Female
100	158 ± 41	98 ± 56	328 ± 42	279 ± 81
250	301 ± 55	170 ± 96	509 ± 110	336 ± 29

From Tucker & Orton, 1995

Following a single intraperitoneal injection to rats of 113 mg/kg bw [^{14}C]clofibrate, 85% of the ^{14}C dose was recovered in the urine within 24 h of administration (70% as clofibryl glucuronide and 15% as clofibric acid) (Emudianughe *et al.*, 1983). In comparison with the same authors' study in humans, a higher dose rate on a mg/kg basis was administered to rats and a different route of administration used. A higher percentage of the dose appeared as unconjugated clofibric acid in the urine of rats than that seen with humans. Odum and Orton (1983) measured hepatic microsomal glucuronyl transferase activity towards clofibric acid in male Alderley Park strain rats, noting an increase in enzyme activity associated with postnatal maturation. Feeding rats with 4000 mg/kg diet (ppm) clofibrate for 14 days did not appear to increase the activity of glucuronyl transferase towards clofibric acid. Bronfman *et al.* (1986) characterized the activity of microsomal fractions from male Sprague-Dawley rats with respect to formation of coenzyme A (CoA) thioesters of clofibric acid *in vitro*. It has been speculated that formation of CoA thioesters of clofibric acid *in vivo* may mediate the pharmacological or toxic effects of clofibrate (Tomaszewski & Melnick, 1994).

Baldwin *et al.* (1980) measured the distribution of ^{14}C following administration of 0.4 mmol/kg bw [^{14}C]clofibrate [97 mg/kg] given either as a single intragastric or intraperitoneal dose (acute) or twice daily for 14 days (chronic) in rats. The units reported were 10^{-5} mmol clofibric acid equivalents per gram of tissue (CFE). Twelve hours after the last dose, levels of radioactivity were similar in liver (6 CFE) and a variety of other tissues for both dosing regimens. Notable exceptions were blood (14 CFE acute versus 7 CFE chronic) and epididymal fat (3 CFE acute versus 11 CFE chronic).

Differences in rates of elimination between humans and rats for clofibric acid have been observed. Baldwin *et al.* (1980) calculated a half-life of 4.1 h in rats, based on elimination of ^{14}C-labelled clofibrate in male Harlan Sprague-Dawley rats given a single dose of 97 mg/kg bw by the intraperitoneal or oral route. The authors attributed the higher elimination rate in rats to the differences in serum protein binding reported by Cayen *et al.* (1977) who found that at concentrations of 10 and 100 µg/mL clofibric acid, the proportions of protein binding in rat serum were 87.2% and 75.4%, respectively, lower than that reported for human serum (see Section 4.1.1).

4.2 Toxic effects

Because clofibrate is readily metabolized to clofibric acid in humans and animals, the toxic effects of clofibric acid are summarized together with those of clofibrate in this section.

4.2.1 *Humans*

Several studies have documented the pharmacological reduction in plasma levels of serum triglycerides and cholesterol in humans treated with clofibrate. Larsen *et al.* (1994) reported the effects of oral clofibrate in 12 human patients with hyperlipoproteinaemia type III treated with clofibrate for eight weeks [1 mg/kg bw est.]. Reductions in circulating total cholesterol (approx. 40%), in VLDL cholesterol (approx. 60%) and triglycerides (approx. 50%) were observed, as was an increase in circulating high-density lipoprotein cholesterol (approx. 9%). The mechanism of this pharmacological effect is unclear.

Various adverse effects have been attributed to the administration of clofibrate. The most common is cholelithiasis. Bateson *et al.* (1978) found a strong association between clofibrate therapy and gallstones in patients with hyperlipidaemia (the prevalence of gallbladder disease was about four times that expected, $p < 0.001$). This effect was associated with the elevated cholesterol concentration of the bile in the clofibrate-treated patients. [The route of exposure was probably oral, but the dose levels and duration of administration were not specified.]

An association of clofibrate therapy with skeletal myopathy has been described in several case reports, summarized in reviews by Rush *et al.* (1986) and London *et al.* (1991). Exposures ranged from 750 to 4000 mg [11–57 mg/kg bw est.] per day and duration of treatment from 3 to 730 days (mean, 56 days). Clofibrate-associated myopathy was characterized by muscle pain, elevated levels of leakage enzymes such as creatine phosphokinase, aspartate aminotransferase and lactate dehydrogenase, and muscle weakness. In some cases, cardiac myopathy accompanied the effect on skeletal muscle (McGarvey, 1973; Smals *et al.*, 1977; Scionti *et al.*, 1984). Single cases of association between clofibrate treatment and eosinophilic pneumonia (Hendrickson & Simpson, 1982), erythema multiforme (Murata *et al.*, 1988) and interstitial nephritis (Cumming, 1980) have been reported.

Because of effects noted in rodents, the effects of clofibrate and clofibric acid on human hepatocytes have been studied following in-vivo and in-vitro exposures. Schwandt *et al.* (1978) studied liver biopsies from 40 patients before and after administration of clofibrate (1.5 g/day in 27 patients and 0.5 g/day in 13 patients). A tendency to decreased fatty infiltration was the only effect noted by light microscopy. Hanefeld *et al.* (1980) also described a regression of fatty infiltration after 3–5 months of clofibrate treatment (2 g/day) [29 mg/kg bw est.]. Ultrastructural evaluation revealed an increase in smooth endoplasmic reticulum as well as increased inner membranes of mitochondria. Selective alterations in microbodies (peroxisomes) were not observed. The effect of longer-term treatment (six months to seven years) with clofibrate elicited similar but more marked ultrastructural alterations, with an increase in microbodies (peroxisomes), although peroxisomal ultrastructural effects were not quantified. A second study (Hanefeld *et al.*, 1983) compared biopsies before and during clofibrate therapy (2 g/day for 3–94 months) [29 mg/kg bw est.]. Volume density and numbers of mitochondria both increased by approximately 30%. The numerical density of peroxisomes (a stereological estimation) was increased by approximately 50%, but there was no statistically significant increase in the volume density of peroxisomes (a direct measurement).

4.2.2 Experimental systems

Many of the pharmacological effects of clofibrate observed in experimental animals are qualitatively similar to those observed in humans. Reductions in serum cholesterol and/or triglyceride levels in rats treated with clofibrate have been reported from several studies (Anthony *et al.*, 1978; Barnard *et al.*, 1980; Watanabe *et al.*, 1987). In the study described in Section 4.1.1 (Tucker & Orton, 1995), in which weanling and mature rats were dosed by gastric instillation with clofibrate, this effect was not statistically significant and measurements other than those of alkaline phosphatase (increase) were not reported. A dose-dependent increase in liver weights and, at the high dose, a loss of glycogen from hepatocytes and hypertrophy and eosinophilia of centrilobular cells were observed.

Hepatic effects of clofibrate treatment in experimental animals include peroxisome proliferation, which is characterized by increases in numbers of hepatocellular peroxisomes and levels of peroxisomal enzymes, and hepatocellular hyperplasia. In one study, male and female Sprague-Dawley rats were given 1500–9000 mg/kg diet (ppm) clofibrate in the diet [90–540 mg/kg bw est.] for up to 13 weeks. Increases in peroxisomal fatty acyl CoA oxidase activity were observed after one week (at all doses in males and at the highest dose in females) and after 13 weeks (at 4500 or 9000 ppm doses in males and females). Increases in relative liver weights and peroxisomal volume densities (measured only after 13 weeks) were observed at similar levels of exposure. In the male rats ingesting 9000 ppm clofibrate for 13 weeks, both peroxisomal fatty acyl CoA oxidase activities and peroxisomal volume densities were increased approximately seven-fold. Hepatocyte nuclear bromodeoxyuridine-labelling indices, an indirect measure of cell replication, were increased at one week of exposure, but decreased at 13 weeks of exposure. These effects of clofibrate did not produce any increase in circulating alanine aminotransferase or aspartate aminotransferase activities, which are markers of hepatocellular injury (Tanaka *et al.*, 1992). Similar effects on liver weights, peroxisomal enzymes and/or cell replication have been reported for male Wistar rats (Price *et al.*, 1986) given clofibrate, as well as male Fischer 344 rats (Eacho *et al.*, 1991; Marsman *et al.*, 1992) and male Sprague-Dawley rats (Barrass *et al.*, 1993) given clofibric acid. Statistically significant increases in peroxisomal β-oxidation and/or lauroyl CoA oxidase activities were observed in male C57Bl/6, ATL/OLA, C3H/He, BALB/c and A/J strain mice but not in male C57Bl/10 or CBA/Ca mice given 5000 ppm clofibrate [625 mg/kg bw est.] in the diet for 10 days. However, peroxisomal catalase activity and relative liver weights were increased in all of the strains examined (Lundgren & DePierre, 1989). In NMRI mice treated similarly for up to 25 days, increased relative liver weights and increased cytoplasmic volume density of peroxisomes were measured (Meijer *et al.*, 1991).

Accumulation of lipofuscin pigment was observed to increase markedly over the duration of exposure in male Fischer 344 rats given 5000 mg/kg diet (ppm) clofibric acid in the diet [300 mg/kg bw est.] for up to 22 weeks (Marsman *et al.*, 1992). In male Sprague-Dawley rats given approximately 500 mg/kg bw clofibrate in the diet for 22 days, increases in hepatic lipofuscin (three to four times control levels) were completely prevented by simultaneous feeding with vitamin E, although no effect on peroxisomal β-oxidation activity was observed (Stanko *et al.*, 1995). However, in male Wistar and Fischer 344 rats given 2500 mg/kg diet (ppm) clofibrate [150 mg/kg bw est.] for 78–79 weeks, only minimal changes in hepatic hydrogen peroxide concentration were observed (Tamura *et al.*, 1990a,b). A slight (two- to three-fold) increase was observed in levels of 8-hydroxydeoxyguanosine, a marker of oxidative DNA damage, in hepatic DNA of male

Fischer 344 rats fed 5000 ppm clofibric acid for 22 weeks in the diet (Cattley & Glover, 1993). Similar feeding with clofibrate gave rise to a two-fold increase in levels of this adduct, compared with controls, after one month. Levels were also slightly elevated at 2, 3, 6, 9 and 12 months, but the increases were statistically significant ($p < 0.05$) only at 2 and 12 months (Takagi et al., 1990). Peroxisomal hydrogen peroxide may injure cellular constituents via the production of hydroxyl radical, as demonstrated in liver fractions prepared from male Alpk/Ap (Wistar-derived) rats given 200 mg/kg bw clofibrate daily by gastric instillation for nine days (Elliott et al., 1986).

The induction of peroxisome proliferation appears to be a direct result of the action of clofibric acid on hepatocytes. Incubation of primary cultures of rat hepatocytes with clofibric acid (50–250 µM) for up to 72 h resulted in an up to six-fold increase in the induction of peroxisomal β-oxidation (Foxworthy & Eacho, 1986). This response is probably mediated by the peroxisome proliferator-activated receptor α (PPARα), a member of the nuclear steroid hormone receptor superfamily. In the presence of clofibric acid, PPARα and retinoic acid-X-receptor α form a heterodimer which binds to the response elements located in the promoter region of several peroxisomal genes, such as that of the rat acyl CoA oxidase gene, and facilitate transcriptional activity (Issemann et al., 1993). The critical role of PPARα in mediating responses to clofibrate has been demonstrated with knockout mice (derived from Sv/129 strain embryonic stem cells) that do not express the receptor (Lee et al., 1995). These mPPARα$^{-/-}$ mice (F2 homozygotes; hybrids of Sv/129×C57Bl/6N), when given 5000 mg/kg diet (ppm) clofibrate in the diet for two weeks [625 mg/kg bw est.], failed to show the increases in liver weight, in peroxisome and in mRNA levels for peroxisomal enzymes, including acyl CoA oxidase, that are seen with wild-type mice.

Because of the difficulty in conducting repeat biopsy studies of hepatic responses in human patients, investigators have studied the response to clofibrate in primary human hepatocytes and in human hepatoma cell lines. Treatment of primary cultures of human hepatocytes with clofibric acid at concentrations of 1–1000 µM for up to 72 h did not induce peroxisomal β-oxidation activity or increase numbers of peroxisomes (Blaauboer et al., 1990). Another marker enzyme of peroxisome proliferation, carnitine acetyltransferase, was not induced in human primary hepatocyte cultures exposed to 500 µM clofibric acid for 48 h (Butterworth et al., 1989). The lack of response in these primary human hepatocyte cultures contrasts with results obtained with human hepatoma cell lines. Treatment of human hepatoma (Hep) EBNA2 cells with 100–1000 µM clofibrate for up to five days resulted in increased peroxisomal acyl CoA oxidase activity and acyl CoA oxidase mRNA content (Scotto et al., 1995). Treatment of human HepG2 cells with 250–1000 µM clofibric acid for two days increased the activities of peroxisomal palmitoyl CoA oxidase and catalase (Chance et al., 1995). The significance of these results is unclear because of the low magnitude of the response ($\leq$ 3-fold) seen and uncertainty about how well these cells model potential responses in human tissues.

The central role of PPARα in mediating the hepatic effects of fibrate drugs in rodents indicated that characterization of human PPARα could be important for the extrapolation of effects in rodents to humans. Tugwood et al. (1996) found generally low (but variable) expression of PPARα mRNA in 10 human liver samples compared with rodent liver samples. They characterized the function of human PPARα cDNA clones isolated from two livers. One had a deleted segment leading to a C-terminal truncation of the receptor; the other had non-conservative codon substitutions at amino acid positions 71 and 123. Both clones failed to activate transcription under conditions in which the mouse wild-type PPARα clone is active, indicating a non-functional human receptor. Thus, the insensitivity of human liver to the adaptive effects of peroxisome proliferators may be attributable to low expression of PPARα and/or genetic variations in the PPARα gene that result in lack of response to peroxisome proliferators.

Comparison of laboratory animal species suggests that sensitivity to induction of peroxisome proliferation is species-dependent. The hepatic effects of 300–350 mg/kg bw clofibrate administered orally for two weeks to male marmosets ($n = 12$), C57Bl/10J mice ($n = 3$) and AP rats ($n = 3$) were reported briefly (Tucker & Orton, 1995). For the mice, the replicate was the pooled livers from five mice per cage. Serum concentrations of clofibric acid were: marmoset, 117 ± 34 μg/mL at 4 h after the final dose; mice, undetectable at autopsy (between 10 h and 12 h); rats, 268 ± 35 μg/mL at autopsy (between 10 h and 12 h). The limit of detection of clofibric acid was 30 μg/mL. The failure to detect clofibric acid in mice may be a function of the time of last consumption of medicated diet and the short half-life (< 4 h) of the compound in this species. The results of the liver analyses are presented in Table 2. No effect upon any of the parameters was observed in marmosets. Liver weight was increased in comparison with concurrent controls by 18% in mice and 54% in rats. The parameters indicative of microsomal oxidase activity and, especially, peroxisomal activity were clearly more strongly affected in rats than in mice. Palmitoyl CoA reduction activity was increased 27.5-fold in rats and 3.9-fold in mice.

A long-term study in marmosets also suggests the relative insensitivity to the hepatic effects of clofibrate of this primate species compared with rodents. Groups of male and female marmosets (*Callithrix jacchus*) were given clofibrate by gastric instillation for up to 343 weeks at doses of 0 (undosed), 0 (vehicle), 94, 157, 213 and 263 mg/kg bw per day (Tucker & Orton, 1995). Initially, there were 20 marmosets of each sex in each control group and 10 of each sex in each dose group. A substantial number of premature deaths occurred. The numbers of survivors at week 343 (sexes combined and controls combined) in each of the groups were 61, 14, 14, 9 and 8. Causes of death were unrelated to clofibrate treatment. Because of the premature deaths, the numbers were supplemented at weeks 30 and 143. An increase in kidney weight was observed in the higher-dose groups, but no corresponding change in renal histopathology to account for this observation. No change in relative liver weight was observed and no histological change in any tissue was attributable to treatment. In particular, there was no evidence of changes in the levels of hepatic peroxisomes (by transmission electron microscopy) on three animals per sex in control and highest-dose groups. [Methods used for the evaluation of this end-point were not described.] Hepatic iron deposits of unknown etiology were observed in all marmosets.

In rodents, modulation of enzyme activities by clofibrate is not limited to peroxisomes, but may also extend to mitochondrial, cytosolic and endoplasmic reticulum enzymes within the cell. For example, clofibrate increases the hepatic expression of an

Table 2. Interspecies comparison of the effect of clofibrate upon parameters of hepatic microsomal and peroxisomal activities

	Marmoset		C57Bl/10J mouse		AP rat	
	Control	Clofibrate	Control	Clofibrate	Control	Clofibrate
Liver weight relative to body weight (%)	4.68 ± 0.41	4.63 ± 0.48	5.91 ± 0.36	6.98 ± 0.54*	4.80 ± 0.50	7.39 ± 0.29***
Cytochrome P450 content (nmol/mg protein)	0.36 ± 0.09	0.41 ± 0.08	0.74 ± 0.14	0.87 ± 0.09	0.37 ± 0.04	0.73 ± 0.02***
Catalase (k.sec/g)	29.5 ± 3.1	36.3 ± 3.1	66.0 ± 16.7	84.3 ± 13.6	76.6 ± 1.3	120.3 ± 2.7**
Palmitoyl coenzyme A oxidase (μmol NAD⁺ reduced/min/mg protein)	0.15 ± 0.03	0.11 ± 0.03	0.34 ± 0.13	1.33 ± 0.23**	0.2 ± 0.0	5.5 ± 0.7***
Crotonyl coenzyme A oxidase (μmol NAD⁺ reduced/min/mg protein)	5.3 ± 0.2	6.0 ± 0.3	15.1 ± 3.4	17.7 ± 3.5	12.1 ± 2.0	28.6 ± 1.2**

From Tucker & Orton (1995)
Results are means ± SD
$*p < 0.05$ $**p < 0.01$ $***p < 0.001$ Student's t test

enzyme of the CYP4A family associated with fatty acid ω-hydroxylase activity. Male Long-Evans rats given 80 mg/kg bw of the enantiomers or racemix mixture of the clofibrate analogue, 2-(4-*para*-chlorophenyloxy)2-phenyl ethanoic acid, by gastric instillation for three consecutive days, had elevated hepatic CYP4A1 and lauric acid 12-hydroxylase activity (Chinje & Gibson, 1990). Clofibrate (730 mg/kg diet (ppm) for 24 weeks) inhibited the expression of γ-glutamyl transpeptidase in liver homogenates of male Fischer 344 rats in which this enzyme activity had been induced by prior feeding of 2-AAF (Numoto et al., 1984).

Some extrahepatic effects of clofibrate in experimental animals are analogous to those observed in the liver. For example, in male but not female Fischer 344 rats given 400 mg/kg bw clofibrate daily by intraperitoneal injection for three consecutive days, increased renal content of CYP4A2 mRNA was observed (Sundseth & Waxman, 1992). Clofibric acid caused an increase in renal peroxisomal palmitoyl CoA oxidase activity in male Wistar rats given 200 mg/kg bw clofibric acid daily by gastric instillation for 10 consecutive days (Chandoga et al., 1994). Administration of 400 mg/kg bw clofibrate per day in the diet to male Wistar rats for 3 months or longer resulted in diminished size of thyroid follicles, with calcium deposition in the colloid and hypertrophy of the Golgi apparatus (Price et al., 1988).

4.3 Reproductive and developmental effects

4.3.1 *Humans*

Schneider and Kaffarnik (1975) reported three cases of male impotence in patients with type IV hyperlipoproteinaemia who were treated with a controlled diet and clofibrate. The complaints of impotence were made within one year of beginning treatment with the drug. Two of the patients reported improvement of the symptoms three and four weeks after interruption of clofibrate therapy; one patient again complained of impotence when clofibrate therapy was resumed.

4.3.2 *Experimental systems*

In a study reported only in abstract, no change in number of resorption sites, litter size, fetal weight or no teratogenic effect was found in rats when dams were given 0.6 mg/kg bw clofibrate per day in feed or 1 or 140 mg/kg bw clofibrate per day by gastric instillation from day 6 to day 20 of gestation (Diener & Hsu, 1966). When doses of 200 mg/kg bw per day were given to both male and female rats by gastric instillation, both before and during gestation, a significant decrease in litter size was observed, and with a dose of 500 mg/kg bw, the number of pregnancies decreased from 7/8 in controls to 0/8 in treated animals. No such effect was found when female rabbits were treated similarly (Pantaleoni & Valeri, 1974). In female albino rats given 50 mg clofibrate per day orally during the entire period of mating, gestation and lactation, the liver weight at birth of the offspring was significantly higher than that of control pups, while there was no difference in birth weight between the groups (Chhabra & Kurup, 1978). The offspring of Wistar rats given 8000 mg/kg diet (ppm) clofibrate in the diet for one week on gestational days 13, 15, 17, 19 or 21 weighed significantly less than the offspring of control rats. Maternal weight gain was reduced in treated animals compared with controls (Cibelli *et al.*, 1988). An abnormal postnatal fetal thrombosis syndrome in rats has been described, consisting of an extension of the normal thrombosis in the umbilical arteries and causing necrosis of the tail or parts of the hindlimbs (Dange *et al.*, 1975). In pregnant Dutch rabbits given 0 or 5000 ppm clofibrate in the diet throughout pregnancy, no effect on fertility or litter size and no skeletal abnormality were detected (Tucker & Orton, 1995). Nishimura and Tanimura (1976) found that the rabbit fetus serum accumulates a higher concentration of clofibrate than maternal serum.

In albino rats, the serum of newborn pups of dams that had received clofibrate (50 mg/day) orally during mating, gestation and lactation contained 93 nmol/mL clofibric acid. This decreased to 48 nmol/mL on day 12 and 31 nmol/mL at the time of weaning. Placenta collected before birth from clofibrate-fed dams contained about 80 nmol/g clofibric acid. This indicates that the drug crosses the placenta. The activity of mitochondrial glycerol phosphate dehydrogenase in hepatic mitochondria isolated from newborn rats of dams that were fed the drug was almost three times the level observed for control offspring. The activity increased and remained at a higher level during lactation but, when the young animals were weaned, it rapidly decreased to about the same level as that seen in control animals. This suggests that the drug may also pass to the offspring via the mother's milk (Chhabra & Kurup, 1978).

Clofibrate (150 mg/kg bw per day) given continuously to female Wistar/H-Riop rats from gestational day 16 to the end of lactation (22nd day post-partum) produced a decrease in birth weight, an increase in perinatal mortality and an increase in liver weight at the age of 22 days. Investigations in which the dam received doses of 150 mg/kg bw per day during four time intervals between gestational day 16 and postnatal day 22 showed that the increase in liver weight was associated with exposure between delivery and postnatal day 15. When the drug was administered in the last week of pregnancy and the young were dissected on postnatal days 1, 8, 15 or 22, increased liver weight was observed in neonates but not subsequently. The authors suggested that this transient increase in liver weight might be related to enzyme induction rather than to hepatotoxicity (Nyitray *et al.*, 1980).

Pregnant Swiss ICR mice were given clofibrate by subcutaneous injections at various dosages (480 and 960 mg/kg bw) and time intervals, and embryos were removed on days 17 or 18 of gestation. In embryos removed on day 17, the level of intestinal catalase activity of the proximal and distal halves did not differ between treated groups and controls. In embryos removed on day 18, a dose-dependent rise in catalase activities in the proximal half of the small intestine in treated groups was observed, but a plateau was attained with repeated injections (Calvert *et al.*, 1979).

Clofibrate treatment of pregnant female rats has been found to increase the number of liver peroxisomes and the levels of fatty acid oxidation enzymes in fetuses, suggesting that the treatment induces fetal peroxisome proliferation (Cibelli *et al.*, 1988; Stefanini *et al.*, 1989). In mice, 400 mg/kg bw oral clofibrate treatment initiated at day 6 of gestation produced a 4–5-fold increase in levels of peroxisomal membrane protein 70, a 1.5-

to 2-fold increase in dihydroxyacetone phosphate acyltransferase specific activity and a 1.2–1.8-fold increase in catalase specific activity in fetal liver of 19 days gestation. Electron microscopy showed amplification of endoplasmic reticulum and peroxisomes in the fetal liver. There was a general increase in peroxisomal proteins between gestational days 13 and 19 in all fetal tissues except the placenta, and the effect of clofibrate in the lung and the placenta was evident by gestational day 13 (Wilson et al. 1991).

4.4 Genetic and related effects

4.4.1 *Humans*

No data were available to the Working Group.

4.4.2 *Experimental systems* (see also Table 3 for references and Appendices 1 and 2)

Clofibrate is not mutagenic in *Salmonella typhimurium* in the presence or absence of microsomal preparations. In the yeast *Saccharomyces cerevisiae*, clofibrate induced neither gene conversion nor mitotic recombination.

In single studies, clofibrate did not induce unscheduled DNA synthesis in cultured hepatocytes or DNA strand breaks in L1210 cells. However, the ability of *N*-ethyl-*N*-nitrosourea to produce single-strand DNA breaks and of *N,N'*-bis(2-chloroethyl)-*N*-nitrosourea to produce both single-strand DNA breaks and interstrand cross-links in L1210 cells was enhanced by prior treatment of the cells with clofibrate (Lawson & Gwilt, 1993).

Clofibrate was not mutagenic in Chinese hamster lung V79 cells, in the presence of a rat hepatocyte metabolic activation system. As reported in an abstract, clofibrate did not induce resistance to 6-thioguanine in the granuloma pouch assay in rats.

Clofibrate did not induce chromosomal aberrations in three studies with cultured mammalian cell lines nor micronucleus formation in a study with cultured rat hepatocytes.

In morphological transformation studies with Syrian hamster embryo (SHE) cells, clofibrate had no effect in one study, but was reported in another study to have increased the frequency of transformation. The administration of clofibrate alone was also without effect in the C3H/10T1/2 C18 cell transformation system, whereas it did enhance the frequency of transformation produced by prior treatment with 3-methylcholanthrene. Weak inhibition of gap-junctional intercellular communication in Chinese hamster V79 cells was reported to occur with high concentrations of clofibrate.

No evidence was seen of DNA adduct formation by clofibrate in the livers of male Fischer 344 rats given three doses of 250 mg/kg at 24-h intervals and killed 2 h after the final dose. DNA was analysed by ^{32}P-postlabelling with an estimated limit of detection of 1 adduct in 10^{10} nucleotides and no adduct was detected in hepatocytes treated *in vitro* with 10^{-3} M clofibrate for 4 h (Gupta et al., 1985).

In vivo, clofibrate did not induce unscheduled DNA synthesis in rat hepatocytes. Neither did it induce sister chromatid exchange in rat peripheral blood lymphocytes or bone marrow cells of Chinese hamsters.

Table 3. Genetic and related effects of clofibrate

Test system	Result[a]		Dose[b] (LED/HID)	Reference
	Without exogenous metabolic system	With exogenous metabolic system		
BSD, *Bacillus subtilis* rec strains, differential toxicity	–	–	NR	Kawachi et al. (1980)
SA0, *Salmonella typhimurium* TA100, reverse mutation	–	–	NR	Kawachi et al. (1980)
SA0, *Salmonella typhimurium* TA100, reverse mutation	–	–	500	Warren et al. (1980)
SA0, *Salmonella typhimurium* TA100, reverse mutation	–	–	100	Dayan et al. (1985)
SA5, *Salmonella typhimurium* TA1535, reverse mutation	–	–	500	Warren et al. (1980)
SA5, *Salmonella typhimurium* TA1535, reverse mutation	–	–	500	Dayan et al. (1985)
SA7, *Salmonella typhimurium* TA1537, reverse mutation	–	–	500	Warren et al. (1980)
SA7, *Salmonella typhimurium* TA1537, reverse mutation	–	–	500	Dayan et al. (1985)
SA8, *Salmonella typhimurium* TA1538, reverse mutation	–	–	500	Warren et al. (1980)
SA9, *Salmonella typhimurium* TA98, reverse mutation	–	–	NR	Kawachi et al. (1980)
SA9, *Salmonella typhimurium* TA98, reverse mutation	–	–	500	Warren et al. (1980)
SA9, *Salmonella typhimurium* TA98, reverse mutation	–	–	500	Dayan et al. (1985)
SA9, *Salmonella typhimurium* TA98, reverse mutation	–	–	500	Dayan et al. (1985)
SAS, *Salmonella typhimurium* TA100Fr1, reverse mutation	–	–	500	Dayan et al. (1985)
SCG, *Saccharomyces cerevisiae*, gene conversion	–	–	20 000	Schiestel & Reddy (1990)
SCH, *Saccharomyces cerevisiae*, mitotic recombination	–	–	20 000	Schiestel & Reddy (1990)
DIA, DNA single-strand breaks, L1210 cells *in vitro*	–	–	3	Lawson & Gwilt (1993)
G9H, Gene mutation, Chinese hamster lung V79 cells, *hprt* locus	–	–	243	Dayan et al. (1985)
G9O, Gene mutation, Chinese hamster lung V79 cells, ouabain	–	–	243	Dayan et al. (1985)
URP, Unscheduled DNA synthesis, rat hepatocytes *in vitro*	–	NT	2400	Williams et al. (1989)
SIC, Sister chromatid exchange, Chinese hamster ovary cells *in vitro*	–	–	243	Linnainmaa (1984)
CIC, Chromosomal aberrations, Chinese hamster CHL cells *in vitro*	–	NT	250	Ishidate et al. (1978)
CIS, Chromosomal aberrations, Syrian hamster lung fibroblasts *in vitro*	–	NT	NR	Kawachi et al. (1980)
CIS, Chromosomal aberrations, Syrian hamster embryo cells *in vitro*	–	NT	72	Tsutsui et al. (1993)
TCM, Cell transformation, C3H 10T½ mouse cells	–	NT	1.2	Lillehaug et al. (1986)

Table 3 (contd)

Test system	Result[a]		Dose[b] (LED/HID)	Reference
	Without exogenous metabolic system	With exogenous metabolic system		
MIA, Micronucleus test, rat hepatocytes in vitro	–	NT	243	Müller et al. (1993)
TCS, Cell transformation, Syrian hamster embryo cells	+	NT	12	Mikalsen et al. (1990)
TCS, Cell transformation, Syrian hamster embryo cells	–	–	72	Tsutsui et al. (1993)
DVA, DNA strand breaks, rat hepatocytes in vivo	–		200 po × 6	Elliott & Elcombe (1987)
DVA, DNA strand breaks, rat hepatocytes in vivo	–		750 diet × 14 d	Nilsson et al. (1991)
DVA, DNA strand breaks, Fischer rat liver in vivo	–		100 diet × 78 wk	Tamura et al. (1991)
UPR, Unscheduled DNA synthesis, rat hepatocytes in vivo	–		750 diet × 14 d	Nilsson et al. (1991)
GVA, Gene mutation, rat granuloma pouch 6-TG resistance in vivo	?		4 sc × 1	Maier (1984) (abstract)
SVA, Sister chromatid exchange, rat peripheral lymphocytes in vivo	–		200 po × 14	Linnainmaa (1984)
SVA, Sister chromatid exchange, Chinese hamster bone-marrow cells in vivo	–		200 po × 14	Linnainmaa (1984)
CBA, Chromosomal aberrations, rat bone marrow in vivo	–		NG	Kawachi et al. (1980)
BID, Binding (covalent) to DNA, male F344 rat hepatocytes in vitro	–	NT	243	Gupta et al. (1985)
BVD, Binding (covalent) to DNA, male F344 rat liver in vivo (^{32}P-postlabelling)	–		250 po × 3	Gupta et al. (1985)
ICR, Inhibition of intercellular communication, V79 cells	(+)	NT	24	Awogi et al. (1984) (abstract)

[a] +, positive; (+), weak positive; –, negative; NT, not tested; ?, inconclusive
[b] LED, lowest effective dose; HID, highest ineffective dose; μg/mL; in-vitro tests, μg/mL; in-vivo tests, mg/kg bw; NG, dose not given

Slightly elevated levels of 8-hydroxydeoxyguanosine have been detected in liver DNA of rats fed diets containing clofibrate (see Section 4.2.2).

Oral treatment of Sprague-Dawley-derived SIV 50 rats with ^{14}C-labelled clofibric acid (225 mg/kg) did not lead to detectable radioactivity associated with liver DNA, although protein binding was clearly demonstrated (von Däniken *et al.*, 1981).

4.5 Mechanistic considerations

The role of data on peroxisome proliferation in evaluating carcinogenicity in humans has been discussed. When the data support the conclusion that a tumour response in mice or rats is secondary only to peroxisome proliferation, this should be considered in addressing the potential carcinogenicity of an agent in humans. The report of the Working Group on Peroxisome Proliferation and its Role in Carcinogenesis (IARC, 1995) indicates that the following issues should be considered:

"(*a*) Information is available to exclude mechanisms of carcinogenesis other than those related to peroxisome proliferation.

(*b*) Peroxisome proliferation (increases in peroxisome volume density or fatty acid β-oxidation activity) and hepatocellular proliferation have been demonstrated under the conditions of the bioassay.

(*c*) Such effects have not been found in adequately designed and conducted investigations of human groups and systems."

The weight of evidence indicates that clofibrate, and peroxisome proliferators in general, do not act as direct DNA-damaging agents and that their mechanism of tumour initiation is indirect. Two responses have been proposed to account for liver carcinogenesis by peroxisome proliferators in rodents. These include (i) induction of peroxisome proliferation and (ii) increased hepatocellular proliferation. These responses are not mutually exclusive with respect to tumour formation.

Chronic administration of peroxisome proliferators produces a sustained oxidative stress in rodent hepatocytes due to overproduction of hydrogen peroxide. This can theoretically generate reactive oxygen species which can attack DNA or may affect cells in other ways. There is also evidence from in-vitro experiments that fatty acid metabolism in peroxisomal fractions can result in hydroxyl radical formation and DNA damage. In-vivo observations in support of this hypothesis include increased lipid peroxidation, increased lipofuscin deposition, the effects on levels of hepatic antioxidants and inhibition of tumour formation by antioxidants (Lake 1995). However, some of the evidence suggests that the level of oxidative damage *in vivo* may be too low to account entirely for the carcinogenicity of peroxisome proliferators.

During the first few days of administration, peroxisome proliferators induce cell division in rodent hepatocytes; in some, but not all, studies sustained stimulation of replicative DNA synthesis has also been observed (Lake, 1995). An enhanced rate of cell proliferation can be a critical effect both in tumour initiation, by increasing the frequency of spontaneous mutations and the rate of conversion of DNA adducts into mutations before they are repaired, and in tumour promotion by facilitating clonal expansion of initiated cells. The promoting activity of clofibrate has been demonstrated in rodent models of multistage hepatocarcinogenesis.

There are clear species differences in the responses of mammalian cells to peroxisome proliferators (Lake, 1995). Biopsy studies have clearly indicated that the responsiveness of human livers to the peroxisome proliferation produced by fibrate drugs is lacking or is much less than that seen in the livers of treated rodents, although similar levels of drug are achieved in the circulation. The striking hepatomegalic effect of peroxisome proliferation is similarly not observed in patients receiving fibrate drugs. In cultures of hepatocytes, peroxisome proliferation and cell proliferation occur with rodent but not human hepatocytes. In rodent liver, hepatomegaly and peroxisome proliferation require expression of functional PPARα, a member of the steroid hormone receptor superfamily. Clofibrate activates rodent PPARα *in vitro*. The insensitivity of human liver to the effects of peroxisome proliferators is consistent with the low level of PPARα in human livers, as well as observations of genetic variations that render the human PPARα receptor inactive as compared to PPARα expressed in rodent liver (Tugwood *et al.*, 1996). In non-human primates, administration of clofibrate and other peroxisome proliferators has also failed to elicit the hepatomegaly and peroxisome proliferation induced in rodent liver.

Clofibrate-induced peroxisome proliferation and cell proliferation have been demonstrated in feeding studies in rats conducted under bioassay conditions. Peroxisome proliferation has not been found in studies of human groups and systems using clofibrate. Taken together, these findings indicate that the increased incidence of liver tumours in rodents treated with clofibrate results from a mechanism that would not be operative in humans.

5. Summary of Data Reported and Evaluation

5.1 Exposure data

Clofibrate was introduced in the 1960s to reduce plasma concentrations of triglycerides and cholesterol in patients at high risk of coronary heart disease. Since the late 1970s, its use has decreased considerably.

5.2 Human carcinogenicity data

In 1978, a randomized trial of the World Health Organization, conducted to determine whether clofibrate treatment would lower the incidence of ischaemic heart disease in men, raised concern over a nonsignificant excess of deaths from cancer in treated subjects.

Subsequently the association between clofibrate and cancer risk was examined in three randomized trials and a small case–control study. A further four-year follow-up of the WHO trial showed no difference in the age-standardized death rates from malignant neoplasms. In two other trials, there was also no difference in cancer deaths between clofibrate-treated patients and a placebo-treated group. A meta-analysis of results from six trials also found no excess cancer mortality due to use of clofibrate as a cholesterol-lowering drug. The case–control study, that had several methodological limitations, showed a nonsignificant excess of soft-tissue sarcoma.

5.3 Animal carcinogenicity data

Clofibrate was tested for carcinogenicity by oral administration in the diet in two experiments in mice and in three experiments in rats, and in one experiment in marmosets by gastric instillation. No increase in incidence of tumours was reported in mice or marmosets. In rats, clofibrate produced hepatocellular carcinomas.

Clofibrate was tested in several experiments by combined administration with other chemicals. It enhanced the hepatocarcinogenicity of *N*-nitrosamines in rats and hamsters. It did not enhance the carcinogenicity of 2-acetylaminofluorene in rat liver.

5.4 Other relevant data

Clofibrate exerts similar pharmacological responses in humans and rodents. Absorption and metabolism of clofibrate are similar in humans and rats. Elimination of clofibric acid, the free acid form of the drug as it appears in the circulation, is more rapid in rats, possibly due to lower binding to plasma proteins.

Clofibrate-induced peroxisome proliferation and cell proliferation have been demonstrated in feeding studies in rats. Peroxisome proliferation has not been found in studies of clofibrate in human livers or hepatocytes.

There are a number of case reports of reversible impotence in men treated with clofibrate. No noteworthy effect on the fetus has been observed in studies in rats or rabbits.

Clofibrate is inactive in most tests for genetic activity, although it induced cell transformation in one study.

Mechanistic considerations

The weight of evidence indicates that clofibrate does not act as a direct DNA-damaging agent and that its mechanism of tumour induction is indirect. Two biological responses have been proposed to account for liver carcinogenesis by peroxisome proliferators in rodents. These are (i) induction of peroxisome proliferation and (ii) increased hepatocellular proliferation. Upon exposure to clofibrate, proliferation of both peroxisomes and cells occurs in rat liver and of peroxisomes in cultured rat hepatocytes, whereas peroxisome proliferation does not occur in human liver or cultured hepatocytes. These observations suggest that the mechanism of liver carcinogenesis in clofibrate-treated rats would not be operative in humans.

5.5 Evaluation[1]

There is *inadequate evidence* in humans for the carcinogenicity of clofibrate.

There is *limited evidence* in experimental animals for the carcinogenicity of clofibrate.

Overall evaluation

Clofibrate is *not classifiable as to its carcinogenicity in humans (Group 3)*.

6. References

Anisimov, V.N., Danetskaya, E.V., Miretsky, G.I., Troitskaya, M.N. & Dilman, V.M. (1981) Influence of miscleron (clofibrate) on carcinogenic effect of 7,12-dimethylbenz[*a*]anthracene and methylnitrosourea in female rats. *Vopr. Onkol.*, **27**, 64–67 (in Russian)

Anthony, L.E., Schmucker, D.L., Mooney, J.S. & Jones, A.L. (1978) A quantitative analysis of fine structure and drug metabolism in livers of clofibrate-treated young adult and retired breeder rats. *J. Lipid Res.*, **19**, 154–165

Awogi, T., Kato, K., Itoh, T. & Tsushimoto, G. (1984) Comparison of inhibiting activity on cell-cell communication between some tumor promoters in Chinese hamster V79 cells (Abstract no. 1). *Mutat. Res.*, **130**, 361

Baldwin, J.R., Witiak, D.T. & Feller, D.R. (1980) Disposition of clofibrate in the rat: acute and chronic administration. *Biochem. Pharmacol.*, **29**, 3143–3154

Barnard, S.D., Molello, J.A., Caldwell, W.J. & LeBeau, J.E. (1980) Comparative ultrastructural study of rat hepatocytes after treatment with the hypolipidemic agents probucol, clofibrate, and fenofibrate. *J. Toxicol. environ. Health*, **6**, 547–557

Barrass, N.C., Price, R.J., Lake, B.G. & Orton, T.C. (1993) Comparison of the acute and chronic mitogenic effects of the peroxisome proliferators methylclofenapate and clofibric acid in rat liver. *Carcinogenesis*, **14**, 1451–1456

Bateson, M.C., Maclean, D., Ross, P.E. & Bouchier, I.A.D. (1978) Clofibrate therapy and gallstone induction. *Digest. Dis.*, **23**, 623–628

Berstein, L.M., Pozharisski, K.M. & Dilman, V.M. (1982) Effects of misclerone (clofibrate) on dimethylhydrazine-induced intestinal carcinogenesis in rats. *Oncology*, **39**, 331–335

Blaauboer, B.J., van Holsteijn, C.W.M., Bleumink, R., Mennes, W.C., van Pelt, F.N.A.M., Yap, S.H., van Pelt, J.F., van Iersel, A.A.J., Timmerman, A. & Schmid, B.P. (1990) The effect of beclobric acid and clofibric acid on peroxisomal β-oxidation and peroxisome proliferation in primary cultures of rat, monkey and human hepatocytes. *Biochem. Pharmacol.*, **40**, 521–528

British Pharmacopoeial Commission (1993) *British Pharmacopoeia 1993*, Vols. I & II, London, Her Majesty's Stationery Office, pp. 167–168, 839–840

Bronfman, M., Amigo, L. & Morales, M.N. (1986) Activation of hypolipidaemic drugs to acyl-coenzyme A thioesters. *Biochem. J.*, **239**, 781–784

---

[1]For definition of the italicized terms, see Preamble, pp. 22–25.

Budavari, S., ed. (1995) *The Merck Index*, 12th Ed., Rahway, NJ, Merck & Co.

Butterworth, B.E., Smith-Oliver, T., Earle, L., Loury, D.J., White, R.D., Doolittle, D.J., Working, P.K., Cattley, R.C., Jirtle, R., Michalopoulos, G. & Strom, S. (1989) Use of primary cultures of human hepatocytes in toxicology studies. *Cancer Res.*, **49**, 1075–1084

Calvert, R., Malka, D. & Ménard, D. (1979) Effect of clofibrate on the small intestine of fetal mice. *Histochemistry*, **63**, 7–14

de Camargo, J.L.V., Tsuda, H., Asamoto, M., Tagawa, Y., Wada, S., Nagase, S. & Ito, N. (1993) Modifying effects of chemicals on the development of liver preneoplastic placental glutathione S-transferase positive foci in analbuminemic and Sprague-Dawley rats. *Toxicol. Pathol.*, **21**, 409–416

Canner, P.L., Berge, K.B., Wenger, N.K., Stamler, J., Friedman, L., Prineas, R.J. & Friedewald, W. (1986) Cooperative studies. Fifteen year mortality in coronary drug project patients: long-term benefit with niacin. *J. Am. Coll. Cardiol.*, **8**, 1245–1255

Carlson, L.A. & Rosenhamer, G. (1988) Reduction of mortality in the Stockholm Ischaemic Heart Disease Secondary Prevention Study by combined treatment with clofibrate and nicotinic acid. *Acta med. scand.*, **223**, 405–418

Cattley, R.C. & Glover, S.E. (1993) Elevated 8-hydroxydeoxyguanosine in hepatic DNA of rats following exposure to peroxisome proliferators: relationship to carcinogenesis and nuclear localization. *Carcinogenesis*, **14**, 2495–2499

Cattley, R.C., Kato, M., Popp, J.A., Teets, V.J. & Voss, K.S. (1994) Initiator-specific promotion of hepatocarcinogenesis by WY-14,643 and clofibrate. *Carcinogenesis*, **15**, 1763–1766

Cayen, M.N., Ferdinandi, E.S., Greselin, E., Robinson, W.T. & Dvornik, D. (1977) Clofibrate and clofibric acid: comparison of the metabolic disposition in rats and dogs. *J. Pharmacol. exp. Ther.*, **200**, 33–43

Chance, D.S., Wu, S.-M. & McIntosh, M.K. (1995) Inverse relationship between peroxisomal and mitochondrial β-oxidation in HepG2 cells treated with dehydroepiandrosterone and clofibric acid (43865). *Proc. Soc. exp. Biol. Med.*, **208**, 378–384

Chandoga, J., Rojeková, I., Hampl, L. & Hocman, G. (1994) Cetaben and fibrates both influence the activities of peroxisomal enzymes in different ways. *Biochem. Pharmacol.*, **47**, 515–519

Chhabra, S. & Kurup, C.K.R. (1978) Maternal transport of chlorophenoxyisobutyrate at the foetal and neonatal stages of development (Short communication). *Biochem. Pharmacol.*, **27**, 2063–2065

Chinje, E.C. & Gibson, G.G. (1990) Stereochemical induction of cytochrome P450IVA1 (P452) and peroxisome proliferation in male rat. *Adv. exp. Med. Biol.*, **283**, 267–270

Cibelli, A., Stefanini, S. & Ceru, M.P. (1988) Peroxisomal β-oxidation and catalase activities in fetal rat liver: effect of maternal treatment with clofibrate. *Cell. mol. Biol..*, **34**, 191–205

Committee of Principal Investigators (1978) A cooperative trial in the primary prevention of ischaemic heart disease using clofibrate. *Br. Heart J.*, **40**, 1069–1118

Committee of Principal Investigators (1980) WHO cooperative trial on primary prevention of ischaemic heart disease using clofibrate to lower serum cholesterol: mortality follow-up. *Lancet*, **ii**, 379–385

Committee of Principal Investigators (1984) WHO cooperative trial on primary prevention of ischaemic heart disease with clofibrate to lower serum cholesterol: final mortality follow-up. *Lancet*, **ii**, 600–604

Coronary Drug Project Research Group (1975) Clofibrate and niacin in coronary heart disease. *J. Am. med. Assoc.*, **231**, 360–381

Council of Europe (1984) *European Pharmacopoeia*, 2nd Ed., Sainte-Ruffine, France, Maisonneuve S.A., pp. 318-1–318-4

Cumming, A. (1980) Acute renal failure and interstitial nephritis after clofibrate treatment. *Br. med. J.*, **281**, 1529–1530

Dange, M., Junghani, J., Nachbaur, J., Perraud, J. & Reinert, H. (1975) Postnatal thrombosis (PNT) in newborn rats by hypolipidemic agents. Preliminary results (Abstract). *Teratology*, **12**, 328

von Däniken, A., Lutz, W.K. & Schlatter, C. (1981) Lack of covalent binding to rat liver DNA of the hypolipidemic drugs clofibrate and fenofibrate. *Toxicol. Lett.*, **7**, 305–310

Dayan, J., Deguingand, S. & Truzman, C. (1985) Study of the mutagenic activity of 6 hepatotoxic pharmaceutical drugs in the *Salmonella typhimurium* microsome test, and the HGPRT and Na^+/K^+ ATPase system in cultured mammalian cells. *Mutat. Res.*, **157**, 1–12

Diener, R.M. & Hsu, B. (1966) Effects of certain aryloxisobutyrates on the rat fetus (Abstract no. 12). *Toxicol. appl. Pharmacol.*, **8**, 338

Dunnigan, M.G. (1992) Should clofibrate still be prescribed? Further trials with harder end points are needed for all lipid lowering drugs. *Br. med. J.*, **305**, 379–380

Eacho, P.I., Lanier, T.L. & Brodhecker, C.A. (1991) Hepatocellular DNA synthesis in rats given the peroxisome proliferating agents: comparison of WY-14,643 to clofibric acid, nafenopin and LY171883. *Carcinogenesis*, **12**, 1557–1561

Elliott, B.M. & Elcombe, C.R. (1987) Lack of DNA damage or lipid peroxidation measured *in vivo* in the rat liver following treatment with peroxisomal proliferators. *Carcinogenesis*, **8**, 1213–1218

Elliott, B.M., Dodd, N.J.F. & Elcombe, C.R. (1986) Increased hydroxyl radical production in liver peroxisomal fractions from rats treated with peroxisome proliferators. *Carcinogenesis*, **7**, 795–799

Emudianughe, T.S., Caldwell, J., Sinclair, K.A. & Smith, R.L. (1983) Species differences in the metabolic conjugation of clofibric acid and clofibrate in laboratory animals and man. *Drug Metab. Dispos.*, **11**, 97–102

Erkul, I., Yavuz, H. & Özel, A. (1991) Clofibrate treatment of neonatal jaundice (Letter to the Editor). *Pediatrics*, **88**, 1292

Expert Panel (1988) Report of the National Cholesterol Education Program Expert Panel on detection, evaluation, and treatment of high blood cholesterol in adults. *Arch. intern. Med.*, **148**, 36–69

Foxworthy, P.S. & Eacho, P.I. (1986) Conditions influencing the induction of peroxisomal β-oxidation in cultured rat hepatocytes. *Toxicol. Lett.*, **30**, 189–196

Gabilan, J.C., Benattar, C. & Lindenbaum, A. (1990) Clofibrate treatment of neonatal jaundice (Letter to the Editor). *Pediatrics*, **86**, 647–648

Gabilan, J.C., Benattar, C. & Lindenbaum, A. (1991) Clofibrate treatment of neonatal jaundice (Letter to the Editor). *Pediatrics*, **88**, 1292–1294

Gennaro, A.R., ed. (1995) *Remington: The Science and Practice of Pharmacy*, 19th Ed., Vol. II, Easton, PA, Mack Publishing Co., p. 967

Goodman Gilman, A., Rall, T.W., Nies, A.S. & Taylor, P., eds (1990) *Goodman and Gilman's. The Pharmacological Basis of Therapeutics*, 8th Ed., New York, Pergamon Press, pp. 886–889

Greaves, P., Irisarri, E. & Monro, A.M. (1986) Hepatic foci of cellular and enzymatic alteration and nodules in rats treated with clofibrate or diethylnitrosamine followed by phenobarbital: their rate of onset and their reversibility. *J. natl Cancer Inst.*, **76**, 475–484

Gugler, R. & Hartlapp, J. (1978) Clofibrate kinetics after single and multiple doses. *Clin. Pharmacol. Ther.*, **24**, 432–438

Gupta, R.C., Goel, S.K., Earley, K., Singh, B. & Reddy, J.K. (1985) ^{32}P-Postlabeling analysis of peroxisome proliferator-DNA adduct formation in rat liver *in vivo* and hepatocytes *in vitro*. *Carcinogenesis*, **6**, 933–936

Hagiwara, A., Tamano, S., Ogiso, T., Asakawa, E. & Fukushima, S. (1990) Promoting effect of the peroxisome proliferator, clofibrate, but not di(2-ethylhexyl)phthalate, on urinary bladder carcinogenesis in F344 rats initiated by *N*-butyl-*N*-(4-hydroxybutyl)nitrosamine. *Jpn. J. Cancer Res.*, **81**, 1232–1238

Hanefeld, M., Kemmer, C., Leonhardt, W., Kunze, K.D., Jaross, W. & Haller, H. (1980) Effects of *p*-chlorophenoxyisobutyric acid (CPIB) on the human liver. *Atherosclerosis*, **36**, 159–172

Hanefeld, M., Kemmer, C. & Kadner, E. (1983) Relationship between morphological changes and lipid-lowering action of *p*-chlorophenoxyisobutyric acid (CPIB) on hepatic mitochondria and peroxisomes in man. *Atherosclerosis*, **46**, 239–246

Harvengt, C. & Desager, J.P. (1976) Pharmacokinetic study and bioavailability of three marketed compounds releasing *p*-chlorophenoxyisobutyric acid (CPIB) in volunteers. *Int. J. clin. Pharmacol.*, **14**, 113–118

Hassan, M.M.A. & Elazzouny, A.A. (1982) Clofibrate. In: Florey, K., ed., *Analytical Profiles of Drug Substances*, Vol. 11, New York, Academic Press, pp. 197–224

Hendrickson, R.M. & Simpson, F. (1982) Clofibrate and eosinophilic pneumonia (Letter to the Editor). *J. Am. med. Assoc.*, **247**, 3082

Hoar Zahm, S., Blair, A., Holmes, F.F., Boysen, C.D., Robel, R.J. & Fraumeni, J.F., Jr (1989) A case–control study of soft-tissue sarcoma. *Am. J. Epidemiol.*, **130**, 665–674

Hosokawa, S., Tatematsu, M., Aoki, T., Nakanowatari, J., Igarashi, T. & Ito, N. (1989) Modulation of diethylnitrosamine-initiated placental glutathione S-transferase positive preneoplastic and neoplastic lesions by clofibrate, a hepatic peroxisome proliferator. *Carcinogenesis*, **10**, 2237–2241

IARC (1980) *IARC Monographs on the Evaluation of the Carcinogenic Risk of Chemicals to Humans*, Vol. 24, *Some Pharmaceutical Drugs*, Lyon, pp. 39–58

IARC (1983) *IARC Monographs on the Evaluation of the Carcinogenic Risk of Chemicals to Humans*, Vol. 31, *Some Food Additives, Feed Additives and Naturally Occurring Substances*, Lyon, pp. 95–132

IARC (1987) *IARC Monographs on the Evaluation of Carcinogenic Risks to Humans*, Suppl. 7, *Overall Evaluations of Carcinogenicity: An Update of* IARC Monographs *Volumes 1 to 42*, Lyon, pp. 171–172

IARC (1995) *Peroxisome Proliferation and its Role in Carcinogenesis* (IARC Technical Report No. 24), Lyon

Ishidate, M., Jr, Hayashi, M., Sawada, M., Matsuoka, A., Yoshikawa, K., Ono, M. & Nakadate, M. (1978) Cytotoxicity test on medical drugs — chromosome aberration tests with Chinese hamster cells *in vitro*. *Eisei Shikenjo Hokoku*, **96**, 55–61 (in Japanese)

Issemann, I., Prince, R.A., Tugwood, J.D. & Green, S. (1993) The peroxisome proliferator-activated receptor:retinoid X receptor heterodimer is activated by fatty acids and fibrate hypolipidaemic drugs. *J. mol. Endocrinol.*, **11**, 37–47

Kawachi, T., Komatsu, T., Kada, T., Ishidate, I., Sasaki, M., Sugiyama, T. & Tazima, Y. (1980) Results of recent studies on the relevance of various short-term screening tests in Japan. *Appl. Methods Oncol.*, **3**, 253–267

Kurokawa, Y., Takamura, N., Matushima, Y., Imazawa, T. & Hayashi, Y. (1988) Promoting effect of peroxisome proliferators in two-stage rat renal tumorigenesis. *Cancer Lett.*, **43**, 145–149

Lake, B.G. (1995) Mechanisms of hepatocarcinogenicity of peroxisome-proliferating drugs and chemicals. *Annu. Rev. Pharmacol. Toxicol.*, **35**, 483–507

Larsen, M.L., Illingworth, D.R. & O'Malley, J.P. (1994) Comparative effects of gemfibrozil and clofibrate in type III hyperlipoproteinemia. *Atherosclerosis*, **106**, 235–240

Law, M.R., Thompson, S.G. & Wald, N.J. (1994) Assessing possible hazards of reducing serum cholesterol. *Br. med. J.*, **308**, 373–379

Lawson, T. & Gwilt, P.R. (1993) Clofibrate enhances the DNA damaging action and cytotoxicity of nitrosoureas. *Cancer Lett.*, **70**, 119–122

Lee, G.-H., Nomura, K. & Kitagawa, T. (1989) Comparative study of diethylnitrosamine-initiated two-stage hepatocarcinogenesis in C3H, C57Bl and BALB mice promoted by various hepatopromoters. *Carcinogenesis*, **10**, 2227–2230

Lee, S.S.-T., Pineau, T., Drago, J., Lee, E.J., Owens, J.W., Kroetz, D.L., Fernandez-Salguero, P.M., Westphal, H. & Gonzalez, F.J. (1995) Targeted disruption of the α isoform of the peroxisome proliferator-activated receptor gene in mice results in abolishment of the pleiotropic effects of peroxisome proliferators. *Mol. cell. Biol.*, **15**, 3012–3022

Lillehaug, J.R., Aarsaether, N., Berge, R.K. & Male, R. (1986) Peroxisome proliferators show tumor-promoting but no direct transforming activity *in vitro*. *Int. J. Cancer*, **37**, 97–100

Linnainmaa, K. (1984) The effects of hypolipidemic peroxisome proliferators on the induction of sister chromatid exchanges. *Basic Life Sci.*, **29B**, 965–974

London, S.F., Gross, K.F. & Ringel, S.P. (1991) Cholesterol-lowering agent myopathy (CLAM). *Neurology*, **41**, 1159–1160

Lundgren, B. & DePierre, J.W. (1989) Proliferation of peroxisomes and induction of cytosolic and microsomal epoxide hydrolases in different strains of mice and rats after dietary treatment with clofibrate. *Xenobiotica*, **19**, 867–881

Maier, P., Schawalder, H.P. & Zbinden, G. (1984) Specific-locus mutations induced with hepatocarcinogens in a subcutaneous granulation tissue in rats (Abstract no. I.3.4). *Mutat. Res.*, **130**, 187

Männistö, P.T., Tuomisto, J., Jounela, A. & Penttilä, O. (1975) Pharmacokinetics of clofibrate and chlorophenoxy isobutyric acid. I. Cross-over studies on human volunteers. *Acta pharmacol. toxicol.*, **36**, 353–365

Marsman, D.S., Goldsworthy, T.L. & Popp, J.A. (1992) Contrasting hepatocytic peroxisome proliferation, lipofuscin accumulation and cell turnover for the hepatocarcinogens Wy-14,643 and clofibric acid. *Carcinogenesis*, **13**, 1011–1017

McGarvey, J.F.X. (1973) Premature contractions and clofibrate (Letter to the Editor). *J. Am. med. Assoc.*, **225**, 638

Medical Economics (1996) *PDR®: Physicians' Desk Reference*, 50th Ed., Montvale, NJ, Medical Economics Data Production Co., pp. 2701–2703

Meijer, J., Starkerud, C., Granell, I. & Afzelius, B.A. (1991) Time-dependent effects of the hypolipidemic agent clofibrate on peroxisomes and mitochondria in mouse hepatocytes. *J. submicrosc. Cytol. Pathol.*, **23**, 185–194

Mikalsen, S.-O., Holen, I. & Sanner, T. (1990) Morphological transformation and catalase activity of Syrian hamster embryo cells treated with hepatic peroxisome proliferators, TPA and nickel sulphate. *Cell Biol. Toxicol.*, **6**, 1–14

Mizumoto, K., Kitazawa, S., Eguchi, T., Nakajima, A., Tsutsumi, M., Ito, S., Danda, A. & Konishi, Y. (1988) Modulation of *N*-nitrosobis(2-hydroxypropyl)amine-induced carcinogenesis by clofibrate in hamsters. *Carcinogenesis*, **9**, 1421–1425

Mochizuki, Y., Furukawa, K. & Sawada, N. (1982) Effects of various concentrations of ethyl-α-p-chlorophenoxyisobutyrate (clofibrate) on diethylnitrosamine-induced hepatic tumorigenesis in the rat. *Carcinogenesis*, **3**, 1027–1029

Mochizuki, Y., Furukawa, K. & Sawada, N. (1983) Effect of simultaneous administration of clofibrate with diethylnitrosamine on hepatic tumorigenesis in the rat. *Cancer Lett.*, **19**, 99–105

Müller, K., Kasper, P. & Müller, L. (1993) An assessment of the in vitro hepatocyte micronucleus assay. *Mutation Res.*, **292**, 213–224

Murata, Y., Tani, M. & Amano, M. (1988) Erythema multiforme due to clofibrate (Letter to the Editor). *J. Am. Acad. Dermatol.*, **18**, 381–382

Mutai, M., Tatematsu, M., Aoki, T., Wada, S. & Ito, N. (1990) Modulatory interaction between initial clofibrate treatment and subsequent administration of 2-acetylaminofluorene or sodium phenobarbital on glutathione *S*-transferase positive lesion development. *Cancer Lett.*, **49**, 127–132

Nilsson, R., Beije, B., Préat, V., Erixon, K. & Ramel, C. (1991) On the mechanism of the hepatocarcinogenicity of peroxisome proliferators. *Chem.-biol. Interactions*, **78**, 235–250

Nishimura, A. & Tanimura, T. (1976) *Clinical Aspects of the Teratogenicity of Drugs*, New York, Excerpta Medica, pp. 256–257

Numoto, S., Furukawa, K., Furuya, K. & Williams, G.M. (1984) Effects of the hepatocarcinogenic peroxisome-proliferating hypolipidemic agents clofibrate and nafenopin on the rat liver cell membrane enzymes γ-glutamyltranspeptidase and alkaline phosphatase and on the early stages of liver carcinogenesis. *Carcinogenesis*, **5**, 1603–1611

Nyitray, M., Szaszovszky, E. & Druga, A. (1980) Clofibrate and the development of rats. *Arch. Toxicol.*, **Suppl. 4**, 463–465

Odum, J. & Orton, T.C. (1983) Hepatic microsomal glucuronidation of clofibric acid in the adult and neonate albino rat. *Biochem. Pharmacol.*, **32**, 3565–3569

Pantaleoni, G.C. & Valeri, P. (1974) Investigation on the interactions of clofibrate with reproductive function. *Clin. Terap.*, **69**, 321–328 (in Italian)

Price, S.C., Hinton, R.H., Mitchell, F.E., Hall, D.E., Grasso, P., Blane, G.F. & Bridges, J.W. (1986) Time and dose study on the response of rats to the hypolipidaemic drug fenofibrate. *Toxicology*, **41**, 169–191

Price, S.C., Chescoe, D., Grasso, P., Wright, M. & Hinton, R.H. (1988) Alterations in the thyroids of rats treated for long periods with di-(2-ethylhexyl)phthalate or with hypolipidaemic agents. *Toxicol. Lett.*, **40**, 37–46

Reddy, J.K. & Qureshi, S.A. (1979) Tumorigenicity of the hypolipidaemic peroxisome proliferator ethyl-α-*p*-chlorophenoxyisobutyrate (clofibrate) in rats. *Br. J. Cancer*, **40**, 476–482

Reddy, J.K. & Rao, M.S. (1978) Enhancement by Wy-14,643, a hepatic peroxisome proliferator, of diethylnitrosamine-initiated hepatic tumorigenesis in the rat. *Br. J. Cancer*, **38**, 537–543

Reynolds, J.E.F., ed. (1993) *Martindale: The Extra Pharmacopoeia*, 30th Ed., London, The Pharmaceutical Press, pp. 986–987

Rush, P., Baron, M. & Kapusta, M. (1986) Clofibrate myopathy: a case report and a review of the literature. *Sem. Arthrit. Rheumat.*, **15**, 226–229

Schiestl, R.H. & Reddy, J.K. (1990) Effect of peroxisome proliferators on intrachromosomal and interchromosomal recombination in yeast. *Carcinogenesis*, **11**, 173–176

Schneider, J. & Kaffarnik, H. (1975) Impotence in patients treated with clofibrate. *Atherosclerosis*, **21**, 455–457

Schwandt, P., Klinge, O. & Immich, H. (1978) Clofibrate and the liver (Letter to the Editor). *Lancet*, **ii**, 325

Scionti, L., Calafiore, R., Coaccioli, S., Bellomo, G., Berrettini, M. & Puxeddu, A. (1984) Clofibrate-induced myocardial injury and disseminated intravascular coagulation in a patient with chronic renal failure. *Pan. Med.*, **26**, 45–47

Scotto, C., Keller, J.-M., Schohn, H. & Dauça, M. (1995) Comparative effects of clofibrate on peroxisomal enzymes of human (Hep EBNA2) and rat (FaO) hepatoma cell lines. *Eur. J. Cell Biol.*, **66**, 375–381

Smals, A.G.H., Beex, L.V.A.M. & Kloppenborg, P.W.C. (1977) Clofibrate-induced muscle damage with myoglobinuria and cardiomyopathy (Letter to the Editor). *New Engl. J. Med.*, **296**, 942

Society of Japanese Pharmacopoeia (1992) *The Pharmacopoeia of Japan JP XII*, 12th Ed., Tokyo, pp. 231–232

Stanko, R.T., Sekas, G., Isaacson, I.A., Clarke, M.R., Billiar, T.R. & Paul, H.S. (1995) Pyruvate inhibits clofibrate-induced hepatic peroxisomal proliferation and free radical production in rats. *Metabolism*, **44**, 166–171

Stefanini, S., Mauriello, A., Farrace, M.G., Cibelli, A. & Ceru, M.P. (1989) Proliferative response of foetal liver peroxisomes to clofibrate treatment of pregnant rats. A quantitive evaluation. *Biol. Cell*, **67**, 299–305

Sundseth, S.S. & Waxman, D.J. (1992) Sex-dependent expression and clofibrate inducibility of cytochrome P450 4A fatty acid ω-hydroxylases. *J. biol. Chem.*, **267**, 3915–3921

Svoboda, D.J. & Azarnoff, D.L. (1979) Tumors in male rats fed ethyl chlorophenoxyisobutyrate, a hypolipidemic drug. *Cancer Res.*, **39**, 3419–3428

Takagi, A., Sai, K., Umemura, T., Hasegawa, R. & Kurokawa, Y. (1990) Relationship between hepatic peroxisome proliferation and 8-hydroxydeoxyguanosine formation in liver DNA of rats following long-term exposure to three peroxisome proliferators; di(2-ethylhexyl)-phthalate, aluminium clofibrate and simfibrate. *Cancer Lett.*, **53**, 33–38

Tamura, H., Iida, T., Watanabe, T. & Suga, T. (1990a) Long-term effects of peroxisome proliferators on the balance between hydrogen peroxide-generating and scavenging capacities in the liver of Fischer-344 rats. *Toxicology*, **63**, 199–213

Tamura, H., Iida, T., Watanabe, T. & Suga, T. (1990b) Long-term effects of hypolipidemic peroxisome proliferator administration of hepatic hydrogen peroxide metabolism in rats. *Carcinogenesis*, **11**, 445–450

Tamura, H., Iida, T., Watanabe, T. & Suga, T. (1991) Lack of induction of hepatic DNA damage on long-term administration of peroxisome proliferators in male F-344 rats. *Toxicology*, **69**, 55–62

Tanaka, K., Smith, P.F., Stromberg, P.C., Eydelloth, R.S., Herold, E.G., Grossman, S.J., Frank, J.D., Hertzog, P.R., Soper, K.A. & Keenan, K.P. (1992) Studies of early hepatocellular proliferation and peroxisomal proliferation in Sprague-Dawley rats treated with tumorigenic doses of clofibrate. *Toxicol. appl. Pharmacol.*, **116**, 71–77

Thomas, J., ed. (1991) *Prescription Products Guide 1991*, 20th Ed., Victoria, Australian Pharmaceutical Publishing Co., pp. 320–321, 333–334

Thorp, J.M. (1962) Experimental evaluation of an orally active combination of androsterone with ethyl chlorophenoxyisobutyrate. *Lancet*, **i**, 1323–1326

Thorp, J.M. & Waring, W.S. (1962) Modification of metabolism and distribution of lipids by ethyl chlorophenoxyisobutyrate. *Nature*, **194**, 948–949

Tomaszewski, K.E. & Melnick, R.L. (1994) In vitro evidence for involvement of CoA thioesters in peroxisome proliferation and hypolipidaemia. *Biochim. biophys. Acta*, **1120**, 118–124

Tsutsui, T., Watanabe, E. & Barrett, J.C. (1993) Ability of peroxisome proliferators to induce cell transformation, chromosome aberrations and peroxisome proliferation in cultured Syrian hamster embryo cells. *Carcinogenesis*, **14**, 611–618

Tucker, M.J. & Orton, T.C. (1995) *Comparative Toxicology of Hypolipidaemic Fibrates*, London, Taylor & Francis, pp. 1–22

Tugwood, J.D., Aldridge, T.C., Lambe, K.G., Macdonald, N. & Woodyatt, N.J. (1996) Peroxisome proliferator-activated receptors — Structures and function. *Ann. N.Y. Acad. Sci.* (in press)

United States Food and Drug Administration (1979) New label restrictions and boxed warning on clofibrate. *FDA Drug Bulletin*, Rockville, MD, August, p. 14

United States National Library of Medicine (1996) *RTEC Database*, Bethesda, MD

United States Pharmacopeial Convention (1994) *The 1995 US Pharmacopeia*, 23rd Rev./*The National Formulary*, 18th Rev., Rockville, MD, pp. 399–400

Vidal (1995) *Dictionnaire Vidal*, 71th Ed., Paris, Editions du Vidal, pp. 837–838

Warren, J.R., Simmon, V.F. & Reddy, J.K. (1980) Properties of hypolipidemic peroxisome proliferators in the lymphocyte [^{3}H]thymidine and *Salmonella* mutagenesis assays. *Cancer Res.*, **40**, 36–41

Watanabe, T., Mitsukawa, M., Horie, S., Suga, T. & Seki, K. (1987) Effects of some hypolipidemic agents on biochemical values and hepatic peroxisomal enzymes in rats: comparison of probucol, CGA, KCD-232, MLM-160, AL-369 and clinofibrate with clofibrate. *J. Pharmacobio-Dyn.*, **10**, 142–147

WHO (1979a) *Drug Information — January–March* (PDT/DI/79.1), Geneva, p. 19

WHO (1979b) *Drug Information — July–September 1979* (PDT/DI/79.3), Geneva, p. 17

Williams, G.M., Mori, H. & McQueen, C.A. (1989) Structure-activity relationships in the rat hepatocyte DNA-repair test for 300 chemicals. *Mutat. Res.*, **221**, 263–286

Wilson, G.N., King, T., Argyle, J.C. & Garcia, R.F. (1991) Maternal clofibrate administration amplifies fetal peroxisomes. *Pediatr. Res.*, **29**, 256–262

Windholz, M., ed. (1976) *The Merck Index*, 9th Ed., Rathway, N.J., Merck & Co., Inc., p. 305

Wysowski, D.K., Kennedy, D.L. & Gross, T.P. (1990) Prescribed use of cholesterol-lowering drugs in the United States, 1978 through 1988. *J. Am. med. Assoc.*, **263**, 2185–2188

Yokoyama, H., Tsuchida, S., Hatayama, I. & Sato, K. (1993) Lack of peroxisomal enzyme inducibility in rat hepatic preneoplastic lesions induced by mutagenic carcinogens: contrasted expression of glutathione S-transferase P form and enoyl CoA hydratase. *Carcinogenesis*, **14**, 393–398

GEMFIBROZIL

1. Exposure Data

1.1 Chemical and physical data

1.1.1 Nomenclature

Chem. Abstr. Serv. Reg. No.: 25812-30-0
Chem. Abstr. Name: 5-(2,5-Dimethylphenoxy)-2,2-dimethylpentanoic acid
IUPAC Systematic Name: 2,2-Dimethyl-5-(2,5-xylyloxy)valeric acid

1.1.2 Structural and molecular formulae and relative molecular mass

$C_{15}H_{22}O_3$ Relative molecular mass: 250.34

1.1.3 Chemical and physical properties of the pure substance

(a) *Description*: White crystals (Gennaro, 1995)
(b) *Boiling-point*: 158–159 °C (at 0.02 mm Hg [2.7 Pa]) (Budavari, 1995)
(c) *Melting-point*: 61–63 °C (Budavari, 1995)
(d) *Solubility*: Practically insoluble in water (19 µg/mL); soluble in ethanol (100 mg/mL) (American Hospital Formulary Service, 1995); slightly soluble in dilute alkali (Gennaro, 1995)
(e) *Dissociation constant*: pK_a = 4.7 (Gennaro, 1995)

1.1.4 Technical products and impurities

Gemfibrozil is available as 300-mg capsules, 600- and 900-mg tablets and 900- and 1200-mg microencapsulated granular powders which also may contain calcium stearate, candelilla wax, colloidal silicon dioxide, gelatin, flavouring, hydroxypropyl cellulose, hydroxypropyl methylcellulose, magnesium stearate, methylparaben, microcrystalline cellulose, Opaspray white, polyethylene glycol, polysorbate 80, precipitated silica, pregelatinized starch, propylparaben, sodium carboxymethylstarch, sorbitol, talc or titanium dioxide (Farmindustria, 1993; British Medical Association/Royal Pharmaceutical Society of Great Britain, 1994; Medical Economics, 1996).

Trade names and designations of the chemical and its pharmaceutical preparations include: Bolutol; CI-719; Decrelip; Elmogan; Fibrocit; GEM; Gemlipid; Genlip; Gevilon; Hipolixan; Ipolipid; Lipozid; Lipur; Lopid; Micolip; Trialmin.

1.1.5 Analysis

The United States Pharmacopeia specifies liquid chromatography as the assay for purity of gemfibrozil, and gas chromatography with flame ionization detection for determining impurities and decomposition products. Assays for water content and heavy metals are also specified. The assay for gemfibrozil in capsules and tablets also applies to liquid chromatography using standards (United States Pharmacopeial Convention, 1994).

Gemfibrozil and its metabolites can be analysed in biological fluids by gas chromatography (Randinitis *et al.*, 1984) and high-performance liquid chromatography (Hengy & Kölle, 1985; Randinitis *et al.*, 1986; Nakagawa *et al.*, 1991).

1.2 Production and use

1.2.1 Production

Gemfibrozil can be prepared by adding lithium to a solution of diisopropylamine in tetrahydrofuran/styrene, followed by addition of 2-methylpropyl 2,2-dimethylacetate and then 1-bromo-3-chloropropane to produce 2-methylpropyl 2,2-dimethyl-5-chloropentanoate. Reaction of this intermediate with a solution of 2,5-dimethylphenol and sodium hydroxide in toluene/dimethyl sulfoxide yields gemfibrozil (Kearney, 1987).

1.2.2 Use

Gemfibrozil was first marketed in the United States of America in 1982 (Wysowski *et al.*, 1990) and in France in 1985 (Vidal, 1994).

Gemfibrozil is used as a hypolipidaemic drug. Like clofibrate (see this volume), gemfibrozil is primarily a triglyceride-lowering agent. It lowers very low-density lipoprotein (VLDL) levels by promoting the lipolysis of VLDL-triglycerides through activation of lipoprotein lipase. Gemfibrozil also inhibits VLDL secretion (Vogt, 1991). It is more active than clofibrate in reducing plasma concentrations of total cholesterol (see IARC, 1983), VLDL-cholesterol and triglycerides (Larsen *et al.*, 1994). Gemfibrozil is recommended in the treatment of type IIa, type IIb, type III, type IV and type V hyperlipoproteinaemia (see Glossary, p. 448) at daily levels of 0.9–1.5 g given as two oral doses 30 min before morning and evening meals (Reynolds, 1993). Gemfibrozil substantially increases plasma concentrations of high-density lipoprotein (HDL)-cholesterol (Goodman Gilman *et al.*, 1990; Miller *et al.*, 1993). In trials in patients with hyperlipoproteinaemia (e.g., the Helsinki Heart Study), gemfibrozil has been shown to reduce coronary heart disease (Grundy, 1988; Manninen *et al.*, 1988).

Gemfibrozil can have a variable effect on low-density lipoprotein (LDL)-cholesterol, with a possible increase in patients with primary hypertriglyceridaemia or mixed hyperlipoproteinaemia (Vogt, 1991; Zimetbaum *et al.*, 1991). In persons with hypercholesterolaemia, however, gemfibrozil produces minor decreases in LDL-cholesterol (Smith *et al.*, 1987).

In patients at high risk for coronary heart disease, gemfibrozil reduces triglyceride levels, lowers production and fractional clearance of LDL and normalizes the composition of LDL. The LDL-cholesterol level usually rises but generally not to abnormally high levels (Vega & Grundy, 1985). Gemfibrozil is one of the drugs that is most effective in raising HDL-cholesterol levels (Miller *et al.*, 1993).

Gemfibrozil is also used, in conjunction with dietary modification (Reynolds, 1993), as a second drug, after nicotinic acid, in persons with high triglyceride levels and increased LDL-cholesterol or LDL-cholesterol : HDL-cholesterol ratio (Smith *et al.*, 1987). The addition of gemfibrozil to lovastatin, a 3-hydroxy-3-methylglutaryl coenzyme A reductase inhibitor (Wysowski *et al.*, 1990), or nicotinic acid usually produces additional lowering of triglycerides, but the effect on the change in LDL-cholesterol levels is quite variable (East *et al.*, 1988; Expert Panel, 1988). For the treatment of combined hyperlipoproteinaemia, a combination of a resin (colestipol, a bile acid sequestant (Wysowski *et al.*, 1990)) with gemfibrozil can be used (Vogt, 1991).

In the United States, gemfibrozil represented 18.1% of prescriptions for cholesterol-lowering medications in 1983 and 29.4% in 1988 (Wysowski *et al.*, 1990).

1.3 Occurrence

Gemfibrozil is not known to occur as a natural product.

1.4 Regulations and guidelines

Gemfibrozil is listed in the French and United States pharmacopoeias (Reynolds, 1993; Vidal, 1995).

Gemfibrozil was originally approved by the United States Food and Drug Administration for lowering triglyceride levels. In 1989, the United States Food and Drug Administration also approved its use for the adjunctive treatment of type IIb hyperlipidaemia (see Glossary, pp. 447–448) patients with low HDL cholesterol levels who had an inadequate response to weight loss, diet, exercise and other pharmacological agents, such as bile acid sequestrants and nicotinic acid (Wysowski *et al.*, 1990).

2. Studies of Cancer in Humans

A randomized, double-blind trial was conducted in Finland to investigate the effect of gemfibrozil on the incidence of coronary heart disease in asymptomatic men, aged 40–55 years, with dyslipidaemia (non-HDL cholesterol level, ≥ 5.2 mmol/L) (Frick *et al.*, 1987). Of 4081 men, 2051 were randomized to receive 600 mg gemfibrozil twice daily for five years and 2030 to receive a placebo. A cholesterol-lowering diet, as well as an increase in physical activity and a reduction in smoking and body weight, were recommended to all participants. A total of 2859 subjects (70%) participated in the trial until its completion; however, all 4081 men were followed for five years. Cancer mortality was identical in the two treatment groups (11 deaths among the treated group and 11 deaths in the placebo group). A borderline statistically significant difference was found in the numbers of basal-cell carcinomas of the skin: five in treated men and none in controls ($p = 0.062$, Fisher's exact test). The expected numbers of basal-cell carcinomas, based on the national cancer statistics of Finland, were 4.8 cases in the gemfibrozil group and 4.7 in the placebo group. No difference was found for other cancers (26 cases, 26 controls).

3. Studies of Cancer in Experimental Animals

3.1 Oral administration

3.1.1 *Mouse*

Groups of 72 male and 72 female non-inbred albino CD-1 mice, eight weeks old, were given 0, 30 or 300 mg/kg of diet (ppm) pharmaceutical-grade gemfibrozil (96.1% pure; mixed with polysorbate 80 on silica) in the diet for 78 weeks, after which time all surviving animals were killed. From graphic presentations, approximately 80% of male mice and 70–80% of female mice survived. Body-weight gain was depressed in gemfibrozil-treated animals [details not given]. All tissues and visually apparent lesions were evaluated histologically. Absolute and relative liver weights in high-dose males and females were increased significantly. Slight hypertrophy and increased cytoplasmic eosinophilia of hepatocytes were observed in high-dose males. The incidence of hepatocellular adenomas in male mice was 10/72 control, 13/72 low-dose and 10/72 high-dose animals, that of hepatocellular carcinomas was 6/72 control, 14/72 low-dose ($p < 0.05$, Fisher's exact test) and 10/72 high-dose animals. The incidence of lung adenomas was decreased in males (19/72 control, 16/72 low-dose and 11/72 high-dose; $p < 0.01$, Fisher's exact test). No increase in tumour incidence was observed in female mice (Fitzgerald *et al.*, 1981) [The Working Group noted that the experiment was terminated at 78 weeks and the lack of a dose–response relationship for hepatocellular carcinomas in males.]

3.1.2 *Rat*

Groups of 50 male and 50 female non-inbred albino CD rats, eight weeks old, were given 0, 30 or 300 mg/kg of diet (ppm) pharmaceutical-grade gemfibrozil (96.1% pure; mixed with polysorbate 80 on silica) in the diet for 104 weeks, after which time all surviving animals were killed. Survival of exposed and control animals was comparable. From graphic presentations, it appeared that approximately 50–60% of rats survived. Body-weight gain was depressed in gemfibrozil-treated animals. All tissues and visually apparent lesions were evaluated histologically. Absolute and relative liver weights in high-dose males and females were increased. Hepatocyte hypertrophy with increased cytoplasmic eosinophilia was observed in treated rats. The incidences of tumours in male rats were: hepatocellular adenomas (neoplastic nodules) — 1/50 control, 2/50 low-dose and 18/50 high-dose ($p < 0.01$; Fisher's exact test); hepatocellular carcinomas — 0/50 control, 4/50 low-dose and 5/50 high-dose; adrenal phaeochromocytomas [malignancy not specified] — 3/50 control, 13/50 low-dose ($p < 0.01$; Fisher's exact test) and 9/50 high-dose; pancreatic acinar adenomas — 0/50 control, 6/50 low-dose and 1/50 high-dose; interstitial-cell tumours of the testis — 1/50 control, 8/50 low-dose ($p < 0.05$; Fisher's exact test) and 17/50 high-dose ($p < 0.01$; Fisher's exact test). In female rats, the incidence of hepatocellular adenomas and carcinomas decreased: 9/50 control, 5/50 (2 carcinomas) low-dose and 3/50 high-dose animals (Fitzgerald et al., 1981). [The Working Group noted the lack of a dose–response relationship for adrenal phaeochromocytomas and pancreatic acinar adenomas.]

4. Other Data Relevant to an Evaluation of Carcinogenicity and its Mechanisms

4.1 Absorption, distribution, metabolism and excretion

4.1.1 *Humans*

The absorption of gemfibrozil in humans following oral exposure has been examined. In six subjects (three men, three women), single oral administration of 900 mg [13 mg/kg bw est.] gemfibrozil resulted in maximal plasma concentrations of 46 ± 16 µg/mL observed between 1 and 4 h after administration (Knauf et al., 1990). In another study, six healthy adult male subjects were given 600 mg [9 mg/kg bw est.] gemfibrozil twice daily for six days followed by an additional dose on day 7 of 600 mg [9 mg/kg bw est.] tritiated gemfibrozil (Okerholm et al., 1976). A maximal plasma concentration of 36 µg gemfibrozil equivalents/mL was observed 1–2 h following administration.

Hamberger et al. (1986) reported that over a clinically relevant range of concentrations (48–504 µM), gemfibrozil was bound approximately 99% to serum protein. In the study of Okerholm et al. (1976), the major route of elimination was urinary, this accounting for 66% of the dose in 5 days. Faecal excretion accounted for an additional 6%.

Gemfibrozil is biotransformed extensively following oral administration (Figure 1). A major pathway of gemfibrozil metabolism is via glucuronidation. Following a single oral administration of 450 mg [6 mg/kg bw est.] gemfibrozil to six male subjects, gemfibrozil glucuronide represented approximately 50% of the total urinary metabolites (32% of the dose) recovered within 24 h (Nakagawa et al., 1991). Very similar results had been obtained in the Okerholm et al. (1976) study (see above), in which 31% of the dose was recovered as urinary gemfibrozil glucuronide over 0–48 h. Among metabolites resulting from phase I biotransformation, 5-(5-carboxy-2-methylphenoxy)-2,2-dimethyl pentanoic acid (M3) was the major metabolite recovered. In the study of Nakagawa et al. (1991), a 24-h urine collection contained both free and conjugated M3 at approximately 15% and

5% of the total dose, respectively, while, in the study of Okerholm et al. (1986), free and conjugated M3 represented approximately 7% and 5% of the recovered radiactivity, respectively. Other minor metabolites identified were the 5-hydroxymethyl derivative (M2, an intermediate in the pathway to M3), a 4-hydroxy derivative (M1) and a 2-hydroxymethyl derivative (M4). In aggregate, urinary and faecal excretion of radio-activity accounted for 66% and 6%, respectively, of the elimination of orally administered gemfibrozil over five days.

Figure 1. Postulated metabolic pathways of gemfibrozil

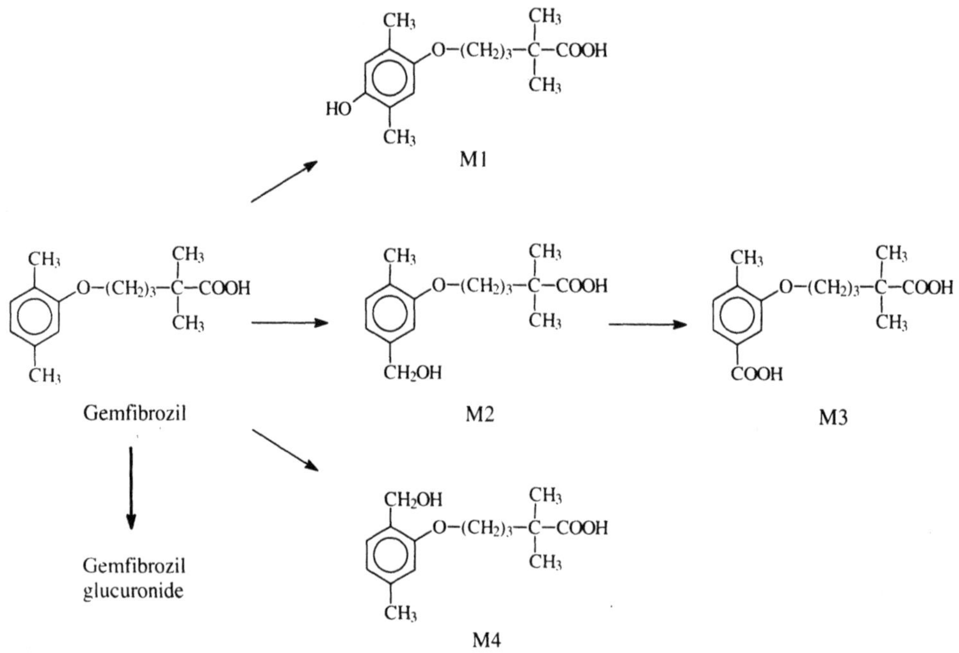

Based upon Nakagawa et al. (1991)

4.1.2 Experimental systems

Information on absorption, distribution, metabolism and excretion of gemfibrozil in animals is extremely limited. In male Fischer 344 rats given 6000–20 000 mg/kg diet (ppm) gemfibrozil in the diet for 42 days, maximal mean serum levels of 19.6–21.2 µg/mL were associated with daily exposure in the range of 522–964 mg/kg, indicating that a plateau in circulating levels of gemfibrozil was achieved (Sausen et al., 1995). In male rats [strain not specified] given 50 mg/kg bw tritiated gemfibrozil as a single oral administration, 47% of the dose was eliminated by the faecal route, while 25% of the dose was recovered in the urine over seven days (Okerholm et al., 1976). The lack of an intravenous formulation of gemfibrozil precludes total plasma clearance determinations in laboratory studies (Knauf et al., 1990).

Okerholm et al. (1976) also studied gemfibrozil metabolism in two beagle dogs and two rhesus monkeys. In dogs given a single oral 25 mg/kg bw dose of tritiated gemfibrozil, 62% was recovered in the faeces in five days, with an additional 7% appearing in the urine. A bile-fistula experiment with one dog indicated that 75% of the dose was excreted in the bile, only 2% and 12% being found in the faeces and urine, respectively. In the monkeys, 62% of the dose was recovered in the urine in 4 days and only 2% was found in the faeces. A bile-fistula experiment with a rhesus monkey demonstrated 41% of the dose was excreted in bile, 7% in faeces and 36% in urine.

4.2 Toxic effects

4.2.1 *Humans*

Several studies have documented the pharmacological reduction in circulating triglycerides and cholesterol in humans treated with gemfibrozil. Larsen et al. (1994) reported the effects of 600 mg [9 mg/kg bw est.] oral gemfibrozil twice daily for eight weeks in patients with hyperlipoproteinaemia type III. Reductions in circulating total cholesterol, VLDL-cholesterol and triglycerides were observed, as was an increase in circulating HDL-cholesterol. In patients with primary familial endogenous hypertriglyceridaemia treated orally with 600 mg [9 mg/kg bw est.] gemfibrozil twice daily for eight weeks, reduction in circulating triglycerides was observed, as was an increase in HDL-cholesterol (Saku et al., 1985). In patients with hyperlipoproteinaemia type IIB treated with 900 mg [13 mg/kg bw est.] gemfibrozil once a day for six weeks gave statistically significant reductions in levels of triglycerides, and cholesterol localized to LDL and VLDL fractions, while HDL-cholesterol content was increased; in patients with hyperlipoproteinaemia type IV, there was a reduction in levels of triglycerides and cholesterol localized to VLDL fractions (but an increase in LDL as well as HDL-cholesterol (Klosiewicz-Latoszek & Szostak, 1991). These pharmacological effects of gemfibrozil in patients with various disorders of lipid metabolism may have several mechanisms of activity, including stimulation of apolipoprotein synthesis (Saku et al., 1985) and stimulation of lipoprotein lipase activities in plasma and adipose tissue (Schwandt, 1991).

Leiss et al. (1985) studied the effect of gemfibrozil on biliary lipid metabolism in eight male volunteers treated for three months with gemfibrozil. The dose was 600 mg per day 12 times over 3 months. Despite the absence of any hyperlipidaemic disease in these volunteers, gemfibrozil reduced plasma concentrations of cholesterol and triglycerides and also increased the HDL-cholesterol levels. Significant increases in biliary output of cholesterol and reduction of bile acid output were observed. The authors suggested that administration of gemfibrozil would enhance the risk of gallstone formation in human subjects, although clear evidence for this was not presented.

Male patients receiving 600 mg [9 mg/kg bw est.] gemfibrozil (twice daily for two months) were examined with respect to effects on the coagulation system (Wilkes et al., 1992). Levels of plasma prothrombin fragment F_{1+2}, a marker of the in-vivo rate of thrombin generation, were reduced by gemfibrozil therapy. A significant reduction in factor VII_c was observed in subjects with elevated cholesterol levels in the circulation.

The authors suggested that the beneficial reduction in the incidence of coronary heart disease associated with gemfibrozil therapy might arise in part through a reduction in procoagulant activity.

A variety of case reports have documented unusual side-effects of gemfibrozil therapy. These include exacerbation of psoriasis (Fisher et al., 1988; Frick, 1989), myopathy (Magarian et al., 1991) and impotence (Bain et al., 1990; Pizzaro et al., 1990) (see Section 4.3.1).

The potential for gemfibrozil to induce structural changes in human liver was examined by percutaneous liver biopsy (de la Iglesia et al., 1982). The subjects included six men and three women with hyperlipoproteinaemia (types IIa, IIb or IV) treated with gemfibrozil for 17–27 months. The dose rate was not defined but may be presumed to approximate therapeutic recommendations (1.2 g per day) [17 mg/kg bw est.]. Light microscopic findings were considered to show no abnormality. The peroxisomes were mostly of normal shape with uniform matrix, but a few were of polyhedral shape on account of marginal plate development. Subjective estimation of the peroxisome population indicated no significant increase in number. The authors concluded that, under the conditions of this study, the lack of a drug-related increase in peroxisomes in humans comparable to that described in rats constituted a real species difference. Results of quantitative ultrastructural analysis of peroxisomes in livers of hyperlipoproteinaemic patients receiving gemfibrozil therapy were described separately (de la Igelsia et al., 1981). Numbers of peroxisomes per hepatocyte ranged from 656 to 1452, with a mean of 850, and the size of peroxisomes varied from 0.059 to 0.129 μm^3. In comparison with normal values reported in the literature, these results show no apparent difference in the gemfibrozil-treated patients.

4.2.2 Experimental systems

Many of the pharmacological effects of gemfibrozil observed in animals are similar to those reported in humans. Treatment of male CDS rats with gemfibrozil (100 mg/kg bw per day by gastric instillation for four weeks) significantly reduced plasma cholesterol and triglyceride levels, with decreases in cholesterol content in the LDL fraction and increased cholesterol content in the HDL fraction (McGuire et al., 1991). Male Sprague-Dawley rats fed diets containing 20% olive oil and 2% cholesterol were treated for two weeks with 50 mg/kg bw per day gemfibrozil by gastric instillation. Gemfibrozil reduced total cholesterol and triglyceride levels, with reduction of LDL-cholesterol and increased HDL-cholesterol (Krause & Newton, 1986). In these rats, circulating levels of apolipoproteins (Apo) were measured. Apo B was decreased, while Apo A-I and Apo E were increased. Male Dahl S rats treated for 12 days with 30 mg/kg bw per day gemfibrozil by gastric instillation also had reduced plasma triglyceride concentrations (Donnelly et al., 1994). In female Swiss OF1 strain mice, treatment with 300 mg/kg bw per day gemfibrozil by gastric instillation for two weeks reduced plasma concentrations of triglycerides but increased HDL-cholesterol (Olivier et al., 1988).

Hepatic peroxisome proliferation, potentially relevant to the mechanism of carcinogenic activity of a variety of agents, has been observed in gemfibrozil-treated animals.

Gray and de la Iglesia (1984) described ultrastructural changes in the livers of male and female CD rats receiving gemfibrozil (300 mg/kg per day) in the diet for one year. Increases in the number of peroxisomes per cell (7-fold) and peroxisomal volume (males only) and in total peroxisomal volume fraction per cell (20-fold) were observed by quantitative analysis. In male CDS albino rats given 100 mg/kg bw per day gemfibrozil by gastric instillation for four weeks, increases in the number of peroxisomes per hepatocyte and number of peroxisomes per gram of tissue were observed. This effect was associated with an increase in the relative liver weights following administration of gemfibrozil (McGuire et al., 1991). Gorgas and Krisans (1989) evaluated the zonal heterogeneity of peroxisomal changes in livers of male Sprague-Dawley rats given 2000 mg/kg diet (ppm) gemfibrozil [120 mg/kg bw est.] in the diet for two weeks. The greatest increases in numbers of peroxisomes were observed in centrilobular hepatocytes. Several studies have documented increases in peroxisomal enzyme activities. In male Fischer 344 rats given gemfibrozil in the diet for 21 days, 20 ppm [150 µg/kg bw est.] was the no-effect level and 50 ppm [375 µg/kg bw est.] was the lowest-effect level. Maximal induction of peroxisomal acyl coenzyme A (CoA) oxidase activity (16–18 fold) was observed in male Fischer 344 rats given 9000–20 000 ppm (522–1179 mg/kg bw per day) gemfibrozil for 42 days. These exposures were associated with a plateau in serum gemfibrozil levels (see Section 4.1.2) (Sausen et al., 1995). In male Fischer 344 rats given 2000 ppm gemfibrozil in the diet for four weeks, activity of two peroxisomal enzyme, palmitoyl-CoA oxidase and enoyl-CoA hydratase, was increased in liver homogenates (Lalwani et al., 1983). Male Wistar rats given 2000 ppm gemfibrozil in the diet for two weeks had increased peroxisomal activities for fatty acyl-CoA β-oxidation and catalase in liver homogenates (Hashimoto et al., 1995). Similar studies in laboratory mice have not been reported. Furthermore, the potential for gemfibrozil to modulate hepatocellular replication in laboratory animals has not been evaluated. While peroxisome proliferation has been hypothesized to contribute to the mechanism of action of gemfibrozil and other agents, no data are available on the induction of oxidative damage to cytoplasmic or nuclear constituents.

Kähönen and Ylikahri (1979) analysed hepatic responses in male Wistar rats rendered hypertriglyceridaemic by adding 10% fructose to the drinking-water. Gemfibrozil was injected subcutaneously at doses of 15–100 mg/kg bw per day for 14 days. Increases in relative liver weights were observed at doses of 15 mg/kg per day or more. Mild but statistically significant increases in mitochondrial activities of carnitine acyltransferases were detected at doses of 15 mg/kg per day or more.

In primary cultures of rat hepatocytes, incubation with 100–500 µM gemfibrozil for up to 72 h resulted in induction of peroxisomal β-oxidation (Foxworthy & Eacho, 1986). This response is probably mediated by the peroxisome proliferator-activated receptor α (PPARα), a member of the nuclear steroid hormone receptor superfamily. In the presence of gemfibrozil, PPARα and retinoid X receptor-α form a heterodimer which binds to response elements located in the promoter regions of several peroxisomal genes, such as that of the rat acyl CoA oxidase gene, and facilitates transcriptional activity (Issemann et al., 1993). The critical role of PPARα in mediating responses to peroxisome proliferating agents has been demonstrated with knockout mice that do not express the receptor (Lee et al., 1995).

No attempt to induce peroxisome proliferation in human cells in vitro, such as primary cultures of human hepatocytes or human hepatoma cell lines, has been reported.

The central role of PPARα in mediating the hepatic effects of fibrate drugs in rodents indicates that characterization of human PPARα could be important for the extrapolation of effects in rodents to humans. Tugwood et al. (1996) found generally low (but variable) expression of PPARα mRNA in 10 human liver samples compared with rodent liver samples. They characterized the function of human PPARα cDNA clones isolated from two livers. One had a deleted segment leading to a C-terminal truncation of the receptor; the other had non-conservative codon substitutions at amino acid positions 71 and 123. Both clones failed to activate transcription under conditions in which the mouse wild-type PPARα clone is active, indicating a non-functional human receptor. Thus, the insensitivity of human liver to the adaptive effects of peroxisome proliferators may be attributable to low expression of PPARα and/or genetic variations in the PPARα gene that result in lack of response to peroxisome proliferators.

4.3 Reproductive and developmental effects

4.3.1 *Humans*

A number of cases of reversible impotence in men being treated with gemfibrozil have been reported (Bain et al., 1990; Pizarro et al., 1990; Bharani, 1992; Figueras et al., 1993).

4.3.2 *Experimental systems*

Groups of pregnant CD rats were given 0, 81 or 281 mg/kg bw gemfibrozil in the diet on gestation days 6–15 (Fitzgerald et al., 1987). Although food intake and body-weight gain were markedly reduced in the high-dose group, no adverse affect on postimplantation loss, litter size or fetal weight was observed. The incidence of fetal malformations and variations was similar between the three groups. Dutch belted rabbits were treated by gastric instillation with 60 or 200 mg/kg bw gemfibrozil or with the vehicle on gestation days 6–18. No significant effect on weight gain, litter size, postimplantation loss, fetal sex ratio, fetal weight or incidence of fetal anomalies occurred. In fertility studies, groups of sexually mature male CD rats were given 93 or 326 mg/kg bw gemfibrozil for 61 days and females were given 94 or 318 mg/kg bw gemfibrozil for 15 days before mating within the treatment groups. Administration of the drug to females continued throughout gestation and weaning of the F_1 offspring. In subsequent fertility experiments, treated male rats were mated with untreated females, while treated females were placed with untreated males. The only apparent drug-related effect was reduced pup weights during the neonatal and weaning periods in the female fertility study. When similar doses of gemfibrozil were given to female rats from gestation day 15 through to weaning, the only apparent drug-related effect was reduced pup weight during the neonatal weaning period.

4.4 Genetic and related effects (see also Table 1 for references and Appendices 1 and 2)

Gemfibrozil was not mutagenic towards five strains of *Salmonella typhimurium* in the presence of rat liver S9 fraction.

Five metabolites were also tested under the same conditions as gemfibrozil, except that the highest dose was 300 µg/plate (approx. 150 µg/mL of soft agar). No mutagenicity was observed with the metabolites that were structures (MI-MIV) (Figure 1) and 2-(2-carboxy-5-hydroxymethylphenoxy)-2,2-dimethyl pentanoic acid (Fitzgerald *et al.*, 1981).

Table 1. Genetic and related effects of gemfibrozil

Test system	Result[a]		Dose[b] (LED/HID)	Reference
	Without exogenous metabolic system	With exogenous metabolic system		
SA0, *Salmonella typhimurium* TA100, reverse mutation	–	–	1250	Fitzgerald *et al.* (1981)
SA5, *Salmonella typhimurium* TA1535, reverse mutation	–	–	1250	Fitzgerald *et al.* (1981)
SA7, *Salmonella typhimurium* TA1537, reverse mutation	–	–	1250	Fitzgerald *et al.* (1981)
SA8, *Salmonella typhimurium* TA1538, reverse mutation	–	–	1250	Fitzgerald *et al.* (1981)
SA9, *Salmonella typhimurium* TA98, reverse mutation	–	–	1250	Fitzgerald *et al.* (1981)

[a] +, positive; (+), weak positive; –, negative; ?, inconclusive
[b] LED, lowest effective dose; HID, highest ineffective dose; in-vitro tests, µg/mL; in-vivo tests, mg/kg bw/day

4.5 Mechanistic considerations

The role of data on peroxisome proliferation in evaluating carcinogenicity in humans has been discussed. When data support the conclusion that a tumour response in mice or rats is secondary only to peroxisome proliferation, this should be considered in addressing the potential carcinogenicity of an agent in humans. The report of the Working Group on Peroxisome Proliferation and its Role in Carcinogenesis (IARC, 1995) indicates that the following issues should be considered:

"(*a*) Information is available to exclude mechanisms of carcinogenesis other than those related to peroxisome proliferation.

(b) Peroxisome proliferation (increases in peroxisome volume density or fatty acid β-oxidation activity) and hepatocellular proliferation have been demonstrated under the conditions of the bioassay.

(c) Such effects have not been found in adequately designed and conducted investigations of human groups and systems."

The weight of evidence, including structural similarities to other fibrates, indicates that gemfibrozil, and peroxisome proliferators in general, do not act as direct DNA-damaging agents and that their mechanism of tumour initiation is indirect. Two responses have been proposed to account for liver carcinogenesis by peroxisome proliferators in rodents. These include (i) induction of peroxisome proliferation and (ii) increased hepatocellular proliferation. These responses are not mutually exclusive with respect to tumour formation.

Chronic administration of peroxisome proliferators produces a sustained oxidative stress in rodent hepatocytes due to overproduction of hydrogen peroxide. This can theoretically generate reactive oxygen species which can attack DNA or may affect cells in other ways. There is also evidence from in vitro experiments that fatty acid metabolism in peroxisomal fractions can result in hydroxyl radical formation and DNA damage. In-vivo observations in support of this hypothesis include increased lipid peroxidation, increased lipofuscin deposition, the effects on levels of hepatic antioxidants and inhibition of tumour formation by antioxidants (Lake, 1995). However, some of the evidence suggests that the level of oxidative damage *in vivo* may be too low to account entirely for the carcinogenicity of peroxisome proliferators.

During the first few days of administration, peroxisome proliferators induce cell division in rodent hepatocytes; in some, but not all, studies, sustained stimulation of replicative DNA synthesis has also been observed (Lake, 1995). An enhanced rate of cell proliferation can be a critical effect in both tumour initiation, by increasing the frequency of spontaneous mutations and the rate of conversion of DNA adducts into mutations before they are repaired, and in tumour promotion by facilitating clonal expansion of initiated cells.

There are clear species differences in the responses of mammalian cells to peroxisome proliferators (Lake, 1995). Biopsy studies have clearly indicated that the responsiveness of human livers to the peroxisome proliferation produced by fibrate drugs is lacking or is much lower than that seen in the livers of treated rodents, although similar levels of drug are achieved in the circulation. The striking hepatomegalic effect of peroxisome proliferation is similarly not observed in patients receiving fibrate drugs. In cultures of hepatocytes, peroxisome proliferation and cell proliferation occur with rodent but not human hepatocytes. In rodent liver, hepatomegaly and peroxisome proliferation require expression of functional PPARα, a member of the steroid hormone receptor superfamily. Gemfibrozil activates rodent PPARα *in vitro*. The insensitivity of human liver to the effects of peroxisome proliferators is consistent with the low level of PPARα in human livers, as well as observations of genetic variations that render the human PPARα receptor inactive compared with PPARα expressed in rodent liver (Tugwood *et al.*,

1996). In non-human primates, administration of peroxisome proliferators has also failed to elicit the hepatomegaly and peroxisome proliferation induced in rodent liver.

Gemfibrozil-induced peroxisome proliferation has been demonstrated under bioassay conditions. An indirect measure of cell proliferation, liver weight, is also increased under bioassay conditions. Peroxisomal proliferation has not been found in studies of human groups and systems using gemfibrozil. Taken together, these findings indicate that the increased incidence of liver tumours in rodents treated with gemfibrozil results from a mechanism that would not be operative in humans.

5. Summary of Data Reported and Evaluation

5.1 Exposure data

Gemfibrozil has been used since the early 1980s to lower serum triglycerides and raise high-density lipoprotein-cholesterol in patients at high risk for coronary heart disease.

5.2 Human carcinogenicity data

In a Finnish trial that aimed to reduce cholesterol concentration with gemfibrozil, no difference was found in cancer incidence or mortality between the treated and control groups.

5.3 Animal carcinogenicity data

Gemfibrozil was tested for carcinogenicity by oral administration in the diet in one experiment in mice and one experiment in rats. There was a slight, not dose-related increase in the incidence of hepatocellular carcinomas in male mice and the incidence of lung adenomas was decreased. In male rats, increases were observed in the incidence of hepatocellular tumours, interstitial-cell tumours of the testis and adrenal phaeochromocytomas; the latter was not dose-related.

5.4 Other relevant data

Gemfibrozil exerts similar pharmacological responses in humans and laboratory rodents. It is readily absorbed, metabolized and eliminated in human subjects. Data are not available to characterize adequately its pharmacokinetic behaviour in animals, although maximal serum levels of gemfibrozil in rats are similar to those in humans receiving therapeutic doses of gemfibrozil.

Gemfibrozil-induced peroxisome proliferation has been demonstrated in rats. An indirect measure of cell proliferation, liver weight, is also increased in rats. Peroxisome proliferation has not been observed in studies of human livers with gemfibrozil.

There are a number of case reports of reversible impotence in men treated with gemfibrozil. No noteworthy effects on the fetus have been observed in studies in rats or rabbits.

Neither gemfibrozil nor its metabolites were mutagenic in bacteria in a single study.

Mechanistic considerations

The data on gemfibrozil are too limited to allow mechanistic assessment. In particular, genotoxicity has not been excluded. Upon exposure to gemfibrozil, proliferation of peroxisomes occurs in rat liver, whereas proliferation of peroxisomes does not occur in human liver. These observations suggest that the mechanism of liver carcinogenesis in gemfibrozil-treated rats would not be operative in humans.

5.5 Evaluation[1]

There is *inadequate evidence* in humans for the carcinogenicity of gemfibrozil.

There is *limited evidence* in experimental animals for the carcinogenicity of gemfibrozil.

Overall evaluation

Gemfibrozil is *not classifiable as to its carcinogenicity in humans (Group 3)*.

6. References

American Hospital Formulary Service (1995) *AHFS Drug Information*® 95, Bethesda, MD, American Society of Health-System Pharmacists, pp. 1168–1173

Bain, S.C., Lemon, M. & Jones, A.F. (1990) Gemfibrozil-induced impotence (Letter to the Editor). *Lancet*, **336**, 1389

Bharani, A. (1992) Sexual dysfunction after gemfibrosil. *Br. med. J.*, **305**, 693

British Medical Association/Royal Pharmaceutical Society of Great Britain (1994) *British National Formulary Number 27 (March 1994)*, London, p. 105

Budavari, S., ed. (1995) *The Merck Index*, 12th Ed., Rahway, NJ, Merck & Co.

Donnelly, R., Plato, P.A., Chang, H. & Reaven, G.M. (1994) Effects of gemfibrozil on triglyceride metabolism in Dahl salt-sensitive rats. *J. Pharmacol. exp. Ther.*, **270**, 809–813

East, C., Bilheimer, D.W. & Grundy, S.M. (1988) Combination drug therapy for familial combined hyperlipidemia. *Ann. intern. Med.*, **109**, 25–32

Expert Panel (1988) Report of the National Cholesterol Education Program Expert Panel on detection, evaluation, and treatment of high blood cholesterol in adults. *Arch. intern. Med.*, **148**, 36–69

---

[1]For definition of the italicized terms, see Preamble, pp. 22–25.

Farmindustria (1993) *Repertorio Farmaceutico Italiano (Italian Pharmaceutical Directory)*, 7th Ed., Milan, Associazione Nazionale dell'Industria Farmaceutica, CEDOF, S.P.A., pp. A-593–A594; A-654–A657; A-874–A875; A-900–A-901

Figueras, A., Castel, J.M., Laporte, J.-R. & Capellà, D. (1993) Gemfibrozil-induced impotence (Letter to the Editor). *Ann. Pharmacol.*, **27**, 982

Fisher, D.A., Elias, P.M. & LeBoit, P.L. (1988) Exacerbation of psoriasis by the hypolipidemic agent, gemfibrozil (Letter to the Editor). *Arch. Dermatol.*, **124**, 854–855

Fitzgerald, J.E., Sanyer, J.L., Schardein, J.L., Lake, R.S., McGuire, E.J. & de la Iglesia, F.A. (1981) Carcinogen bioassay and mutagenicity studies with the hypolipidemic agent gemfibrozil. *J. natl Cancer Inst.*, **67**, 1105–1116

Fitzgerald, J.E., Petrere, J.A. & de la Iglesia, F.A. (1987) Experimental studies on reproduction with the lipid-regulating agent gemfibrozil. *Fundam. appl. Toxicol.*, **8**, 454–464

Foxworthy, P.S. & Eacho, P.I. (1986) Conditions influencing the induction of peroxisomal β-oxidation in cultured rat hepatocytes. *Toxicol. Lett.*, **30**, 189–196

Frick, M.H. (1989) Exacerbation of psoriasis (Letter to the Editor). *Arch. Dermatol.*, **125**, 132

Frick, M.H., Elo, O., Haapa, K., Heinonen, O.P., Heinsalmi, P., Helo, P., Huttunen, J.K., Kaitaniemi, P., Koskinen, P., Manninen, V., Mäenpää, H., Mälkönen, M., Mänttäri, M., Norola, S., Pasternack, A., Pikkarainen, J., Romo, M., Sjöblom, T. & Nikkilä, E.A. (1987) Helsinki Heart Study: primary-prevention trial with gemfibrozil in middle-aged men with dyslipidemia. Safety of treatment, changes in risk factors, and incidence of coronary breast disease. *New Engl. J. Med.*, **317**, 1237–1245

Gennaro, A.R., ed. (1995) *Remington: The Science and Practice of Pharmacy*, 19th Ed., Vol. II, Easton, PA, Mack Publishing Co., p. 968

Goodman Gilman, A., Rall, T.W., Nies, A.S. & Taylor, P., eds (1990) *Goodman and Gilman's. The Pharmacological Basis of Therapeutics*, 8th Ed., New York, Pergamon Press, pp. 886–889

Gorgas, K. & Krisans, S.K. (1989) Zonal heterogeneity of peroxisome proliferation and morphology in rat liver after gemfibrozil treatment. *J. Lipid Res.*, **30**, 1859–1875

Gray, R.H. & de la Iglesia, F.A. (1984) Quantitative microscopy comparison of peroxisome proliferation by the lipid-regulating agent gemfibrozil in several species. *Hepatology*, **4**, 520–530

Grundy, S.M. (1988) Lessons from the Helsinki Heart Study. Fibric acid therapy for dyslipidemia. *Postgrad. Med.*, **84**, 217–234

Hamberger, C., Barre, J., Zini, R., Taiclet, A., Houin, G. & Tillement, J.P. (1986) In vitro binding study of gemfibrozil to human serum proteins and erythrocytes: interactions with other drugs. *Int. clin. pharm. Res.*, **6**, 441–449

Hashimoto, F., Ishikawa, T., Hamada, S. & Hayashi, H. (1995) Effect of gemfibrozil on lipid biosynthesis from acetyl-CoA derived from peroxisomal β-oxidation. *Biochem. Pharmacol.*, **49**, 1213–1221

Hengy, H. & Kölle, E.U. (1985) Determination of gemfibrozil in plasma by high performance liquid chromatography. *Arzneimittel Forsch./Drug Res.*, **35**, 1637–1639

IARC (1983) *IARC Monographs on the Evaluation of the Carcinogenic Risk of Chemicals to Humans*, Vol. 31, *Some Food Additives, Feed Additives and Naturally Occurring Substances*, Lyon, pp. 95–132

IARC (1995) *Peroxisome Proliferation and its Role in Carcinogenesis* (IARC Technical Report No. 24), Lyon

de la Iglesia, F.A., Pinn, S.M., Lucas, J. & McGuire, E.J. (1981) Quantitative stereology of peroxisomes in hepatocytes from hyperlipoproteinemic patients receiving gemfibrozil. *Micron*, **12**, 97–98

de la Iglesia, F.A., Lewis, J.E., Buchanan, R.A., Marcus, E.L. & McMahon, G. (1982) Light and electron microscopy of liver in hyperlipoproteinemic patients under long-term gemfibrozil treatment. *Atherosclerosis*, **43**, 19–37

Issemann, I., Prince, R.A., Tugwood, J.D. & Green, S. (1993) The peroxisome proliferator-activated receptor:retinoid X receptor heterodimer is activated by fatty acids and fibrate hypolipidaemic drugs. *J. mol. Endocrinol.*, **11**, 37–47

Kähönen, M.T. & Ylikahri, R.H. (1979) Effect of clofibrate and gemfibrozil on the activities of mitochondrial carnitine acyltransferases in rat liver. Dose-response relations. *Atherosclerosis*, **32**, 47–56

Kearney, F.R. (1987) *Process for Preparing 5-(2,5-Dimethylphenoxy)-2,2-dimethylpentanoic Acid as an Agent for Treatment or Prevention of Arteriosclerosis*. US Patent 4,665,226-A; Patent Assignee: Warner-Lambert Co.

Klosiewicz-Latoszek, L. & Szostak, W.B. (1991) Comparative studies on the influence of different fibrates on serum lipoproteins in endogenous hyperlipoproteinemia. *Eur. J. clin. Pharmacol.*, **40**, 33–41

Knauf, H., Kölle, E.U. & Mutschler, E. (1990) Gemfibrozil absorption and elimination in kidney and liver disease. *Klin. Wochenschr.*, **68**, 692–698

Krause, B.R. & Newton, R.S. (1986) Gemfibrozil increases both Apo A-I and Apo E concentrations. Comparison to other lipid regulators in cholesterol-fed rats. *Atherosclerosis*, **59**, 95–98

Lake, B.G. (1995) Mechanisms of hepatocarcinogenicity of peroxisome-proliferating drugs and chemicals. *Annu. Rev. Pharmacol. Toxicol.*, **35**, 483–507

Lalwani, N.D., Reddy, M.K., Qureshi, S.A., Sirtori, C.R., Abiko, Y. & Reddy, J.K. (1983) Evaluation of selected hypolipidemic agents for the induction of peroxisomal enzymes and peroxisome proliferation in the rat liver. *Human Toxicol.*, **2**, 27–48

Larsen, M.L., Illingworth, D.R. & O'Malley, J.P. (1994) Comparative effects of gemfibrozil and clofibrate in type III hyperlipoproteinemia. *Atherosclerosis*, **106**, 235–240

Lee, S.S.-T., Pineau, T., Drago, J., Lee, E.J., Owens, J.W., Kroetz, D.L., Fernandez-Salguero, P.M., Westphal, H. & Gonzalez, F.J. (1995) Targeted disruption of the α isoform of the peroxisome proliferator-activated receptor gene in mice results in abolishment of the pleiotropic effects of peroxisome proliferators. *Mol. cell. Biol.*, **15**, 3012–3022

Leiss, O., von Bergmann, K., Gnasso, A. & Augustin, J. (1985) Effect of gemfibrozil on biliary lipid metabolism in normolipemic subjects. *Metabolism*, **34**, 74–82

Magarian, G.J., Lucas, L.M. & Colley, C. (1991) Gemfibrozil-induced myopathy. *Arch. intern. Med.*, **151**, 1873–1874

Manninen, V., Elo, M.O., Frick, M.H., Haapa, K., Heinonen, O.P., Heinsalmi, P., Helo, P., Huttunen, J.K., Kaitaniemi, P., Koskinen, P., Mäenpää, H., Mälkönen, M., Mänttäri, M., Norola, S., Pasternack, A., Pikkarainen, J., Romo, M., Sjöblom, T. & Nikkilä, E.A. (1988) Lipid alterations and decline in the incidence of coronary heart disease in the Helsinki Heart Study. *J. Am. med. Assoc.*, **260**, 641–651

McGuire, E.J., Lucas, J.A., Gray, R.H. & de la Iglesia, F.A. (1991) Peroxisome induction potential and lipid-regulating activity in rats. Quantitative microscopy and chemical structure-activity relationships. *Am. J. Pathol.*, **139**, 217–229

Medical Economics (1996) *PDR®: Physicians' Desk Reference*, 50th Ed., Montvale, NJ, Medical Economics Data Production Co., pp. 1917–1919

Miller, M., Bachorik, P.S., McCrindle, B.W. & Kwiterovich, P.O., Jr (1993) Effect of gemfibrozil in men with primary isolated low high-density lipoprotein cholesterol: a randomized double-blind, placebo-controlled, crossover study. *Am. J. Med.*, **94**, 7–12

Nakagawa, A., Shigeta, A., Iwabuchi, H., Horiguchi, M., Nakamura, K.-I. & Takahagi, H. (1991) Simultaneous determination of gemfibrozil and its metabolites in plasma and urine by a fully automated high performance liquid chromatographic system. *Biomed. Chromatogr.*, **5**, 68–73

Okerholm, R.A., Keeley, F.J., Peterson, F.E. & Glazko, A.J. (1976) The metabolism of gemfibrozil. *Proc. R. Soc. Med.*, **69** (Suppl. 2), 11–14

Olivier, P., Plancke, M.O., Marzin, D., Clavey, V., Sauzieres, J. & Fruchart, J.C. (1988) Effects of fenofibrate, gemfibrozil and nicotinic acid on plasma lipoprotein levels in normal and hyperlipidemic mice. *Atherosclerosis*, **70**, 107–114

Pizzaro, S., Bargay, J. & D'Agosto, P. (1990) Gemfibrozil-induced impotence (Letter to the Editor). *Lancet*, **336**, 1135

Randinitis, E.J., Kinkel, A.W., Nelson, C. & Parker, T.D., III (1984) Gas chromatographic determination of gemfibrozil and its metabolites in plasma and urine. *J. Chromatogr.*, **307**, 210–215

Randinitis, E.J., Parker, T.D., III & Kinkel, A.W. (1986) Liquid chromatographic determination of gemfibrozil and its metabolites in plasma. *J. Chromatogr.*, **383**, 444–448

Reynolds, J.E.F., ed. (1993) *Martindale: The Extra Pharmacopoeia*, 30th Ed., London, The Pharmaceutical Press, pp. 989–990

Saku, K., Gartside, P.S., Hynd, B.A. & Kashyap, M.L. (1985) Mechanism of action of gemfibrozil on lipoprotein metabolism. *J. clin. Invest.*, **75**, 1702–1712

Sausen, P.J., Teets, V.J., Voss, K.S., Miller, R.T. & Cattley, R.C. (1995) Gemofibrozil-induced peroxisome proliferation and hepatomegaly in male F344 rats. *Cancer Lett.*, **97**, 263–268

Schwandt, P. (1991) Fibrates and triglyceride metabolism. *Eur. J. clin. Pharmacol.*, **40** (Suppl. 1), S41–S43

Smith, D.A., Karmally, W. & Brown, W.V. (1987) Treating hyperlipidemia, Part III: drug therapy. *Geriatrics*, **42**, 55–62

Tugwood, J.D., Aldridge, T.C., Lambe, K.G., Macdonald, N. & Woodyatt, N.J. (1996) Peroxisome proliferator-activated receptors — Structures and function. *Ann. N.Y. Acad. Sci.* (in press)

United States Pharmacopeial Convention (1994) *The 1995 US Pharmacopeia*, 23rd rev./*The National Formulary*, 18th rev., Rockville, MD, pp. 701–702

Vega, G.L. & Grundy, S.M. (1985) Gemfibrozil therapy in primary hypertriglyceridemia associated with coronary heart disease. Effects on metabolism of low-density lipoproteins. *J. Am. med. Assoc.*, **253**, 2398–2403

Vidal (1994) *Dictionnaire Vidal*, 70th Ed., Paris, Editions du Vidal, pp. 819–820

Vidal (1995) *Dictionnaire Vidal*, 71st Ed., Paris, Editions du Vidal, pp. 838–839

Vogt, H.B. (1991) Hyperlipoproteinemias: Part IV: Drug regimens. *S. Dakota J. Med.*, **44**, 117–120

Wilkes, H.C., Meade, T.W., Barzegar, S., Foley, A.J., Hughes, L.O., Bauer, K.A., Rosenberg, R.D. & Miller, G.J. (1992) Gemfibrozil reduces plasma prothrombin fragment F_{1+2} concentration, a marker of coagulability, in patients with coronary heart disease. *Thromb. Haemost.*, **67**, 503–506

Wysowski, D.K., Kennedy, D.L. & Gross, T.P. (1990) Prescribed use of cholesterol-lowering drugs in the United States, 1978 through 1988. *J. Am. med. Assoc.*, **263**, 2185–2188

Zimetbaum, P., Frishman, W.H. & Kahn, S. (1991) Effects of gemfibrozil and other fibric acid derivatives on blood lipids and lipoproteins. *J. clin. Pharmacol.*, **31**, 25–37

SUMMARY OF FINAL EVALUATIONS

Agent	Degree of evidence of carcinogenicity		Overall evaluation of carcinogenicity to humans
	Human	Animal	
Clofibrate	I	L	3
Diazepam	ESL (breast cancer)	I	3
	I (other sites)		
Doxefazepam	I	L	3
Droloxifene	I	I	3
Estazolam	I	ESL	3
Gemfibrozil	I	L	3
Oxazepam	I	S	2B
Phenytoin	I	S	2B
Prazepam	I	I	3
Rifazepam	I	L	3
Tamoxifen	S* (endometrial cancer)	S	1*
	I (other sites)		
Temazepam	I	I	3
Toremifene	I	I	3

I, inadequate evidence; L, limited evidence; ESL, evidence suggesting lack of carcinogenicity; S, sufficient evidence; for definitions of criteria for degrees of evidence and groups, see preamble, pp. 22–25.

*and there is conclusive evidence that tamoxifen reduces the risk of contralateral breast cancer.

Glossary

Adjuvant therapy

Therapy given in addition to or following surgery or other primary therapy to reduce the risk of recurrence

Antiarrhythmic drug

Drug given to combat irregularity of heartbeat, classified according to mechanism of action:
- Class I: Sodium channel blockade
    A. Moderate phase-0 depression and slow conduction (2+); usually prolong repolarization
    B. Minimal phase-0 depression and slow conduction (0 to 1+); usually shorten repolarization
    C. Marked phase-0 depression and slow conduction (3+ to 4+); little effect on repolarization
- Class II: β-adrenergic blockade
- Class III: Prolong repolarization
- Class IV: Ca^{2+}-channel blockade

Axillary node-positive

Axillary lymph node involvement in breast cancer patients. Following apparently curative surgery for the primary tumour, the strongest prognostic indicator of recurrence or death from breast cancer is histological involvement of axillary nodes at surgery.

Hyperlipidaemia (also referred to as hyperlipaemia or lipaemia)

The presence of abnormally large amounts of lipid in the circulating blood. Primary hyperlipidaemia may be classified according to the genetic and metabolic disorder, resulting in the following categories:

Familial hypercholesteroluemia, which is usually heterozygous but very rarely may be homozygous, is characterized by a type IIa pattern (see hyperlipoproteinaemia) but occasionally a type IIb pattern may be present;

Familial hypertriglyceridaemia is usually associated with a type IV or type V pattern;

Familial combined hyperlipidaemia may be characterized by elevated cholesterol only, elevated triglyceride only or elevated cholesterol and triglyceride, and type IIa, type IV or type IIb patterns may be found;

Familial dysbetalipoproteinaemia (remnant hyperlipoproteinaemia or broad-β disease) shows the type III pattern;

Lipoprotein lipase deficiency or *apolipoprotein C-II deficiency* show a type I or type V pattern.

Hyperlipoproteinaemia

An increase in the lipoprotein concentration of the blood. The classification proposed by WHO (1970) is based solely on the patterns of the particular lipoproteins that are elevated; it reflects neither clinical status nor genetic or metabolic characteristics and should not be used as a diagnostic classification.

Type I (hyperchylomicronaemia) is characterized by the presence of chylomicrons and by normal or only slightly increased concentrations of very low-density lipoproteins (VLDLs);

Type IIa (hyper-β-lipoproteinaemia) is characterized by an elevation in the concentration of low-density lipoproteins (LDLs);

Type IIb is characterized by an elevation in the concentration of LDLs and VLDLs;

Type III ('floating β' or 'broad β' pattern) is characterized by the presence of VLDLs having an abnormally high cholesterol content and an abnormal electrophoretic mobility;

Type IV (hyperpre-β-lipoproteinaemia) is characterized by an elevation in the concentration of VLDLs, by no increase in the concentration of LDLs and by the absence of chylomicrons;

Type V (hyperpre-β-lipoproteinaemia and chylomicronaemia) is characterized by an elevation in the concentration of VLDLs and the presence of chylomicrons.

Lipoproteins

Water- (or plasma-) soluble complexes or compounds of lipids with proteins

Chylomicrons (from the intestine) and **very low-density lipoproteins** (VLDLs; produced in the liver) are composed largely of triglycerides and function to transport triglycerides to tissues for metabolic use or storage. VLDLs contain only 10–15% of total serum cholesterol.

Low-density lipoproteins (LDLs; from intravascular metabolism of VLDLs) and **high-density lipoproteins** (HDLs; from intestine, liver and intravascular metabolism) transport cholesterol, with LDL being the major cholesterol carrying lipoprotein in normal human plasma (60–70% of total serum cholesterol).

Oestrogen and progesterone receptors

Cytoplasmic receptors which can be measured in breast cancer and other cells. Tumours that are oestrogen- or progesterone-receptor-positive are more likely to respond to hormonal therapies such as tamoxifen or other anti-oestrogens

GLOSSARY

Phase I trial

A trial in which a pharmaceutical is given for the first time to humans. The aim of a phase I trial is to determine the maximal tolerated dose of a drug and to describe its toxicity. Such a trial is usually done in a group of patients whose disease has failed to respond to all standard therapy.

Phase II trial

A trial in which a drug which has already passed through phase I testing is tested to determine its degree of activity.

Phase III trial

A randomized comparative trial in which two drugs or therapies are compared. This may be carried out for patients with metastatic disease, or in the adjuvant setting.

Recurrence

After surgical removal or other therapy for cancer, there may be no visible or measurable disease (by X-ray, clinical or other means) if a tumour then reappears, either at the site of the original primary or elsewhere, this constitutes a recurrence.

Response

In cancer patients, this is generally defined as a shrinkage of a measurable tumour by $\geq 50\%$ (partial response) or a complete disappearance of all measurable or visible tumour (complete response).

Reference

WHO (1970) Classification of hyperlipidaemias and hyperlipoproteinaemias. *Bull. WHO*, **43**, 891–915

APPENDIX 1

SUMMARY TABLES OF
GENETIC AND RELATED EFFECTS

APPENDIX 1

Summary table of genetic and related effects of diazepam

Non-mammalian systems				Mammalian systems			
Prokaryotes	Lower eukaryotes	Plants	Insects	In vitro		In vivo	
				Animal cells	Human cells	Animals	Humans
D G	D R G A	D G C	R G C A	D G S M C A T I	D G S M C A T I	D G S M C DL A	D S M C A
– –	– – – –			– – + ? + +	–¹ + + – ? –¹	–¹ ? – ? ?ª	? –¹ ? +¹

A, aneuploidy; C, chromosomal aberrations; D, DNA damage; DL, dominant lethal mutation; G, gene mutation; I, inhibition of intercellular communication; M, micronuclei; R, mitotic recombination and gene conversion; S, sister chromatid exchange; T, cell transformation

In completing the table, the following symbols indicate the consensus of the Working Group with regard to the results for each end-point:

+ considered to be positive for the specific end-point and level of biological complexity
+¹ considered to be positive, but only one valid study was available to the Working Group
– considered to be negative
–¹ considered to be negative, but only one valid study was available to the Working Group
? considered to be equivocal or inconclusive (e.g. there were contradictory results from different laboratories; there were confounding exposures; the results were equivocal)

ªSomatic cell, –; germ cells: sperm, +; oocyte, –

Summary table of genetic and related effects of doxefazepam

Non-mammalian systems				Mammalian systems			
Proka-ryotes	Lower eukaryotes	Plants	Insects	In vitro		In vivo	
				Animal cells	Human cells	Animals	Humans
D G	D R G A	D G C	R G C A	D G S M C A T I	D G S M C A T I	D G S M C DL A	D S M C A
– –	– –					– – –	

A, aneuploidy; C, chromosomal aberrations; D, DNA damage; DL, dominant lethal mutation; G, gene mutation; I, inhibition of intercellular communication; M, micronuclei; R, mitotic recombination and gene conversion; S, sister chromatid exchange; T, cell transformation

In completing the table, the following symbols indicate the consensus of the Working Group with regard to the results for each end-point:

+ considered to be positive for the specific end-point and level of biological complexity
+¹ considered to be positive, but only one valid study was available to the Working Group
– considered to be negative
–¹ considered to be negative, but only one valid study was available to the Working Group
? considered to be equivocal or inconclusive (e.g. there were contradictory results from different laboratories; there were confounding exposures; the results were equivocal)

APPENDIX 1

Summary table of genetic and related effects of estazolam

Non-mammalian systems				Mammalian systems			
				In vitro		*In vivo*	
Proka-ryotes	Lower eukaryotes	Plants	Insects	Animal cells	Human cells	Animals	Humans
D G	D R G A	D G C	R G C A	D G S M C A T I	D G S M C A T I	D G S M C DL A	D S M C A
–¹						–¹ –¹ –¹	

A, aneuploidy; C, chromosomal aberrations; D, DNA damage; DL, dominant lethal mutation; G, gene mutation; I, inhibition of intercellular communication; M, micronuclei; R, mitotic recombination and gene conversion; S, sister chromatid exchange; T, cell transformation

In completing the table, the following symbols indicate the consensus of the Working Group with regard to the results for each end-point:

+   considered to be positive for the specific end-point and level of biological complexity
+¹ considered to be positive, but only one valid study was available to the Working Group
–   considered to be negative
–¹ considered to be negative, but only one valid study was available to the Working Group
?   considered to be equivocal or inconclusive (e.g. there were contradictory results from different laboratories; there were confounding exposures; the results were equivocal)

Summary table of genetic and related effects of oxazepam

Non-mammalian systems				Mammalian systems			
Proka-ryotes	Lower eukaryotes	Plants	Insects	In vitro		In vivo	
				Animal cells	Human cells	Animals	Humans
D G	D R G A	D G C	R G C A	D G S M C A T I	D G S M C A T I	D G S M C DL A	D S M C A
– –	– – – –	– – –		– – – +¹ +¹	+¹ +¹ +¹	– – – –¹ –¹	

A, aneuploidy; C, chromosomal aberrations; D, DNA damage; DL, dominant lethal mutation; G, gene mutation; I, inhibition of intercellular communication; M, micronuclei; R, mitotic recombination and gene conversion; S, sister chromatid exchange; T, cell transformation

In completing the table, the following symbols indicate the consensus of the Working Group with regard to the results for each end-point:

+ considered to be positive for the specific end-point and level of biological complexity
+¹ considered to be positive, but only one valid study was available to the Working Group
– considered to be negative
–¹ considered to be negative, but only one valid study was available to the Working Group
? considered to be equivocal or inconclusive (e.g. there were contradictory results from different laboratories; there were confounding exposures; the results were equivocal)

APPENDIX 1

Summary table of genetic and related effects of prazepam

Non-mammalian systems				Mammalian systems			
Prokaryotes	Lower eukaryotes	Plants	Insects	In vitro		In vivo	
				Animal cells	Human cells	Animals	Humans
D G	D R G A	D G C	R G C A	D G S M C A T I	D G S M C A T I	D G S M C DL A	D S M C A
	–¹					–¹	

A, aneuploidy; C, chromosomal aberrations; D, DNA damage; DL, dominant lethal mutation; G, gene mutation; I, inhibition of intercellular communication; M, micronuclei; R, mitotic recombination and gene conversion; S, sister chromatid exchange; T, cell transformation

In completing the table, the following symbols indicate the consensus of the Working Group with regard to the results for each end-point:

+ considered to be positive for the specific end-point and level of biological complexity
+¹ considered to be positive, but only one valid study was available to the Working Group
– considered to be negative
–¹ considered to be negative, but only one valid study was available to the Working Group
? considered to be equivocal or inconclusive (e.g. there were contradictory results from different laboratories; there were confounding exposures; the results were equivocal)

Summary table of genetic and related effects of temazepam

Non-mammalian systems				Mammalian systems			
Proka-ryotes	Lower eukaryotes	Plants	Insects	In vitro			In vivo
				Animal cells	Human cells		Animals	Humans
D G	D R G A	D G C	R G C A	D G S M C A T I	D G S M C A T I		D G S M C DL A	D S M C A
	–						–[1]	

A, aneuploidy; C, chromosomal aberrations; D, DNA damage; DL, dominant lethal mutation; G, gene mutation; I, inhibition of intercellular communication; M, micronuclei; R, mitotic recombination and gene conversion; S, sister chromatid exchange; T, cell transformation

In completing the table, the following symbols indicate the consensus of the Working Group with regard to the results for each end-point:

+   considered to be positive for the specific end-point and level of biological complexity
+[1]   considered to be positive, but only one valid study was available to the Working Group
–   considered to be negative
–[1] considered to be negative, but only one valid study was available to the Working Group
?   considered to be equivocal or inconclusive (e.g. there were contradictory results from different laboratories; there were confounding exposures; the results were equivocal)

Summary table of genetic and related effects of phenytoin

Non-mammalian systems				Mammalian systems			
Proka- ryotes	Lower eukaryotes	Plants	Insects	In vitro		In vivo	
				Animal cells	Human cells	Animals	Humans
D G	D R G A	D G C	R G C A	D G S M C A T I	D G S M C A T I	D G S M C DL A	D S M C A
–			–	– – – –⁺¹ – ⁺ ⁺ ⁺	⁺¹ ? ? ⁺¹	– ? – ⁺¹ ?	? – – –

A, aneuploidy; C, chromosomal aberrations; D, DNA damage; DL, dominant lethal mutation; G, gene mutation; I, inhibition of intercellular communication; M, micronuclei; R, mitotic recombination and gene conversion; S, sister chromatid exchange; T, cell transformation

In completing the table, the following symbols indicate the consensus of the Working Group with regard to the results for each end-point:

+ considered to be positive for the specific end-point and level of biological complexity
+¹ considered to be positive, but only one valid study was available to the Working Group
– considered to be negative
–¹ considered to be negative, but only one valid study was available to the Working Group
? considered to be equivocal or inconclusive (e.g. there were contradictory results from different laboratories; there were confounding exposures; the results were equivocal)

Summary table of genetic and related effects of droloxifene

Non-mammalian systems				Mammalian systems			
Proka-ryotes	Lower eukaryotes	Plants	Insects	In vitro		In vivo	
				Animal cells	Human cells	Animals	Humans
D G	D R G A	D G C	R G C A	D G S M C A T I	D G S M C A T I	D G S M C DL A	D S M C A
				–¹		–¹	

A, aneuploidy; C, chromosomal aberrations; D, DNA damage; DL, dominant lethal mutation; G, gene mutation; I, inhibition of intercellular communication; M, micronuclei; R, mitotic recombination and gene conversion; S, sister chromatid exchange; T, cell transformation

In completing the table, the following symbols indicate the consensus of the Working Group with regard to the results for each end-point:

+ considered to be positive for the specific end-point and level of biological complexity
+¹ considered to be positive, but only one valid study was available to the Working Group
– considered to be negative
–¹ considered to be negative, but only one valid study was available to the Working Group
? considered to be equivocal or inconclusive (e.g. there were contradictory results from different laboratories; there were confounding exposures; the results were equivocal)

APPENDIX 1

Summary table of genetic and related effects of tamoxifen

Non-mammalian systems				Mammalian systems			
Proka-ryotes	Lower eukaryotes	Plants	Insects	In vitro		In vivo	
				Animal cells	Human cells	Animals	Humans
D G	D R G A	D G C	R G C A	D G S M C A T I	D G S M C A T I	D G S M C DL A	D S M C A
				$-$ $+^1$	$+$	$+$ $+^1$ $+^1$	$-$

A, aneuploidy; C, chromosomal aberrations; D, DNA damage; DL, dominant lethal mutation; G, gene mutation; I, inhibition of intercellular communication; M, micronuclei; R, mitotic recombination and gene conversion; S, sister chromatid exchange; T, cell transformation

In completing the table, the following symbols indicate the consensus of the Working Group with regard to the results for each end-point:

+ considered to be positive for the specific end-point and level of biological complexity
$+^1$ considered to be positive, but only one valid study was available to the Working Group
− considered to be negative
$−^1$ considered to be negative, but only one valid study was available to the Working Group
? considered to be equivocal or inconclusive (e.g.: there were contradictory results from different laboratories; there were confounding exposures; the results were equivocal)

461

Summary table of genetic and related effects of toremifene

Non-mammalian systems				Mammalian systems			
Proka-ryotes	Lower eukaryotes	Plants	Insects	In vitro			In vivo
				Animal cells	Human cells	Animals	Humans
D G	D R G A	D G C	R G C A	D G S M C A T I	D G S M C A T I	D G S M C DL A	D S M C A
					+[-] +	?	

A, aneuploidy; C, chromosomal aberrations; D, DNA damage; DL, dominant lethal mutation; G, gene mutation; I, inhibition of intercellular communication; M, micronuclei; R, mitotic recombination and gene conversion; S, sister chromatid exchange; T, cell transformation

In completing the table, the following symbols indicate the consensus of the Working Group with regard to the results for each end-point:

+   considered to be positive for the specific end-point and level of biological complexity
+[-]   considered to be positive, but only one valid study was available to the Working Group
−   considered to be negative
−[-]   considered to be negative, but only one valid study was available to the Working Group
?   considered to be equivocal or inconclusive (e.g. there were contradictory results from different laboratories; there were confounding exposures; the results were equivocal)

APPENDIX 1

Summary table of genetic and related effects of clofibrate

Non-mammalian systems				Mammalian systems			
				In vitro			*In vivo*
Proka-ryotes	Lower eukaryotes	Plants	Insects	Animal cells	Human cells	Animals	Humans
D G	D R G A	D G C	R G C A	D G S M C A T I	D G S M C A T I	D G S M C DL A	D S M C A
– –	–			– – – – – ?		– – – – – –	

A, aneuploidy; C, chromosomal aberrations; D, DNA damage; DL, dominant lethal mutation; G, gene mutation; I, inhibition of intercellular communication; M, micronuclei; R, mitotic recombination and gene conversion; S, sister chromatid exchange; T, cell transformation

In completing the table, the following symbols indicate the consensus of the Working Group with regard to the results for each end-point:

+ considered to be positive for the specific end-point and level of biological complexity
+¹ considered to be positive, but only one valid study was available to the Working Group
– considered to be negative
–¹ considered to be negative, but only one valid study was available to the Working Group
? considered to be equivocal or inconclusive (e.g. there were contradictory results from different laboratories; there were confounding exposures; the results were equivocal)

Summary table of genetic and related effects of gemfibrozil

Non-mammalian systems				Mammalian systems			
Proka-ryotes	Lower eukaryotes	Plants	Insects	In vitro		In vivo	
				Animal cells	Human cells	Animals	Humans
D G	D R G A	D G C	R G C A	D G S M C A T I	D G S M C A T I	D G S M C DL A	D S M C A
$-^1$							

A, aneuploidy; C, chromosomal aberrations; D, DNA damage; DL, dominant lethal mutation; G, gene mutation; I, inhibition of intercellular communication; M, micronuclei; R, mitotic recombination and gene conversion; S, sister chromatid exchange; T, cell transformation

In completing the table, the following symbols indicate the consensus of the Working Group with regard to the results for each end-point:

+   considered to be positive for the specific end-point and level of biological complexity
+^{1} considered to be positive, but only one valid study was available to the Working Group
−   considered to be negative
−^{1} considered to be negative, but only one valid study was available to the Working Group
?   considered to be equivocal or inconclusive (e.g. there were contradictory results from different laboratories; there were confounding exposures; the results were equivocal)

APPENDIX 2

ACTIVITY PROFILES FOR GENETIC AND RELATED EFFECTS

APPENDIX 2

ACTIVITY PROFILES FOR GENETIC AND RELATED EFFECTS

Methods

The x-axis of the activity profile (Waters *et al.*, 1987, 1988) represents the bioassays in phylogenetic sequence by end-point, and the values on the y-axis represent the logarithmically transformed lowest effective doses (LED) and highest ineffective doses (HID) tested. The term 'dose', as used in this report, does not take into consideration length of treatment or exposure and may therefore be considered synonymous with concentration. In practice, the concentrations used in all the in-vitro tests were converted to µg/ml, and those for in-vivo tests were expressed as mg/kg bw. Because dose units are plotted on a log scale, differences in the relative molecular masses of compounds do not, in most cases, greatly influence comparisons of their activity profiles. Conventions for dose conversions are given below.

Profile-line height (the magnitude of each bar) is a function of the LED or HID, which is associated with the characteristics of each individual test system — such as population size, cell-cycle kinetics and metabolic competence. Thus, the detection limit of each test system is different, and, across a given activity profile, responses will vary substantially. No attempt is made to adjust or relate responses in one test system to those of another.

Line heights are derived as follows: for negative test results, the highest dose tested without appreciable toxicity is defined as the HID. If there was evidence of extreme toxicity, the next highest dose is used. A single dose tested with a negative result is considered to be equivalent to the HID. Similarly, for positive results, the LED is recorded. If the original data were analysed statistically by the author, the dose recorded is that at which the response was significant ($p < 0.05$). If the available data were not analysed statistically, the dose required to produce an effect is estimated as follows: when a dose-related positive response is observed with two or more doses, the lower of the doses is taken as the LED; a single dose resulting in a positive response is considered to be equivalent to the LED.

In order to accommodate both the wide range of doses encountered and positive and negative responses on a continuous scale, doses are transformed logarithmically, so that effective (LED) and ineffective (HID) doses are represented by positive and negative numbers, respectively. The response, or logarithmic dose unit (LDUij), for a given test system i and chemical j is represented by the expressions

$LDU_{ij} = -\log_{10}$ (dose), for HID values; LDU ≤ 0

and (1)

$LDU_{ij} = -\log_{10}$ (dose $\times 10^{-5}$), for LED values; LDU ≥ 0.

These simple relationships define a dose range of 0 to –5 logarithmic units for ineffective doses (1–100 000 µg/mL or mg/kg bw) and 0 to +8 logarithmic units for effective doses (100 000–0.001 µg/mL or mg/kg bw). A scale illustrating the LDU values is shown in Figure 1. Negative responses at doses less than 1 µg/mL (mg/kg bw) are set equal to 1. Effectively, an LED value $\geq$ 100 000 or an HID value $\leq$ 1 produces an LDU = 0; no quantitative information is gained from such extreme values. The dotted lines at the levels of log dose units 1 and –1 define a 'zone of uncertainty' in which positive results are reported at such high doses (between 10 000 and 100 000 mg/mL or mg/kg bw) or negative results are reported at such low doses (1 to 10 mg/ml or mg/kg bw) as to call into question the adequacy of the test.

Fig. 1. Scale of log dose units used on the y-axis of activity profiles

Positive (µg/mL or mg/kg bw)		Log dose units
0.001		8 ----
0.01		7 --
0.1		6 --
1.0		5 --
10		4 --
100		3 --
1000		2 --
10 000		1 --
100 000	1	0 ----
	10	–1 --
	100	–2 --
	1000	–3 --
	10 000	–4 --
	100 000	–5 ----

Negative
(µg/mL or mg/kg bw)

In practice, an activity profile is computer generated. A data entry programme is used to store abstracted data from published reports. A sequential file (in ASCII) is created for each compound, and a record within that file consists of the name and Chemical Abstracts Service number of the compound, a three-letter code for the test system (see below), the qualitative test result (with and without an exogenous metabolic system), dose (LED or HID), citation number and additional source information. An abbreviated citation for each publication is stored in a segment of a record accessing both the test data file and the citation file. During processing of the data file, an average of the logarithmic values of the data subset is calculated, and the length of the profile line represents this average value. All dose values are plotted for each profile line, regardless of whether results are positive or negative. Results obtained in the absence of an exogenous metabolic system are indicated by a bar (–), and results obtained in the presence of an exogenous metabolic system are indicated by an upward-directed arrow (↑). When all results for a given assay are either positive or negative, the mean of the LDU values is plotted as a solid line; when conflicting data are reported for the same assay (i.e. both positive and negative results), the majority data are shown by a solid line and the minority data by a dashed line (drawn to the extreme conflicting response). In the few cases in which the numbers of positive and negative results are equal, the solid line is drawn in the positive direction and the maximal negative response is indicated with a dashed line. Profile lines are identified by three-letter code words representing the commonly used tests. Code words for most of the test systems in current use in genetic toxicology were defined for the US Environmental Protection Agency's GENE-TOX Program (Waters, 1979; Waters & Auletta, 1981). For *IARC Monographs* Supplement 6, Volume 44 and subsequent volumes, including this publication, codes were redefined in a manner that should facilitate inclusion of additional tests. Naming conventions are described below.

Data listings are presented in the text and include end-point and test codes, a short test code definition, results, either with (M) or without (NM) an exogenous activation system, the associated LED or HID value and a short citation. Test codes are organized phylogenetically and by end-point from left to right across each activity profile and from top to bottom of the corresponding data listing. End-points are defined as follows: A, aneuploidy; C, chromosomal aberrations; D, DNA damage; F, assays of body fluids; G, gene mutation; H, host-mediated assays; I, inhibition of intercellular communication; M, micronuclei; P, sperm morphology; R, mitotic recombination or gene conversion; S, sister chromatid exchange; and T, cell transformation.

Dose conversions for activity profiles

Doses are converted to µg/mL for in-vitro tests and to mg/kg bw per day for in-vivo experiments.

1. In-vitro test systems
   (a) Weight/volume converts directly to µg/ml.
   (b) Molar (M) concentration × molecular weight = mg/mL = 10^3 mg/mL; mM concentration × molecular weight = µg/mL.
   (c) Soluble solids expressed as % concentration are assumed to be in units of mass per volume (i.e. 1% = 0.01 g/mL = 10 000 µg/mL; also, 1 ppm = 1 µg/mL).
   (d) Liquids and gases expressed as % concentration are assumed to be given in units of volume per volume. Liquids are converted to weight per volume using the density (D) of the solution (D = g/mL). Gases are converted from volume to mass using the ideal gas law, PV = nRT. For exposure at 20–37 °C at standard

atmospheric pressure, 1% (v/v) = 0.4 µg/ml × molecular weight of the gas. Also, 1 ppm (v/v) = 4 × 10^5 µg/mL × molecular weight.

(e) In microbial plate tests, it is usual for the doses to be reported as weight/plate, whereas concentrations are required to enter data on the activity profile chart. While remaining cognisant of the errors involved in the process, it is assumed that a 2-ml volume of top agar is delivered to each plate and that the test substance remains in solution within it; concentrations are derived from the reported weight/plate values by dividing by this arbitrary volume. For spot tests, a 1-ml volume is used in the calculation.

(f) Conversion of particulate concentrations given in µg/cm^2 is based on the area (A) of the dish and the volume of medium per dish; i.e. for a 100-mm dish: $A = \pi R^2 = \pi \times (5 \text{ cm})^2 = 78.5 \text{ cm}^2$. If the volume of medium is 10 mL, then 78.5 cm^2 = 10 mL and 1 cm^2 = 0.13 mL.

2. In-vitro systems using in-vivo activation

For the body fluid-urine (BF-) test, the concentration used is the dose (in mg/kg bw) of the compound administered to test animals or patients.

3. In-vivo test systems

(a) Doses are converted to mg/kg bw per day of exposure, assuming 100% absorption. Standard values are used for each sex and species of rodent, including body weight and average intake per day, as reported by Gold *et al.* (1984). For example, in a test using male mice fed 50 ppm of the agent in the diet, the standard food intake per day is 12% of body weight, and the conversion is dose = 50 ppm × 12% = 6 mg/kg bw per day.

Standard values used for humans are: weight—males, 70 kg; females, 55 kg; surface area, 1.7 m^2; inhalation rate, 20 L/min for light work, 30 L/min for mild exercise.

(b) When reported, the dose at the target site is used. For example, doses given in studies of lymphocytes of humans exposed *in vivo* are the measured blood concentrations in µg/mL.

Codes for test systems

For specific nonmammalian test systems, the first two letters of the three-symbol code word define the test organism (e.g. SA- for *Salmonella typhimurium*, EC- for *Escherichia coli*). If the species is not known, the convention used is -S-. The third symbol may be used to define the tester strain (e.g. SA8 for *S. typhimurium* TA1538, ECW for *E. coli* WP2*uvr*A). When strain designation is not indicated, the third letter is used to define the specific genetic end-point under investigation (e.g. --D for differential toxicity, --F for forward mutation, --G for gene conversion or genetic crossing-over, --N for aneuploidy, --R for reverse mutation, --U for unscheduled DNA synthesis). The third letter may also be used to define the general end-point under investigation when a more complete definition is not possible or relevant (e.g. --M for mutation, --C for chromosomal aberration). For mammalian test systems, the first letter of the three-letter code word defines the genetic end-point under investigation: A-- for aneuploidy, B-- for binding, C-- for chromosomal aberration, D-- for DNA strand breaks, G-- for gene mutation, I-- for inhibition of intercellular communication, M-- for micronucleus formation, R-- for DNA repair, S-- for sister chromatid exchange, T-- for cell transformation and U-- for unscheduled DNA synthesis.

For animal (i.e. non-human) test systems *in vitro*, when the cell type is not specified, the code letters -IA are used. For such assays *in vivo*, when the animal species is not specified, the code letters -VA are used. Commonly used animal species are identified by the third letter (e.g. --C for Chinese hamster, --M for mouse, --R for rat, --S for Syrian hamster).

For test systems using human cells *in vitro*, when the cell type is not specified, the code letters -IH are used. For assays on humans *in vivo*, when the cell type is not specified, the code letters -VH are used. Otherwise, the second letter specifies the cell type under investigation (e.g. -BH for bone marrow, -LH for lymphocytes).

Some other specific coding conventions used for mammalian systems are as follows: BF- for body fluids, HM- for host-mediated, --L for leukocytes or lymphocytes *in vitro* (-AL, animals; -HL, humans), -L- for leukocytes *in vivo* (-LA, animals; -LH, humans), --T for transformed cells.

Note that these are examples of major conventions used to define the assay code words. The alphabetized listing of codes must be examined to confirm a specific code word. As might be expected from the limitation to three symbols, some codes do not fit the naming conventions precisely. In a few cases, test systems are defined by first-letter code words, for example: MST, mouse spot test; SLP, mouse specific locus mutation, postspermatogonia; SLO, mouse specific locus mutation, other stages; DLM, dominant lethal mutation in mice; DLR, dominant lethal mutation in rats; MHT, mouse heritable translocation.

The genetic activity profiles and listings were prepared in collaboration with Environmental Health Research and Testing Inc. (EHRT) under contract to the United States Environmental Protection Agency; EHRT also determined the doses used. The references cited in each genetic activity profile listing can be found in the list of references in the appropriate monograph.

References

Garrett, N.E., Stack, H.F., Gross, M.R. & Waters, M.D. (1984) An analysis of the spectra of genetic activity produced by known or suspected human carcinogens. *Mutat. Res.*, **134**, 89–111

Gold, L.S., Sawyer, C.B., Magaw, R., Backman, G.M., de Veciana, M., Levinson, R., Hooper, N.K., Havender, W.R., Bernstein, L., Peto, R., Pike, M.C. & Ames, B.N. (1984) A carcinogenic potency database of the standardized results of animal bioassays. *Environ. Health Perspect.*, **58**, 9–319

Waters, M.D. (1979) *The GENE-TOX program*. In: Hsie, A.W., O'Neill, J.P. & McElheny, V.K., eds, *Mammalian Cell Mutagenesis: The Maturation of Test Systems* (Banbury Report 2), Cold Spring Harbor, NY, CSH Press, pp. 449–467

Waters, M.D. & Auletta, A. (1981) The GENE-TOX program: genetic activity evaluation. *J. chem. Inf. comput. Sci.*, **21**, 35–38

Waters, M.D., Stack, H.F., Brady, A.L., Lohman, P.H.M., Haroun, L. & Vainio, H. (1987) Appendix 1: Activity profiles for genetic and related tests. In: *IARC Monographs on the Evaluation of the Carcinogenic Risk of Chemicals to Humans*, Suppl. 6, *Genetic and Related Effects: An Updating of Selected* IARC Monographs *from Volumes 1 to 42*, Lyon, IARC, pp. 687–696

Waters, M.D., Stack, H.F., Brady, A.L., Lohman, P.H.M., Haroun, L. & Vainio, H. (1988) Use of computerized data listings and activity profiles of genetic and related effects in the review of 195 compounds. *Mutat. Res.*, **205**, 295–312

APPENDIX 2

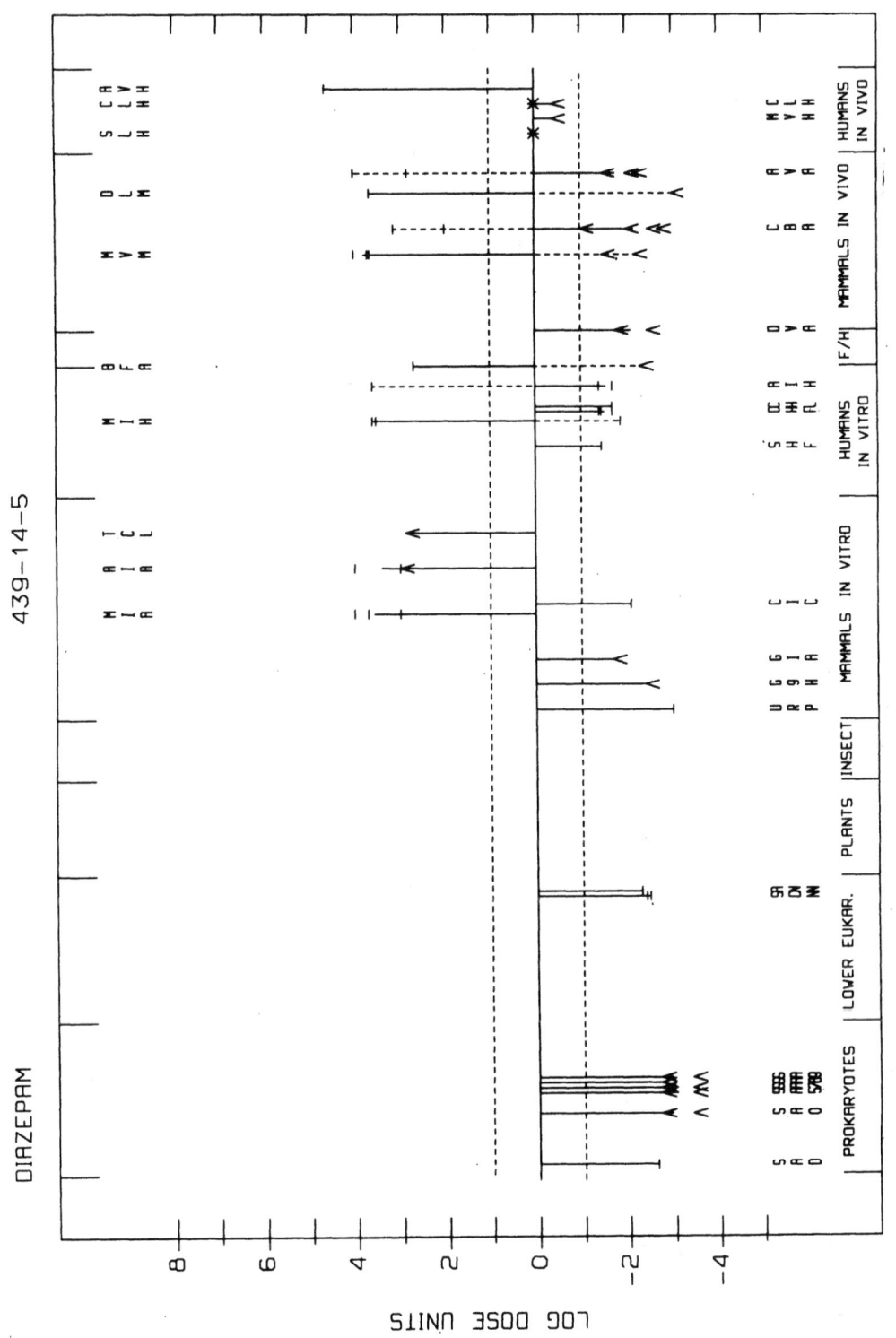

474

IARC MONOGRAPHS VOLUME 66

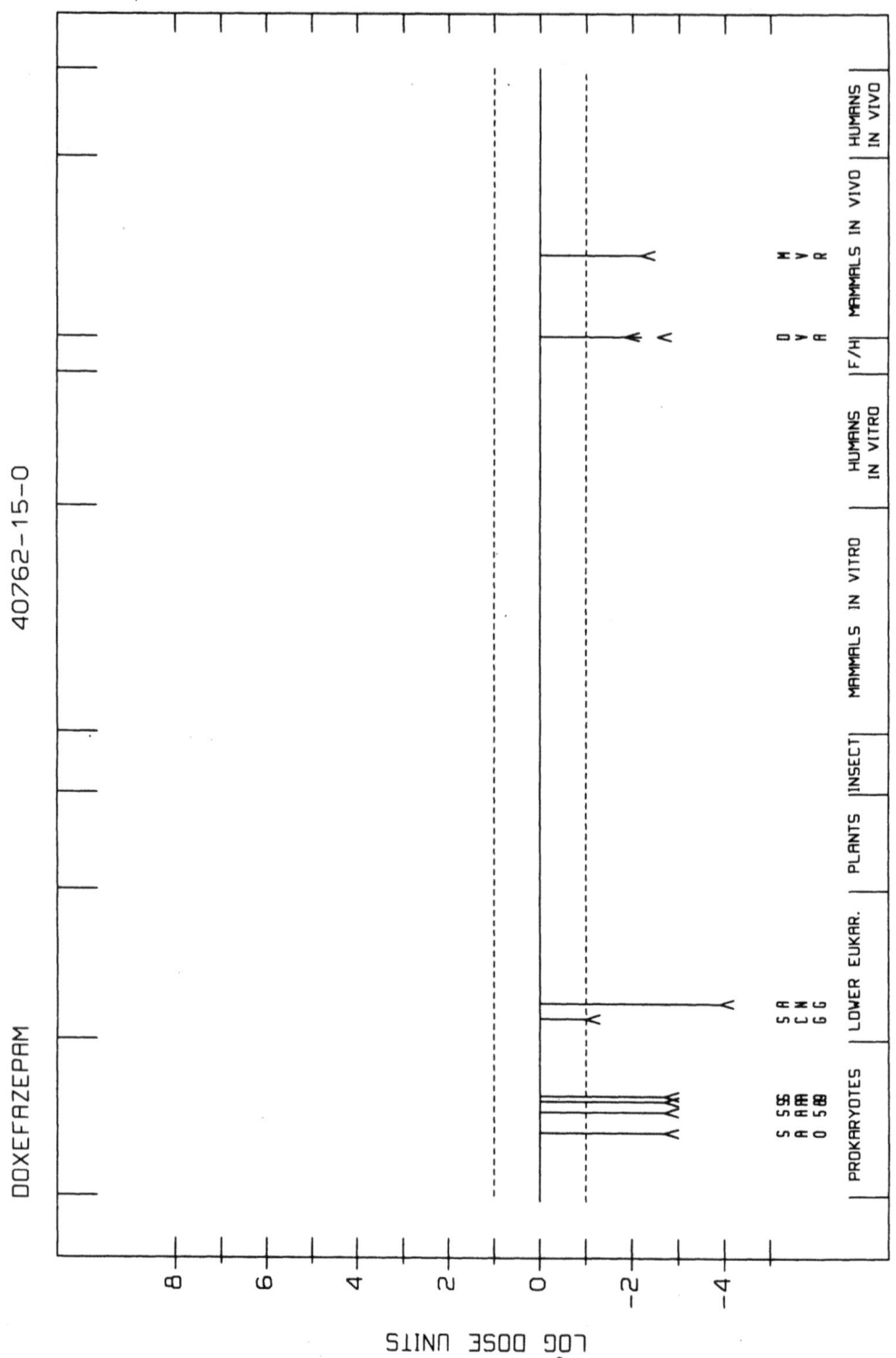

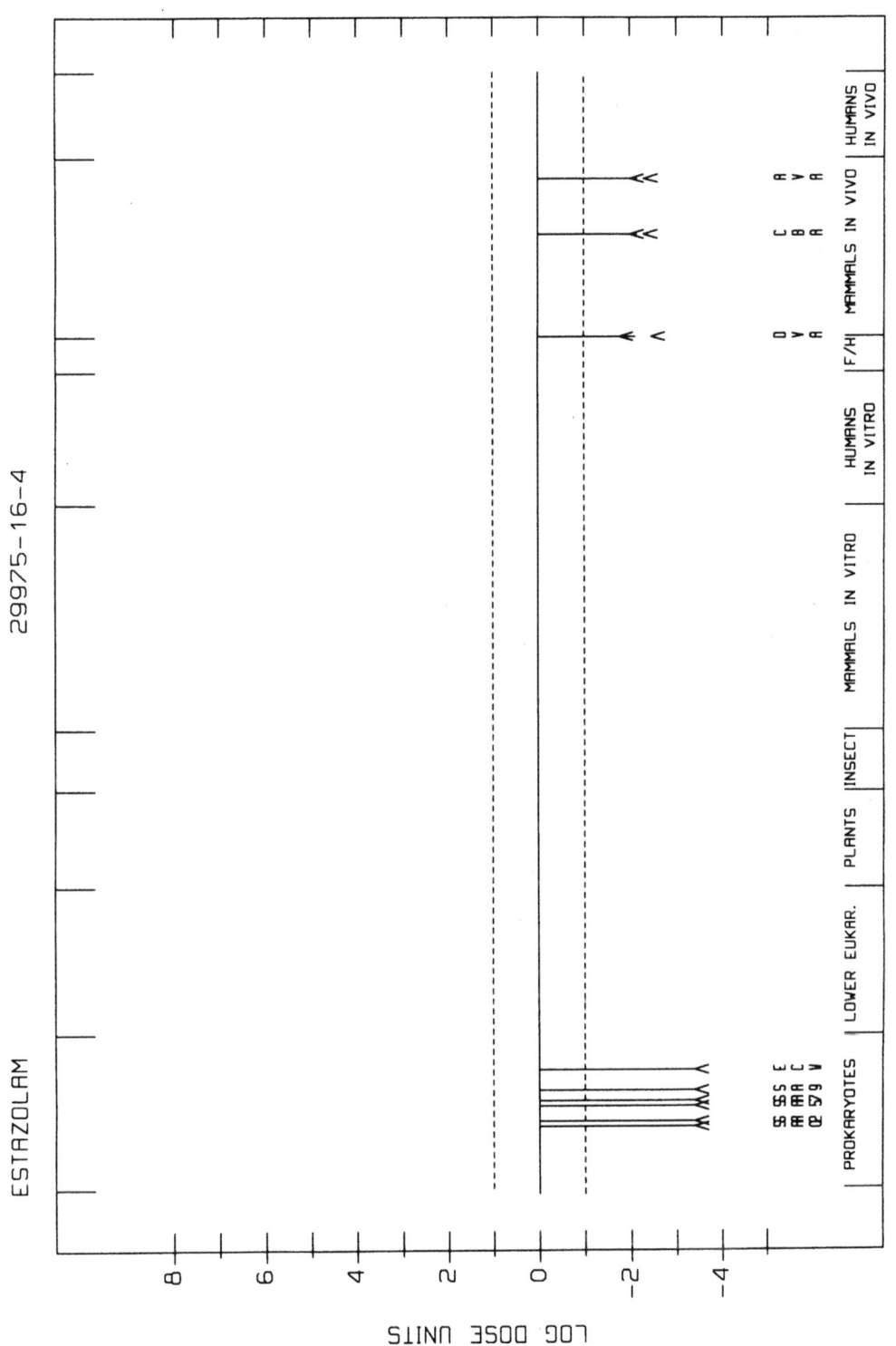

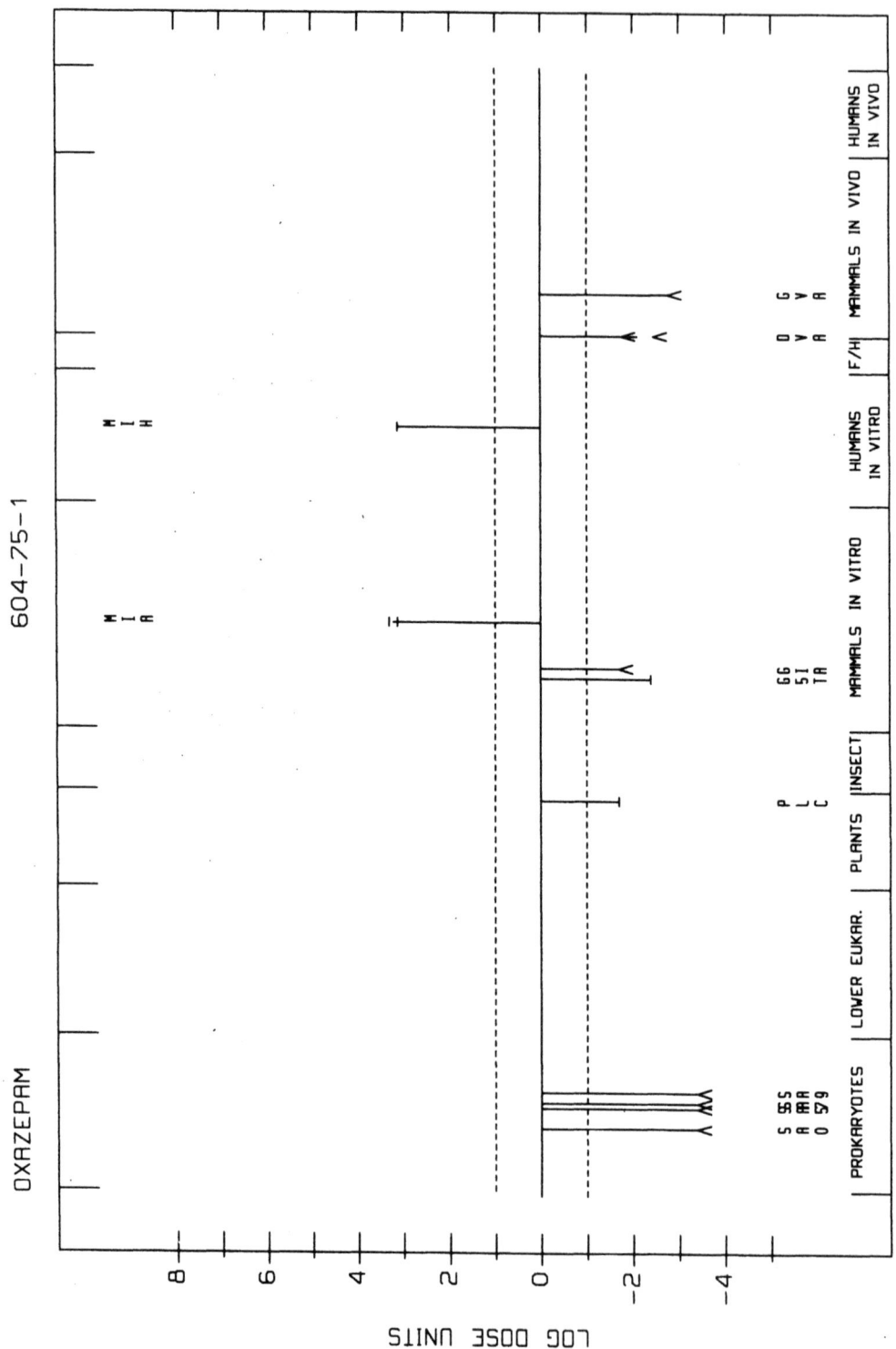

APPENDIX 2

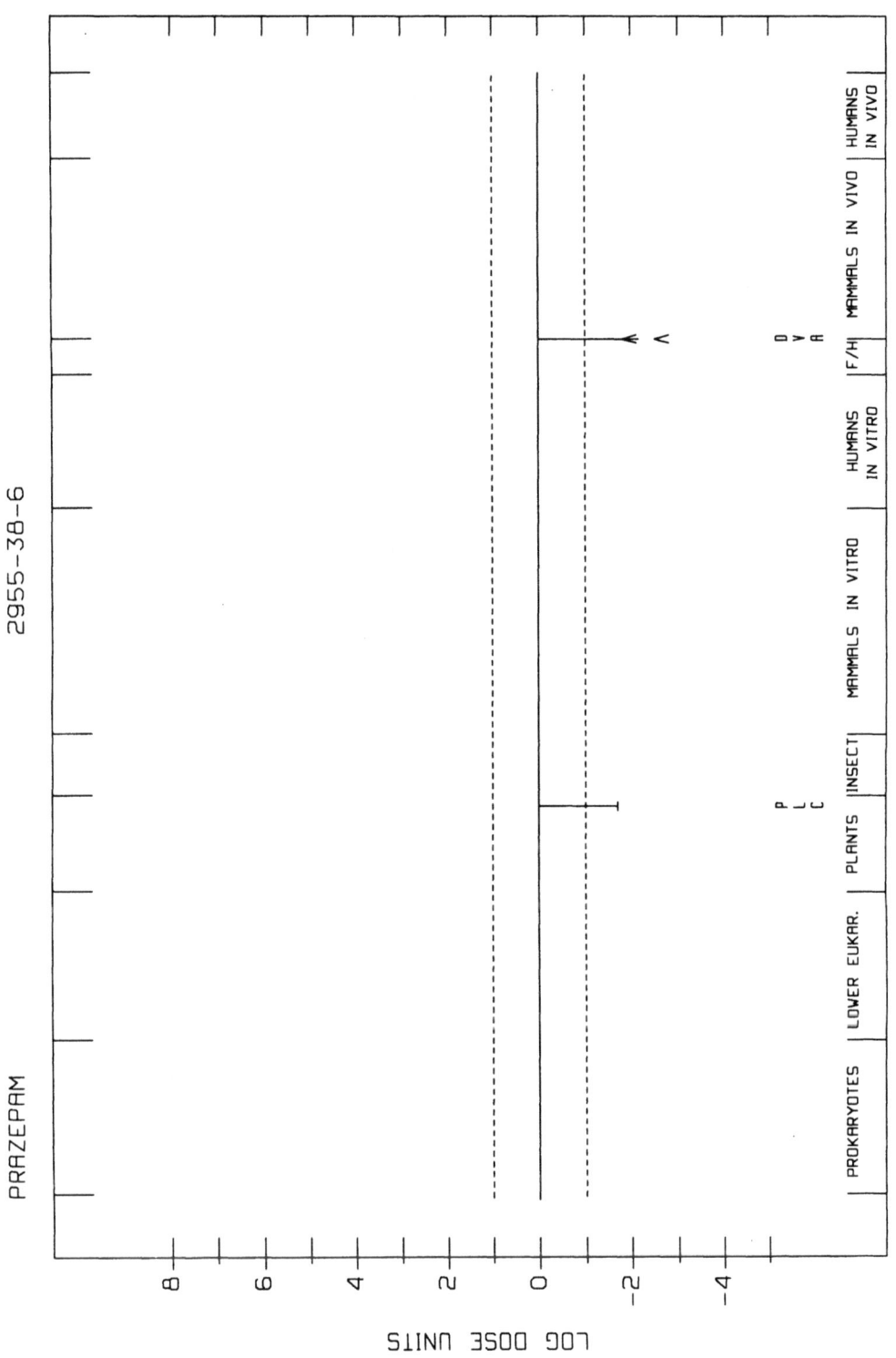

478 IARC MONOGRAPHS VOLUME 66

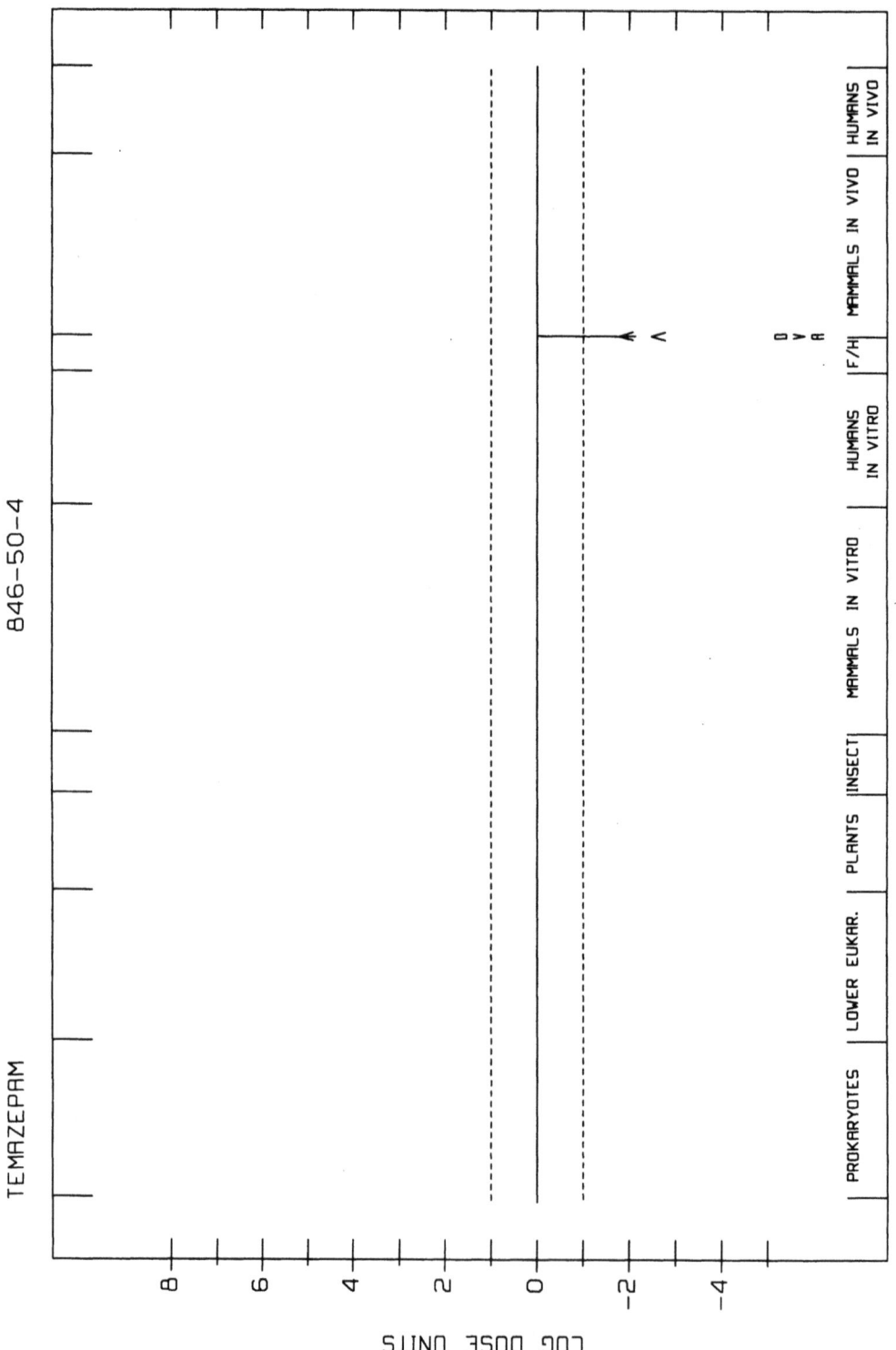

APPENDIX 2

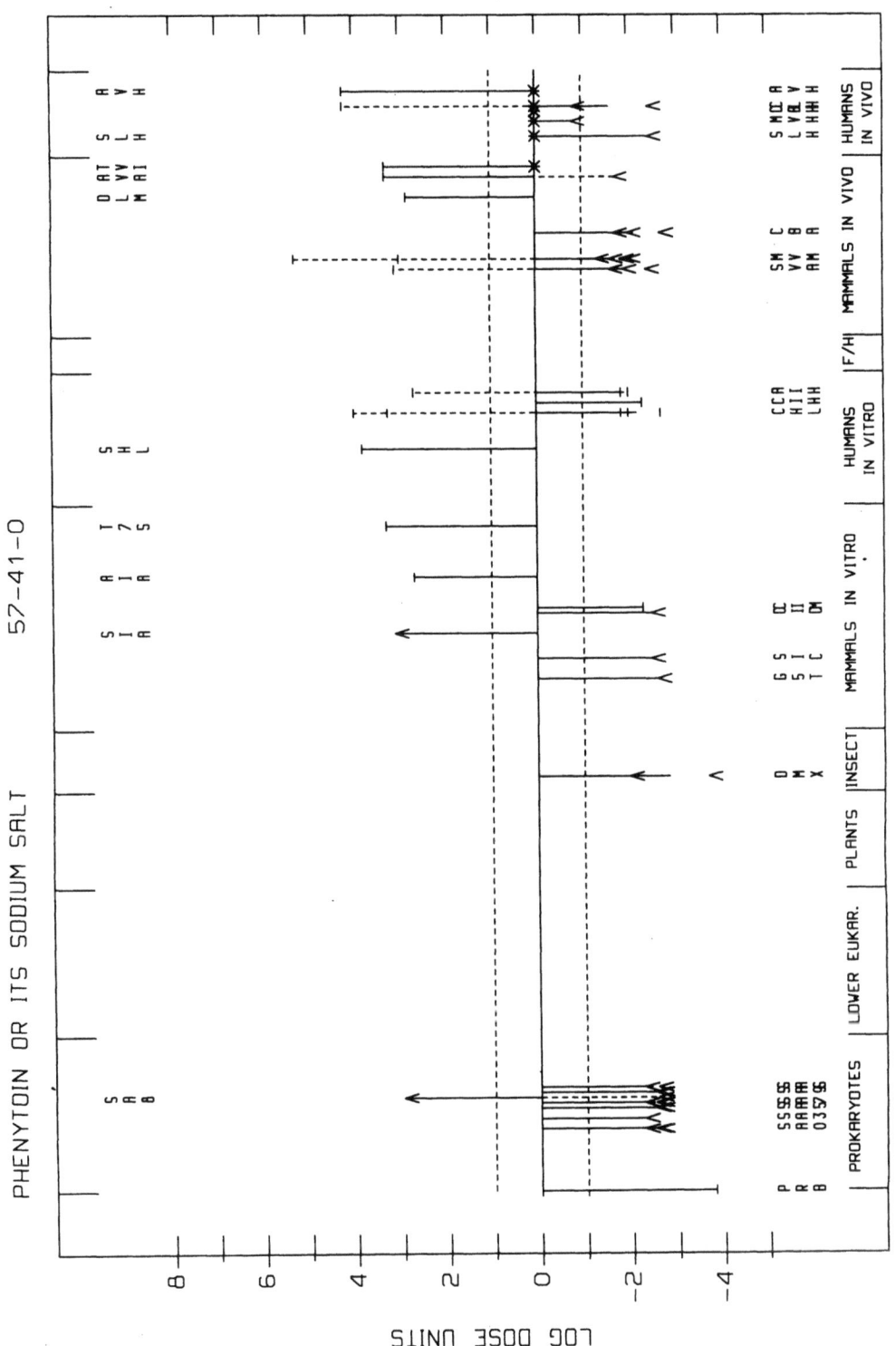

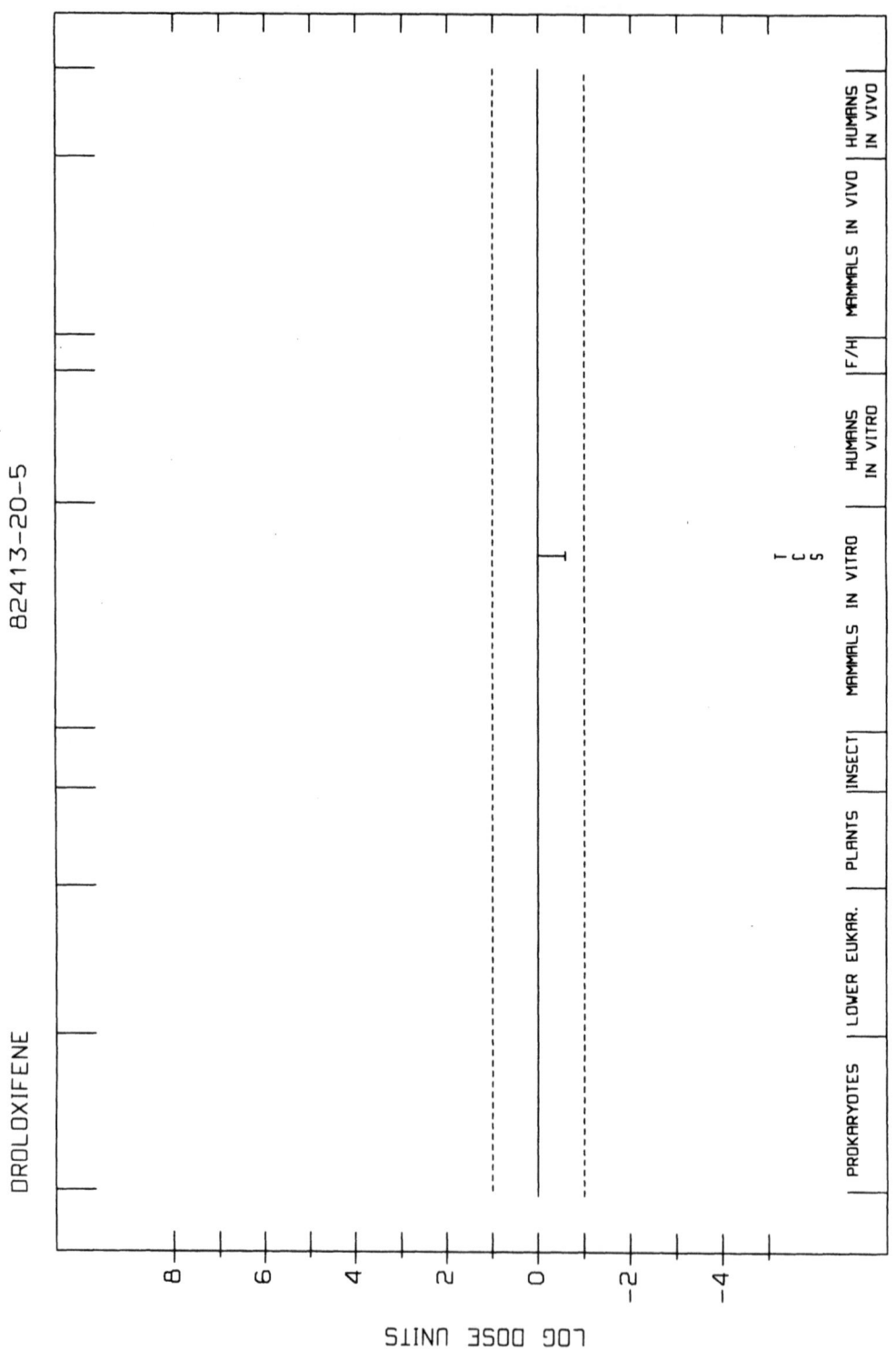

APPENDIX 2

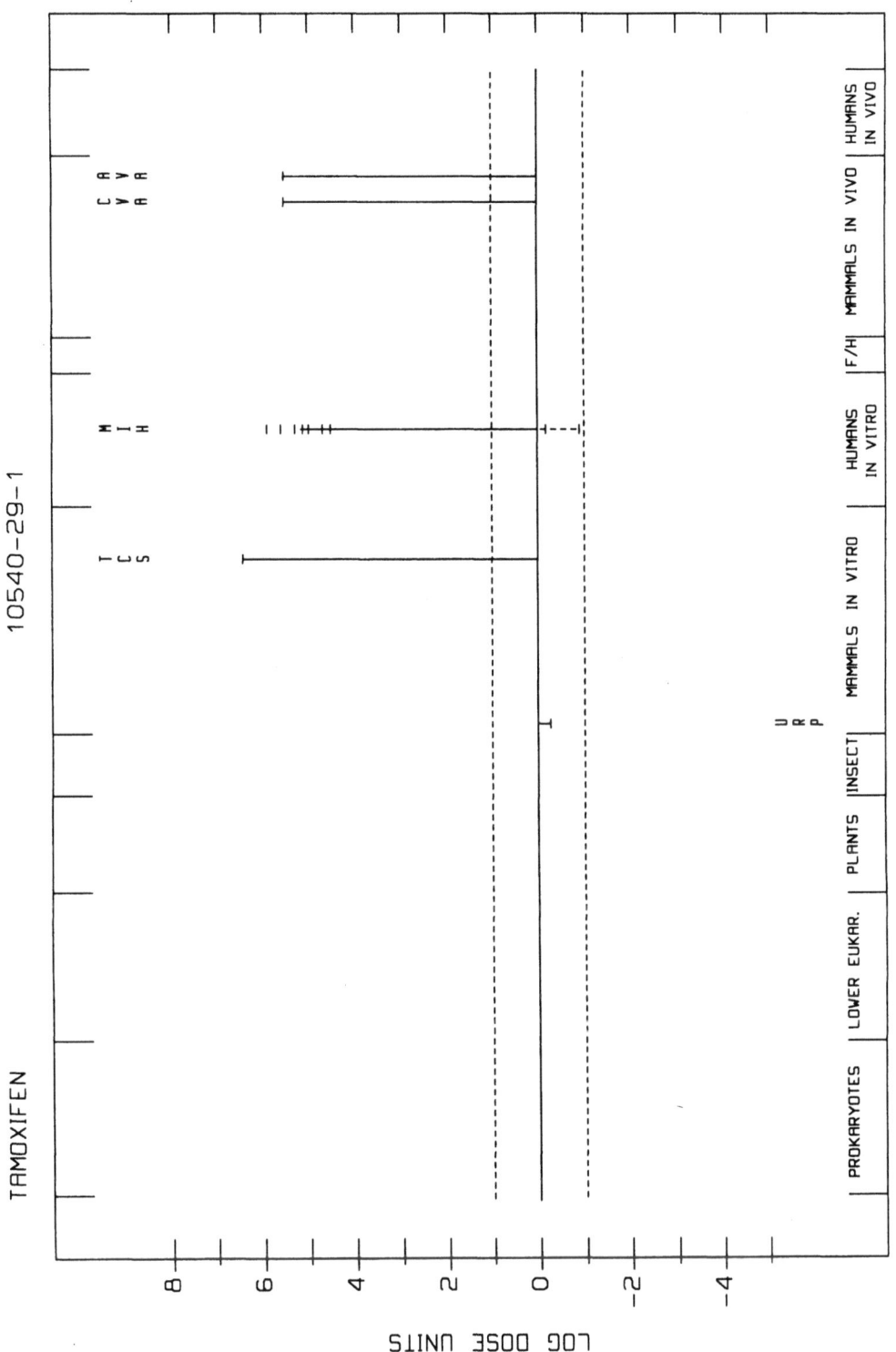

482   IARC MONOGRAPHS VOLUME 66

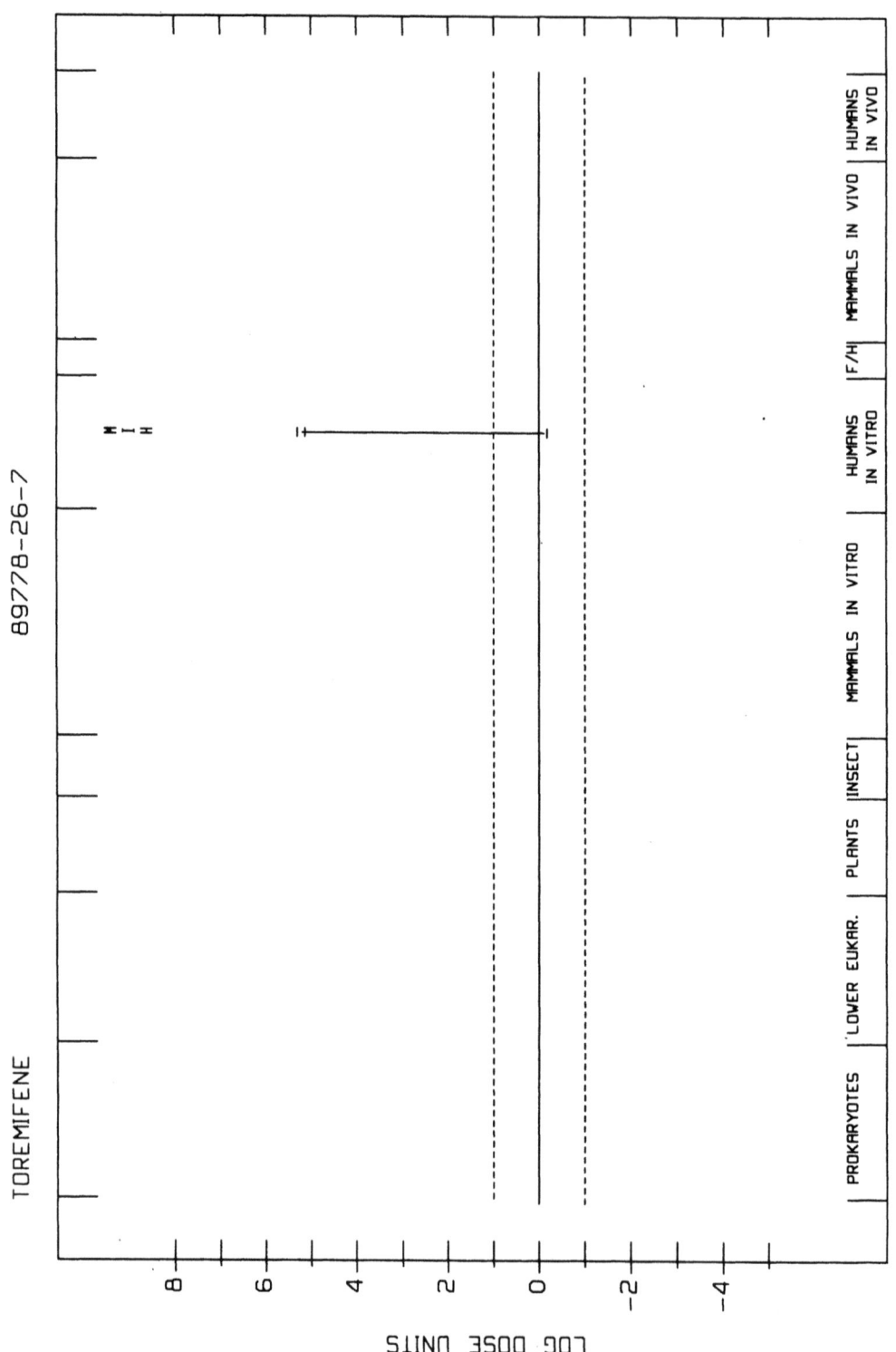

APPENDIX 2

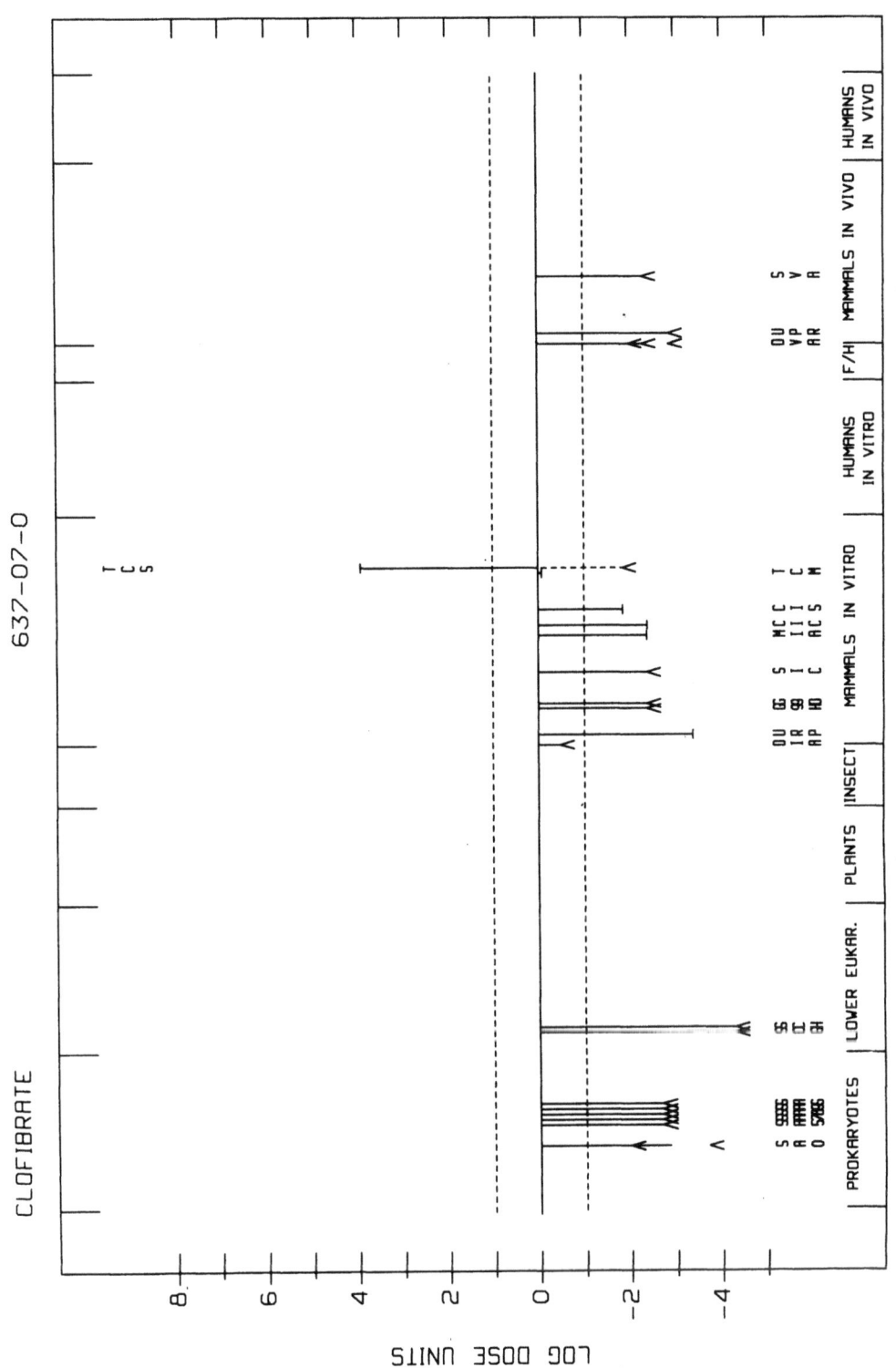

484

IARC MONOGRAPHS VOLUME 66

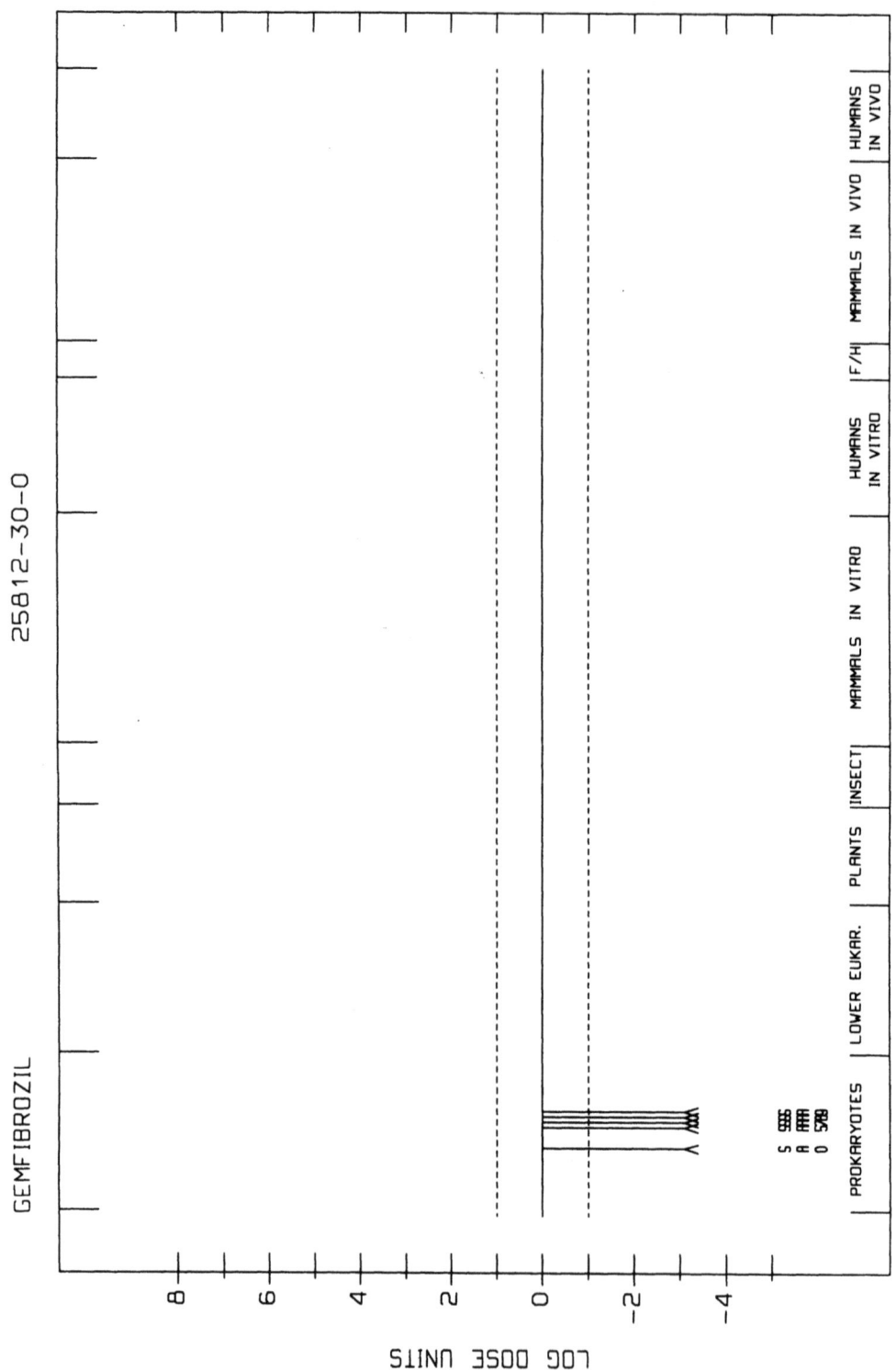

SUPPLEMENTARY CORRIGENDA TO VOLUMES 1–65

Volume 62

p. 218, footnote, *replace* (103.5 kPa) *by* (101.3 kPa)

Volume 64

p. 52, 3rd paragraph, *replace* in section 3.2 *by* in section 2.4(c)

p. 57, last paragraph, 2nd line, *replace* in section 1.2 and 3.2 *by* in section 1.2 and 2.4(c)

p. 86, last line, *replace* (1995) *by* (1995a)

p. 100, Figure 15, title, *replace* HP-16 *by* HPV-16

p. 142:

2.4.1 Cervical cancer, 1st paragraph, two last lines, *replace* Bosch *et al.*, 1992 *by* Bosch & Muñoz, 1989 *and add* Muñoz *et al.*, 1994.

(*a*) title, *replace* CIN III *by* CIN I–III

p. 173, 2nd paragraph, last line, *replace* Muñoz *et al.*, 1994 *by* Muñoz *et al.*, 1992

p. 174, before last two lines, *add* heading (*c*) *HPV antibodies in CIN and invasive carcinoma*

p. 195, 2nd paragraph, last line, *replace* Muñoz *et al.*, 1994 *by* Muñoz *et al.*, 1995b; 6th paragraph, last line, add Muñoz *et al.*, 1995b

p. 342, Muñoz *et al.*, 1995 *is* 1995a. Also *add* Muñoz, N., Kato, I., Bosch, F.X., De Sanjosé, S., Sundquist, V.-A., Izarzugaza, I., Gonzalez, L.C., Tafur, L., Gili, M., Viladiu, P., Navarro, C., Moreo, P., Guerrero, E., Shah, K.V. & Wahren, B. (1995b) Cervical cancer and herpes simplex virus type 2: case–control studies in Spain and Colombia, with special reference to immunoglobulin-G sub-classes. *Int. J. Cancer*, **60**, 438–442

Volume 65

p. 348 *should be* p. 351

p. 351 *should be* p. 348

CUMULATIVE CROSS INDEX TO *IARC MONOGRAPHS ON THE EVALUATION OF CARCINOGENIC RISKS TO HUMANS*

The volume, page and year of publication are given. References to corrigenda are given in parentheses.

A

A-α-C	*40*, 245 (1986); *Suppl. 7*, 56 (1987)
Acetaldehyde	*36*, 101 (1985) (*corr. 42*, 263); *Suppl. 7*, 77 (1987)
Acetaldehyde formylmethylhydrazone (*see* Gyromitrin)	
Acetamide	*7*, 197 (1974); *Suppl. 7*, 389 (1987)
Acetaminophen (*see* Paracetamol)	
Acridine orange	*16*, 145 (1978); *Suppl. 7*, 56 (1987)
Acriflavinium chloride	*13*, 31 (1977); *Suppl. 7*, 56 (1987)
Acrolein	*19*, 479 (1979); *36*, 133 (1985); *Suppl. 7*, 78 (1987); *63*, 337 (1995) (*corr. 65*, 549)
Acrylamide	*39*, 41 (1986); *Suppl. 7*, 56 (1987); *60*, 389 (1994)
Acrylic acid	*19*, 47 (1979); *Suppl. 7*, 56 (1987)
Acrylic fibres	*19*, 86 (1979); *Suppl. 7*, 56 (1987)
Acrylonitrile	*19*, 73 (1979); *Suppl. 7*, 79 (1987)
Acrylonitrile-butadiene-styrene copolymers	*19*, 91 (1979); *Suppl. 7*, 56 (1987)
Actinolite (*see* Asbestos)	
Actinomycins	*10*, 29 (1976) (*corr. 42*, 255); *Suppl. 7*, 80 (1987)
Adriamycin	*10*, 43 (1976); *Suppl. 7*, 82 (1987)
AF-2	*31*, 47 (1983); *Suppl. 7*, 56 (1987)
Aflatoxins	*1*, 145 (1972) (*corr. 42*, 251); *10*, 51 (1976); *Suppl. 7*, 83 (1987); *56*, 245 (1993)
Aflatoxin B$_1$ (*see* Aflatoxins)	
Aflatoxin B$_2$ (*see* Aflatoxins)	
Aflatoxin G$_1$ (*see* Aflatoxins)	
Aflatoxin G$_2$ (*see* Aflatoxins)	
Aflatoxin M$_1$ (*see* Aflatoxins)	
Agaritine	*31*, 63 (1983); *Suppl. 7*, 56 (1987)
Alcohol drinking	*44* (1988)
Aldicarb	*53*, 93 (1991)
Aldrin	*5*, 25 (1974); *Suppl. 7*, 88 (1987)
Allyl chloride	*36*, 39 (1985); *Suppl. 7*, 56 (1987)
Allyl isothiocyanate	*36*, 55 (1985); *Suppl. 7*, 56 (1987)
Allyl isovalerate	*36*, 69 (1985); *Suppl. 7*, 56 (1987)
Aluminium production	*34*, 37 (1984); *Suppl. 7*, 89 (1987)

Amaranth	8, 41 (1975); Suppl. 7, 56 (1987)
5-Aminoacenaphthene	16, 243 (1978); Suppl. 7, 56 (1987)
2-Aminoanthraquinone	27, 191 (1982); Suppl. 7, 56 (1987)
para-Aminoazobenzene	8, 53 (1975); Suppl. 7, 390 (1987)
ortho-Aminoazotoluene	8, 61 (1975) (corr. 42, 254); Suppl. 7, 56 (1987)
para-Aminobenzoic acid	16, 249 (1978); Suppl. 7, 56 (1987)
4-Aminobiphenyl	1, 74 (1972) (corr. 42, 251); Suppl. 7, 91 (1987)
2-Amino-3,4-dimethylimidazo[4,5-f]quinoline (see MeIQ)	
2-Amino-3,8-dimethylimidazo[4,5-f]quinoxaline (see MeIQx)	
3-Amino-1,4-dimethyl-5H-pyrido[4,3-b]indole (see Trp-P-1)	
2-Aminodipyrido[1,2-a:3',2'-d]imidazole (see Glu-P-2)	
1-Amino-2-methylanthraquinone	27, 199 (1982); Suppl. 7, 57 (1987)
2-Amino-3-methylimidazo[4,5-f]quinoline (see IQ)	
2-Amino-6-methyldipyrido[1,2-a:3',2'-d]imidazole (see Glu-P-1)	
2-Amino-1-methyl-6-phenylimidazo[4,5-b]pyridine (see PhIP)	
2-Amino-3-methyl-9H-pyrido[2,3-b]indole (see MeA-α-C)	
3-Amino-1-methyl-5H-pyrido[4,3-b]indole (see Trp-P-2)	
2-Amino-5-(5-nitro-2-furyl)-1,3,4-thiadiazole	7, 143 (1974); Suppl. 7, 57 (1987)
2-Amino-4-nitrophenol	57, 167 (1993)
2-Amino-5-nitrophenol	57, 177 (1993)
4-Amino-2-nitrophenol	16, 43 (1978); Suppl. 7, 57 (1987)
2-Amino-5-nitrothiazole	31, 71 (1983); Suppl. 7, 57 (1987)
2-Amino-9H-pyrido[2,3-b]indole (see A-α-C)	
11-Aminoundecanoic acid	39, 239 (1986); Suppl. 7, 57 (1987)
Amitrole	7, 31 (1974); 41, 293 (1986) (corr. 52, 513; Suppl. 7, 92 (1987)
Ammonium potassium selenide (see Selenium and selenium compounds)	
Amorphous silica (see also Silica)	42, 39 (1987); Suppl. 7, 341 (1987)
Amosite (see Asbestos)	
Ampicillin	50, 153 (1990)
Anabolic steroids (see Androgenic (anabolic) steroids)	
Anaesthetics, volatile	11, 285 (1976); Suppl. 7, 93 (1987)
Analgesic mixtures containing phenacetin (see also Phenacetin)	Suppl. 7, 310 (1987)
Androgenic (anabolic) steroids	Suppl. 7, 96 (1987)
Angelicin and some synthetic derivatives (see also Angelicins)	40, 291 (1986)
Angelicin plus ultraviolet radiation (see also Angelicin and some synthetic derivatives)	Suppl. 7, 57 (1987)
Angelicins	Suppl. 7, 57 (1987)
Aniline	4, 27 (1974) (corr. 42, 252); 27, 39 (1982); Suppl. 7, 99 (1987)
ortho-Anisidine	27, 63 (1982); Suppl. 7, 57 (1987)
para-Anisidine	27, 65 (1982); Suppl. 7, 57 (1987)
Anthanthrene	32, 95 (1983); Suppl. 7, 57 (1987)
Anthophyllite (see Asbestos)	
Anthracene	32, 105 (1983); Suppl. 7, 57 (1987)
Anthranilic acid	16, 265 (1978); Suppl. 7, 57 (1987)
Antimony trioxide	47, 291 (1989)
Antimony trisulfide	47, 291 (1989)
ANTU (see 1-Naphthylthiourea)	
Apholate	9, 31 (1975); Suppl. 7, 57 (1987)
Aramite®	5, 39 (1974); Suppl. 7, 57 (1987)
Areca nut (see Betel quid)	
Arsanilic acid (see Arsenic and arsenic compounds)	

CUMULATIVE INDEX

Arsenic and arsenic compounds	*1*, 41 (1972); *2*, 48 (1973); *23*, 39 (1980); *Suppl. 7*, 100 (1987)
Arsenic pentoxide (*see* Arsenic and arsenic compounds)	
Arsenic sulfide (*see* Arsenic and arsenic compounds)	
Arsenic trioxide (*see* Arsenic and arsenic compounds)	
Arsine (*see* Arsenic and arsenic compounds)	
Asbestos	*2*, 17 (1973) (*corr. 42*, 252); *14* (1977) (*corr. 42*, 256); *Suppl. 7*, 106 (1987) (*corr. 45*, 283)
Atrazine	*53*, 441 (1991)
Attapulgite	*42*, 159 (1987); *Suppl. 7*, 117 (1987)
Auramine (technical-grade)	*1*, 69 (1972) (*corr. 42*, 251); *Suppl. 7*, 118 (1987)
Auramine, manufacture of (*see also* Auramine, technical-grade)	*Suppl. 7*, 118 (1987)
Aurothioglucose	*13*, 39 (1977); *Suppl. 7*, 57 (1987)
Azacitidine	*26*, 37 (1981); *Suppl. 7*, 57 (1987); *50*, 47 (1990)
5-Azacytidine (*see* Azacitidine)	
Azaserine	*10*, 73 (1976) (*corr. 42*, 255); *Suppl. 7*, 57 (1987)
Azathioprine	*26*, 47 (1981); *Suppl. 7*, 119 (1987)
Aziridine	*9*, 37 (1975); *Suppl. 7*, 58 (1987)
2-(1-Aziridinyl)ethanol	*9*, 47 (1975); *Suppl. 7*, 58 (1987)
Aziridyl benzoquinone	*9*, 51 (1975); *Suppl. 7*, 58 (1987)
Azobenzene	*8*, 75 (1975); *Suppl. 7*, 58 (1987)

B

Barium chromate (*see* Chromium and chromium compounds)	
Basic chromic sulfate (*see* Chromium and chromium compounds)	
BCNU (*see* Bischloroethyl nitrosourea)	
Benz[*a*]acridine	*32*, 123 (1983); *Suppl. 7*, 58 (1987)
Benz[*c*]acridine	*3*, 241 (1973); *32*, 129 (1983); *Suppl. 7*, 58 (1987)
Benzal chloride (*see also* α-Chlorinated toluenes)	*29*, 65 (1982); *Suppl. 7*, 148 (1987)
Benz[*a*]anthracene	*3*, 45 (1973); *32*, 135 (1983); *Suppl. 7*, 58 (1987)
Benzene	*7*, 203 (1974) (*corr. 42*, 254); *29*, 93, 391 (1982); *Suppl. 7*, 120 (1987)
Benzidine	*1*, 80 (1972); *29*, 149, 391 (1982); *Suppl. 7*, 123 (1987)
Benzidine-based dyes	*Suppl. 7*, 125 (1987)
Benzo[*b*]fluoranthene	*3*, 69 (1973); *32*, 147 (1983); *Suppl. 7*, 58 (1987)
Benzo[*j*]fluoranthene	*3*, 82 (1973); *32*, 155 (1983); *Suppl. 7*, 58 (1987)
Benzo[*k*]fluoranthene	*32*, 163 (1983); *Suppl. 7*, 58 (1987)
Benzo[*ghi*]fluoranthene	*32*, 171 (1983); *Suppl. 7*, 58 (1987)
Benzo[*a*]fluorene	*32*, 177 (1983); *Suppl. 7*, 58 (1987)
Benzo[*b*]fluorene	*32*, 183 (1983); *Suppl. 7*, 58 (1987)
Benzo[*c*]fluorene	*32*, 189 (1983); *Suppl. 7*, 58 (1987)
Benzofuran	*63*, 431 (1995)
Benzo[*ghi*]perylene	*32*, 195 (1983); *Suppl. 7*, 58 (1987)
Benzo[*c*]phenanthrene	*32*, 205 (1983); *Suppl. 7*, 58 (1987)

Benzo[a]pyrene	3, 91 (1973); 32, 211 (1983); Suppl. 7, 58 (1987)
Benzo[e]pyrene	3, 137 (1973); 32, 225 (1983); Suppl. 7, 58 (1987)
para-Benzoquinone dioxime	29, 185 (1982); Suppl. 7, 58 (1987)
Benzotrichloride (see also α-Chlorinated toluenes)	29, 73 (1982); Suppl. 7, 148 (1987)
Benzoyl chloride	29, 83 (1982) (corr. 42, 261); Suppl. 7, 126 (1987)
Benzoyl peroxide	36, 267 (1985); Suppl. 7, 58 (1987)
Benzyl acetate	40, 109 (1986); Suppl. 7, 58 (1987)
Benzyl chloride (see also α-Chlorinated toluenes)	11, 217 (1976) (corr. 42, 256); 29, 49 (1982); Suppl. 7, 148 (1987)
Benzyl violet 4B	16, 153 (1978); Suppl. 7, 58 (1987)
Bertrandite (see Beryllium and beryllium compounds)	
Beryllium and beryllium compounds	1, 17 (1972); 23, 143 (1980) (corr. 42, 260); Suppl. 7, 127 (1987); 58, 41 (1993)
Beryllium acetate (see Beryllium and beryllium compounds)	
Beryllium acetate, basic (see Beryllium and beryllium compounds)	
Beryllium-aluminium alloy (see Beryllium and beryllium compounds)	
Beryllium carbonate (see Beryllium and beryllium compounds)	
Beryllium chloride (see Beryllium and beryllium compounds)	
Beryllium-copper alloy (see Beryllium and beryllium compounds)	
Beryllium-copper-cobalt alloy (see Beryllium and beryllium compounds)	
Beryllium fluoride (see Beryllium and beryllium compounds)	
Beryllium hydroxide (see Beryllium and beryllium compounds)	
Beryllium-nickel alloy (see Beryllium and beryllium compounds)	
Beryllium oxide (see Beryllium and beryllium compounds)	
Beryllium phosphate (see Beryllium and beryllium compounds)	
Beryllium silicate (see Beryllium and beryllium compounds)	
Beryllium sulfate (see Beryllium and beryllium compounds)	
Beryl ore (see Beryllium and beryllium compounds)	
Betel quid	37, 141 (1985); Suppl. 7, 128 (1987)
Betel-quid chewing (see Betel quid)	
BHA (see Butylated hydroxyanisole)	
BHT (see Butylated hydroxytoluene)	
Bis(1-aziridinyl)morpholinophosphine sulfide	9, 55 (1975); Suppl. 7, 58 (1987)
Bis(2-chloroethyl)ether	9, 117 (1975); Suppl. 7, 58 (1987)
N,N-Bis(2-chloroethyl)-2-naphthylamine	4, 119 (1974) (corr. 42, 253); Suppl. 7, 130 (1987)
Bischloroethyl nitrosourea (see also Chloroethyl nitrosoureas)	26, 79 (1981); Suppl. 7, 150 (1987)
1,2-Bis(chloromethoxy)ethane	15, 31 (1977); Suppl. 7, 58 (1987)
1,4-Bis(chloromethoxymethyl)benzene	15, 37 (1977); Suppl. 7, 58 (1987)
Bis(chloromethyl)ether	4, 231 (1974) (corr. 42, 253); Suppl. 7, 131 (1987)
Bis(2-chloro-1-methylethyl)ether	41, 149 (1986); Suppl. 7, 59 (1987)
Bis(2,3-epoxycyclopentyl)ether	47, 231 (1989)
Bisphenol A diglycidyl ether (see Glycidyl ethers)	
Bisulfites (see Sulfur dioxide and some sulfites, bisulfites and metabisulfites)	
Bitumens	35, 39 (1985); Suppl. 7, 133 (1987)
Bleomycins	26, 97 (1981); Suppl. 7, 134 (1987)
Blue VRS	16, 163 (1978); Suppl. 7, 59 (1987)
Boot and shoe manufacture and repair	25, 249 (1981); Suppl. 7, 232 (1987)
Bracken fern	40, 47 (1986); Suppl. 7, 135 (1987)

Brilliant Blue FCF, disodium salt	*16*, 171 (1978) (*corr. 42*, 257); *Suppl. 7*, 59 (1987)
Bromochloroacetonitrile (*see* Halogenated acetonitriles)	
Bromodichloromethane	*52*, 179 (1991)
Bromoethane	*52*, 299 (1991)
Bromoform	*52*, 213 (1991)
1,3-Butadiene	*39*, 155 (1986) (*corr. 42*, 264 *Suppl. 7*, 136 (1987); *54*, 237 (1992)
1,4-Butanediol dimethanesulfonate	*4*, 247 (1974); *Suppl. 7*, 137 (1987)
n-Butyl acrylate	*39*, 67 (1986); *Suppl. 7*, 59 (1987)
Butylated hydroxyanisole	*40*, 123 (1986); *Suppl. 7*, 59 (1987)
Butylated hydroxytoluene	*40*, 161 (1986); *Suppl. 7*, 59 (1987)
Butyl benzyl phthalate	*29*, 193 (1982) (*corr. 42*, 261); *Suppl. 7*, 59 (1987)
β-Butyrolactone	*11*, 225 (1976); *Suppl. 7*, 59 (1987)
γ-Butyrolactone	*11*, 231 (1976); *Suppl. 7*, 59 (1987)

C

Cabinet-making (*see* Furniture and cabinet-making)	
Cadmium acetate (*see* Cadmium and cadmium compounds)	
Cadmium and cadmium compounds	*2*, 74 (1973); *11*, 39 (1976) (*corr. 42*, 255); *Suppl. 7*, 139 (1987); *58*, 119 (1993)
Cadmium chloride (*see* Cadmium and cadmium compounds)	
Cadmium oxide (*see* Cadmium and cadmium compounds)	
Cadmium sulfate (*see* Cadmium and cadmium compounds)	
Cadmium sulfide (*see* Cadmium and cadmium compounds)	
Caffeic acid	*56*, 115 (1993)
Caffeine	*51*, 291 (1991)
Calcium arsenate (*see* Arsenic and arsenic compounds)	
Calcium chromate (see Chromium and chromium compounds)	
Calcium cyclamate (*see* Cyclamates)	
Calcium saccharin (*see* Saccharin)	
Cantharidin	*10*, 79 (1976); *Suppl. 7*, 59 (1987)
Caprolactam	*19*, 115 (1979) (*corr. 42*, 258); *39*, 247 (1986) (*corr. 42*, 264); *Suppl. 7*, 390 (1987)
Captafol	*53*, 353 (1991)
Captan	*30*, 295 (1983); *Suppl. 7*, 59 (1987)
Carbaryl	*12*, 37 (1976), *Suppl. 7*, 59 (1987)
Carbazole	*32*, 239 (1983); *Suppl. 7*, 59 (1987)
3-Carbethoxypsoralen	*40*, 317 (1986); *Suppl. 7*, 59 (1987)
Carbon black	*3*, 22 (1973); *33*, 35 (1984); *Suppl. 7*, 142 (1987); *65*, 149 (1996)
Carbon tetrachloride	*1*, 53 (1972); *20*, 371 (1979); *Suppl. 7*, 143 (1987)
Carmoisine	*8*, 83 (1975); *Suppl. 7*, 59 (1987)
Carpentry and joinery	*25*, 139 (1981); *Suppl. 7*, 378 (1987)
Carrageenan	*10*, 181 (1976) (*corr. 42*, 255); *31*, 79 (1983); *Suppl. 7*, 59 (1987)
Catechol	*15*, 155 (1977); *Suppl. 7*, 59 (1987)
CCNU (*see* 1-(2-Chloroethyl)-3-cyclohexyl-1-nitrosourea)	
Ceramic fibres (see Man-made mineral fibres)	

Chemotherapy, combined, including alkylating agents (see MOPP and
  other combined chemotherapy including alkylating agents)
Chloral   63, 245 (1995)
Chloral hydrate   63, 245 (1995)
Chlorambucil   9, 125 (1975); 26, 115 (1981);
                                                                 Suppl. 7, 144 (1987)

Chloramphenicol   10, 85 (1976); Suppl. 7, 145 (1987);
                                                                 50, 169 (1990)
Chlordane (see also Chlordane/Heptachlor)   20, 45 (1979) (corr. 42, 258)
Chlordane/Heptachlor   Suppl. 7, 146 (1987); 53, 115 (1991)
Chlordecone   20, 67 (1979); Suppl. 7, 59 (1987)
Chlordimeform   30, 61 (1983); Suppl. 7, 59 (1987)
Chlorendic acid   48, 45 (1990)
Chlorinated dibenzodioxins (other than TCDD)   15, 41 (1977); Suppl. 7, 59 (1987)
Chlorinated drinking-water   52, 45 (1991)
Chlorinated paraffins   48, 55 (1990)
α-Chlorinated toluenes   Suppl. 7, 148 (1987)
Chlormadinone acetate (see also Progestins; Combined oral   6, 149 (1974); 21, 365 (1979)
  contraceptives)
Chlornaphazine (see N,N-Bis(2-chloroethyl)-2-naphthylamine)
Chloroacetonitrile (see Halogenated acetonitriles)
para-Chloroaniline   57, 305 (1993)
Chlorobenzilate   5, 75 (1974); 30, 73 (1983);
                                                                 Suppl. 7, 60 (1987)
Chlorodibromomethane   52, 243 (1991)
Chlorodifluoromethane   41, 237 (1986) (corr. 51, 483);
                                                                 Suppl. 7, 149 (1987)
Chloroethane   52, 315 (1991)
1-(2-Chloroethyl)-3-cyclohexyl-1-nitrosourea (see also Chloroethyl   26, 137 (1981) (corr. 42, 260);
  nitrosoureas)   Suppl. 7, 150 (1987)
1-(2-Chloroethyl)-3-(4-methylcyclohexyl)-1-nitrosourea (see also   Suppl. 7, 150 (1987)
  Chloroethyl nitrosoureas)
Chloroethyl nitrosoureas   Suppl. 7, 150 (1987)
Chlorofluoromethane   41, 229 (1986); Suppl. 7, 60 (1987)
Chloroform   1, 61 (1972); 20, 401 (1979)
                                                                 Suppl. 7, 152 (1987)
Chloromethyl methyl ether (technical-grade) (see also   4, 239 (1974); Suppl. 7, 131 (1987)
  Bis(chloromethyl)ether)
(4-Chloro-2-methylphenoxy)acetic acid (see MCPA)
1-Chloro-2-methylpropene   63, 315 (1995)
3-Chloro-2-methylpropene   63, 325 (1995)
2-Chloronitrobenzene   65, 263 (1996)
3-Chloronitrobenzene   65, 263 (1996)
4-Chloronitrobenzene   65, 263 (1996)
Chlorophenols   Suppl. 7, 154 (1987)
Chlorophenols (occupational exposures to)   41, 319 (1986)
Chlorophenoxy herbicides   Suppl. 7, 156 (1987)
Chlorophenoxy herbicides (occupational exposures to)   41, 357 (1986)
4-Chloro-ortho-phenylenediamine   27, 81 (1982); Suppl. 7, 60 (1987)
4-Chloro-meta-phenylenediamine   27, 82 (1982); Suppl. 7, 60 (1987)
Chloroprene   19, 131 (1979); Suppl. 7, 160 (1987)
Chloropropham   12, 55 (1976); Suppl. 7, 60 (1987)
Chloroquine   13, 47 (1977); Suppl. 7, 60 (1987)
Chlorothalonil   30, 319 (1983); Suppl. 7, 60 (1987)

para-Chloro-*ortho*-toluidine and its strong acid salts (*see also* Chlordimeform)	*16*, 277 (1978); *30*, 65 (1983); *Suppl. 7*, 60 (1987); *48*, 123 (1990)
Chlorotrianisene (*see also* Nonsteroidal oestrogens)	*21*, 139 (1979)
2-Chloro-1,1,1-trifluoroethane	*41*, 253 (1986); *Suppl. 7*, 60 (1987)
Chlorozotocin	*50*, 65 (1990)
Cholesterol	*10*, 99 (1976); *31*, 95 (1983); *Suppl. 7*, 161 (1987)
Chromic acetate (*see* Chromium and chromium compounds)	
Chromic chloride (*see* Chromium and chromium compounds)	
Chromic oxide (*see* Chromium and chromium compounds)	
Chromic phosphate (*see* Chromium and chromium compounds)	
Chromite ore (*see* Chromium and chromium compounds)	
Chromium and chromium compounds	*2*, 100 (1973); *23*, 205 (1980); *Suppl. 7*, 165 (1987); *49*, 49 (1990) (*corr. 51*, 483)
Chromium carbonyl (*see* Chromium and chromium compounds)	
Chromium potassium sulfate (*see* Chromium and chromium compounds)	
Chromium sulfate (*see* Chromium and chromium compounds)	
Chromium trioxide (*see* Chromium and chromium compounds)	
Chrysazin (*see* Dantron)	
Chrysene	*3*, 159 (1973); *32*, 247 (1983); *Suppl. 7*, 60 (1987)
Chrysoidine	*8*, 91 (1975); *Suppl. 7*, 169 (1987)
Chrysotile (*see* Asbestos)	
CI Acid Orange 3	*57*, 121 (1993)
CI Acid Red 114	*57*, 247 (1993)
CI Basic Red 9	*57*, 215 (1993)
Ciclosporin	*50*, 77 (1990)
CI Direct Blue 15	*57*, 235 (1993)
CI Disperse Yellow 3 (see Disperse Yellow 3)	
Cimetidine	*50*, 235 (1990)
Cinnamyl anthranilate	*16*, 287 (1978); *31*, 133 (1983); *Suppl. 7*, 60 (1987)
CI Pigment Red 3	*57*, 259 (1993)
CI Pigment Red 53:1 (*see* D&C Red No. 9)	
Cisplatin	*26*, 151 (1981); *Suppl. 7*, 170 (1987)
Citrinin	*40*, 67 (1986); *Suppl. 7*, 60 (1987)
Citrus Red No. 2	*8*, 101 (1975) (*corr. 42*, 254) *Suppl. 7*, 60 (1987)
Clofibrate	*24*, 39 (1980); *Suppl. 7*, 171 (1987); *66*, 391 (1996)
Clomiphene citrate	*21*, 551 (1979); *Suppl. 7*, 172 (1987)
Clonorchis sinensis (infection with)	*61*, 121 (1994)
Coal gasification	*34*, 65 (1984); *Suppl. 7*, 173 (1987)
Coal-tar pitches (*see also* Coal-tars)	*35*, 83 (1985); *Suppl. 7*, 174 (1987)
Coal-tars	*35*, 83 (1985); *Suppl. 7*, 175 (1987)
Cobalt[III] acetate (*see* Cobalt and cobalt compounds)	
Cobalt-aluminium-chromium spinel (*see* Cobalt and cobalt compounds)	
Cobalt and cobalt compounds	*52*, 363 (1991)
Cobalt[II] chloride (*see* Cobalt and cobalt compounds)	
Cobalt-chromium alloy (*see* Chromium and chromium compounds)	
Cobalt-chromium-molybdenum alloys (*see* Cobalt and cobalt compounds)	
Cobalt metal powder (*see* Cobalt and cobalt compounds)	
Cobalt naphthenate (*see* Cobalt and cobalt compounds)	
Cobalt[II] oxide (*see* Cobalt and cobalt compounds)	

Cobalt[II,III] oxide (see Cobalt and cobalt compounds)
Cobalt[II] sulfide (see Cobalt and cobalt compounds)
Coffee   51, 41 (1991) (corr. 52, 513)
Coke production   34, 101 (1984); Suppl. 7, 176 (1987)
Combined oral contraceptives (see also Oestrogens, progestins   Suppl. 7, 297 (1987)
    and combinations)
Conjugated oestrogens (see also Steroidal oestrogens)   21, 147 (1979)
Contraceptives, oral (see Combined oral contraceptives;
    Sequential oral contraceptives)
Copper 8-hydroxyquinoline   15, 103 (1977); Suppl. 7, 61 (1987)
Coronene   32, 263 (1983); Suppl. 7, 61 (1987)
Coumarin   10, 113 (1976); Suppl. 7, 61 (1987)
Creosotes (see also Coal-tars)   35, 83 (1985); Suppl. 7, 177 (1987)
meta-Cresidine   27, 91 (1982); Suppl. 7, 61 (1987)
para-Cresidine   27, 92 (1982); Suppl. 7, 61 (1987)
Crocidolite (see Asbestos)
Crotonaldehyde   63, 373 (1995) (corr. 65, 549)
Crude oil   45, 119 (1989)
Crystalline silica (see also Silica)   42, 39 (1987); Suppl. 7, 341 (1987)
Cycasin   1, 157 (1972) (corr. 42, 251); 10,
                                                                                        121 (1976); Suppl. 7, 61 (1987)
Cyclamates   22, 55 (1980); Suppl. 7, 178 (1987)
Cyclamic acid (see Cyclamates)
Cyclochlorotine   10, 139 (1976); Suppl. 7, 61 (1987)
Cyclohexanone   47, 157 (1989)
Cyclohexylamine (see Cyclamates)
Cyclopenta[cd]pyrene   32, 269 (1983); Suppl. 7, 61 (1987)
Cyclopropane (see Anaesthetics, volatile)
Cyclophosphamide   9, 135 (1975); 26, 165 (1981);
                                                                                        Suppl. 7, 182 (1987)

D

2,4-D (see also Chlorophenoxy herbicides; Chlorophenoxy   15, 111 (1977)
    herbicides, occupational exposures to)
Dacarbazine   26, 203 (1981); Suppl. 7, 184 (1987)
Dantron   50, 265 (1990) (corr. 59, 257)
D&C Red No. 9   8, 107 (1975); Suppl. 7, 61 (1987);
                                                                                        57, 203 (1993)
Dapsone   24, 59 (1980); Suppl. 7, 185 (1987)
Daunomycin   10, 145 (1976); Suppl. 7, 61 (1987)
DDD (see DDT)
DDE (see DDT)
DDT   5, 83 (1974) (corr. 42, 253);
                                                                                        Suppl. 7, 186 (1987); 53, 179 (1991)
Decabromodiphenyl oxide   48, 73 (1990)
Deltamethrin   53, 251 (1991)
Deoxynivalenol (see Toxins derived from Fusarium graminearum,
    F. culmorum and F. crookwellense)
Diacetylaminoazotoluene   8, 113 (1975); Suppl. 7, 61 (1987)
N,N'-Diacetylbenzidine   16, 293 (1978); Suppl. 7, 61 (1987)
Diallate   12, 69 (1976); 30, 235 (1983);
                                                                                        Suppl. 7, 61 (1987)
2,4-Diaminoanisole   16, 51 (1978); 27, 103 (1982);
                                                                                        Suppl. 7, 61 (1987)

4,4'-Diaminodiphenyl ether	*16*, 301 (1978); *29*, 203 (1982); Suppl. *7*, 61 (1987)
1,2-Diamino-4-nitrobenzene	*16*, 63 (1978); Suppl. *7*, 61 (1987)
1,4-Diamino-2-nitrobenzene	*16*, 73 (1978); Suppl. *7*, 61 (1987); *57*, 185 (1993)
2,6-Diamino-3-(phenylazo)pyridine (*see* Phenazopyridine hydrochloride)	
2,4-Diaminotoluene (*see also* Toluene diisocyanates)	*16*, 83 (1978); Suppl. *7*, 61 (1987)
2,5-Diaminotoluene (*see also* Toluene diisocyanates)	*16*, 97 (1978); Suppl. *7*, 61 (1987)
ortho-Dianisidine (*see* 3,3'-Dimethoxybenzidine)	
Diazepam	*13*, 57 (1977); Suppl. *7*, 189 (1987); *66*, 37 (1996)
Diazomethane	*7*, 223 (1974); Suppl. *7*, 61 (1987)
Dibenz[*a,h*]acridine	*3*, 247 (1973); *32*, 277 (1983); Suppl. *7*, 61 (1987)
Dibenz[*a,j*]acridine	*3*, 254 (1973); *32*, 283 (1983); Suppl. *7*, 61 (1987)
Dibenz[*a,c*]anthracene	*32*, 289 (1983) (*corr. 42*, 262); Suppl. *7*, 61 (1987)
Dibenz[*a,h*]anthracene	*3*, 178 (1973) (*corr. 43*, 261); *32*, 299 (1983); Suppl. *7*, 61 (1987)
Dibenz[*a,j*]anthracene	*32*, 309 (1983); Suppl. *7*, 61 (1987)
7*H*-Dibenzo[*c,g*]carbazole	*3*, 260 (1973); *32*, 315 (1983); Suppl. *7*, 61 (1987)
Dibenzodioxins, chlorinated (other than TCDD) [*see* Chlorinated dibenzodioxins (other than TCDD)]	
Dibenzo[*a,e*]fluoranthene	*32*, 321 (1983); Suppl. *7*, 61 (1987)
Dibenzo[*h,rst*]pentaphene	*3*, 197 (1973); Suppl. *7*, 62 (1987)
Dibenzo[*a,e*]pyrene	*3*, 201 (1973); *32*, 327 (1983); Suppl. *7*, 62 (1987)
Dibenzo[*a,h*]pyrene	*3*, 207 (1973); *32*, 331 (1983); Suppl. *7*, 62 (1987)
Dibenzo[*a,i*]pyrene	*3*, 215 (1973); *32*, 337 (1983); Suppl. *7*, 62 (1987)
Dibenzo[*a,l*]pyrene	*3*, 224 (1973); *32*, 343 (1983); Suppl. *7*, 62 (1987)
Dibromoacetonitrile (*see* Halogenated acetonitriles)	
1,2-Dibromo-3-chloropropane	*15*, 139 (1977); *20*, 83 (1979); Suppl. *7*, 191 (1987)
Dichloroacetic acid	*63*, 271 (1995)
Dichloroacetonitrile (*see* Halogenated acetonitriles)	
Dichloroacetylene	*39*, 369 (1986); Suppl. *7*, 62 (1987)
ortho-Dichlorobenzene	*7*, 231 (1974); *29*, 213 (1982); Suppl. *7*, 192 (1987)
para-Dichlorobenzene	*7*, 231 (1974); *29*, 215 (1982); Suppl. *7*, 192 (1987)
3,3'-Dichlorobenzidine	*4*, 49 (1974); *29*, 239 (1982); Suppl. *7*, 193 (1987)
trans-1,4-Dichlorobutene	*15*, 149 (1977); Suppl. *7*, 62 (1987)
3,3'-Dichloro-4,4'-diaminodiphenyl ether	*16*, 309 (1978); Suppl. *7*, 62 (1987)
1,2-Dichloroethane	*20*, 429 (1979); Suppl. *7*, 62 (1987)
Dichloromethane	*20*, 449 (1979); *41*, 43 (1986); Suppl. *7*, 194 (1987)
2,4-Dichlorophenol (*see* Chlorophenols; Chlorophenols, occupational exposures to)	
(2,4-Dichlorophenoxy)acetic acid (*see* 2,4-D)	

2,6-Dichloro-*para*-phenylenediamine	*39*, 325 (1986); *Suppl. 7*, 62 (1987)
1,2-Dichloropropane	*41*, 131 (1986); *Suppl. 7*, 62 (1987)
1,3-Dichloropropene (technical-grade)	*41*, 113 (1986); *Suppl. 7*, 195 (1987)
Dichlorvos	*20*, 97 (1979); *Suppl. 7*, 62 (1987); *53*, 267 (1991)
Dicofol	*30*, 87 (1983); *Suppl. 7*, 62 (1987)
Dicyclohexylamine (*see* Cyclamates)	
Dieldrin	*5*, 125 (1974); *Suppl. 7*, 196 (1987)
Dienoestrol (*see also* Nonsteroidal oestrogens)	*21*, 161 (1979)
Diepoxybutane	*11*, 115 (1976) (*corr. 42*, 255); *Suppl. 7*, 62 (1987)
Diesel and gasoline engine exhausts	*46*, 41 (1989)
Diesel fuels	*45*, 219 (1989) (*corr. 47*, 505)
Diethyl ether (*see* Anaesthetics, volatile)	
Di(2-ethylhexyl)adipate	*29*, 257 (1982); *Suppl. 7*, 62 (1987)
Di(2-ethylhexyl)phthalate	*29*, 269 (1982) (*corr. 42*, 261); *Suppl. 7*, 62 (1987)
1,2-Diethylhydrazine	*4*, 153 (1974); *Suppl. 7*, 62 (1987)
Diethylstilboestrol	*6*, 55 (1974); *21*, 173 (1979) (*corr. 42*, 259); *Suppl. 7*, 273 (1987)
Diethylstilboestrol dipropionate (*see* Diethylstilboestrol)	
Diethyl sulfate	*4*, 277 (1974); *Suppl. 7*, 198 (1987); *54*, 213 (1992)
Diglycidyl resorcinol ether	*11*, 125 (1976); *36*, 181 (1985); *Suppl. 7*, 62 (1987)
Dihydrosafrole	*1*, 170 (1972); *10*, 233 (1976) *Suppl. 7*, 62 (1987)
1,8-Dihydroxyanthraquinone (*see* Dantron)	
Dihydroxybenzenes (*see* Catechol; Hydroquinone; Resorcinol)	
Dihydroxymethylfuratrizine	*24*, 77 (1980); *Suppl. 7*, 62 (1987)
Diisopropyl sulfate	*54*, 229 (1992)
Dimethisterone (*see also* Progestins; Sequential oral contraceptives	*6*, 167 (1974); *21*, 377 (1979))
Dimethoxane	*15*, 177 (1977); *Suppl. 7*, 62 (1987)
3,3′-Dimethoxybenzidine	*4*, 41 (1974); *Suppl. 7*, 198 (1987)
3,3′-Dimethoxybenzidine-4,4′-diisocyanate	*39*, 279 (1986); *Suppl. 7*, 62 (1987)
para-Dimethylaminoazobenzene	*8*, 125 (1975); *Suppl. 7*, 62 (1987)
para-Dimethylaminoazobenzenediazo sodium sulfonate	*8*, 147 (1975); *Suppl. 7*, 62 (1987)
trans-2-[(Dimethylamino)methylimino]-5-[2-(5-nitro-2-furyl)-vinyl]-1,3,4-oxadiazole	*7*, 147 (1974) (*corr. 42*, 253); *Suppl. 7*, 62 (1987)
4,4′-Dimethylangelicin plus ultraviolet radiation (*see also* Angelicin and some synthetic derivatives)	*Suppl. 7*, 57 (1987)
4,5′-Dimethylangelicin plus ultraviolet radiation (*see also* Angelicin and some synthetic derivatives)	*Suppl. 7*, 57 (1987)
2,6-Dimethylaniline	*57*, 323 (1993)
N,N-Dimethylaniline	*57*, 337 (1993)
Dimethylarsinic acid (*see* Arsenic and arsenic compounds)	
3,3′-Dimethylbenzidine	*1*, 87 (1972); *Suppl. 7*, 62 (1987)
Dimethylcarbamoyl chloride	*12*, 77 (1976); *Suppl. 7*, 199 (1987)
Dimethylformamide	*47*, 171 (1989)
1,1-Dimethylhydrazine	*4*, 137 (1974); *Suppl. 7*, 62 (1987)
1,2-Dimethylhydrazine	*4*, 145 (1974) (*corr. 42*, 253); *Suppl. 7*, 62 (1987)
Dimethyl hydrogen phosphite	*48*, 85 (1990)
1,4-Dimethylphenanthrene	*32*, 349 (1983); *Suppl. 7*, 62 (1987)
Dimethyl sulfate	*4*, 271 (1974); *Suppl. 7*, 200 (1987)

3,7-Dinitrofluoranthene	*46*, 189 (1989); *65*, 297 (1996)
3,9-Dinitrofluoranthene	*46*, 195 (1989); *65*, 297 (1996)
1,3-Dinitropyrene	*46*, 201 (1989)
1,6-Dinitropyrene	*46*, 215 (1989)
1,8-Dinitropyrene	*33*, 171 (1984); *Suppl. 7*, 63 (1987); *46*, 231 (1989)
Dinitrosopentamethylenetetramine	*11*, 241 (1976); *Suppl. 7*, 63 (1987)
2,4-Dinitrotoluene	*65*, 309 (1996) (*corr. 66*, 485)
2,6-Dinitrotoluene	*65*, 309 (1996) (*corr. 66*, 485)
3,5-Dinitrotoluene	*65*, 309 (1996)
1,4-Dioxane	*11*, 247 (1976); *Suppl. 7*, 201 (1987)
2,4′-Diphenyldiamine	*16*, 313 (1978); *Suppl. 7*, 63 (1987)
Direct Black 38 (*see also* Benzidine-based dyes)	*29*, 295 (1982) (*corr. 42*, 261)
Direct Blue 6 (*see also* Benzidine-based dyes)	*29*, 311 (1982)
Direct Brown 95 (*see also* Benzidine-based dyes)	*29*, 321 (1982)
Disperse Blue 1	*48*, 139 (1990)
Disperse Yellow 3	*8*, 97 (1975); *Suppl. 7*, 60 (1987); *48*, 149 (1990)
Disulfiram	*12*, 85 (1976); *Suppl. 7*, 63 (1987)
Dithranol	*13*, 75 (1977); *Suppl. 7*, 63 (1987)
Divinyl ether (*see* Anaesthetics, volatile)	
Doxefazepam	*66*, 97 (1996)
Droloxifene	*66*, 241 (1996)
Dry cleaning	*63*, 33 (1995)
Dulcin	*12*, 97 (1976); *Suppl. 7*, 63 (1987)

E

Endrin	*5*, 157 (1974); *Suppl. 7*, 63 (1987)
Enflurane (*see* Anaesthetics, volatile)	
Eosin	*15*, 183 (1977); *Suppl. 7*, 63 (1987)
Epichlorohydrin	*11*, 131 (1976) (*corr. 42*, 256); *Suppl. 7*, 202 (1987)
1,2-Epoxybutane	*47*, 217 (1989)
1-Epoxyethyl-3,4-epoxycyclohexane (*see* 4-Vinylcyclohexene diepoxide)	
3,4-Epoxy-6-methylcyclohexylmethyl-3,4-epoxy-6-methylcyclohexane carboxylate	*11*, 147 (1976); *Suppl. 7*, 63 (1987)
cis-9,10-Epoxystearic acid	*11*, 153 (1976); *Suppl. 7*, 63 (1987)
Erionite	*42*, 225 (1987); *Suppl. 7*, 203 (1987)
Estazolam	*66*, 105 (1996)
Ethinyloestradiol (*see also* Steroidal oestrogens)	*6*, 77 (1974); *21*, 233 (1979)
Ethionamide	*13*, 83 (1977); *Suppl. 7*, 63 (1987)
Ethyl acrylate	*19*, 57 (1979); *39*, 81 (1986); *Suppl. 7*, 63 (1987)
Ethylene	*19*, 157 (1979); *Suppl. 7*, 63 (1987); *60*, 45 (1994)
Ethylene dibromide	*15*, 195 (1977); *Suppl. 7*, 204 (1987)
Ethylene oxide	*11*, 157 (1976); *36*, 189 (1985) (*corr. 42*, 263); *Suppl. 7*, 205 (1987); *60*, 73 (1994)
Ethylene sulfide	*11*, 257 (1976); *Suppl. 7*, 63 (1987)
Ethylene thiourea	*7*, 45 (1974); *Suppl. 7*, 207 (1987)
2-Ethylhexyl acrylate	*60*, 475 (1994)
Ethyl methanesulfonate	*7*, 245 (1974); *Suppl. 7*, 63 (1987)

N-Ethyl-N-nitrosourea   1, 135 (1972); 17, 191 (1978);
                                                                               Suppl. 7, 63 (1987)
Ethyl selenac (see also Selenium and selenium compounds)   12, 107 (1976); Suppl. 7, 63 (1987)
Ethyl tellurac   12, 115 (1976); Suppl. 7, 63 (1987)
Ethynodiol diacetate (see also Progestins; Combined oral   6, 173 (1974); 21, 387 (1979)
    contraceptives)
Eugenol   36, 75 (1985); Suppl. 7, 63 (1987)
Evans blue   8, 151 (1975); Suppl. 7, 63 (1987)

F

Fast Green FCF   16, 187 (1978); Suppl. 7, 63 (1987)
Fenvalerate   53, 309 (1991)
Ferbam   12, 121 (1976) (corr. 42, 256);
                                                                               Suppl. 7, 63 (1987)
Ferric oxide   1, 29 (1972); Suppl. 7, 216 (1987)
Ferrochromium (see Chromium and chromium compounds)
Fluometuron   30, 245 (1983); Suppl. 7, 63 (1987)
Fluoranthene   32, 355 (1983); Suppl. 7, 63 (1987)
Fluorene   32, 365 (1983); Suppl. 7, 63 (1987)
Fluorescent lighting (exposure to) (see Ultraviolet radiation)
Fluorides (inorganic, used in drinking-water)   27, 237 (1982); Suppl. 7, 208 (1987)
5-Fluorouracil   26, 217 (1981); Suppl. 7, 210 (1987)
Fluorspar (see Fluorides)
Fluosilicic acid (see Fluorides)
Fluroxene (see Anaesthetics, volatile)
Formaldehyde   29, 345 (1982); Suppl. 7, 211 (1987);
                                                                               62, 217 (1995) (corr. 65, 549;
                                                                               corr. 66, 485)
2-(2-Formylhydrazino)-4-(5-nitro-2-furyl)thiazole   7, 151 (1974) (corr. 42, 253);
                                                                               Suppl. 7, 63 (1987)
Frusemide (see Furosemide)
Fuel oils (heating oils)   45, 239 (1989) (corr. 47, 505)
Fumonisin B_1 (see Toxins derived from Fusarium moniliforme)
Fumonisin B_2 (see Toxins derived from Fusarium moniliforme)
Furan   63, 393 (1995)
Furazolidone   31, 141 (1983); Suppl. 7, 63 (1987)
Furfural   63, 409 (1995)
Furniture and cabinet-making   25, 99 (1981); Suppl. 7, 380 (1987)
Furosemide   50, 277 (1990)
2-(2-Furyl)-3-(5-nitro-2-furyl)acrylamide (see AF-2)
Fusarenon-X (see Toxins derived from Fusarium graminearum,
    F. culmorum and F. crookwellense)
Fusarenone-X (see Toxins derived from Fusarium graminearum,
    F. culmorum and F. crookwellense)
Fusarin C (see Toxins derived from Fusarium moniliforme)

G

Gasoline   45, 159 (1989) (corr. 47, 505)
Gasoline engine exhaust (see Diesel and gasoline engine exhausts)
Gemfibrozil   66, 427 (1996)
Glass fibres (see Man-made mineral fibres)

Glass manufacturing industry, occupational exposures in	58, 347 (1993)
Glasswool (see Man-made mineral fibres)	
Glass filaments (see Man-made mineral fibres)	
Glu-P-1	40, 223 (1986); Suppl. 7, 64 (1987)
Glu-P-2	40, 235 (1986); Suppl. 7, 64 (1987)
L-Glutamic acid, 5-[2-(4-hydroxymethyl)phenylhydrazide] (see Agaritine)	
Glycidaldehyde	11, 175 (1976); Suppl. 7, 64 (1987)
Glycidyl ethers	47, 237 (1989)
Glycidyl oleate	11, 183 (1976); Suppl. 7, 64 (1987)
Glycidyl stearate	11, 187 (1976); Suppl. 7, 64 (1987)
Griseofulvin	10, 153 (1976); Suppl. 7, 391 (1987)
Guinea Green B	16, 199 (1978); Suppl. 7, 64 (1987)
Gyromitrin	31, 163 (1983); Suppl. 7, 391 (1987)

H

Haematite	1, 29 (1972); Suppl. 7, 216 (1987)
Haematite and ferric oxide	Suppl. 7, 216 (1987)
Haematite mining, underground, with exposure to radon	1, 29 (1972); Suppl. 7, 216 (1987)
Hairdressers and barbers (occupational exposure as)	57, 43 (1993)
Hair dyes, epidemiology of	16, 29 (1978); 27, 307 (1982);
Halogenated acetonitriles	52, 269 (1991)
Halothane (see Anaesthetics, volatile)	
HC Blue No. 1	57, 129 (1993)
HC Blue No. 2	57, 143 (1993)
α-HCH (see Hexachlorocyclohexanes)	
β-HCH (see Hexachlorocyclohexanes)	
γ-HCH (see Hexachlorocyclohexanes)	
HC Red No. 3	57, 153 (1993)
HC Yellow No. 4	57, 159 (1993)
Heating oils (see Fuel oils)	
Helicobacter pylori (infection with)	61, 177 (1994)
Hepatitis B virus	59, 45 (1994)
Hepatitis C virus	59, 165 (1994)
Hepatitis D virus	59, 223 (1994)
Heptachlor (see also Chlordane/Heptachlor)	5, 173 (1974); 20, 129 (1979)
Hexachlorobenzene	20, 155 (1979); Suppl. 7, 219 (1987)
Hexachlorobutadiene	20, 179 (1979); Suppl. 7, 64 (1987)
Hexachlorocyclohexanes	5, 47 (1974); 20, 195 (1979) (corr. 42, 258), Suppl. 7, 220 (1987)
Hexachlorocyclohexane, technical-grade (see Hexachlorocyclohexanes)	
Hexachloroethane	20, 467 (1979); Suppl. 7, 64 (1987)
Hexachlorophene	20, 241 (1979); Suppl. 7, 64 (1987)
Hexamethylphosphoramide	15, 211 (1977); Suppl. 7, 64 (1987)
Hexoestrol (see Nonsteroidal oestrogens)	
Human papillomaviruses	64 (1995) (corr. 66, 485)
Hycanthone mesylate	13, 91 (1977); Suppl. 7, 64 (1987)
Hydralazine	24, 85 (1980); Suppl. 7, 222 (1987)
Hydrazine	4, 127 (1974); Suppl. 7, 223 (1987)
Hydrochloric acid	54, 189 (1992)
Hydrochlorothiazide	50, 293 (1990)
Hydrogen peroxide	36, 285 (1985); Suppl. 7, 64 (1987)
Hydroquinone	15, 155 (1977); Suppl. 7, 64 (1987)

4-Hydroxyazobenzene   8, 157 (1975); *Suppl. 7*, 64 (1987)
17α-Hydroxyprogesterone caproate (*see also* Progestins)   21, 399 (1979) (*corr. 42*, 259)
8-Hydroxyquinoline   13, 101 (1977); *Suppl. 7*, 64 (1987)
8-Hydroxysenkirkine   10, 265 (1976); *Suppl. 7*, 64 (1987)
Hypochlorite salts   52, 159 (1991)

I

Indeno[1,2,3-*cd*]pyrene   3, 229 (1973); 32, 373 (1983);
                                                            Suppl. 7, 64 (1987)

Inorganic acids (*see* Sulfuric acid and other strong inorganic acids,
   occupational exposures to mists and vapours from)
Insecticides, occupational exposures in spraying and application of   53, 45 (1991)
IQ   40, 261 (1986); *Suppl. 7*, 64 (1987);
                                                            56, 165 (1993)
Iron and steel founding   34, 133 (1984); *Suppl. 7*, 224 (1987)
Iron-dextran complex   2, 161 (1973); *Suppl. 7*, 226 (1987)
Iron-dextrin complex   2, 161 (1973) (*corr. 42*, 252);
                                                            Suppl. 7, 64 (1987)

Iron oxide (*see* Ferric oxide)
Iron oxide, saccharated (*see* Saccharated iron oxide)
Iron sorbitol-citric acid complex   2, 161 (1973); *Suppl. 7*, 64 (1987)
Isatidine   10, 269 (1976); *Suppl. 7*, 65 (1987)
Isoflurane (*see* Anaesthetics, volatile)
Isoniazid (*see* Isonicotinic acid hydrazide)
Isonicotinic acid hydrazide   4, 159 (1974); *Suppl. 7*, 227 (1987)
Isophosphamide   26, 237 (1981); *Suppl. 7*, 65 (1987)
Isoprene   60, 215 (1994)
Isopropanol   15, 223 (1977); *Suppl. 7*, 229 (1987)
Isopropanol manufacture (strong-acid process)   *Suppl. 7*, 229 (1987)
   (*see also* Isopropanol; Sulfuric acid and other strong inorganic
   acids, occupational exposures to mists and vapours from)
Isopropyl oils   15, 223 (1977); *Suppl. 7*, 229 (1987)
Isosafrole   1, 169 (1972); 10, 232 (1976);
                                                            Suppl. 7, 65 (1987)

J

Jacobine   10, 275 (1976); *Suppl. 7*, 65 (1987)
Jet fuel   45, 203 (1989)
Joinery (*see* Carpentry and joinery)

K

Kaempferol   31, 171 (1983); *Suppl. 7*, 65 (1987)
Kepone (*see* Chlordecone)

L

Lasiocarpine   10, 281 (1976); *Suppl. 7*, 65 (1987)
Lauroyl peroxide   36, 315 (1985); *Suppl. 7*, 65 (1987)
Lead acetate (*see* Lead and lead compounds)

Lead and lead compounds	*1*, 40 (1972) (*corr. 42*, 251); *2*, 52, 150 (1973); *12*, 131 (1976); *23*, 40, 208, 209, 325 (1980); *Suppl. 7*, 230 (1987)
Lead arsenate (*see* Arsenic and arsenic compounds)	
Lead carbonate (*see* Lead and lead compounds)	
Lead chloride (*see* Lead and lead compounds)	
Lead chromate (*see* Chromium and chromium compounds)	
Lead chromate oxide (*see* Chromium and chromium compounds)	
Lead naphthenate (*see* Lead and lead compounds)	
Lead nitrate (*see* Lead and lead compounds)	
Lead oxide (*see* Lead and lead compounds)	
Lead phosphate (*see* Lead and lead compounds)	
Lead subacetate (*see* Lead and lead compounds)	
Lead tetroxide (*see* Lead and lead compounds)	
Leather goods manufacture	*25*, 279 (1981); *Suppl. 7*, 235 (1987)
Leather industries	*25*, 199 (1981); *Suppl. 7*, 232 (1987)
Leather tanning and processing	*25*, 201 (1981); *Suppl. 7*, 236 (1987)
Ledate (*see also* Lead and lead compounds)	*12*, 131 (1976)
Light Green SF	*16*, 209 (1978); *Suppl. 7*, 65 (1987)
d-Limonene	*56*, 135 (1993)
Lindane (*see* Hexachlorocyclohexanes)	
Liver flukes (*see* Clonorchis sinensis, Opisthorchis felineus and Opisthorchis viverrini)	
Lumber and sawmill industries (including logging)	*25*, 49 (1981); *Suppl. 7*, 383 (1987)
Luteoskyrin	*10*, 163 (1976); *Suppl. 7*, 65 (1987)
Lynoestrenol (*see also* Progestins; Combined oral contraceptives)	*21*, 407 (1979)

M

Magenta	*4*, 57 (1974) (*corr. 42*, 252); *Suppl. 7*, 238 (1987); *57*, 215 (1993)
Magenta, manufacture of (*see also* Magenta)	*Suppl. 7*, 238 (1987); *57*, 215 (1993)
Malathion	*30*, 103 (1983); *Suppl. 7*, 65 (1987)
Maleic hydrazide	*4*, 173 (1974) (*corr. 42*, 253); *Suppl. 7*, 65 (1987)
Malonaldehyde	*36*, 163 (1985); *Suppl. 7*, 65 (1987)
Maneb	*12*, 137 (1976); *Suppl. 7*, 65 (1987)
Man-made mineral fibres	*43*, 39 (1988)
Mannomustine	*9*, 157 (1975); *Suppl. 7*, 65 (1987)
Mate	*51*, 273 (1991)
MCPA (*see also* Chlorophenoxy herbicides; Chlorophenoxy herbicides, occupational exposures to)	*30*, 255 (1983)
MeA-α-C	*40*, 253 (1986); *Suppl. 7*, 65 (1987)
Medphalan	*9*, 168 (1975); *Suppl. 7*, 65 (1987)
Medroxyprogesterone acetate	*6*, 157 (1974); *21*, 417 (1979) (*corr. 42*, 259); *Suppl. 7*, 289 (1987)
Megestrol acetate (*see also* Progestins; Combined oral contraceptives)	
MeIQ	*40*, 275 (1986); *Suppl. 7*, 65 (1987); *56*, 197 (1993)
MeIQx	*40*, 283 (1986); *Suppl. 7*, 65 (1987); *56*, 211 (1993)
Melamine	*39*, 333 (1986); *Suppl. 7*, 65 (1987)
Melphalan	*9*, 167 (1975); *Suppl. 7*, 239 (1987)

6-Mercaptopurine   26, 249 (1981); Suppl. 7, 240 (1987)
Mercuric chloride (see Mercury and mercury compounds)
Mercury and mercury compounds   58, 239 (1993)
Merphalan   9, 169 (1975); Suppl. 7, 65 (1987)
Mestranol (see also Steroidal oestrogens)   6, 87 (1974); 21, 257 (1979)
                                                  (corr. 42, 259)
Metabisulfites (see Sulfur dioxide and some sulfites, bisulfites
    and metabisulfites)
Metallic mercury (see Mercury and mercury compounds)
Methanearsonic acid, disodium salt (see Arsenic and arsenic compounds)
Methanearsonic acid, monosodium salt (see Arsenic and arsenic
    compounds
Methotrexate   26, 267 (1981); Suppl. 7, 241 (1987)
Methoxsalen (see 8-Methoxypsoralen)
Methoxychlor   5, 193 (1974); 20, 259 (1979);
                                                  Suppl. 7, 66 (1987)
Methoxyflurane (see Anaesthetics, volatile)
5-Methoxypsoralen   40, 327 (1986); Suppl. 7, 242 (1987)
8-Methoxypsoralen (see also 8-Methoxypsoralen plus ultraviolet   24, 101 (1980)
    radiation)
8-Methoxypsoralen plus ultraviolet radiation   Suppl. 7, 243 (1987)
Methyl acrylate   19, 52 (1979); 39, 99 (1986);
                                                  Suppl. 7, 66 (1987)
5-Methylangelicin plus ultraviolet radiation (see also Angelicin
    and some synthetic derivatives)   Suppl. 7, 57 (1987)
2-Methylaziridine   9, 61 (1975); Suppl. 7, 66 (1987)
Methylazoxymethanol acetate   1, 164 (1972); 10, 131 (1976);
                                                  Suppl. 7, 66 (1987)
Methyl bromide   41, 187 (1986) (corr. 45, 283);
                                                  Suppl. 7, 245 (1987)
Methyl carbamate   12, 151 (1976); Suppl. 7, 66 (1987)
Methyl-CCNU [see 1-(2-Chloroethyl)-3-(4-methylcyclohexyl)-
    1-nitrosourea]
Methyl chloride   41, 161 (1986); Suppl. 7, 246 (1987)
1-, 2-, 3-, 4-, 5- and 6-Methylchrysenes   32, 379 (1983); Suppl. 7, 66 (1987)
N-Methyl-N,4-dinitrosoaniline   1, 141 (1972); Suppl. 7, 66 (1987)
4,4'-Methylene bis(2-chloroaniline)   4, 65 (1974) (corr. 42, 252);
                                                  Suppl. 7, 246 (1987); 57, 271 (1993)
4,4'-Methylene bis(N,N-dimethyl)benzenamine   27, 119 (1982); Suppl. 7, 66 (1987)
4,4'-Methylene bis(2-methylaniline)   4, 73 (1974); Suppl. 7, 248 (1987)
4,4'-Methylenedianiline   4, 79 (1974) (corr. 42, 252);
                                                  39, 347 (1986); Suppl. 7, 66 (1987)
4,4'-Methylenediphenyl diisocyanate   19, 314 (1979); Suppl. 7, 66 (1987)
2-Methylfluoranthene   32, 399 (1983); Suppl. 7, 66 (1987)
3-Methylfluoranthene   32, 399 (1983); Suppl. 7, 66 (1987)
Methylglyoxal   51, 443 (1991)
Methyl iodide   15, 245 (1977); 41, 213 (1986);
                                                  Suppl. 7, 66 (1987)
Methylmercury chloride (see Mercury and mercury compounds)
Methylmercury compounds (see Mercury and mercury compounds)
Methyl methacrylate   19, 187 (1979); Suppl. 7, 66 (1987);
                                                  60, 445 (1994)
Methyl methanesulfonate   7, 253 (1974); Suppl. 7, 66 (1987)
2-Methyl-1-nitroanthraquinone   27, 205 (1982); Suppl. 7, 66 (1987)
N-Methyl-N'-nitro-N-nitrosoguanidine   4, 183 (1974); Suppl. 7, 248 (1987)

3-Methylnitrosaminopropionaldehyde [*see* 3-(*N*-Nitrosomethylamino)-
propionaldehyde]
3-Methylnitrosaminopropionitrile [*see* 3-(*N*-Nitrosomethylamino)-
propionitrile]
4-(Methylnitrosamino)-4-(3-pyridyl)-1-butanal [*see* 4-(*N*-Nitrosomethyl-
amino)-4-(3-pyridyl)-1-butanal]
4-(Methylnitrosamino)-1-(3-pyridyl)-1-butanone [*see* 4-(-Nitrosomethyl-
amino)-1-(3-pyridyl)-1-butanone]

N-Methyl-*N*-nitrosourea	*1*, 125 (1972); *17*, 227 (1978); *Suppl. 7*, 66 (1987)
N-Methyl-*N*-nitrosourethane	*4*, 211 (1974); *Suppl. 7*, 66 (1987)
N-Methylolacrylamide	*60*, 435 (1994)
Methyl parathion	*30*, 131 (1983); *Suppl. 7*, 392 (1987)
1-Methylphenanthrene	*32*, 405 (1983); *Suppl. 7*, 66 (1987)
7-Methylpyrido[3,4-*c*]psoralen	*40*, 349 (1986); *Suppl. 7*, 71 (1987)
Methyl red	*8*, 161 (1975); *Suppl. 7*, 66 (1987)
Methyl selenac (*see also* Selenium and selenium compounds)	*12*, 161 (1976); *Suppl. 7*, 66 (1987)
Methylthiouracil	*7*, 53 (1974); *Suppl. 7*, 66 (1987)
Metronidazole	*13*, 113 (1977); *Suppl. 7*, 250 (1987)
Mineral oils	*3*, 30 (1973); *33*, 87 (1984) (*corr. 42*, 262); *Suppl. 7*, 252 (1987)
Mirex	*5*, 203 (1974); *20*, 283 (1979) (*corr. 42*, 258); *Suppl. 7*, 66 (1987)
Mists and vapours from sulfuric acid and other strong inorganic acids	*54*, 41 (1992)
Mitomycin C	*10*, 171 (1976); *Suppl. 7*, 67 (1987)

MNNG [*see N*-Methyl-*N'*-nitro-*N*-nitrosoguanidine]
MOCA [*see* 4,4'-Methylene bis(2-chloroaniline)]

Modacrylic fibres	*19*, 86 (1979); *Suppl. 7*, 67 (1987)
Monocrotaline	*10*, 291 (1976); *Suppl. 7*, 67 (1987)
Monuron	*12*, 167 (1976); *Suppl. 7*, 67 (1987); *53*, 467 (1991)
MOPP and other combined chemotherapy including alkylating agents	*Suppl. 7*, 254 (1987)
Morpholine	*47*, 199 (1989)
5-(Morpholinomethyl)-3-[(5-nitrofurfurylidene)amino]-2-oxazolidinone	*7*, 161 (1974); *Suppl. 7*, 67 (1987)
Musk ambrette	*65*, 477 (1996)
Musk xylene	*65*, 477 (1996)
Mustard gas	*9*, 181 (1975) (*corr. 42*, 254); *Suppl. 7*, 259 (1987)

Myleran (*see* 1,4-Butanediol dimethanesulfonate)

N

Nafenopin	*24*, 125 (1980); *Suppl. 7*, 67 (1987)
1,5-Naphthalenediamine	*27*, 127 (1982); *Suppl. 7*, 67 (1987)
1,5-Naphthalene diisocyanate	*19*, 311 (1979); *Suppl. 7*, 67 (1987)
1-Naphthylamine	*4*, 87 (1974) (*corr. 42*, 253); *Suppl. 7*, 260 (1987)
2-Naphthylamine	*4*, 97 (1974); *Suppl. 7*, 261 (1987)
1-Naphthylthiourea	*30*, 347 (1983); *Suppl. 7*, 263 (1987)

Nickel acetate (*see* Nickel and nickel compounds)
Nickel ammonium sulfate (*see* Nickel and nickel compounds)

Nickel and nickel compounds	2, 126 (1973) (*corr. 42*, 252); *11*, 75 (1976); *Suppl. 7*, 264 (1987) (*corr. 45*, 283); *49*, 257 (1990)
Nickel carbonate (*see* Nickel and nickel compounds)	
Nickel carbonyl (*see* Nickel and nickel compounds)	
Nickel chloride (*see* Nickel and nickel compounds)	
Nickel-gallium alloy (*see* Nickel and nickel compounds)	
Nickel hydroxide (*see* Nickel and nickel compounds)	
Nickelocene (*see* Nickel and nickel compounds)	
Nickel oxide (*see* Nickel and nickel compounds)	
Nickel subsulfide (*see* Nickel and nickel compounds)	
Nickel sulfate (*see* Nickel and nickel compounds)	
Niridazole	*13*, 123 (1977); *Suppl. 7*, 67 (1987)
Nithiazide	*31*, 179 (1983); *Suppl. 7*, 67 (1987)
Nitrilotriacetic acid and its salts	*48*, 181 (1990)
5-Nitroacenaphthene	*16*, 319 (1978); *Suppl. 7*, 67 (1987)
5-Nitro-*ortho*-anisidine	*27*, 133 (1982); *Suppl. 7*, 67 (1987)
2-Nitroanisole	*65*, 369 (1996)
9-Nitroanthracene	*33*, 179 (1984); *Suppl. 7*, 67 (1987)
7-Nitrobenz[*a*]anthracene	*46*, 247 (1989)
Nitrobenzene	*65*, 381 (1996)
6-Nitrobenzo[*a*]pyrene	*33*, 187 (1984); *Suppl. 7*, 67 (1987); *46*, 255 (1989)
4-Nitrobiphenyl	*4*, 113 (1974); *Suppl. 7*, 67 (1987)
6-Nitrochrysene	*33*, 195 (1984); *Suppl. 7*, 67 (1987); *46*, 267 (1989)
Nitrofen (technical-grade)	*30*, 271 (1983); *Suppl. 7*, 67 (1987)
3-Nitrofluoranthene	*33*, 201 (1984); *Suppl. 7*, 67 (1987)
2-Nitrofluorene	*46*, 277 (1989)
Nitrofural	*7*, 171 (1974); *Suppl. 7*, 67 (1987); *50*, 195 (1990)
5-Nitro-2-furaldehyde semicarbazone (*see* Nitrofural)	
Nitrofurantoin	*50*, 211 (1990)
Nitrofurazone (*see* Nitrofural)	
1-[(5-Nitrofurfurylidene)amino]-2-imidazolidinone	*7*, 181 (1974); *Suppl. 7*, 67 (1987)
N-[4-(5-Nitro-2-furyl)-2-thiazolyl]acetamide	*1*, 181 (1972); *7*, 185 (1974); *Suppl. 7*, 67 (1987)
Nitrogen mustard	*9*, 193 (1975); *Suppl. 7*, 269 (1987)
Nitrogen mustard *N*-oxide	*9*, 209 (1975); *Suppl. 7*, 67 (1987)
1-Nitronaphthalene	*46*, 291 (1989)
2-Nitronaphthalene	*46*, 303 (1989)
3-Nitroperylene	*46*, 313 (1989)
2-Nitro-*para*-phenylenediamine (*see* 1,4-Diamino-2-nitrobenzene)	
2-Nitropropane	*29*, 331 (1982); *Suppl. 7*, 67 (1987)
1-Nitropyrene	*33*, 209 (1984); *Suppl. 7*, 67 (1987); *46*, 321 (1989)
2-Nitropyrene	*46*, 359 (1989)
4-Nitropyrene	*46*, 367 (1989)
N-Nitrosatable drugs	*24*, 297 (1980) (*corr. 42*, 260)
N-Nitrosatable pesticides	*30*, 359 (1983)
N'-Nitrosoanabasine	*37*, 225 (1985); *Suppl. 7*, 67 (1987)
N'-Nitrosoanatabine	*37*, 233 (1985); *Suppl. 7*, 67 (1987)
N-Nitrosodi-*n*-butylamine	*4*, 197 (1974); *17*, 51 (1978); *Suppl. 7*, 67 (1987)
N-Nitrosodiethanolamine	*17*, 77 (1978); *Suppl. 7*, 67 (1987)

N-Nitrosodiethylamine	*1*, 107 (1972) (*corr. 42*, 251); *17*, 83 (1978) (*corr. 42*, 257); *Suppl. 7*, 67 (1987)
N-Nitrosodimethylamine	*1*, 95 (1972); *17*, 125 (1978) (*corr. 42*, 257); *Suppl. 7*, 67 (1987)
N-Nitrosodiphenylamine	*27*, 213 (1982); *Suppl. 7*, 67 (1987)
para-Nitrosodiphenylamine	*27*, 227 (1982) (*corr. 42*, 261); *Suppl. 7*, 68 (1987)
N-Nitrosodi-*n*-propylamine	*17*, 177 (1978); *Suppl. 7*, 68 (1987)
N-Nitroso-*N*-ethylurea (*see N*-Ethyl-*N*-nitrosourea)	
N-Nitrosofolic acid	*17*, 217 (1978); *Suppl. 7*, 68 (1987)
N-Nitrosoguvacine	*37*, 263 (1985); *Suppl. 7*, 68 (1987)
N-Nitrosoguvacoline	*37*, 263 (1985); *Suppl. 7*, 68 (1987)
N-Nitrosohydroxyproline	*17*, 304 (1978); *Suppl. 7*, 68 (1987)
3-(*N*-Nitrosomethylamino)propionaldehyde	*37*, 263 (1985); *Suppl. 7*, 68 (1987)
3-(*N*-Nitrosomethylamino)propionitrile	*37*, 263 (1985); *Suppl. 7*, 68 (1987)
4-(*N*-Nitrosomethylamino)-4-(3-pyridyl)-1-butanal	*37*, 205 (1985); *Suppl. 7*, 68 (1987)
4-(*N*-Nitrosomethylamino)-1-(3-pyridyl)-1-butanone	*37*, 209 (1985); *Suppl. 7*, 68 (1987)
N-Nitrosomethylethylamine	*17*, 221 (1978); *Suppl. 7*, 68 (1987)
N-Nitroso-*N*-methylurea (*see N*-Methyl-*N*-nitrosourea)	
N-Nitroso-*N*-methylurethane (*see N*-Methyl-*N*-nitrosourethane)	
N-Nitrosomethylvinylamine	*17*, 257 (1978); *Suppl. 7*, 68 (1987)
N-Nitrosomorpholine	*17*, 263 (1978); *Suppl. 7*, 68 (1987)
N'-Nitrosonornicotine	*17*, 281 (1978); *37*, 241 (1985); *Suppl. 7*, 68 (1987)
N-Nitrosopiperidine	*17*, 287 (1978); *Suppl. 7*, 68 (1987)
N-Nitrosoproline	*17*, 303 (1978); *Suppl. 7*, 68 (1987)
N-Nitrosopyrrolidine	*17*, 313 (1978); *Suppl. 7*, 68 (1987)
N-Nitrososarcosine	*17*, 327 (1978); *Suppl. 7*, 68 (1987)
Nitrosoureas, chloroethyl (*see* Chloroethyl nitrosoureas)	
5-Nitro-*ortho*-toluidine	*48*, 169 (1990)
2-Nitrotoluene	*65*, 409 (1996)
3-Nitrotoluene	*65*, 409 (1996)
4-Nitrotoluene	*65*, 409 (1996)
Nitrous oxide (*see* Anaesthetics, volatile)	
Nitrovin	*31*, 185 (1983); *Suppl. 7*, 68 (1987)
Nivalenol (*see* Toxins derived from *Fusarium graminearum*, *F. culmorum* and *F. crookwellense*)	
NNA [*see* 4-(*N*-Nitrosomethylamino)-4-(3-pyridyl)-1-butanal]	
NNK [*see* 4-(*N*-Nitrosomethylamino)-1-(3-pyridyl)-1-butanone]	
Nonsteroidal oestrogens (*see also* Oestrogens, progestins and combinations)	*Suppl. 7*, 272 (1987)
Norethisterone (*see also* Progestins; Combined oral contraceptives)	*6*, 179 (1974); *21*, 461 (1979)
Norethynodrel (*see also* Progestins; Combined oral contraceptives	*6*, 191 (1974); *21*, 461 (1979) (*corr. 42*, 259)
Norgestrel (*see also* Progestins, Combined oral contraceptives)	*6*, 201 (1974); *21*, 479 (1979)
Nylon 6	*19*, 120 (1979); *Suppl. 7*, 68 (1987)

O

Ochratoxin A	*10*, 191 (1976); *31*, 191 (1983) (*corr. 42*, 262); *Suppl. 7*, 271 (1987); *56*, 489 (1993)
Oestradiol-17β (*see also* Steroidal oestrogens)	*6*, 99 (1974); *21*, 279 (1979)

Oestradiol 3-benzoate (*see* Oestradiol-17β)
Oestradiol dipropionate (*see* Oestradiol-17β)
Oestradiol mustard   9, 217 (1975); *Suppl. 7*, 68 (1987)
Oestradiol-17β-valerate (*see* Oestradiol-17β)
Oestriol (*see also* Steroidal oestrogens)   6, 117 (1974); 21, 327 (1979);
                                                                 Suppl. 7, 285 (1987)
Oestrogen-progestin combinations (*see* Oestrogens, progestins
    and combinations)
Oestrogen-progestin replacement therapy (*see also* Oestrogens, *Suppl. 7*, 308 (1987)
    progestins and combinations)
Oestrogen replacement therapy (*see also* Oestrogens, progestins *Suppl. 7*, 280 (1987)
    and combinations)
Oestrogens (*see* Oestrogens, progestins and combinations)
Oestrogens, conjugated (*see* Conjugated oestrogens)
Oestrogens, nonsteroidal (*see* Nonsteroidal oestrogens)
Oestrogens, progestins and combinations   6 (1974); 21 (1979);
                                                                 Suppl. 7, 272 (1987)
Oestrogens, steroidal (*see* Steroidal oestrogens)
Oestrone (*see* also Steroidal oestrogens)   6, 123 (1974); 21, 343 (1979)
                                                                 (*corr.* 42, 259)
Oestrone benzoate (*see* Oestrone)
Oil Orange SS   8, 165 (1975); *Suppl. 7*, 69 (1987)
Opisthorchis felineus (infection with)   61, 121 (1994)
Opisthorchis viverrini (infection with)   61, 121 (1994)
Oral contraceptives, combined (*see* Combined oral contraceptives)
Oral contraceptives, investigational (*see* Combined oral contraceptives)
Oral contraceptives, sequential (*see* Sequential oral contraceptives)
Orange I   8, 173 (1975); *Suppl. 7*, 69 (1987)
Orange G   8, 181 (1975); *Suppl. 7*, 69 (1987)
Organolead compounds (*see also* Lead and lead compounds)   *Suppl. 7*, 230 (1987)
Oxazepam   13, 58 (1977); *Suppl. 7*, 69 (1987);
                                                                 66, 115 (1996)
Oxymetholone [*see also* Androgenic (anabolic) steroids]   13, 131 (1977)
Oxyphenbutazone   13, 185 (1977); *Suppl. 7*, 69 (1987)

P

Paint manufacture and painting (occupational exposures in)   47, 329 (1989)
Panfuran S (*see also* Dihydroxymethylfuratrizine)   24, 77 (1980); *Suppl. 7*, 69 (1987)
Paper manufacture (*see* Pulp and paper manufacture)
Paracetamol   50, 307 (1990)
Parasorbic acid   10, 199 (1976) (*corr.* 42, 255);
                                                                 Suppl. 7, 69 (1987)
Parathion   30, 153 (1983); *Suppl. 7*, 69 (1987)
Patulin   10, 205 (1976); 40, 83 (1986);
                                                                 Suppl. 7, 69 (1987)
Penicillic acid   10, 211 (1976); *Suppl. 7*, 69 (1987)
Pentachloroethane   41, 99 (1986); *Suppl. 7*, 69 (1987)
Pentachloronitrobenzene (see Quintozene)
Pentachlorophenol (*see also* Chlorophenols; Chlorophenols,   20, 303 (1979); 53, 371 (1991)
    occupational exposures to)
Permethrin   53, 329 (1991)
Perylene   32, 411 (1983); *Suppl. 7*, 69 (1987)
Petasitenine   31, 207 (1983); *Suppl. 7*, 69 (1987)

Petasites japonicus (see Pyrrolizidine alkaloids)	
Petroleum refining (occupational exposures in)	45, 39 (1989)
Petroleum solvents	47, 43 (1989)
Phenacetin	13, 141 (1977); 24, 135 (1980); Suppl. 7, 310 (1987)
Phenanthrene	32, 419 (1983); Suppl. 7, 69 (1987)
Phenazopyridine hydrochloride	8, 117 (1975); 24, 163 (1980) (corr. 42, 260); Suppl. 7, 312 (1987)
Phenelzine sulfate	24, 175 (1980); Suppl. 7, 312 (1987)
Phenicarbazide	12, 177 (1976); Suppl. 7, 70 (1987)
Phenobarbital	13, 157 (1977); Suppl. 7, 313 (1987)
Phenol	47, 263 (1989) (corr. 50, 385)
Phenoxyacetic acid herbicides (see Chlorophenoxy herbicides)	
Phenoxybenzamine hydrochloride	9, 223 (1975); 24, 185 (1980); Suppl. 7, 70 (1987)
Phenylbutazone	13, 183 (1977); Suppl. 7, 316 (1987)
meta-Phenylenediamine	16, 111 (1978); Suppl. 7, 70 (1987)
para-Phenylenediamine	16, 125 (1978); Suppl. 7, 70 (1987)
Phenyl glycidyl ether (see Glycidyl ethers)	
N-Phenyl-2-naphthylamine	16, 325 (1978) (corr. 42, 257); Suppl. 7, 318 (1987)
ortho-Phenylphenol	30, 329 (1983); Suppl. 7, 70 (1987)
Phenytoin	13, 201 (1977); Suppl. 7, 319 (1987); 66, 175 (1996)
PhIP	56, 229 (1993)
Pickled vegetables	56, 83 (1993)
Picloram	53, 481 (1991)
Piperazine oestrone sulfate (see Conjugated oestrogens)	
Piperonyl butoxide	30, 183 (1983); Suppl. 7, 70 (1987)
Pitches, coal-tar (see Coal-tar pitches)	
Polyacrylic acid	19, 62 (1979); Suppl. 7, 70 (1987)
Polybrominated biphenyls	18, 107 (1978); 41, 261 (1986); Suppl. 7, 321 (1987)
Polychlorinated biphenyls	7, 261 (1974); 18, 43 (1978) (corr. 42, 258); Suppl. 7, 322 (1987)
Polychlorinated camphenes (see Toxaphene)	
Polychloroprene	19, 141 (1979); Suppl. 7, 70 (1987)
Polyethylene	19, 164 (1979); Suppl. 7, 70 (1987)
Polymethylene polyphenyl isocyanate	19, 314 (1979); Suppl. 7, 70 (1987)
Polymethyl methacrylate	19, 195 (1979); Suppl. 7, 70 (1987)
Polyoestradiol phosphate (see Oestradiol-17β)	
Polypropylene	19, 218 (1979); Suppl. 7, 70 (1987)
Polystyrene	19, 245 (1979); Suppl. 7, 70 (1987)
Polytetrafluoroethylene	19, 288 (1979); Suppl. 7, 70 (1987)
Polyurethane foams	19, 320 (1979); Suppl. 7, 70 (1987)
Polyvinyl acetate	19, 346 (1979); Suppl. 7, 70 (1987)
Polyvinyl alcohol	19, 351 (1979); Suppl. 7, 70 (1987)
Polyvinyl chloride	7, 306 (1974); 19, 402 (1979); Suppl. 7, 70 (1987)
Polyvinyl pyrrolidone	19, 463 (1979); Suppl. 7, 70 (1987)
Ponceau MX	8, 189 (1975); Suppl. 7, 70 (1987)
Ponceau 3R	8, 199 (1975); Suppl. 7, 70 (1987)
Ponceau SX	8, 207 (1975); Suppl. 7, 70 (1987)
Potassium arsenate (see Arsenic and arsenic compounds)	
Potassium arsenite (see Arsenic and arsenic compounds)	

Potassium bis(2-hydroxyethyl)dithiocarbamate	12, 183 (1976); *Suppl. 7*, 70 (1987)
Potassium bromate	40, 207 (1986); *Suppl. 7*, 70 (1987)
Potassium chromate (*see* Chromium and chromium compounds)	
Potassium dichromate (*see* Chromium and chromium compounds)	
Prazepam	66, 143 (1996)
Prednimustine	50, 115 (1990)
Prednisone	26, 293 (1981); *Suppl. 7*, 326 (1987)
Printing processes and printing inks	65, 33 (1996)
Procarbazine hydrochloride	26, 311 (1981); *Suppl. 7*, 327 (1987)
Proflavine salts	24, 195 (1980); *Suppl. 7*, 70 (1987)
Progesterone (*see also* Progestins; Combined oral contraceptives)	6, 135 (1974); 21, 491 (1979) (*corr. 42*, 259)
Progestins (*see also* Oestrogens, progestins and combinations)	*Suppl. 7*, 289 (1987)
Pronetalol hydrochloride	13, 227 (1977) (*corr. 42*, 256); *Suppl. 7*, 70 (1987)
1,3-Propane sultone	4, 253 (1974) (*corr. 42*, 253); *Suppl. 7*, 70 (1987)
Propham	12, 189 (1976); *Suppl. 7*, 70 (1987)
β-Propiolactone	4, 259 (1974) (*corr. 42*, 253); *Suppl. 7*, 70 (1987)
n-Propyl carbamate	12, 201 (1976); *Suppl. 7*, 70 (1987)
Propylene	19, 213 (1979); *Suppl. 7*, 71 (1987); 60, 161 (1994)
Propylene oxide	11, 191 (1976); 36, 227 (1985) (*corr. 42*, 263); *Suppl. 7*, 328 (1987); 60, 181 (1994)
Propylthiouracil	7, 67 (1974); *Suppl. 7*, 329 (1987)
Ptaquiloside (*see also* Bracken fern)	40, 55 (1986); *Suppl. 7*, 71 (1987)
Pulp and paper manufacture	25, 157 (1981); *Suppl. 7*, 385 (1987)
Pyrene	32, 431 (1983); *Suppl. 7*, 71 (1987)
Pyrido[3,4-*c*]psoralen	40, 349 (1986); *Suppl. 7*, 71 (1987)
Pyrimethamine	13, 233 (1977); *Suppl. 7*, 71 (1987)
Pyrrolizidine alkaloids (*see* Hydroxysenkirkine; Isatidine; Jacobine; Lasiocarpine; Monocrotaline; Retrorsine; Riddelliine; Seneciphylline; Senkirkine)	

Q

Quercetin (*see also* Bracken fern)	31, 213 (1983); *Suppl. 7*, 71 (1987)
para-Quinone	15, 255 (1977); *Suppl. 7*, 71 (1987)
Quintozene	5, 211 (1974); *Suppl. 7*, 71 (1987)

R

Radon	43, 173 (1988) (*corr. 45*, 283)
Reserpine	10, 217 (1976); 24, 211 (1980) (*corr. 42*, 260); *Suppl. 7*, 330 (1987)
Resorcinol	15, 155 (1977); *Suppl. 7*, 71 (1987)
Retrorsine	10, 303 (1976); *Suppl. 7*, 71 (1987)
Rhodamine B	16, 221 (1978); *Suppl. 7*, 71 (1987)
Rhodamine 6G	16, 233 (1978); *Suppl. 7*, 71 (1987)
Riddelliine	10, 313 (1976); *Suppl. 7*, 71 (1987)
Rifampicin	24, 243 (1980); *Suppl. 7*, 71 (1987)

Ripazepam	66, 157 (1996)
Rockwool (see Man-made mineral fibres)	
Rubber industry	28 (1982) (corr. 42, 261); Suppl. 7, 332 (1987)
Rugulosin	40, 99 (1986); Suppl. 7, 71 (1987)

S

Saccharated iron oxide	2, 161 (1973); Suppl. 7, 71 (1987)
Saccharin	22, 111 (1980) (corr. 42, 259); Suppl. 7, 334 (1987)
Safrole	1, 169 (1972); 10, 231 (1976); Suppl. 7, 71 (1987)
Salted fish	56, 41 (1993)
Sawmill industry (including logging) [see Lumber and sawmill industry (including logging)]	
Scarlet Red	8, 217 (1975); Suppl. 7, 71 (1987)
Schistosoma haematobium (infection with)	61, 45 (1994)
Schistosoma japonicum (infection with)	61, 45 (1994)
Schistosoma mansoni (infection with)	61, 45 (1994)
Selenium and selenium compounds	9, 245 (1975) (corr. 42, 255); Suppl. 7, 71 (1987)
Selenium dioxide (see Selenium and selenium compounds)	
Selenium oxide (see Selenium and selenium compounds)	
Semicarbazide hydrochloride	12, 209 (1976) (corr. 42, 256); Suppl. 7, 71 (1987)
Senecio jacobaea L. (see Pyrrolizidine alkaloids)	
Senecio longilobus (see Pyrrolizidine alkaloids)	
Seneciphylline	10, 319, 335 (1976); Suppl. 7, 71 (1987)
Senkirkine	10, 327 (1976); 31, 231 (1983); Suppl. 7, 71 (1987)
Sepiolite	42, 175 (1987); Suppl. 7, 71 (1987)
Sequential oral contraceptives (see also Oestrogens, progestins and combinations)	Suppl. 7, 296 (1987)
Shale-oils	35, 161 (1985); Suppl. 7, 339 (1987)
Shikimic acid (see also Bracken fern)	40, 55 (1986); Suppl. 7, 71 (1987)
Shoe manufacture and repair (see Boot and shoe manufacture and repair)	
Silica (see also Amorphous silica; Crystalline silica)	42, 39 (1987)
Simazine	53, 495 (1991)
Slagwool (see Man-made mineral fibres)	
Sodium arsenate (see Arsenic and arsenic compounds)	
Sodium arsenite (see Arsenic and arsenic compounds)	
Sodium cacodylate (see Arsenic and arsenic compounds)	
Sodium chlorite	52, 145 (1991)
Sodium chromate (see Chromium and chromium compounds)	
Sodium cyclamate (see Cyclamates)	
Sodium dichromate (see Chromium and chromium compounds)	
Sodium diethyldithiocarbamate	12, 217 (1976); Suppl. 7, 71 (1987)
Sodium equilin sulfate (see Conjugated oestrogens)	
Sodium fluoride (see Fluorides)	
Sodium monofluorophosphate (see Fluorides)	
Sodium oestrone sulfate (see Conjugated oestrogens)	

Sodium *ortho*-phenylphenate (*see also* ortho-Phenylphenol)	*30*, 329 (1983); *Suppl. 7*, 392 (1987)
Sodium saccharin (*see* Saccharin)	
Sodium selenate (*see* Selenium and selenium compounds)	
Sodium selenite (*see* Selenium and selenium compounds)	
Sodium silicofluoride (*see* Fluorides)	
Solar radiation	*55* (1992)
Soots	*3*, 22 (1973); *35*, 219 (1985); *Suppl. 7*, 343 (1987)
Spironolactone	*24*, 259 (1980); *Suppl. 7*, 344 (1987)
Stannous fluoride (*see* Fluorides)	
Steel founding (*see* Iron and steel founding)	
Sterigmatocystin	*1*, 175 (1972); *10*, 245 (1976); *Suppl. 7*, 72 (1987)
Steroidal oestrogens (*see also* Oestrogens, progestins and combinations)	*Suppl. 7*, 280 (1987)
Streptozotocin	*4*, 221 (1974); *17*, 337 (1978); *Suppl. 7*, 72 (1987)
Strobane* (*see* Terpene polychlorinates)	
Strong-inorganic-acid mists containing sulfuric acid (*see* Mists and vapours from sulfuric acid and other strong inorganic acids)	
Strontium chromate (*see* Chromium and chromium compounds)	
Styrene	*19*, 231 (1979) (*corr. 42*, 258); *Suppl. 7*, 345 (1987); *60*, 233 (1994) (*corr. 65*, 549)
Styrene-acrylonitrile-copolymers	*19*, 97 (1979); *Suppl. 7*, 72 (1987)
Styrene-butadiene copolymers	*19*, 252 (1979); *Suppl. 7*, 72 (1987)
Styrene-7,8-oxide	*11*, 201 (1976); *19*, 275 (1979); *36*, 245 (1985); *Suppl. 7*, 72 (1987); *60*, 321 (1994)
Succinic anhydride	*15*, 265 (1977); *Suppl. 7*, 72 (1987)
Sudan I	*8*, 225 (1975); *Suppl. 7*, 72 (1987)
Sudan II	*8*, 233 (1975); *Suppl. 7*, 72 (1987)
Sudan III	*8*, 241 (1975); *Suppl. 7*, 72 (1987)
Sudan Brown RR	*8*, 249 (1975); *Suppl. 7*, 72 (1987)
Sudan Red 7B	*8*, 253 (1975); *Suppl. 7*, 72 (1987)
Sulfafurazole	*24*, 275 (1980); *Suppl. 7*, 347 (1987)
Sulfallate	*30*, 283 (1983); *Suppl. 7*, 72 (1987)
Sulfamethoxazole	*24*, 285 (1980); *Suppl. 7*, 348 (1987)
Sulfites (*see* Sulfur dioxide and some sulfites, bisulfites and metabisulfites)	
Sulfur dioxide and some sulfites, bisulfites and metabisulfites	*54*, 131 (1992)
Sulfur mustard (*see* Mustard gas)	
Sulfuric acid and other strong inorganic acids, occupational exposures to mists and vapours from	*54*, 41 (1992)
Sulfur trioxide	*54*, 121 (1992)
Sulphisoxazole (*see* Sulfafurazole)	
Sunset Yellow FCF	*8*, 257 (1975); *Suppl. 7*, 72 (1987)
Symphytine	*31*, 239 (1983); *Suppl. 7*, 72 (1987)

T

2,4,5-T (*see also* Chlorophenoxy herbicides; Chlorophenoxy herbicides, occupational exposures to)	*15*, 273 (1977)
Talc	*42*, 185 (1987); *Suppl. 7*, 349 (1987)
Tamoxifen	*66*, 253 (1996)

Tannic acid	10, 253 (1976) (corr. 42, 255); Suppl. 7, 72 (1987)
Tannins (see also Tannic acid)	10, 254 (1976); Suppl. 7, 72 (1987)
TCDD (see 2,3,7,8-Tetrachlorodibenzo-*para*-dioxin)	
TDE (see DDT)	
Tea	51, 207 (1991)
Temazepam	66, 161 (1996)
Terpene polychlorinates	5, 219 (1974); Suppl. 7, 72 (1987)
Testosterone (see also Androgenic (anabolic) steroids)	6, 209 (1974); 21, 519 (1979)
Testosterone oenanthate (see Testosterone)	
Testosterone propionate (see Testosterone)	
2,2′,5,5′-Tetrachlorobenzidine	27, 141 (1982); Suppl. 7, 72 (1987)
2,3,7,8-Tetrachlorodibenzo-*para*-dioxin	15, 41 (1977); Suppl. 7, 350 (1987)
1,1,1,2-Tetrachloroethane	41, 87 (1986); Suppl. 7, 72 (1987)
1,1,2,2-Tetrachloroethane	20, 477 (1979); Suppl. 7, 354 (1987)
Tetrachloroethylene	20, 491 (1979); Suppl. 7, 355 (1987); 63, 159 (1995) (corr. 65, 549)
2,3,4,6-Tetrachlorophenol (see Chlorophenols; Chlorophenols, occupational exposures to)	
Tetrachlorvinphos	30, 197 (1983); Suppl. 7, 72 (1987)
Tetraethyllead (see Lead and lead compounds)	
Tetrafluoroethylene	19, 285 (1979); Suppl. 7, 72 (1987)
Tetrakis(hydroxymethyl) phosphonium salts	48, 95 (1990)
Tetramethyllead (see Lead and lead compounds)	
Tetranitromethane	65, 437 (1996)
Textile manufacturing industry, exposures in	48, 215 (1990) (corr. 51, 483)
Theobromine	51, 421 (1991)
Theophylline	51, 391 (1991)
Thioacetamide	7, 77 (1974); Suppl. 7, 72 (1987)
4,4′-Thiodianiline	16, 343 (1978); 27, 147 (1982); Suppl. 7, 72 (1987)
Thiotepa	9, 85 (1975); Suppl. 7, 368 (1987); 50, 123 (1990)
Thiouracil	7, 85 (1974); Suppl. 7, 72 (1987)
Thiourea	7, 95 (1974); Suppl. 7, 72 (1987)
Thiram	12, 225 (1976); Suppl. 7, 72 (1987); 53, 403 (1991)
Titanium dioxide	47, 307 (1989)
Tobacco habits other than smoking (see Tobacco products, smokeless)	
Tobacco products, smokeless	37 (1985) (corr. 42, 263; 52, 513); Suppl. 7, 357 (1987)
Tobacco smoke	38 (1986) (corr. 42, 263); Suppl. 7, 357 (1987)
Tobacco smoking (see Tobacco smoke)	
ortho-Tolidine (see 3,3′-Dimethylbenzidine)	
2,4-Toluene diisocyanate (see also Toluene diisocyanates)	19, 303 (1979); 39, 287 (1986)
2,6-Toluene diisocyanate (see also Toluene diisocyanates)	19, 303 (1979); 39, 289 (1986)
Toluene	47, 79 (1989)
Toluene diisocyanates	39, 287 (1986) (corr. 42, 264); Suppl. 7, 72 (1987)
Toluenes, α-chlorinated (see α-Chlorinated toluenes)	
ortho-Toluenesulfonamide (see Saccharin)	
ortho-Toluidine	16, 349 (1978); 27, 155 (1982); Suppl. 7, 362 (1987)

Toremifene	66, 367 (1996)
Toxaphene	20, 327 (1979); Suppl. 7, 72 (1987)
T-2 Toxin (see Toxins derived from *Fusarium sporotrichioides*)	
Toxins derived from *Fusarium graminearum*, *F. culmorum* and *F. crookwellense*	11, 169 (1976); 31, 153, 279 (1983); Suppl. 7, 64, 74 (1987); 56, 397 (1993)
Toxins derived from *Fusarium moniliforme*	56, 445 (1993)
Toxins derived from *Fusarium sporotrichioides*	31, 265 (1983); Suppl. 7, 73 (1987); 56, 467 (1993)
Tremolite (see Asbestos)	
Treosulfan	26, 341 (1981); Suppl. 7, 363 (1987)
Triaziquone [see Tris(aziridinyl)-*para*-benzoquinone]	
Trichlorfon	30, 207 (1983); Suppl. 7, 73 (1987)
Trichlormethine	9, 229 (1975); Suppl. 7, 73 (1987); 50, 143 (1990)
Trichloroacetic acid	63, 291 (1995) (corr. 65, 549)
Trichloroacetonitrile (see Halogenated acetonitriles)	
1,1,1-Trichloroethane	20, 515 (1979); Suppl. 7, 73 (1987)
1,1,2-Trichloroethane	20, 533 (1979); Suppl. 7, 73 (1987); 52, 337 (1991)
Trichloroethylene	11, 263 (1976); 20, 545 (1979); Suppl. 7, 364 (1987); 63, 75 (1995) (corr. 65, 549)
2,4,5-Trichlorophenol (see also Chlorophenols; Chlorophenols occupational exposures to)	20, 349 (1979)
2,4,6-Trichlorophenol (see also Chlorophenols; Chlorophenols, occupational exposures to)	20, 349 (1979)
(2,4,5-Trichlorophenoxy)acetic acid (see 2,4,5-T)	
1,2,3-Trichloropropane	63, 223 (1995)
Trichlorotriethylamine-hydrochloride (see Trichlormethine)	
T_2-Trichothecene (see Toxins derived from *Fusarium sporotrichioides*)	
Triethylene glycol diglycidyl ether	11, 209 (1976); Suppl. 7, 73 (1987)
Trifluralin	53, 515 (1991)
4,4',6-Trimethylangelicin plus ultraviolet radiation (see also Angelicin and some synthetic derivatives)	Suppl. 7, 57 (1987)
2,4,5-Trimethylaniline	27, 177 (1982); Suppl. 7, 73 (1987)
2,4,6-Trimethylaniline	27, 178 (1982); Suppl. 7, 73 (1987)
4,5',8-Trimethylpsoralen	40, 357 (1986); Suppl. 7, 366 (1987)
Trimustine hydrochloride (see Trichlormethine)	
2,4,6-Trinitrotoluene	65, 449 (1996)
Triphenylene	32, 447 (1983); Suppl. 7, 73 (1987)
Tris(aziridinyl)-*para*-benzoquinone	9, 67 (1975); Suppl. 7, 367 (1987)
Tris(1-aziridinyl)phosphine-oxide	9, 75 (1975); Suppl. 7, 73 (1987)
Tris(1-aziridinyl)phosphine-sulphide (see Thiotepa)	
2,4,6-Tris(1-aziridinyl)-*s*-triazine	9, 95 (1975); Suppl. 7, 73 (1987)
Tris(2-chloroethyl) phosphate	48, 109 (1990)
1,2,3-Tris(chloromethoxy)propane	15, 301 (1977); Suppl. 7, 73 (1987)
Tris(2,3-dibromopropyl)phosphate	20, 575 (1979); Suppl. 7, 369 (1987)
Tris(2-methyl-1-aziridinyl)phosphine-oxide	9, 107 (1975); Suppl. 7, 73 (1987)
Trp-P-1	31, 247 (1983); Suppl. 7, 73 (1987)
Trp-P-2	31, 255 (1983); Suppl. 7, 73 (1987)
Trypan blue	8, 267 (1975); Suppl. 7, 73 (1987)
Tussilago farfara L. (see Pyrrolizidine alkaloids)	

U

Ultraviolet radiation	*40*, 379 (1986); *55* (1992)
Underground haematite mining with exposure to radon	*1*, 29 (1972); *Suppl. 7*, 216 (1987)
Uracil mustard	*9*, 235 (1975); *Suppl. 7*, 370 (1987)
Urethane	*7*, 111 (1974); *Suppl. 7*, 73 (1987)

V

Vat Yellow 4	*48*, 161 (1990)
Vinblastine sulfate	*26*, 349 (1981) (*corr. 42*, 261); *Suppl. 7*, 371 (1987)
Vincristine sulfate	*26*, 365 (1981); *Suppl. 7*, 372 (1987)
Vinyl acetate	*19*, 341 (1979); *39*, 113 (1986); *Suppl. 7*, 73 (1987); *63*, 443 (1995)
Vinyl bromide	*19*, 367 (1979); *39*, 133 (1986); *Suppl. 7*, 73 (1987)
Vinyl chloride	*7*, 291 (1974); *19*, 377 (1979) (*corr. 42*, 258); *Suppl. 7*, 373 (1987)
Vinyl chloride-vinyl acetate copolymers	*7*, 311 (1976); *19*, 412 (1979) (*corr. 42*, 258); *Suppl. 7*, 73 (1987)
4-Vinylcyclohexene	*11*, 277 (1976); *39*, 181 (1986) *Suppl. 7*, 73 (1987); *60*, 347 (1994)
4-Vinylcyclohexene diepoxide	*11*, 141 (1976); *Suppl. 7*, 63 (1987); *60*, 361 (1994)
Vinyl fluoride	*39*, 147 (1986); *Suppl. 7*, 73 (1987); *63*, 467 (1995)
Vinylidene chloride	*19*, 439 (1979); *39*, 195 (1986); *Suppl. 7*, 376 (1987)
Vinylidene chloride-vinyl chloride copolymers	*19*, 448 (1979) (*corr. 42*, 258); *Suppl. 7*, 73 (1987)
Vinylidene fluoride	*39*, 227 (1986); *Suppl. 7*, 73 (1987)
N-Vinyl-2-pyrrolidone	*19*, 461 (1979); *Suppl. 7*, 73 (1987)
Vinyl toluene	*60*, 373 (1994)

W

Welding	*49*, 447 (1990) (*corr. 52*, 513)
Wollastonite	*42*, 145 (1987); *Suppl. 7*, 377 (1987)
Wood dust	*62*, 35 (1995)
Wood industries	*25* (1981); *Suppl. 7*, 378 (1987)

X

Xylene	*47*, 125 (1989)
2,4-Xylidine	*16*, 367 (1978); *Suppl. 7*, 74 (1987)
2,5-Xylidine	*16*, 377 (1978); *Suppl. 7*, 74 (1987)
2,6-Xylidine (*see* 2,6-Dimethylaniline)	

Y

Yellow AB	8, 279 (1975); *Suppl. 7*, 74 (1987)
Yellow OB	8, 287 (1975); *Suppl. 7*, 74 (1987)

Z

Zearalenone (*see* Toxins derived from *Fusarium graminearum*, *F. culmorum* and *F. crookwellense*)
Zectran   *12*, 237 (1976); *Suppl. 7*, 74 (1987)
Zinc beryllium silicate (*see* Beryllium and beryllium compounds)
Zinc chromate (*see* Chromium and chromium compounds)
Zinc chromate hydroxide (*see* Chromium and chromium compounds)
Zinc potassium chromate (*see* Chromium and chromium compounds)
Zinc yellow (*see* Chromium and chromium compounds)
Zineb   *12*, 245 (1976); *Suppl. 7*, 74 (1987)
Ziram   *12*, 259 (1976); *Suppl. 7*, 74 (1987); *53*, 423 (1991)

IARC Scientific Publications

No. 1
Liver Cancer
1971; 176 pages; ISBN 0 19 723000 8

No. 2
Oncogenesis and Herpesviruses
Edited by P.M. Biggs, G. de Thé and
L.N. Payne
1972; 515 pages; ISBN 0 19 723001 6

No. 3
N-Nitroso Compounds: Analysis and
Formation
Edited by P. Bogovski, R. Preussman
and E.A. Walker
1972; 140 pages; ISBN 0 19 723002 4

No. 4
Transplacental Carcinogenesis
Edited by L. Tomatis and U. Mohr
1973; 181 pages; ISBN 0 19 723003 2

No. 5/6
Pathology of Tumours in Laboratory
Animals. Volume 1: Tumours of the Rat
Edited by V.S. Turusov
1973/1976; 533 pages;
ISBN 92 832 1410 2

No. 7
Host Environment Interactions in the
Etiology of Cancer in Man
Edited by R. Doll and I. Vodopija
1973; 464 pages; ISBN 0 19 723006 7

No. 8
Biological Effects of Asbestos
Edited by P. Bogovski, J.C. Gilson,
V. Timbrell and J.C. Wagner
1973; 346 pages; ISBN 0 19 723007 5

No. 9
N-Nitroso Compounds in the
Environment
Edited by P. Bogovski and E.A. Walker
1974; 243 pages; ISBN 0 19 723008 3

No. 10
Chemical Carcinogenesis Essays
Edited by R. Montesano and L. Tomatis
1974; 230 pages; ISBN 0 19 723009 1

No. 11
Oncogenesis and Herpes-viruses II
Edited by G. de-Thé, M.A. Epstein
and H. zur Hausen
1975; Two volumes, 511 pages; and
403 pages; ISBN 0 19 723010 5

No. 12
Screening Tests in Chemical
Carcinogenesis
Edited by R. Montesano, H. Bartsch
and L. Tomatis
1976; 666 pages; ISBN 0 19 723051 2

No. 13
Environmental Pollution and
Carcinogenic Risks
Edited by C. Rosenfeld and W. Davis
1975; 441 pages; ISBN 0 19 723012 1

No. 14
Environmental N-Nitroso Compounds.
Analysis and Formation
Edited by E.A. Walker, P. Bogovski and
L. Griciute
1976; 512 pages; ISBN 0 19 723013 X

No. 15
Cancer Incidence in Five Continents,
Volume III
Edited by J.A.H. Waterhouse, C. Muir,
P. Correa and J. Powell
1976; 584 pages; ISBN 0 19 723014 8

No. 16
Air Pollution and Cancer in Man
Edited by U. Mohr, D. Schmähl and
L. Tomatis
1977; 328 pages; ISBN 0 19 723015 6

No. 17*
Directory of On-Going Research in
Cancer Epidemiology 1977
Edited by C.S. Muir and G. Wagner
1977; 599 pages; ISBN 92 832 1117 0

No. 18
Environmental Carcinogens. Selected
Methods of Analysis. Volume 1: Analysis of Volatile Nitrosamines in Food
Editor-in-Chief: H. Egan
1978; 212 pages; ISBN 0 19 723017 2

No. 19
Environmental Aspects of N-Nitroso
Compounds
Edited by E.A. Walker, M. Castegnaro,
L. Griciute and R.E. Lyle
1978; 561 pages; ISBN 0 19 723018 0

No. 20
Nasopharyngeal Carcinoma:
Etiology and Control
Edited by G. de Thé and Y. Ito
1978; 606 pages; ISBN 0 19 723019 9

No. 21
Cancer Registration and its Techniques
Edited by R. MacLennan, C. Muir,
R. Steinitz and A. Winkler
1978; 235 pages; ISBN 0 19 723020 2

No. 22
Environmental Carcinogens: Selected
Methods of Analysis. Volume 2:
Methods for the Measurement of Vinyl
Chloride in Poly(vinyl chloride), Air,
Water and Foodstuffs
Editor-in-Chief: H. Egan
1978; 142 pages; ISBN 0 19 723021 0

No. 23
Pathology of Tumours in Laboratory
Animals.
Volume II: Tumours of the Mouse
Editor-in-Chief: V.S. Turusov
1979; 669 pages; ISBN 0 19 723022 9

No. 24
Oncogenesis and Herpesviruses III
Edited by G. de-Thé, W. Henle and
F. Rapp
1978; Part I: 580 pages;
Part II: 512 pages; ISBN 0 19 723023 7

No. 25
Carcinogenic Risk: Strategies for
Intervention
Edited by W. Davis and C. Rosenfeld
1979; 280 pages; ISBN 0 19 723025 3

No. 26*
Directory of On-going Research in
Cancer Epidemiology 1978
Edited by C.S. Muir and G. Wagner
1978; 550 pages; ISBN 0 19 723026 1

No. 27
Molecular and Cellular Aspects of
Carcinogen Screening Tests
Edited by R. Montesano, H. Bartsch
and L. Tomatis
1980; 372 pages; ISBN 0 19 723027 X

No. 28*
Directory of On-going Research in
Cancer Epidemiology 1979
Edited by C.S. Muir and G. Wagner
1979; 672 pages; ISBN 92 832 1128 6

No. 29
Environmental Carcinogens. Selected
Methods of Analysis. Volume 3:
Analysis of Polycyclic Aromatic Hydrocarbons in Environmental Samples
Editor-in-Chief: H. Egan
1979; 240 pages; ISBN 0 19 723028 8

No. 30
Biological Effects of Mineral Fibres
Editor-in-Chief: J.C. Wagner
1980; Two volumes, 494 pages & 513
pages; ISBN 0 19 723030 X

No. 31
N-Nitroso Compounds: Analysis,
Formation and Occurrence
Edited by E.A. Walker, L. Griciute,
M. Castegnaro and M. Börzsönyi
1980; 835 pages; ISBN 0 19 723031 8

No. 32
Statistical Methods in Cancer Research.
Volume 1: The Analysis of Case-control Studies
By N.E. Breslow and N.E. Day
1980; 338 pages; ISBN 92 832 0132 9

*(out of print)

Publications list: Scientific Publications

No. 33*
Handling Chemical Carcinogens in the Laboratory
Edited by R. Montesano, H. Bartsch, E. Boyland, G. Della Porta, L. Fishbein, R.A. Griesemer, A.B. Swan and L. Tomatis
1979; 32 pages; ISBN 0 19 723033 4

No. 34
Pathology of Tumours in Laboratory Animals.
Volume III: Tumours of the Hamster
Editor-in-Chief: V.S. Turusov
1982; 461 pages; ISBN 0 19 723034 2

No. 35*
Directory of On-going Research in Cancer Epidemiology 1980
Edited by C.S. Muir and G. Wagner
1980; 660 pages; ISBN 0 19 723035 0

No. 36
Cancer Mortality by Occupation and Social Class 1851–1971
Edited by W.P.D. Logan
1982; 253 pages; ISBN 0 19 723036 9

No. 37
Laboratory Decontamination and Destruction of Aflatoxins B1, B2, G1, G2 in Laboratory Wastes
Edited by M. Castegnaro, D.C. Hunt, E.B. Sansone, P.L. Schuller, M.G. Siriwardana, G.M. Telling, H.P. van Egmond and E.A. Walker
1980; 56 pages; ISBN 0 19 723037 7

No. 38*
Directory of On-going Research in Cancer Epidemiology 1981
Edited by C.S. Muir and G. Wagner
1981; 696 pages; ISBN 0 19 723038 5

No. 39
Host Factors in Human Carcinogenesis
Edited by H. Bartsch and B. Armstrong
1982; 583 pages; ISBN 0 19 723039 3

No. 40
Environmental Carcinogens: Selected Methods of Analysis. Volume 4: Some Aromatic Amines and Azo Dyes in the General and Industrial Environment
Edited by L. Fishbein, M. Castegnaro, I.K. O'Neill and H. Bartsch
1981; 347 pages; ISBN 0 19 723040 7

No. 41
N-Nitroso Compounds: Occurrence and Biological Effects
Edited by H. Bartsch, I.K. O'Neill, M. Castegnaro and M. Okada
982; 755 pages; ISBN 0 19 723041 5

No. 42
Cancer Incidence in Five Continents Volume IV
Edited by J. Waterhouse, C. Muir, K. Shanmugaratnam and J. Powell
1982; 811 pages; ISBN 0 19 723042 3

No. 43
Laboratory Decontamination and Destruction of Carcinogens in Laboratory Wastes: Some N-Nitrosamines
Edited by M. Castegnaro, G. Eisenbrand, G. Ellen, L. Keefer, D. Klein, E.B. Sansone, D. Spincer, G. Telling and K. Webb
1982; 73 pages; ISBN 0 19 723043 1

No. 44
Environmental Carcinogens: Selected Methods of Analysis.
Volume 5: Some Mycotoxins
Edited by L. Stoloff, M. Castegnaro, P. Scott, I.K. O'Neill and H. Bartsch
1983; 455 pages; ISBN 0 19 723044 X

No. 45
Environmental Carcinogens: Selected Methods of Analysis.
Volume 6: N-Nitroso Compounds
Edited by R. Preussmann, I.K. O'Neill, G. Eisenbrand, B. Spiegelhalder and H. Bartsch 1983;
508 pages; ISBN 0 19 723045 8

No. 46*
Directory of On-going Research in Cancer Epidemiology 1982
Edited by C.S. Muir and G. Wagner
1982; 722 pages; ISBN 0 19 723046 6

No. 47
Cancer Incidence in Singapore 1968–1977
Edited by K. Shanmugaratnam, H.P. Lee and N.E. Day
1983; 171 pages; ISBN 0 19 723047 4

No. 48
Cancer Incidence in the USSR (2nd Revised Edition)
Edited by N.P. Napalkov, G.F. Tserkovny, V.M. Merabishvili, D.M. Parkin, M. Smans and C.S. Muir
1983; 75 pages; ISBN 0 19 723048 2

No. 49
Laboratory Decontamination and Destruction of Carcinogens in Laboratory Wastes: Some Polycyclic Aromatic Hydrocarbons
Edited by M. Castegnaro, G. Grimmer, O. Hutzinger, W. Karcher, H. Kunte, M. Lafontaine, H.C. Van der Plas, E.B. Sansone and S.P. Tucker
1983; 87 pages; ISBN 0 19 723049 0

No. 50*
Directory of On-going Research in Cancer Epidemiology 1983
Edited by C.S. Muir and G. Wagner
1983; 731 pages; ISBN 0 19 723050 4

No. 51
Modulators of Experimental Carcinogenesis
Edited by V. Turusov and R. Montesano
1983; 307 pages; ISBN 0 19 723060 1

No. 52
Second Cancers in Relation to Radiation Treatment for Cervical Cancer: Results of a Cancer Registry Collaboration.
Edited by N.E. Day and J.C. Boice, Jr
1984; 207 pages; ISBN 0 19 723052 0

No. 53
Nickel in the Human Environment
Editor-in-Chief: F.W. Sunderman, Jr
1984; 529 pages; ISBN 0 19 723059 8

No. 54
Laboratory Decontamination and Destruction of Carcinogens in Laboratory Wastes: Some Hydrazines
Edited by M. Castegnaro, G. Ellen, M. Lafontaine, H.C. van der Plas, E.B. Sansone and S.P. Tucker
1983; 87 pages; ISBN 0 19 723053

No. 55
Laboratory Decontamination and Destruction of Carcinogens in Laboratory Wastes: Some N-Nitrosamides
Edited by M. Castegnaro, M. Bernard, L.W. van Broekhoven, D. Fine, R. Massey, E.B. Sansone, P.L.R. Smith, B. Spiegelhalder, A. Stacchini, G. Telling and J.J. Vallon
1984; 66 pages; ISBN 0 19 723054 7

No. 56
Models, Mechanisms and Etiology of Tumour Promotion
Edited by M. Börzsönyi, N.E. Day, K. Lapis and H. Yamasaki
1984; 532 pages; ISBN 0 19 723058 X

No. 57
N-Nitroso Compounds: Occurrence, Biological Effects and Relevance to Human Cancer
Edited by I.K. O'Neill, R.C. von Borstel, C.T. Miller, J. Long and H. Bartsch
1984; 1013 pages; ISBN 0 19 723055 5

No 58
Age-related Factors in Carcinogenesis
Edited by A. Likhachev, V. Anisimov and R. Montesano
1985; 288 pages; ISBN 92 832 1158 8

No. 59
Monitoring Human Exposure to Carcinogenic and Mutagenic Agents
Edited by A. Berlin, M. Draper, K. Hemminki and H. Vainio
1984; 457 pages; ISBN 0 19 723056 3

*(out of print)

No. 60
Burkitt's Lymphoma: A Human Cancer Model
Edited by G. Lenoir, G. O'Conor and C.L.M. Olweny
1985; 484 pages; ISBN 0 19 723057 1

No. 61
Laboratory Decontamination and Destruction of Carcinogens in Laboratory Wastes: Some Haloethers
Edited by M. Castegnaro, M. Alvarez, M. Iovu, E.B. Sansone, G.M. Telling and D.T. Williams
1985; 55 pages; ISBN 0 19 723061 X

No. 62*
Directory of On-going Research in Cancer Epidemiology 1984
Edited by C.S. Muir and G. Wagner
1984; 717 pages; ISBN 0 19 723062 8

No. 63
Virus-associated Cancers in Africa
Edited by A.O. Williams, G.T. O'Conor, G.B. de Thé and C.A. Johnson
1984; 773 pages; ISBN: 0 19 723063 6

No. 64
Laboratory Decontamination and Destruction of Carcinogens in Laboratory Wastes: Some Aromatic Amines and 4-Nitrobiphenyl
Edited by M. Castegnaro, J. Barek, J. Dennis, G. Ellen, M. Klibanov, M. Lafontaine, R. Mitchum, P. van Roosmalen, E.B. Sansone, L.A. Sternson and M. Vahl
1985; 84 pages; ISBN: 92 832 1164 2

No. 65
Interpretation of Negative Epidemiological Evidence for Carcinogenicity
Edited by N.J. Wald and R. Doll
1985; 232 pages; ISBN 92 832 1165 0

No. 66
The Role of the Registry in Cancer Control
Edited by D.M. Parkin, G. Wagner and C.S. Muir
1985; 152 pages; ISBN 92 832 0166 3

No. 67
Transformation Assay of Established Cell Lines: Mechanisms and Application
Edited by T. Kakunaga and H. Yamasaki
1985; 225 pages; ISBN 92 832 1167 7

No. 68
Environmental Carcinogens: Selected Methods of Analysis.
Volume 7: Some Volatile Halogenated Hydrocarbons
Edited by L. Fishbein and I.K. O'Neill
1985; 479 pages; ISBN 92 832 1168 5

No. 69*
Directory of On-going Research in Cancer Epidemiology 1985
Edited by C.S. Muir and G. Wagner
1985; 745 pages; ISBN 92 823 1169 3

No. 70
The Role of Cyclic Nucleic Acid Adducts in Carcinogenesis and Mutagenesis
Edited by B. Singer and H. Bartsch
1986; 467 pages; ISBN 92 832 1170 7

No. 71
Environmental Carcinogens: Selected Methods of Analysis. Volume 8: Some Metals: As, Be, Cd, Cr, Ni, Pb, Se, Zn
Edited by I.K. O'Neill, P. Schuller and L. Fishbein
1986; 485 pages; ISBN 92 832 1171 5

No. 72
Atlas of Cancer in Scotland, 1975–1980: Incidence and Epidemiological Perspective
Edited by I. Kemp, P. Boyle, M. Smans and C.S. Muir
1985; 285 pages; ISBN 92 832 1172 3

No. 73
Laboratory Decontamination and Destruction of Carcinogens in Laboratory Wastes:Some Antineoplastic Agents
Edited by M. Castegnaro, J. Adams, M.A. Armour, J. Barek, J. Benvenuto, C. Confalonieri, U. Goff, G. Telling
1985; 163 pages; ISBN 92 832 1173 1

No. 74
Tobacco: A Major International Health Hazard
Edited by D. Zaridze and R. Peto
1986; 324 pages; ISBN 92 832 1174 X

No. 75
Cancer Occurrence in Developing Countries
Edited by D.M. Parkin
1986; 339 pages; ISBN 92 832 1175 8

No. 76
Screening for Cancer of the Uterine Cervix
Edited by M. Hakama, A.B. Miller and N.E. Day
1986; 315 pages; ISBN 92 832 1176 6

No. 77
Hexachlorobenzene: Proceedings of an International Symposium
Edited by C.R. Morris and J.R.P. Cabral
1986; 668 pages; ISBN 92 832 1177 4

No. 78
Carcinogenicity of Alkylating Cytostatic Drugs
Edited by D. Schmähl and J.M. Kaldor
1986; 337 pages; ISBN 92 832 1178 2

No. 79
Statistical Methods in Cancer Research Volume III: The Design and Analysis of Long-term Animal Experiments
By J.J. Gart, D. Krewski, P.N. Lee, R.E. Tarone and J. Wahrendorf
1986; 213 pages; ISBN 92 832 1179 0

No. 80*
Directory of On-going Research in Cancer Epidemiology 1986
Edited by C.S. Muir and G. Wagner
1986; 805 pages; ISBN 92 832 1180 4

No. 81
Environmental Carcinogens: Methods of Analysis and Exposure Measurement. Volume 9: Passive Smoking
Edited by I.K. O'Neill, K.D. Brunnemann, B. Dodet and D. Hoffmann
1987; 383 pages; ISBN 92 832 1181 2

No. 82
Statistical Methods in Cancer Research. Volume II: The Design and Analysis of Cohort Studies
By N.E. Breslow and N.E. Day
1987; 404 pages; ISBN 92 832 0182 5

No. 83
Long-term and Short-term Assays for Carcinogens: A Critical Appraisal
Edited by R. Montesano, H. Bartsch, H. Vainio, J. Wilbourn and H. Yamasaki
1986; 575 pages; ISBN 92 832 1183 9

No. 84
The Relevance of N-Nitroso Compounds to Human Cancer: Exposure and Mechanisms
Edited by H. Bartsch, I.K. O'Neill and R. Schulte-Hermann
1987; 671 pages; ISBN 92 832 1184 7

No. 85
Environmental Carcinogens: Methods of Analysis and Exposure Measurement. Volume 10: Benzene and Alkylated Benzenes
Edited by L. Fishbein and I.K. O'Neill
1988; 327 pages; ISBN 92 832 1185 5

No. 86*
Directory of On-going Research in Cancer Epidemiology 1987
Edited by D.M. Parkin and J. Wahrendorf
1987; 685 pages; ISBN: 92 832 1186 3

No. 87*
International Incidence of Childhood Cancer
Edited by D.M. Parkin, C.A. Stiller, C.A. Bieber, G.J. Draper. B. Terracini and J.L. Young
1988; 401 pages; ISBN 92 832 1187 1

*(out of print)

Publications list: Scientific Publications

No. 88
Cancer Incidence in Five Continents, Volume V
Edited by C. Muir, J. Waterhouse, T. Mack, J. Powell and S. Whelan
1987; 1004 pages; ISBN 92 832 1188 X

No. 89*
Methods for Detecting DNA Damaging Agents in Humans: Applications in Cancer Epidemiology and Prevention
Edited by H. Bartsch, K. Hemminki and I.K. O'Neill
1988; 518 pages; ISBN 92 832 1189 8

No. 90
Non-occupational Exposure to Mineral Fibres
Edited by J. Bignon, J. Peto and R. Saracci
1989; 500 pages; ISBN 92 832 1190 1

No. 91
Trends in Cancer Incidence in Singapore 1968–1982
Edited by H.P. Lee, N.E. Day and K. Shanmugaratnam
1988; 160 pages; ISBN 92 832 1191 X

No. 92
Cell Differentiation, Genes and Cancer
Edited by T. Kakunaga, T. Sugimura, L. Tomatis and H. Yamasaki
1988; 204 pages; ISBN 92 832 1192 8

No. 93*
Directory of On-going Research in Cancer Epidemiology 1988
Edited by M. Coleman and J. Wahrendorf
1988; 662 pages; ISBN 92 832 1193 6

No. 94
Human Papillomavirus and Cervical Cancer
Edited by N. Muñoz, F.X. Bosch and O.M. Jensen
1989; 154 pages; ISBN 92 832 1194 4

No. 95
Cancer Registration: Principles and Methods
Edited by O.M. Jensen, D.M. Parkin, R. MacLennan, C.S. Muir and R. Skeet
1991; 296 pages; ISBN 92 832 1195 2

No. 96
Perinatal and Multigeneration Carcinogenesis
Edited by N.P. Napalkov, J.M. Rice, L. Tomatis and H. Yamasaki
1989; 436 pages; ISBN 92 832 1196 0

No. 97
Occupational Exposure to Silica and Cancer Risk
Edited by L. Simonato, A.C. Fletcher, R. Saracci and T. Thomas
1990; 124 pages; ISBN 92 832 1197 9

No. 98
Cancer Incidence in Jewish Migrants to Israel, 1961-1981
Edited by R. Steinitz, D.M. Parkin, J.L. Young, C.A. Bieber and L. Katz
1989; 320 pages; ISBN 92 832 1198 7

No. 99
Pathology of Tumours in Laboratory Animals, Second Edition, Volume 1, Tumours of the Rat
Edited by V.S. Turusov and U. Mohr
1990; 740 pages; ISBN 92 832 1199 5

No. 100
Cancer: Causes, Occurrence and Control
Editor-in-Chief: L. Tomatis
1990; 352 pages; ISBN 92 832 0110 8

No. 101
Directory of On-going Research in Cancer Epidemiology 1989/90
Edited by M. Coleman and J. Wahrendorf
1989; 828 pages; ISBN 92 832 2101 X

No. 102
Patterns of Cancer in Five Continents
Edited by S.L. Whelan, D.M. Parkin and E. Masuyer
1990; 160 pages; ISBN 92 832 2102 8

No. 103
Evaluating Effectiveness of Primary Prevention of Cancer
Edited by M. Hakama, V. Beral, J.W. Cullen and D.M. Parkin
1990; 206 pages; ISBN 92 832 2103 6

No. 104
Complex Mixtures and Cancer Risk
Edited by H. Vainio, M. Sorsa and A.J. McMichael
1990; 441 pages; ISBN 92 832 2104 4

No. 105
Relevance to Human Cancer of N-Nitroso Compounds, Tobacco Smoke and Mycotoxins
Edited by I.K. O'Neill, J. Chen and H. Bartsch
1991; 614 pages; ISBN 92 832 2105 2

No. 106
Atlas of Cancer Incidence in the Former German Democratic Republic
Edited by W.H. Mehnert, M. Smans, C.S. Muir, M. Möhner and D. Schön
1992; 384 pages; ISBN 92 832 2106 0

No. 107
Atlas of Cancer Mortality in the European Economic Community
Edited by M. Smans, C. Muir and P. Boyle
1992; 213 pages +44 coloured maps; ISBN 92 832 2107 9

No. 108
Environmental Carcinogens: Methods of Analysis and Exposure Measurement. Volume 11: Polychlorinated Dioxins and Dibenzofurans
Edited by C. Rappe, H.R. Buser, B. Dodet and I.K. O'Neill
1991; 400 pages; ISBN 92 832 2108 7

No. 109
Environmental Carcinogens: Methods of Analysis and Exposure Measurement. Volume 12: Indoor Air
Edited by B. Seifert, H. van de Wiel, B. Dodet and I.K. O'Neill
1993; 385 pages; ISBN 92 832 2109 5

No. 110
Directory of On-going Research in Cancer Epidemiology 1991
Edited by M.P. Coleman and J. Wahrendorf
1991; 753 pages; ISBN 92 832 2110 9

No. 111
Pathology of Tumours in Laboratory Animals, Second Edition. Volume 2: Tumours of the Mouse
Edited by V. Turusov and U. Mohr
1994; 800 pages; ISBN 92 832 2111 1

No. 112
Autopsy in Epidemiology and Medical Research
Edited by E. Riboli and M. Delendi
1991; 288 pages; ISBN 92 832 2112 5

No. 113
Laboratory Decontamination and Destruction of Carcinogens in Laboratory Wastes: Some Mycotoxins
Edited by M. Castegnaro, J. Barek, J.M. Frémy, M. Lafontaine, M. Miraglia, E.B. Sansone and G.M. Telling
1991; 63 pages; ISBN 92 832 2113 3

No. 114
Laboratory Decontamination and Destruction of Carcinogens in Laboratory Wastes: Some Polycyclic Heterocyclic Hydrocarbons
Edited by M. Castegnaro, J. Barek, J. Jacob, U. Kirso, M. Lafontaine, E.B. Sansone, G.M. Telling and T. Vu Duc
1991; 50 pages; ISBN 92 832 2114 1

No. 115
Mycotoxins, Endemic Nephropathy and Urinary Tract Tumours
Edited by M. Castegnaro, R. Plestina, G. Dirheimer, I.N. Chernozemsky and H. Bartsch
1991; 340 pages; ISBN 92 832 2115 X

*(out of print)

No. 116
Mechanisms of Carcinogenesis in Risk Identification
Edited by H. Vainio, P. Magee, D. McGregor and A.J. McMichael
1992; 615 pages; ISBN 92 832 2116 8

No. 117
Directory of On-going Research in Cancer Epidemiology 1992
Edited by M. Coleman, E. Demaret and J. Wahrendorf
1992; 773 pages; ISBN 92 832 2117 6

No. 118
Cadmium in the Human Environment: Toxicity and Carcinogenicity
Edited by G.F. Nordberg, R.F.M. Herber and L. Alessio
1992; 470 pages; ISBN 92 832 2118 4

No. 119
The Epidemiology of Cervical Cancer and Human Papillomavirus
Edited by N. Muñoz, F.X. Bosch, K.V. Shah and A. Meheus
1992; 288 pages; ISBN 92 832 2119 2

No. 120
Cancer Incidence in Five Continents, Vol. VI
Edited by D.M. Parkin, C.S. Muir, S.L. Whelan, Y.T. Gao, J. Ferlay and J. Powell
1992; 1020 pages; ISBN 92 832 2120 6

No. 121
Time Trends in Cancer Incidence and Mortality
By M. Coleman, J. Estève P. Damiecki, A. Arslan and H. Renard
1993; 820 pages; ISBN 92 832 2121 4

No. 122
International Classification of Rodent Tumours. Part I. The Rat
Editor-in-Chief: U. Mohr
1992-1996; 10 fascicles of 60–100 pages; ISBN 92 832 2122 2

No. 123
Cancer in Italian Migrant Populations
Edited by M. Geddes, D.M. Parkin, M. Khlat, D. Balzi and E. Buiatti
1993; 292 pages; ISBN 92 832 2123 0

No. 124
Postlabelling Methods for the Detection of DNA Damage
Edited by D.H. Phillips, M. Castegnaro and H. Bartsch 1993; 392 pages; ISBN 92 832 2124 9

No. 125
DNA Adducts: Identification and Biological Significance
Edited by K. Hemminki, A. Dipple, D.E.G. Shuker, F.F. Kadlubar, D. Segerbäck and H. Bartsch
1994; 478 pages; ISBN 92 832 2125 7

No. 126
Pathology of Tumours in Laboratory Animals, Second Edition. Volume 3: Tumours of the Hamster
Edited by V.S. Turusov and U. Mohr
1966; 465 pages; ISBN 92 836 2126 5

No. 127
Butadiene and Styrene: Assessment of Health Hazards
Edited by M. Sorsa, K. Peltonen, H. Vainio and K. Hemminki
1993; 412 pages; ISBN 92 832 2127 3

No. 128
Statistical Methods in Cancer Research. Volume IV. Descriptive Epidemiology
By J. Estève, E. Benhamou and L. Raymond
1994; 302 pages; ISBN 92 832 2128 1

No. 129
Occupational Cancer in Developing Countries
Edited by N. Pearce, E. Matos, H. Vainio, P. Boffetta and M. Kogevinas
1994; 191 pages; ISBN 92 832 2129 X

No. 130
Directory of On-going Research in Cancer Epidemiology 1994
Edited by R. Sankaranarayanan, J. Wahrendorf and E. Démaret
1994; 800 pages; ISBN 92 832 2130 3

No. 132
Survival of Cancer Patients in Europe: The EUROCARE Study
Edited by F. Berrino, M. Sant, A. Verdecchia, R. Capocaccia, T. Hakulinen and J. Estève
1995; 463 pages; ISBN 92 832 2132 X

No. 134
Atlas of Cancer Mortality in Central Europe
W. Zatonski, J. Estève, M. Smans, J. Tyczynski and P. Boyle
1996; 175 pages + 40 coloured maps
ISBN 92 832 2134 6

No. 136
Chemoprevention in Cancer Control
Edited by M. Hakama, V. Beral, E. Buiatti, J. Faivre and D.M. Parkin
1996; 160 pages; ISBN 93 832 2136 2

No. 137
Directory of On-Going Research in Cancer Epidemiology 1996
Edited by R. Sankaranarayanan, J. Wahrendorf and E. Démaret
1996; 810 pages; ISBN 93 832 2137 0

IARC Monographs on the Evaluation of Carcinogenic Risks to Humans

Volume 1*
Some Inorganic Substances, Chlorinated Hydrocarbons, Aromatic Amines, N-Nitroso Compounds, and Natural Products
1972; 184 pages; ISBN 92 832 1201 0

Volume 2*
Some Inorganic and Organometallic Compounds
1973; 181 pages; ISBN 92 832 1202 9

Volume 3*
Certain Polycyclic Aromatic Hydrocarbons and Heterocyclic Compounds
1973; 271 pages; ISBN 92 832 1203 7

Volume 4
Some Aromatic Amines, Hydrazine and Related Substances, N-Nitroso Compounds and Miscellaneous Alkylating Agents
1974; 286 pages; ISBN 92 832 1204 5

Volume 5*
Some Organochlorine Pesticides
1974; 241 pages; ISBN 92 832 1205 3

Volume 6*
Sex Hormones
1974; 243 pages; ISBN 92 832 1206 1

Volume 7*
Some Anti-Thyroid and Related Substances, Nitrofurans and Industrial Chemicals
1974; 326 pages; ISBN 92 832 1207 X

Volume 8
Some Aromatic Azo Compounds
1975; 357 pages; ISBN 92 832 1208 8

Volume 9
Some Aziridines, N-, S- and O-Mustards and Selenium
1975; 268 pages; ISBN 92 832 1209 6

Volume 10*
Some Naturally Occurring Substances
1976; 353 pages; ISBN 92 832 1210 X

Volume 11*
Cadmium, Nickel, Some Epoxides, Miscellaneous Industrial Chemicals and General Considerations on Volatile Anaesthetics
1976; 306 pages; ISBN 92 832 1211 8

Volume 12
Some Carbamates, Thiocarbamates and Carbazides
1976; 282 pages; ISBN 92 832 1212 6

Volume 13
Some Miscellaneous Pharmaceutical Substances
1977; 255 pages; ISBN 92 832 1213 4

Volume 14*
Asbestos
1977; 106 pages; ISBN 92 832 1214 2

Volume 15*
Some Fumigants, the Herbicides 2,4-D and 2,4,5-T, Chlorinated Dibenzodioxins and Miscellaneous Industrial Chemicals
1977; 354 pages; ISBN 92 832 1215 0

Volume 16
Some Aromatic Amines and Related Nitro Compounds – Hair Dyes, Colouring Agents and Miscellaneous Industrial Chemicals
1978; 400 pages; ISBN 92 832 1216 9

Volume 17
Some N-Nitroso Compounds
1978; 365 pages; ISBN 92 832 1217 7

Volume 18
Polychlorinated Biphenyls and Polybrominated Biphenyls
1978; 140 pages; ISBN 92 832 1218 5

Volume 19*
Some Monomers, Plastics and Synthetic Elastomers, and Acrolein
1979; 513 pages; ISBN 92 832 1219 3

Volume 20*
Some Halogenated Hydrocarbons
1979; 609 pages; ISBN 92 832 1220 7

Volume 21
Sex Hormones (II)
1979; 583 pages; ISBN 92 832 1521 4

Volume 22
Some Non-Nutritive Sweetening Agents
1980; 208 pages; ISBN 92 832 1522 2

Volume 23*
Some Metals and Metallic Compounds
1980; 438 pages; ISBN 92 832 1523 0

Volume 24
Some Pharmaceutical Drugs
1980; 337 pages; ISBN 92 832 1524 9

Volume 25
Wood, Leather and Some Associated Industries.
1981; 412 pages; ISBN 92 832 1525 7

Volume 26
Some Antineoplastic and Immuno-suppressive Agents.
1981; 411 pages; ISBN 92 832 1526 5

Volume 27
Some Aromatic Amines, Anthraquinones and Nitroso Compounds, and Inorganic Fluorides Used in Drinking Water and Dental Preparations
1982; 341 pages; ISBN 92 832 1527 3

Volume 28
The Rubber Industry
1982; 486 pages; ISBN 92 832 1528 1

Volume 29
Some Industrial Chemicals and Dyestuffs
1982; 416 pages; ISBN 92 832 1529 X

Volume 30
Miscellaneous Pesticides
1983; 424 pages; ISBN 92 832 1530 3

Volume 31
Some Food Additives, Feed Additives and Naturally Occurring Substances
1983; 314 pages; ISBN 92 832 1531 1

Volume 32
Polynuclear Aromatic Compounds, Part 1: Chemical, Environmental and Experimental Data.
1983; 477 pages; ISBN 92 832 1532 X

Volume 33*
Polynuclear Aromatic Compounds, Part 2: Carbon Blacks, Mineral Oils and Some Nitroarenes
1984; 245 pages; ISBN 92 832 1533 8

Volume 34
Polynuclear Aromatic Compounds, Part 3: Industrial Exposures in Aluminium Production, Coal Gasification, Coke Production, and Iron and Steel Founding
1984; 219 pages; ISBN 92 832 1534 6

Volume 35
Polynuclear Aromatic Compounds: Part 4: Bitumens, Coal-Tars and Derived Products, Shale-Oils and Soots
1985; 271 pages; ISBN 92 832 1535 4

Volume 36
Allyl Compounds, Aldehydes, Epoxides and Peroxides
1985; 369 pages; ISBN 92 832 1536 2

Volume 37
Tobacco Habits Other than Smoking; Betel-Quid and Areca-Nut Chewing; and Some Related Nitrosamines
1985; 291 pages; ISBN 92 832 1537 0

*(out of print)

Publications list: Monographs

Volume 38
Tobacco Smoking
1986; 421 pages; ISBN 92 832 1538 9

Volume 39
Some Chemicals Used in Plastics and Elastomers
1986; 403 pages; ISBN 92 832 1239 8

Volume 40
Some Naturally Occurring and Synthetic Food Components, Furocoumarins and Ultraviolet Radiation
1986; 444 pages; ISBN 92 832 1240 1

Volume 41
Some Halogenated Hydrocarbons and Pesticide Exposures
1986; 434 pages; ISBN 92 832 1241 X

Volume 42
Silica and Some Silicates
1987; 289 pages; ISBN 92 832 1242 8

Volume 43
Man-Made Mineral Fibres and Radon
1988; 300 pages; ISBN 92 832 1243 6

Volume 44
Alcohol Drinking.
1988; 416 pages; ISBN 92 832 1244 4

Volume 45
Occupational Exposures in Petroleum Refining; Crude Oil and Major Petroleum Fuels.
1989; 322 pages; ISBN 92 832 1245 2

Volume 46
Diesel and Gasoline Engine Exhausts and Some Nitroarenes
1989; 458 pages; ISBN 92 832 1246 0

Volume 47
Some Organic Solvents, Resin Monomers and Related Compounds, Pigments and Occupational Exposures in Paint Manufacture and Painting
1989; 535 pages; ISBN 92 832 1247 9

Volume 48
Some Flame Retardants and Textile Chemicals, and Exposures in the Textile Manufacturing Industry
1990; 345 pages; ISBN: 92 832 1248 7

Volume 49
Chromium, Nickel and Welding
1990; 677 pages; ISBN: 92 832 1249 5

Volume 50
Some Pharmaceutical Drugs
1990; 415 pages; ISBN: 92 832 1259 9

Volume 51
Coffee, Tea, Mate, Methylxanthines and Methylglyoxal
1991; 513 pages; ISBN: 92 832 1251 7

Volume 52
Chlorinated Drinking-Water; Chlorination By-products; Some other Halogenated Compounds; Cobalt and Cobalt Compounds
1991; 544 pages; ISBN: 92 832 1252 5

Volume 53
Occupational Exposures in Insecticide Application, and Some Pesticides
1991; 612 pages; ISBN 92 832 1253 3

Volume 54
Occupational Exposures to Mists and Vapours from Strong Inorganic Acids; and other Industrial Chemicals
1992; 336 pages; ISBN 92 832 1254 1

Volume 55
Solar and Ultraviolet Radiation
1992; 316 pages; ISBN 92 832 1255 X

Volume 56
Some Naturally Occurring Substances: Food Items and Constituents, Heterocyclic Aromatic Amines and Mycotoxins
1993; 600 pages; ISBN 92 832 1256 8

Volume 57
Occupational Exposures of Hairdressers and Barbers and Personal Use of Hair Colourants; Some Hair Dyes, Cosmetic Colourants, Industrial Dyestuffs and Aromatic Amines
1993; 428 pages; ISBN 92 832 1257 6

Volume 58
Beryllium, Cadmium, Mercury and Exposures in the Glass Manufacturing Industry
1994; 444 pages; ISBN 92 832 1258 4

Volume 59
Hepatitis Viruses
1994; 286 pages; ISBN 92 832 1259 2

Volume 60
Some Industrial Chemicals
1994; 560 pages; ISBN 92 832 1260 6

Volume 61
Schistosomes, Liver Flukes and *Helicobacter pylori*
1994; 270 pages; ISBN 92 832 1261 4

Volume 62
Wood Dusts and Formaldehyde
1995; 405 pages; ISBN 92 832 1262 2

Volume 63
Dry cleaning, Some chlorinated Solvents and Other Industrial Chemicals
1995; 551 pages; ISBN 92 832 1263 0

Volume 64
Human Papillomaviruses
1995; 409 pages; ISBN 92 832 1264 9

Volume 65
Printing Processes, Printing Inks, Carbon Blacks and Some Nitro Compounds
1996; 578 pages; ISBN 92 832 1265 7

Supplements to Monographs

Supplement No. 1*
Chemicals and Industrial Processes Associated with Cancer in Humans (IARC Monographs, Volumes 1 to 20)
1979; 71 pages; ISBN 92 832 1402 1

Supplement No. 2
Long-Term and Short-Term Screening Assays for Carcinogens: A Critical Appraisal
1980; 426 pages; ISBN 92 832 1404 8

Supplement No. 3*
Cross Index of Synonyms and Trade Names in Volumes 1 to 26
1982; 199 pages; ISBN 92 832 1405 6

Supplement No. 4*
Chemicals, Industrial Processes and Industries Associated with Cancer in Humans (IARC Monographs, Volumes 1 to 29)
1982; 292 pages; ISBN 92 832 1407 2

Supplement No. 5*
Cross Index of Synonyms and Trade Names in Volumes 1 to 36
1985; 259 pages; ISBN 92 832 1408 0

Supplement No. 6
Genetic and Related Effects: An Updating of Selected IARC Monographs from Volumes 1 to 42
1987; 729 pages; ISBN 92 832 1409 9

Supplement No. 7
Overall Evaluations of Carcinogenicity: An Updating of IARC Monographs Volumes 1 to 42
1987; 440 pages; ISBN 92 832 1411 0

Supplement No. 8
Cross Index of Synonyms and Trade Names in Volumes 1 to 46
1989; 346 pages; ISBN 92 832 1417 X

*(out of print)

IARC Technical Reports

No. 1
Cancer in Costa Rica
Edited by R. Sierra, R. Barrantes,
G. Muñoz Leiva, D.M. Parkin, C.A.
Bieber and N. Muñoz Calero
1988; 124 pages; ISBN 92 832 1412 9

No. 2*
SEARCH: A Computer Package to
Assist the Statistical Analysis of
Case-Control Studies
Edited by G.J. Macfarlane, P. Boyle
and P. Maisonneuve
1991; 80 pages; ISBN 92 832 1413 7

No. 3
Cancer Registration in the European
Economic Community
Edited by M.P. Coleman and E.
Démaret
1988; 188 pages; ISBN 92 832 1414 5

No. 4
Diet, Hormones and Cancer: Methodological Issues for Prospective Studies
Edited by E. Riboli and R. Saracci
1988; 156 pages; ISBN 92 832 1415 3

No. 5
Cancer in the Philippines
Edited by A.V. Laudico, D. Esteban and
D.M. Parkin
1989; 186 pages; ISBN 92 832 1416 1

No. 6
La genèse du Centre international de
recherche sur le cancer
By R. Sohier and A.G.B. Sutherland
1990, 102 pages; ISBN 92 832 1418 8

No. 7
Epidémiologie du cancer dans les
pays de langue latine
1990, 292 pages; ISBN 92 832 1419 6

No. 8
Comparative Study of Anti-smoking
Legislation in Countries of the
European Economic Community
By A. J. Sasco, P. Dalla-Vorgia and
P. Van der Elst
1992; 82 pages; ISBN: 92 832 1421 8
Also available in French
(ISBN 92 832 2402 7)

No. 9
Epidémiologie du cancer dans les
pays de langue latine
1991; 346 pages; ISBN 92 832 1423 4

No. 10
Manual for Cancer Registry Personnel
Edited by D. Esteban, S. Whelan,
A. Laudico and D.M. Parkin
1995; 400 pages; ISBN 92 832 1424 2

No. 11
Nitroso Compounds: Biological
Mechanisms, Exposures and Cancer
Etiology
Edited by I. O'Neill and H. Bartsch
1992; 150 pages; ISBN 92 832 1425 X

No. 12
Epidémiologie du cancer dans les
pays de langue latine
1992; 375 pages; ISBN 92 832 1426 9

No. 13
Health, Solar UV Radiation and
Environmental Change
By A. Kricker, B.K. Armstrong, M.E.
Jones and R.C. Burton
1993; 213 pages; ISBN 92 832 1427 7

No. 14
Epidémiologie du cancer dans les
pays de langue latine
1993; 400 pages; ISBN 92 832 1428 5

No. 15
Cancer in the African Population of
Bulawayo, Zimbabwe, 1963–1977
By M.E.G. Skinner, D.M. Parkin,
A.P. Vizcaino and A. Ndhlovu
1993; 120 pages; ISBN 92 832 1429 3

No. 16
Cancer in Thailand 1984–1991
By V. Vatanasapt, N. Martin, H. Sriplung,
K. Chindavijak, S. Sontipong,
S. Sriamporn, D.M. Parkin and J. Ferlay
1993; 164 pages; ISBN 92 832 1430 7

No. 18
Intervention Trials for Cancer
Prevention
By E. Buiatti
1994; 52 pages; ISBN 92 832 1432 3

No. 19
Comparability and Quality Control in
Cancer Registration
By D.M. Parkin, V.W. Chen, J. Ferlay,
J. Galceran, H.H. Storm and
S.L. Whelan
1994; 110 pages; plus diskette;
ISBN 92 832 1433 1
Also available in French
(ISBN 92 832 2403 5)
and Spanish
(ISBN 92 832 0402 6)

No. 20
Epidémiologie du cancer dans les
pays de langue latine
1994; 346 pages; ISBN 92 832 1434 X

No. 21
ICD Conversion Programs for Cancer
By J Ferlay
1994; 24 pages plus diskette;
ISBN 92 832 1435 8

No. 22
Cancer in Tianjin
By Q.S. Wang, P. Boffetta, M. Kogevinas
and D.M. Parkin
1994; 96 pages; ISBN 92 832 1433 1

No. 23
An Evaluation Programme for Cancer
Preventive Agents
By Bernard W. Stewart
1995; 40 pages; ISBN 92 832 1438 2

No. 24
Peroxisome Proliferation and its
Role in Carcinogenesis. Views and
expert opinions of an IARC Working
Group
1995; 85 pages; ISBN 92 832 1439 0

No. 25
Combined Analysis of Cancer Mortality
in Nuclear Workers in Canada, the
United Kingdom and the United States
of America
By E. Cardis, E.S. Gilbert, L. Carpenter, G. Howe, I. Kato, J. Fix, L. Salmon,
G. Cowper, B.K. Armstrong, V. Beral,
A. Douglas, S.A. Fry, J. Kaldor, C. Lavé,
P.G. Smith, G. Voelz and L. Wiggs
1995; 160 pages; ISBN 92 832 1440 4

*(out of print)

Directories of Agents being Tested for Carcinogenicity

No. 14
Edited by M.-J. Ghess, J.D. Wilbourn and H. Vainio
1990; 369 pages; ISBN 92 832 1314 9

No. 15
Edited by M.-J. Ghess, J.D. Wilbourn and H. Vainio
1992; 317 pages; ISBN 92 832 1315 7

No. 16
Edited by M.-J. Ghess, J.D. Wilbourn and H. Vainio
1994; 294 pages; ISBN 92 832 1316 5

No. 17
Edited by A. Meneghel and J.D. Wilbourn
1996; 360 pages; ISBN 92 832 1317 3

Non-serial publications

Alcool et Cancer
By A. Tuyns
1978; 48 pages; ISBN 92 832 2401 9

Cancer Morbidity and Causes of Death among Danish Brewery Workers
By O.M. Jensen
1980; 143 pages; ISBN 92 832 1403 X

Directory of Computer Systems Used in Cancer Registries
By H.R. Menck and D.M. Parkin
1986; 236 pages

Facts and Figures of Cancer in the European Community
By J. Estève, A. Kricker, J. Ferlay and D.M. Parkin
1993; 52 pages; ISBN 92 832 1437 4

IARC Monographs and Technical Reports are available from the
World Health Organization Distribution and Sales, CH-1211 Geneva 27
(Fax: +41 22 791 4857)
and from WHO Sales Agents worldwide.

IARC Scientific Publications are available from
Oxford University Press,
Walton Street, Oxford, UK OX2 6DP
(Fax: +44 1865 267782).

All IARC Publications are also available directly from
IARC*Press*, 150 Cours Albert Thomas, F-69372 Lyon cedex 08, France
(Fax: +33 72 73 83 02; E-mail: press@iarc.fr).

www.ingramcontent.com/pod-product-compliance
Ingram Content Group UK Ltd.
Pitfield, Milton Keynes, MK11 3LW, UK
UKHW051258180426
11947UKWH00020B/1770